Digestive Physiology and Nutrition of Ruminants

Volume I - Digestive Physiology

Second Edition

by **D. C. Church**, Ph.D.
Professor of Ruminant Nutrition
Department of Animal Science
Oregon State University
Corvallis, Oregon 97331
United States of America

II

ISBN 0-9601586-4-2

Third printing June, 1979

Published by **D.C. Church**

Distributed by **O & B Books**
          1215 NW Kline Place
          Corvallis, Oregon 97330
          USA

Printed by Oxford Press, Inc.
          1427 SE Stark
          Portland, Oregon 97214

TABLE OF CONTENTS

Tables of Contents of Other Volumes of DIGESTIVE PHYSIOLOGY AND NUTRITION OF RUMINANTS

Other Books Published by O & B Books, Inc.

Basic Animal Nutrition and Feeding by D.C. Church and W.G. Pond, 1974

Livestock Feeds and Feeding by D.C. Church et al, 1977

Supplementary Sources of Information

As you progress through this book you will find that it is far from being complete with respect to coverage of nutritional physiology of ruminants. Due to the diversity of subject matter and the great number of research papers available, the data reviewed are intended in most instances to be selective rather than exhaustive. Additional reference books are listed below for the reader desiring more information. These books are, for the most part, excellent sources of additional information on specific topics. Many of them will be referred to frequently during discussions that follow.

Benzie, D. and A.T. Phillipson. 1957. The Alimentary Tract of the Ruminant. Oliver and Boyd. (X-ray studies of the GIT)

Blaxter, K.L. 1967. The Energy Metabolism of Ruminants. 2nd ed. Hutchinson Pub. Co.

Blood, D.C. and J.A. Henderson. 1968. Veterinary Medicine. 3rd ed. Williams & Wilkins Co.

Briggs, M.H. (ed.). 1967. Urea as a Protein Supplement. Pergamon Press.

Brody, S. 1945. Bioenergetics and Growth. Reinhold Pub. Co. (reprinted in 1964 by Hafner Pub. Co.).

Church, D.C. and W.G. Pond. 1974. Basic Animal Nutrition and Feeding. O & B Books, Corvallis, Oregon.

Cuthbertson, D. (ed.). 1969. Nutrition of Animals of Agricultural Importance. Part I. The Science of Nutrition of Farm Livestock. Part II. Assessment of and Factors Affecting Requirements of Farm Livestock. Pergamon Press.

Dougherty, R.W., et al (eds.). 1965. Physiology of Digestion in the Ruminant. Butterworths Pub. Co. (proceedings)

Hafez, E.S.E. and I.A. Dyer (eds.). 1969. Animal Growth and Nutrition. Lea & Febiger.

Hungate, R.E. 1966. The Rumen and Its Microbes. Academic Press.

Lewis, D. (ed.). 1961. Digestive Physiology and Nutrition of the Ruminant. Butterworths Pub. Co. (proceedings)

Maynard, L.A. and J.K. Loosli. 1969. Animal Nutrition. 6th ed. McGraw-Hill Co.

McDonald, P., R.A. Edwards and J.F.D. Greenhalgh. 1973. Animal Nutrition. 2nd ed. Oliver & Boyd.

Mitchell, H.H. 1962, 1964. Comparative Nutrition of Man and Domestic Animals. Vol. 1 & 2. Academic Press.

Phillipson, A.T. (ed.). 1970. Physiology of Digestion and Metabolism in the Ruminant. Oriel Press. (proceedings)

Sisson, S. and J.D. Grossman. 1953. The Anatomy of the Domestic Animals. 4th ed. W.B. Saunders Co.

Swenson, M.J. (ed.). 1970. Dukes' Physiology of Domestic Animals. 8th ed. Comstock Pub. Assoc.

Underwood, E.J. 1966. The Mineral Nutrition of Livestock. FAO & Commonwealth Agricultural Bureaux.

Underwood, E.J. 1971. Trace Elements in Human and Animal Nutrition. 3rd ed. Academic Press.

Credits on Cover Illustrations

The cartoons on the back cover were done by Chuck Sharman, Olympia, Washington.

Foreword to Second Edition

In the intervening years since this book was first published the author is older and wiser (I hope), the latter partly because of involvement in writing and publishing three other books. In the meantime, the abstracts and reprints pile up faster and faster and it becomes more difficult each year to stay reasonably abreast of this total field. However, one of the fringe benefits of this type of writing is the continual learning that is forced on the writer and, in the process, the development of a good overall understanding of a wide scope of subject matter.

The subject of digestive physiology and nutrition of ruminants is a fascinating field dealing with most interesting animals. With the extensive research going on world-wide, even in the face of restricted research budgets, we are gradually accumulating more and more data which continually gives us a better understanding of these interesting animals. Thus, it is towards a better understanding of these species and the facilitation of it by interested readers that encourages the revision of this book.

D.C. Church

CHAPTER 1 — THE IMPORTANCE OF RUMINANTS AND THEIR SYSTEMATIC CLASSIFICATION

Ruminant animals include those classified in the order *Artiodactyla,* which are even-toed, hooved mammals, and the suborder ruminantia. The word, ruminant, comes from the Latin word *ruminare* and means to chew over again; thus ruminants are "cud-chewing," even-toed, hooved mammals.

Ruminant species currently make a very important contribution to man's welfare primarily in the form of meat, milk and fiber, but also for work in some less mechanized countries and for recreation of various types such as hunting and sporting events (rodeo, bull fighting). Not only is this the case now, but it has been this way in numerous societies in the near and distant past. Examples from the past of the extreme dependence of some societies on ruminants are the many nomadic American Indian tribes which depended on the bison (buffalo) and other lesser ruminant species. The bison yielded meat, clothing, shelter, weapons and utensils which were the staff of life to some of the plains tribes. Today, the Masai tribes found in East Africa are almost as dependent upon their domestic cattle which provide meat, milk and blood to drink, as well as artifacts of use to these primitive people.

All developed countries are quite dependent on ruminant animals for many food or industrial items. For example, current (1974) per capita beef consumption in the USA is about 120 lb and lamb and mutton about 6 lb. Data indicate a whole milk equivalent consumption of 565 lb in the USA (16th on the world list), of which fluid milk accounted for 273 lb, cheese 10.6 and butter 4.7 lb/year. Wool consumption (1973) is about ¾ lb per capita in the USA. These various statistics, of course, will vary from year to year and are quite different for different countries, but give some indication of the importance of ruminant animals in our current society.

Various by-products are also of considerable importance. Hides are an important industrial product and leather is used in many different ways. Other packing house products, particularly fats, find uses in a wide variety of foods and industrial chemicals (Price and Schweigert, 1971). Other animal by-products — meat meals, meat and bone meal — are used extensively in animal feeds. Intestines are used for sausage casings and surgical suture, for example, and a wide variety of pharmaceutical products are prepared from blood, liver, adrenal glands, pancreas and other glands and tissues.

The importance of ruminant species (and other herbivorous animals) is, perhaps, more properly emphasized when we look at the total world land area. Approximately ⅓ of the earth's surface is land — about 34 billion acres or a little more than 53 million square miles. Of this, about 3-4% is utilized for urban and industrial purposes, while about 10% is under cultivation. Nonproductive lands comprise about 15% of the earth's land area. These lands, termed nonproductive because plant photosynthetic activity is relatively unimportant, include the very high mountain areas, barren deserts and land areas covered by glaciers or permanent snow. Forest lands, some of which may be utilized by grazing animals, cover 28-30% of the land. The land remaining, which includes 40% or more of the earth's land area, is comprised of rangeland, which is more suitable to grazing than cultivation. Rangelands include natural grasslands, savannas, shrublands, most deserts, tundra, alpine communities, coastal marshes, and wet meadows (Anonymous). Thus, it is obvious, that productivity of products useful to man from a large majority of the earth's surface would be greatly reduced if grazing animals were not available to utilize the plants to some degree.

Of the herbivorous animals, ruminants represent by far the most important group in terms of the numbers of mammals existing today, either domestic or feral (wild). Judging by fossil remains, ruminants abounded in large numbers of a very diverse nature in prehistoric eras. Simpson (1945) gives some estimates of the number of extinct and living genera of herbivorous animals derived from fossil finds. For the order *Artiodactyla,* he estimated that 333 genera are extinct and 86 living, as compared to 1,932 extinct and 932 living genera for all mammals. He estimated that about 180 genera of ruminants are extinct and that 68 genera have survived to this time. Only a few primitive ruminants [*Tragulina*] have survived. Domesticated ruminants, represented by only a few genera, undoubtedly outnumber all of the wild ruminants at the present time.

The geographical distribution of ruminants in prehistoric times is open to question because of incomplete fossil records. In recent geological times it is certainly true in the western hemisphere that a larger variety and more total numbers abounded in temperate climates. In the Afro-European area many more diverse genera currently exist in the semitropical and tropical areas than in Europe. Whether the diversity in Africa is due to the climate and geography or to geological phenomena that allowed existing species to survive ice invasions or other drastic climatic changes in times past is an unresolved question. Certainly, the mountain ranges of southern Europe and Asia, the Mediterranean Sea, or surrounding deserts would be formidable barriers for many species to overcome following a period of ice invasion or extreme cold in the northern areas of Europe and Asia.

Existing species inhabit climates varying from arctic (yak, caribou, musk ox mountain goats and sheep, etc.) to tropical climates (mostly African species), and from swampy environments (moose, water buffalo, swamp deer) to deserts (antelope, sheep, various African and Asian species). Consequently, the dietary habits or food preferences of ruminants vary tremendously. Extremes in food preference vary from those ruminants such as the caribou which consumes arctic lichens to the giraffe's predilection for the leaves of tropical trees. The moose, for example, is a heavy consumer of water plants. The antelope and most deer prefer browse (woody plants) or forbes to grasses. Animals such as the water buffalo do well on coarse reeds and grasses that would not sustain many domestic cattle. The American bison and domestic cattle, as well as many other species, prefer grasses. However, data (for species on which it is available) demonstrate that ruminants will consume a varied diet if they have the opportunity to do so. The geneticist might say that this natural preference for certain plant types is the outcome of evolution, resulting from development of the animal in a given environment. Pressure of other species or

overpopulation of a species may have also been factors. Undoubtedly, physiological differences are also involved, but comparative data to establish this point are lacking on most wild species and, for that matter, even on domestic species.

For the benefit of readers interested in classification, a partial systematic classification is shown (Simpson, 1945; Mochi and Carter, 1971):

Kingdom — Animal
 Phylum — Chordata
  Subphylum — Veterbrata
  Superclass — Tetrapoda
   Class — Mammalia
    Order — Artiodactyla (even-toed, hooved mammals)
    Suborder — Ruminantia
    Infraorder
    Family
     Subfamilies
     Tribe
      Genus and Subgenus
      Species and Subspecies

Existing ruminant animals are divided into five families: Giraffidae (2 genera), the giraffes and okapi, characterized by having short horns covered with hair-bearing skin; Cervidae (16 genera), deer, animals carrying solid antlers comprised of bone which are shed and renewed annually (two exceptions where the male has canine tusks instead of antlers); Antilocapridae (1 genera), the pronghorn antelope, in which the horns carry a prong, grow over a bony core and are renewed each year; Bovidae (47 genera), the antelopes, goat-antelopes, musk oxen, takins, goats, sheep, cattle, bison and buffalo in which the horns grow over a bony core and are never shed; and Tragulidae (2 genera), the chevrotains, small primitive species similar to the Pecora (true ruminants) in not having upper incisors and in chewing their cud, but different in that the stomach has only three compartments and, for males, in having long tusk-like canines (Mochi and Carter, 1971). The Camelidae (3 genera), camels and camelids (llama and related species), are animals which walk on broad fleshy pads and have two toes on each foot. They are generally classed as pseudo-ruminants because the stomach has only three compartments as opposed to four compartments in true ruminants.

A listing follows of scientific names, most common name, and general area where wild ruminants are found. Many subspecies names are not given, but may be found in sources such as that of Mochi and Carter (1971).

Infraorder Tragulina (most primitive surviving ruminants)
  Family Traguilade
    Tragulus napu. Large Malayan Chevrotain. Maylay.
    T. javanicus. Small Malayan Chevrotain. Malay. Over 50 subspecies of these two species
      are known.
    T. meminna. Indian Chevrotain. India, Ceylon.
    T. nigricans. Philippine Chevrotain. Philippine Islands.
    Hyemoschus aquaticus. Water Chevrotai; 3 subspecies. Africa.
Infraorder Pecora (true ruminants)
  Family Cervidae — deer and allied animals
    Subfamily Moschinae
      Moschus moschiferus. Musk deer. Himalayan Mountains.

    Subfamily Muntiacinae
      Muntiacus muntjak. Javan and Indian Muntjac.
      M. feae. Tenasserim Muntjac. Burma.
      M. crinifrons. Hairy-fronted Muntjac. Rare.
      Elaphodus cephalophus. West China Tufted Deer. China.
    Subfamily Cervinae
      Dama dama. Fallow Deer. Europe.
      D. mesopotamica. Mesopotamian Fallow Deer. Asia Minor.
      Elaphurus davidianus. Pere David's Deer. China. In captivity only.
      Axis axis. Axis Deer. India, Ceylon.
      A. procinus. Hog Deer. Southeastern Asia.
      Cervus elaphus. Red Deer; 11 subspecies found in Europe, Africa, Asia.
      C. canadensis. Wapiti, elk; 7 subspecies found in North America and Asia.
      C. albirostris. Thorold's or White-lipped Deer. China, Tibet.
      C. duvauceli. Barasingha or Swamp Deer. India.
      C. eldi. Thamin, Eld's Deer. SE Asia.
      C. schomburgki. Schomburkg's Deer. Probably extinct.
      C. nippon. Sika Deer; 3 subspecies found in Asian countries.
      C. alfredi. Philippine Spotted Deer. Philippine Islands.
      C. unicolor. Sambar; 4 subspecies found in India, SE Asia, Philippines.
      C. timoriensis. Rusa; 2 subspecies found in Java, Celebes, Moluccas.

    Subfamily Odocoileinae
      Odocoileus virginianus. White-tailed Deer; 4 subspecies in the US, Canada.
      O. couesi. Arizona White-tailed Deer. Mexico, SE USA.
      O. mexicanus. Mexican White-tailed Deer. Mexico.
      O. gymnotis. Savannah Deer. S. America.
      O. heminonus. Black-tailed Deer; Mule Deer (different subspecies). Pacific side of
        Rocky Mountains.
      Blastocerus bezoarticus. Pampas Deer. S. America.
      B. dichotomus. S. Amer. Marsh Deer. S. America.
      Hippocamelus antisensis. Peruvian Guemal or Taruga. S. America.
      H. bisulcus. Chilean Guemal. Argentina, Chile.
      Mazama simplicicornis. Brown Brocket. S. America.
      M. americana. Red Brocket. S. America.
      Pudu pudu. Chilean Pudu. Chile.
      Capreolus capreolus. Roe Buck; 4 subspecies found in Europe and northern Asia.
      Hydropotes inermis. Chinese Water Deer. China, Korea.
      Rangifer tarandus. Reindeer; 2 subspecies found in Norway, Siberia.
      R. arcticus. Caribou; 7 subspecies found in N. America, Greenland.
      R. caribou. Woodland Caribou. Northern parts of N. America.
      R. terraenovae. Newfoundland Caribou. Newfoundland.

R. montanus.   Mountain Caribou. Believed to be extinct.
Alces alces.   European Elk; 2 subspecies in Northern Europe, Siberia.
A. americana.   American and Alaskan Moose (2 subspecies).

Family Giraffidae
Subfamily Palaeotraginae
Akapia johnstoni.   Okapi. Congo.
Subfamily Giraffinae
Giraffa camelopardalis.   Giraffe; 12 subspecies found in central, eastern and southern Africa.

Superfamily Bovoidae (hollow horned animals)
Subfamily Antilocaprinae
Antilocapra americana.   Pronghorn Antelope; 3 subspecies in the plains of N. America.
Subfamily Bovinae
Boselaphus tragocamelus.   Nilgai. India.
Tragelaphus stepsiceros.   Greater Kudu. Africa.
T. imberbis.   Lesser Kudu. Africa.
T. angasii.   Nyala. Africa.
T. buxtoni.   Mountain Nyala. Ethiopia.
T. scriptus.   Bushbuck; 2 subspecies. Africa.
T. spekii.   Sitatunga. Africa.
Taurotragus oryx.   Common Eland. Africa.
T. derbianus.   Giant Eland. West African Coast.
Boocercus eurycerus.   Bongo. West and central Africa.

Tribe Bovini
Anoa depressicornis.   Anoa. Celebes.
A. mindorensis.   Tamarou. Mindoro Island, Philippines.
Bos taurus.   Domestic European Cattle.
Bos indicus.   Domestic brahman or humped cattle.
Bos grunniens.   Yak. Northern Asia.
Bos gaurus.   Gaur. India, southeastern Asia.
Bos frontalis.   Gayal. Assam, Burma.
Bos sauveli.   Kouprey or Forest Ox. Cambodia.
Bos banteng.   Banting; 2 subspecies in Burma, Java, Maylay Peninsula.
Bison bison.   American Bison (Buffalo). Formerly over most of N. America.
B. bonasus.   European Bison or Wisent. Formerly most of central Europe.
Syncerus caffer.   Cape Buffalo. Central Africa.
S. nanus.   Buffalo; 2 subspecies (Chad or Red); central or west Africa.
Bubalus bubalis.   Indian Buffalo. India and neighboring countries.

Subfamily Hippotraginae
Kobus ellipsiprymnus.   Common Waterbuck. Africa.
K. defassa.   Defassa Waterbuck. Central Africa.
K. leche.   Lechwe; 2 subspecies. Central Africa.
K. megaceros.   Nile Lechwe. Southern Sudan.
K. kob.   Kob; 3 subspecies. Central Africa.
K. vardoni.   Puku. Zambia, Malawi.
Redunca arundinum.   Common Reedbuck. South to Central Africa.
R. redunca.   Behor Reedbuck. Central Africa.
R. fulvorufula.   Mountain Reedbuck. East Africa.
Damaliscus hunteri.   Hunter's Hartebeest. Central Africa.
D. lunatus. 4 subspecies — Senegal Hartebeest, Topi, Tiang, Sassaby. Central Africa.
D. dorcas. 2 subspecies — Bontebok, Blesbok. Central Africa.
Alcelaphus buselaphus.   Hartebeest; 5 subspecies. Africa.

A. caama. Cape Hartebeest. Africa.
A. lichtensteini. Lichtenstein's Hartebeest. Africa.
Connochoetes gnou. White-tailed Gnu. Central Africa.
C. taurinus. 2 subspecies — Brindled and White-bearded Gnu. Central Africa.
Pelea capreolus. Vaal Rhebok. South Africa.
Hippotragus niger. 2 subspecies — Sable and Giant Sable Antelope. Central Africa.
H. equinus. Roan Antelope. Central to southern Africa.
H. leucophoeus. Bluebok. Southern Africa.
Oryx gazella. 2 subspecies — Gemsbok, Beisa Oryx. Central and SW Africa.
O. leucoryx. Arabian Oryx. Arabia.
O. dammah. White Oryx. Deserts of N. Africa.
Addax nasomaculatus. Addax. Deserts of N. Africa.

Subfamily Antilopinae
Ammodorcas clarkei. Dibatag. Somali, Ethiopia.
Antidorcas marsupialis. Springbuck or Springbok. South Africa.
Aepyceros melampus. Impalla. East Africa.
Litocranius walleri. Gerenuk. Somali, Ethiopia, Tanzania.
Gazella dama. Addra Gazelle. Deserts of N. Africa.
G. dorcas. Dorcas Gazelle. Deserts of N. Africa.
G. muscatensis. Muscat Gazelle. Eastern Arabia.
G. spekei. Speke's Gazelle. Somalia.
G. leptoceros. Loder's Gazelle. Deserts of N. Africa.
G. soemmerringii. Soemmerring's Gazelle. Somalia, Ethiopia.
G. rufifrons. Red-fronted Gazelle. Central Africa.
G. thomsonii. Thompson's Gazelle. West and southern Africa.
G. arabica. Arabian Gazelle. West and southern Arabia.
G. cuvieri. Edmi Gazelle. Morocco, Algeria, Tunisia.
G. bennetti. Indian Gazelle. India.
G. granti. Grant's Gazelle. Central Africa.
G. subgutturosa. Goitered Gazelle. Gobi Desert in Asia.
Procapra gutturosa. Zeren Gazelle. Mongolia.
P. picticudata. 2 subspecies. Goa and Prezewalski's Gazelles. Tibetan plateau, Mongolia.
Antilope cervicapra. Blackbuck. Plains of India.
Tetracerus quadricornis. Chousingha. India.
Saiga tatarica. Saiga. Central Asia.
Pantholops hodgsoni. Chiru or Tibetan Antelope. Tibet.
Sylvicapra grimmia. 3 subspecies — Gray Crowned and Athi Gray Duiker. Central and southern Africa.
Cephalophus dorsalis. 2 subspecies — Bay and Chestnut Duiker. Central Africa.
C. natalensis. Weyn's Duiker. Central Africa.
C. silvicultor. Yellow-backed Duiker. Central Africa.
C. spadix. Abbott's Duiker. Tanzania.
C. leucogaster. Gaboon Duiker. Gabon, Congo.
C. maxwelli. Maxwell's Blue Duiker. West Coast of Africa.
C. zebra. Zebra Antelope. Liberia, Sierra Leone.
C. monticolo. 2 subspecies — Equatorial Blue Duiker and Simpson's Duiker. Central Africa.
Ourebia ourebi. Uasin Gishu Oribi. Central Africa.
Raphicerus campestris. Masailand Steinbok. Tanzania, N. Kenya.
R. melanotis. Grysbok. South to Central Africa.
Oreotragus oreotragus. 2 subspecies of Klipspringers. Kenya.
Neotragus pygmaeus. Royal Pygmy Antelope. Sierra Leone, Ghana.
N. moschatus. Suni or Zanzibar Antelope. Central Africa.
Dorcatragus megalotis. Beira. Somalia.
Madoqua phillipsi. Phillip's Dik-Dik. Somalia, Ethiopia.
M. guentheri. Long-snouted Dik-Dik. Somalia, Ethiopia.

Subfamily Caprinae
  Tribe Rupicaprini (goat-antelopes)
    Oreamnos americanus.   Rocky Mountain Goat. Rocky Mtn. of N. America.
    Rupicapra rupicapra.   Chamois. Mountains of southern Europe.
    Capricornis sumatraensis.   Serow. Mtn. of southeastern Asia.
    C. crispus.   Japanese Serow. Mtn. of Japan.
    Noemorhedus goral.   Goral. Himalayan Mtn.

  Tribe Ovibovini (Muskox and Takin)
    Ovibos muschatus.   Muskox. Arctic areas of N. America.
    Budorcas taxicolor.   Takin. Mountains of southeast Asia.

  Tribe Caprini (Ibex, Goats, Tahr, Sheep)
    Capra ibex.   Ibex or Steinbock. Mtn. of southern Europe.
    C. pyrenaica.   Spanish Ibex or Spanish Tur. Pyrenees Mtn.
    C. hircus aegagrus.   Persian Ibex or Pasang. Mtn. of southeast Asia.
    C. ibex.   3 subspecies — Asiatic Ibex, Himalayan Ibex and Nubian Ibex found respectively in the Mtn. of central Asia, Himalayan or N. Africa.
    C. walie.   Abyssinian Ibex. Mtn. of Ethiopia.
    C. falconeri.   2 subspecies — Astor and Cabul Makhor. Mtn. of Kashmir and of Afghanistan.
    C. caucasica.   Caucasian Tur. Caucasus.
    C. hircus nana.   African Pygmy Goat. Central Africa.
    C. hircus hircus.   Domestic Goats.
    Hemitragus jemlahicus.   Tahr, Himalayan Tahr. Himalayan Mtn.
    H. hylocrius.   Milgiri Tahr. Mtn. of India.
    H. jayakaari.   Arabian Tahr. Mtn. of southern Arabia.
    Ovis musimon.   Muflon. Corsica, Sardinia.
    O. orientalis.   3 subspecies — Red Sheep, Punjab Urial, Afghan Urial found in Asia Minor and N. Asia.
    O. canadensis.   Rocky Mountain Sheep or Bighorn Sheep. Mtn. of western N. America.
    O. dalli.   White Sheep, Dall's Sheep. Alaska south through British Columbia.
    O. ammon.   3 subspecies — Siberian, Alatau and Marco Polo's Argali, found respectively in Siberia, Tien Shan Mtn. and Pamir Plateau.
    O. aries.   Domestic Sheep.
    Pseudois nayaur.   Bharal, Burrel or Blue Sheep. Highlands of N. Asia.
    Ammotragus lervia.   Aoudad or Barbary Sheep. Mtn. of N. Africa.

Pseudoruminants (Camels and Their Relatives)
    Camelus bactrianus.   Bactrian Camel. Asia.
    C. dromedarius.   Arabian Camel. Probably originated in Arabia.
    Lama glama huanacus.   Guanaco. Western S. America.
    L. g. glama.   Llama. Andes Mtn.
    L. g. pacas.   Alpaca. High plateaus of Peru, Bolivia.
    Vicugna vicugna.   Vicuna. Andes Mtn.

References Cited

Anonymous. Undated. Benchmarks: A statement of Concepts and Positions. Soc. for Range Mgmt., Denver, Colo.
Mochi, Ugo and T.D. Carter. 1971. Hoofed Mammals of the World. 2nd ed. Chas. Scribner's Sons, N.Y.
Price, J.F. and B.S. Schweigert. 1971. The Science of Meat and Meat Products. W.H. Freeman & Co.
Simpson, G.G. 1945. Bul. Amer. Museum of Natural History. 85:1-350.

Part I

CHAPTER 2 — ANATOMY OF THE STOMACH OF RUMINANTS AND PSEUDORUMINANTS

The principal function of the gastrointestinal tract (GIT) of animals is to provide for the digestion and absorption of nutrients and the excretion of certain waste products. Although the functions may be similar in very diverse species, the nature of their food differs markedly as does their GIT. Most carnivorous (meat eaters) and omnivorous (meat-plant eaters) animals have relatively simple stomachs referred to as **monogastric** stomachs. In such animals the stomach is essentially a pouch-like structure which contains glands that secrete HCl and pepsinogen, the precursor of pepsin. In the young mammal, rennin (coagulates milk) and gastric lipase (hydrolyzes fat) are also secreted. In contrast, the stomach of most birds is considerably different in structure in that it is divided into 3 different parts — namely the crop (storage and possibly some fermentation), the proventriculus (gastric secretions), and the gizzard (mechanical reduction). These three organs combine, to some degree, the functions of the teeth and stomach in monogastric species; the type of digestion that takes place is similar to that in mammals.

Herbivorous species, however, have developed stomachs and/or intestinal modifications which enable them to utilize cellulose and other plant polysaccharides such as hemicellulose and xylan. Cellulose is a basic structural carbohydrate in nearly all plants and it is one of the more abundant organic compounds available to terrestrial animals. Utilization of such a large potential source of energy is desirable and necessary to support many different animal species. For some unknown reason during the evolutionary development of vertebrates they did not develop the capacity to produce in the GIT enzymes capable of hydrolyzing the β, 1-4 glucosidic linkage which binds glucose molecules together to form cellulose.

Many bacteria and fungi produce cellulolytic enzymes capable of hydrolyzing cellulose to cellobiose or glucose. Since herbivorous animals apparently could not produce cellulolytic enzymes themselves, they have developed a variety of ways to utilize cellulose and related plant polysaccharides indirectly by playing host to symbiotic microorganisms. The ruminant stomach represents one modification of the GIT which allows the animals to utilize large amounts of cellulose. The GIT's of the horse and rabbit represent another modification in which there is a large cecum where microbial activity occurs which is believed to be similar to that in the rumen. Some herbivorous species, such as rabbits, practice coprophagy (ingestion of feces), and thereby may get additional benefits from fermentation in the cecum and large gut in that they obtain a supply of nutrients that are not normally absorbed by this part of the GIT (particularly vitamins). Other animals such as rats have similar habits.

The ruminant stomach, in contrast, has developed into an organ that provides for extensive pregastric microbial fermentation. Microbial fermentation takes place in the gut, primarily the cecum and colon of all animals, but pregastric fermentation is restricted to ruminants, pseudoruminants and a few other isolated species.

It is interesting to speculate on the evolutionary development of the GIT of animals as represented by carnivorous, omnivorous and herbivorous animals. In the case of carnivores, the GIT is relatively short and simple. Omnivores usually have a relatively longer gut, perhaps a more complex stomach, and may have slight to moderate development of the cecum. As mentioned, herbivores have provided for either pre- or postgastric fermentation, and the gut is usually relatively longer and more complex. With respect to evolutionary development, it seems that two possibilities are apparent. In one case we might suggest that the animal developed a GIT suited to the type of food which was available; in the other, perhaps the animal must seek out food that is suited to its digestive organs. Of the two possibilities, the author is inclined to choose the first, although this is like speculating on whether the chicken or the egg arrived first on the scene.

Anatomy of the Stomach

The stomach of the ruminant animal is divided into four compartments, namely **reticulum, rumen, omasum** and **abomasum.** The reticulum and the rumen are joined by a fold of tissue, the **reticulo-rumen fold,** with the result that ingesta may flow freely from one to the other. It is in the reticulo-rumen* that most microbial activity takes place. With respect to the other two parts of the stomach, the function of the omasum has not been clearly defined; functions of the abomasum appears to be similar to the simple stomach of monogastric species.

In view of the complexity of the ruminant stomach, its marked effect on the nutrition and physiology of the animal, and in order to provide a readily available description, a relatively detailed description of the anatomy of the ruminant stomach is included in this chapter. For more detailed descriptions and pictorial illustrations, the reader is referred to Sisson and Grossman (1953) or other references on anatomy of domestic animals, such as that of Habel (1964). The reader is also referred to the figures and pictures showing various parts of the stomach and the drawings illustrating the blood supply (Fig. 2-1 through 2-17; Plates 2-1 through 2-8).

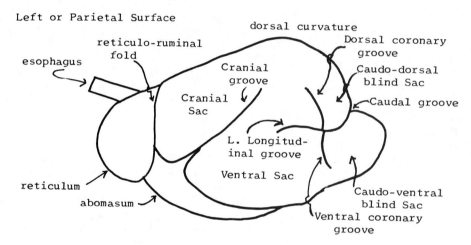

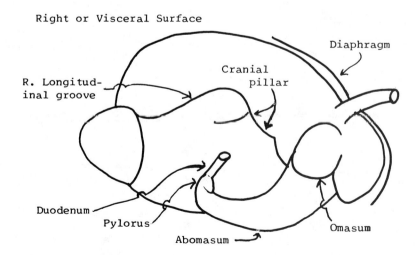

Figure 2-1. Diagramatic sketch of a sheep's stomach.

*Preferred nomenclature is said to be rumino-reticulum, but the author chooses to use this terminology, partly because it has been used for some time.

Exterior of the Stomach

The stomach of ruminant species is very large in proportion to body size and occupies nearly ¾ of the abdominal cavity. It fills the left half of the abdominal cavity except for a small space occupied by part of the spleen (cattle) and a few coils of the small intestine (see Fig. 2-2, 3). The rumen extends over the median plane ventrally and its long axis reaches from a point opposite the ventral part of the 7th or 8th rib almost to the pelvis. It is somewhat compressed from side to side. The parietal (left) surface rests against the diaphragm, left wall of the abdomen, and spleen. The visceral (right) surface is more irregular and is related to the omasum and abomasum, the intestines, liver, pancreas, left kidney, the aorta and posterior vena cava. The dorsal curvature follows the curve of the diaphragm and sublumbar muscles and is firmly attached to these structures by peritoneum and connective tissue as far caudal as the 4th lumbar vertebra (Sisson and Grossman, 1953).

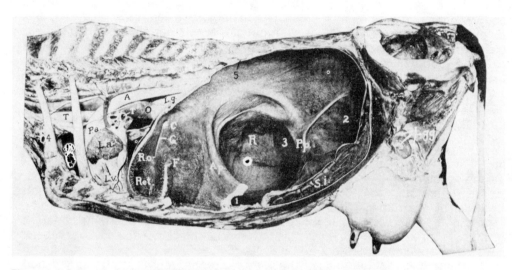

Figure 2-2. Internal placement of the bovine stomach, left view in a partially dissected cow. Ro is the reticulo-omasal orifice; Ret, the reticulum; F, reticulo-ruminal fold; C, cardia; G, reticular groove; Ap, cranial pillar; Pp, caudal pillar; Si, small intestines. From Sisson and Grossman [1953]. Courtesy of Saunders Pub. Co.

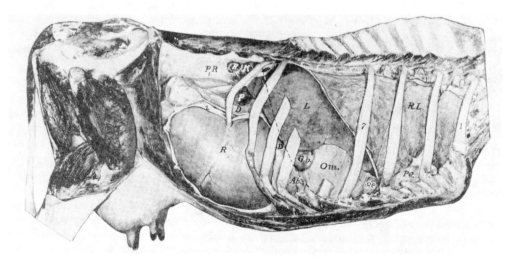

Figure 2-3. Internal placement of the bovine stomach, right view. R, rumen [ventral sac]; Ab, abomasum [pyloric part]; Gb, gall bladder; Om, omasum; L, liver; P, pancreas; D, duodenum; K, kidney; RL, right lung. From Sisson and Grossman [1943]. Courtesy of Saunders Pub. Co.

The reticulum rests against the diaphragm opposite the 6-8th ribs (cattle) on the left of the median plane. It is flattened more or less by pressure of the other compartments and by contact with the diaphragm and the liver and the omasum and abomasum on the right side. The omasum is connected to the reticulum by a short, narrow neck (Fig. 2-6). It is more or less spherical in form and lies to the right of the median plane, opposite the 7-11 ribs in cattle. The abomasum is an elongated sac, variable in form, which lies chiefly on the abdominal floor. The cranial blind end, the fundus, is much the larger part. The smaller pyloric part joins the duodenum at the pylorus, usually situated near the 9-10th rib in cattle (Sisson and Grossman, 1953). The duodenum of the small intestine is attached to the right side of the rumen as is the pancreas.

The exterior surfaces of the reticulo-rumen are marked by **grooves** which are structures separating the organ into sacs and are synonymous with pillars on the interior. The most conspicuous of these grooves on the exterior surface is the reticulo-ruminal fold, which separates the reticulum from the cranial (or anterior) sac of the rumen (Fig. 2-1). Dorsally, there is no natural separation between the reticulum and rumen with the result that these two structures join together to form the cardia, a dome-like vestibule at which the esophagus terminates (Sisson and Grossman, 1953). Of the other grooves, the transversely directed cranial groove divides the cranial sac from the ventral sac. The left and right longitudinal grooves run into the caudal (posterior) groove at the rear of the rumen. The caudo-dorsal (dorsal blind) and caudo-ventral (ventral blind) blind sacs are marked off from the dorsal and ventral sacs by the dorsal coronary and ventral coronary grooves, respectively (Fig. 2-1). In the case of sheep, the right dorsal coronary groove is absent.

Interior of the Stomach

The interior of the reticulo-rumen is partially divided into sacs by the reticulo-ruminal fold and by the various pillars (Fig. 2-1, 2). The greatest restriction of flow of ingesta would be between the reticulum and rumen, but there still remains a relatively large opening between these two compartments (Fig. 2-4). The pillars are composed of thick, muscular bundles of tissue that project into the rumen. The cranial, longi-

tudinal, and caudal pillars form a large and almost complete ring in the rumen (cattle). The cranial pillar in the cow is very large in comparison to the reticulo-ruminal fold. In the sheep the reticulo-ruminal fold is the more prominent of the two structures (Stevens and Stettler, 1966). The pillars, as explained in a subsequent chapter (Ch. 6), aid in the contraction of the various sacs and in circulation of ingesta in the reticulo-rumen.

The **cardia** is the terminal end of the esophagus in the rumen (Fig. 2-2, 4, 5). The opening (cattle) is usually slit-like and about an inch in height. The cardia is also the point of origin of the **reticular groove.** The reticular (or esophageal) groove begins at the cardia and passes ventrally, ending at the **reticulo-omasal orifice.** In cattle, it is about 7-8 in. long. The groove is twisted in a spiral fashion so that its thickened edges project first backward, then to the left, and finally forward (Sisson and Grossman, 1953).

It was once thought that the reticulum, rumen, and omasum were derived embryologically from the same common tissue, probably esophageal, since the tissue lining these compartments is similar in some respects. However, subsequent information has shown that this is not the case (Lambert, 1958; Warner, 1958). The type of cells lining these three compartments (commonly called the **forestomach**) is classified histologically as keratinized, stratified squamous epithelial cells (Lavker et al, 1969), a type that does not produce mucus and which is nonglandular. Although some authors refer to this type of cell lining as mucosa, this is improper use of the word; consequently, the lining of the stomach will be referred to here as epithelia, not as mucosa. The epithelia of the reticulum is raised into folds forming cells with four, five or six sides, thus giving rise to the scientific name as well as the common term, honeycomb (Fig. 2-4, 5, Plate 2-1). The cells are subdivided by smaller folds and the bottom of the cells have numerous pointed, horny papillae (Plate 2-1; Ch. 3, Plate 3-1). The cells are smaller and gradually disappear near the reticular groove and the edge of the reticulo-ruminal fold. In some species the cells reach maximal height in the ventral portions of the reticulum. At the reticulo-omasal orifice there are peculiar horny papillae, termed unguliform, which resemble the claws of a small bird (Fig. 2-5). The reticulo-omasal orifice is situated in the

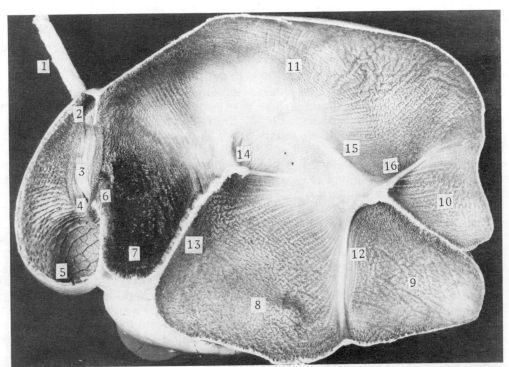

Figure 2-4. A dried bovine stomach preparation which illustrates the position of the reticular groove, 3, the space between [from 6 to 6] the reticulum and cranial sac, 7, and the relative size of the cranial sac. Other landmarks are: cardia, 2; cranial pillar, 13; longitudinal pillar, 15; dorsal [16] and ventral [12] coronary pillars. From Benevenga et al [1969].

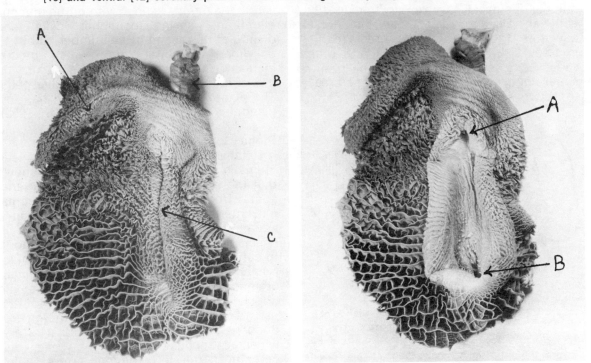

Figure 2-5. The reticulum and reticular groove of the bovine. Left. A, the dorsal aspect of the reticulo-ruminal fold; B, the esophagus; C, the reticular groove in a closed position. The cardia is at the upper end of the groove and the reticulo-omasal orifice at the lower end. Right. The groove is pinned in an open position to show its interior, the opening into the esophagus or cardia, A, and the reticulo-omasal orifice, B.

lesser curvature (right side), 5 to 6 in. above the bottom of the reticulum and to the right of the median plane (Sisson and Grossman, 1953).

In cattle the epithelia in the reticulum, rumen and omasum is rather dark brown in color except on the margins of the pillars and the upper part of the dorsal sac where the color gradually turns to a pale brown shade. The papillae (Plates 2-1 through 2-9) are most dense in the ventral parts of the cranial and ventral sacs; areas where, presumably, the most absorption occurs. Papillae from the various sacs can be distinguished from one another on the basis of shape and/or size, varying from large ones nearly half an inch long to small, sparse, horny papillae in the dorsal sac. Some are foliate, others are narrow or filiform and others are conical or club-shaped.

The interior of the omasum is partially filled by a variable number of longitudinal folds or leaves, the laminae omasi (Fig. 2-6, 7, 8), giving rise to use of the lay term, "the book." There is a series of large leaves which have a convex attached edge and a concave free edge. A second, third and fourth order (in terms of size) are also present. Becker et al (1963) found, in Jersey cattle, the total number of omasal leaves to vary from 89-192, with an average of 152 at the dorsal curvature. The sequence of the orders (cattle) is 1, 2, 1, 3, 1, 2, 1, 4. The fourth order varies considerably in size, ranging from a small ridge, just preceptible in some areas, to about ½ inch in height.

A cross section of a full organ (Fig. 2-7) shows that the spaces between the leaves are tightly packed with rather finely ground ingesta. The leaves have only a relatively few small horny papillae (Fig. 2-9). It has been calculated that the omasal leaves in bovines provide a surface area equivalent to about ⅓ of the total forestomach (Stevens and Stettler, 1966).

The reticulo-omasal orifice opens into the neck of the omasum from which ingesta may either pass between the leaves or into the abomasum through the neck of the omasum (Fig. 2-6). A groove, the **sulcus omasi**, extends from the reticulo-omasal opening to the omaso-abomasal opening and is presumed to provide a direct pathway for finely divided solids and liquids from the reticulum to the abomasum. The neck of the abomasum is short and a relatively large part of the omasal body projects across the omaso-abomasal orifice which is really not an orifice in the true meaning since there is no evidence of a sphincter. It is apparently open most of the time (Sisson and Grossman, 1953; Sellers and Stevens, 1966).

The interior of the abomasum is divided by a constriction into the fundus (proximal or cranial position) and the pyloric region (Fig. 2-10). The fundus is lined with a true mucous membrane having columnar cells and glandular tissue and has a number (about 12 or more) of spiral folds which greatly increase the surface area (Fig. 2-10, 11) available for proliferation of glandular cells. The pyloric region is narrower and has few glandular cells (Sisson and Grossman, 1953).

Blood Supply to the Stomach

Relatively recent information on the sheep stomach (Anderson and Weber, 1969) shows that the stomach receives its entire arterial supply from a single artery, the celiac-cranial mesenteric trunk, which in turn arises from a common trunk of the abdominal aorta in sheep or from separate branches of the aorta in cattle (Habel, 1964). There are four major branches of the celiac artery to the ruminant stomach (Plate 2-10): the common hepatic artery, which in turn branches to the pancreas, liver, gall bladder and the gastro-duodenal branch; the right ruminal artery, which branches to the pancreas and omentum; the left ruminal artery which branches to the reticulum and esophagus; and the left gastric artery which branches to the omasum and abomasum.

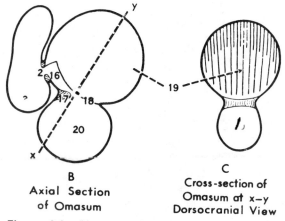

B
Axial Section of Omasum

C
Cross-section of Omasum at x–y Dorsocranial View

Figure 2-6. Diagrammatic section of the bovine omasum showing [2] the reticulo-omasal orifice, [16] omasal canal, [17] omasal pillar, [18] omasal-abomasal orifice, [19] omasal leaves [lamina], and [20] the abomasum. From Sellers and Stevens [1966].

Cattle

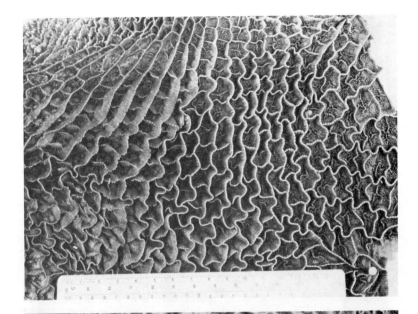

Sheep

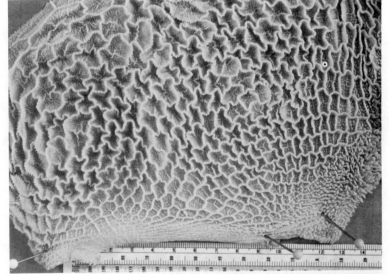

Black-tailed deer

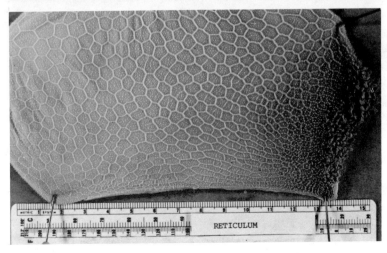

Plate 2-1. The reticulum of cattle, sheep and black-tailed deer. Note typical 'honeycombed' cell structure. Also note the difference in cell depth, particularly for the deer.

Cattle

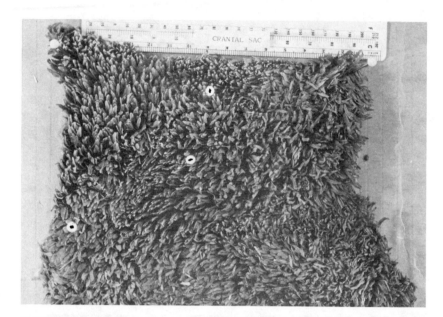

Sheep

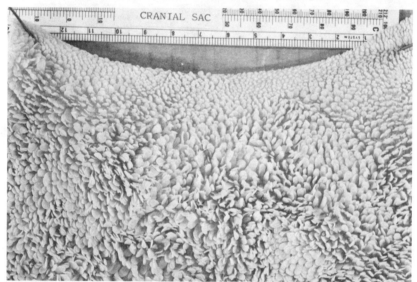

Black-tailed deer

Plate 2-2. Tissue from the cranial sac taken immediately adjacent to the reticulo-ruminal fold. Note the difference in shape, color and length of the papillae between the different species.

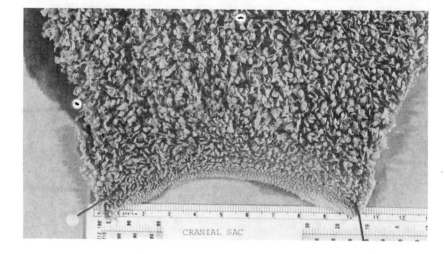

Cattle

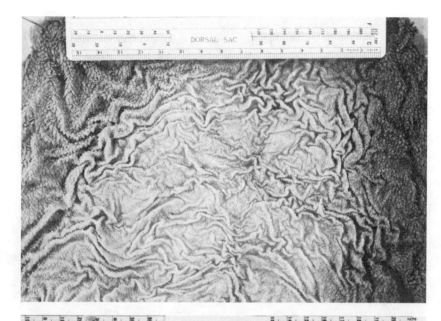

Sheep

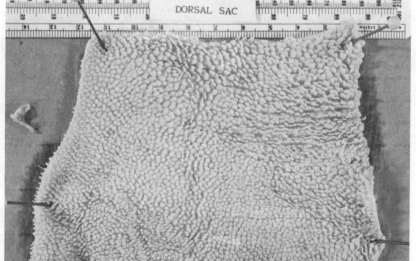

Black-tailed deer

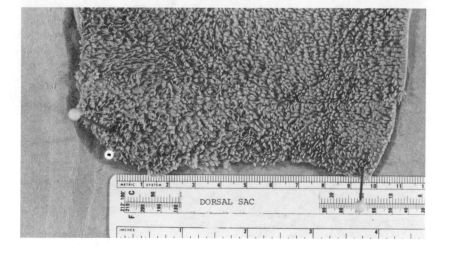

Plate 2-3. The dorsal rumen sac epithelia. Note that the dorsal sac of cattle, in the center of the photograph, that the papillae are small and sparce as compared to the other species.

Cattle

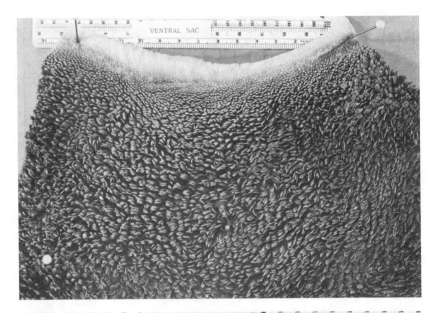

Sheep

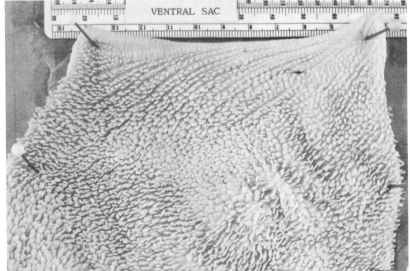

Black-tailed deer

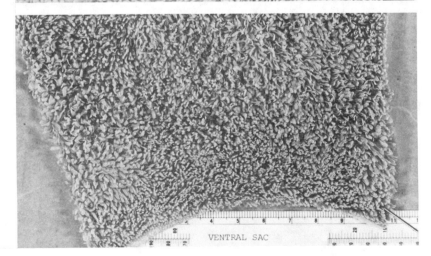

Plate 2-4. Epithelia from the ventral sac. Samples taken immediately adjacent to the cranial pillar [nearest to the ruler].

Cattle

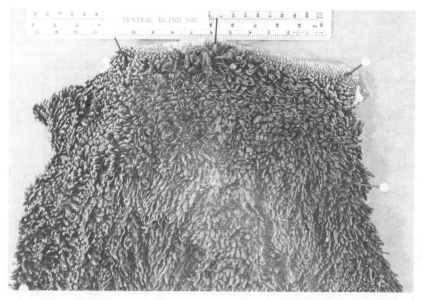

Sheep

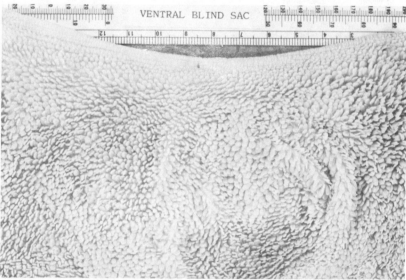

Black-tailed deer

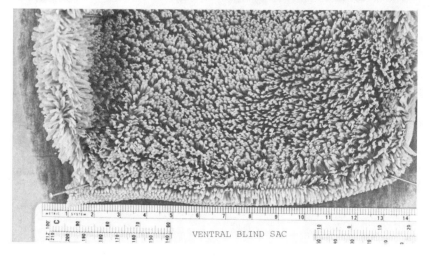

Plate 2-5. Epithelia of the caudo-ventral blind sac. Samples taken immediately adjacent to the caudal pillar.

Cattle

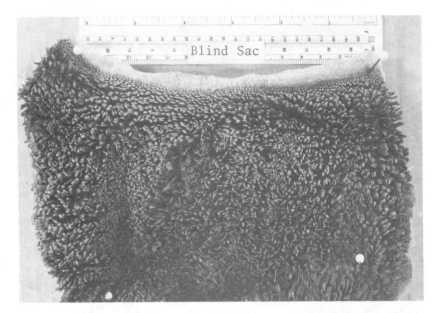

Sheep

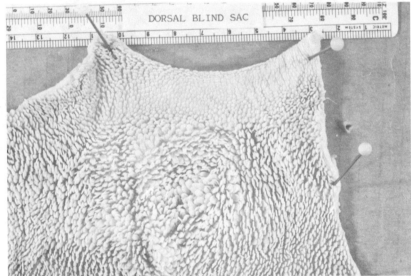

Black-tailed deer

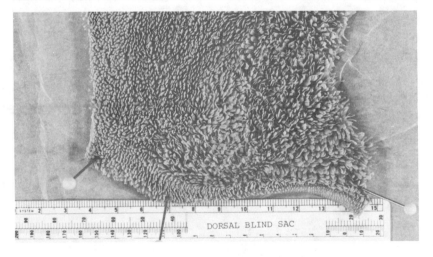

Plate 2-6. Epithelia of the caudo-dorsal blind sac. Samples taken immediately adjacent to the caudal pillar.

Cattle

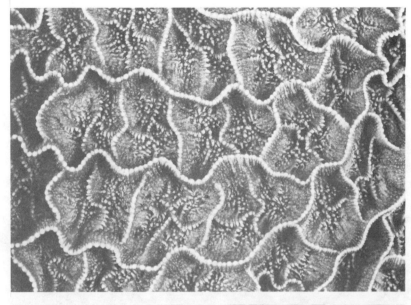

Sheep

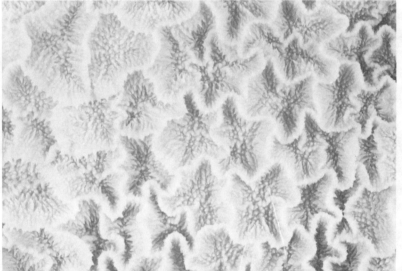

Goat

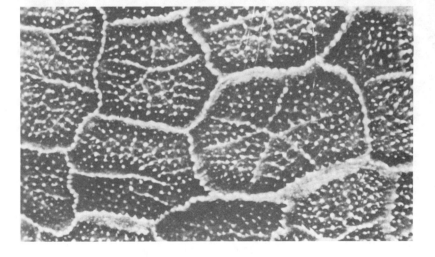

Plate 2-7. Reticular tissue of cattle, sheep and goat enlarged to show the secondary cells within the larger cells.

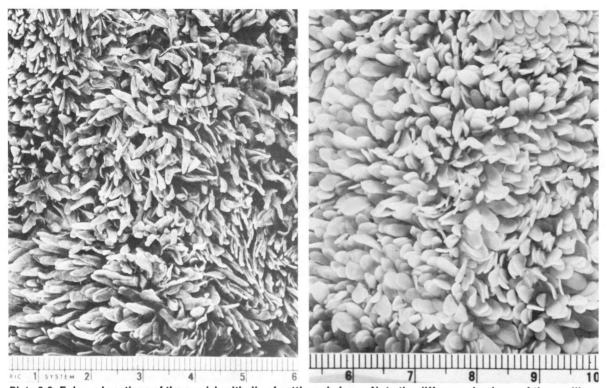

Plate 2-8. Enlarged sections of the cranial epithelia of cattle and sheep. Note the difference in shape of the papillae.

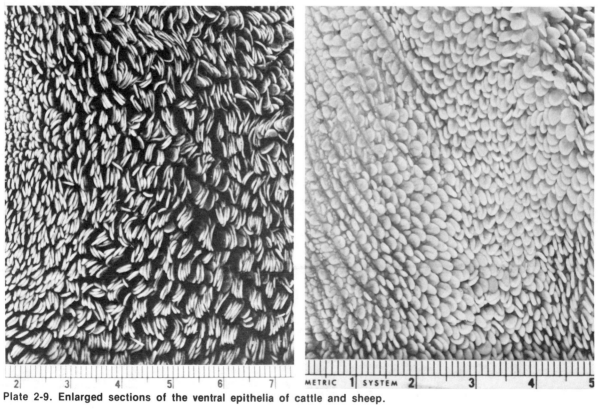

Plate 2-9. Enlarged sections of the ventral epithelia of cattle and sheep.

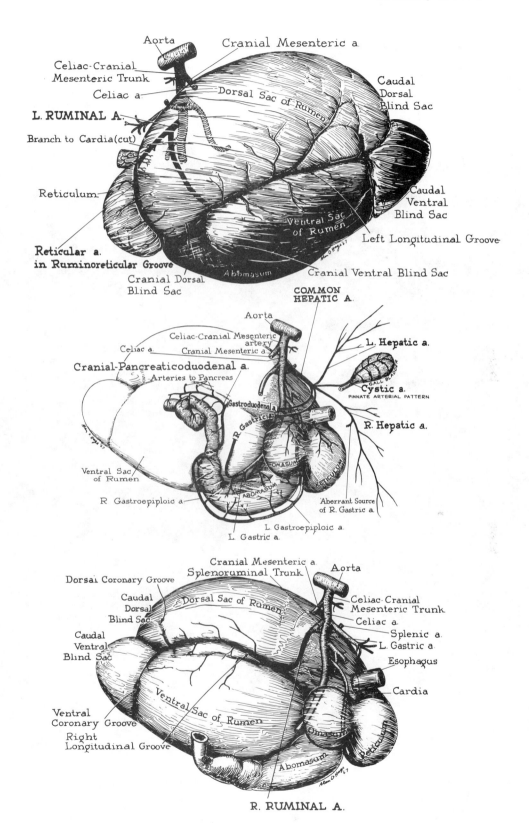

Plate 2-10. Semidiagrammatic drawings showing ovine rumen blood supply. Top, left surface of the course of the left ruminal artery; Center, right surface showing distribution of common hepatic artery; Bottom, origin and distribution of right ruminal artery. From Anderson and Weber [1969].

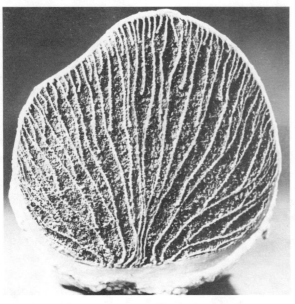
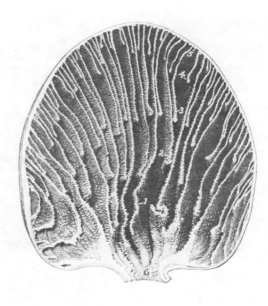

Figure 2-7. Left. Cross section of the bovine omasum showing how tightly packed the organ is with ingesta. Right. Cross section with the ingesta washed out. The various numbers refer to the laminae of different orders. No. 6 refers to the neck of the omasum. Left, courtesy of R.B. Becker, Fla. Agr. Expt. Sta. Right, from Sisson and Grossman [1943]. Courtesy of Saunders Pub. Co.

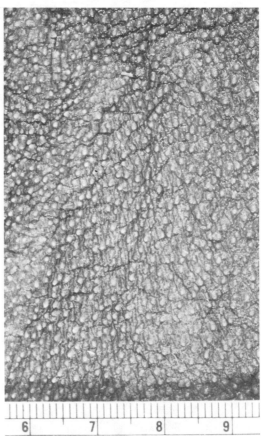

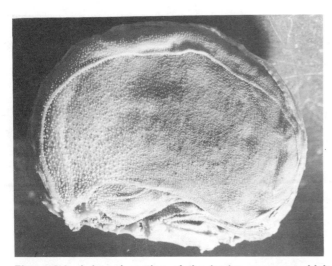

Figure 2-8. A lateral section of the bovine omasum which illustrates the sizes of two of the four different orders and shows the nature of the free edge of the leaves. Courtesy of R.B. Becker, Univ. of Florida.

Figure 2-9. A close-up of the surface of the bovine omasal leaf.

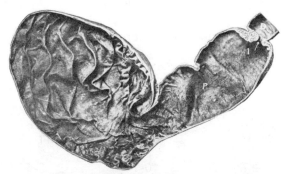

Figure 2-10. The interior of the bovine abomasum. F is the fundus gland region with large spiral folds; P, pyloric region; D, duodenum; 1, pylorus. From Sisson and Grossman [1953]. Courtesy of Saunders Pub. Co.

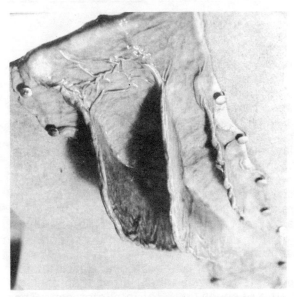

Figure 2-11. A picture illustrating the spiral folds in the abomasum of the sheep. A section of the abomasum was tacked to a board so that the folds would hang vertically.

Blood from the stomach area is drained into the portal vein which goes directly to the liver. One of the large veins, the gastric vein, receives blood from the right ruminal vein and from the left ruminal, omaso-abomasal, and reticular veins. The anterior mesenteric vein receives blood from three other veins which drain blood from the intestines (Sisson and Grossman, 1953).

Relative Size of Various Parts of the Stomach

The true relative size of the various compartments of the stomach is difficult to determine. In the live animal, estimates have been made by filling the reticulo-rumen with water and then measuring the water. Other methods involve the use of various markers that can be added to stomach contents, allowing the time for adequate dilution and equilibration and then sampling and analyzing for the marker, thus giving an estimate of quantity of liquid. Measurements on stomachs of slaughtered animals have been carried out by filling them with water, measurement of the normal stomach contents, or by determining the wet or dry tissue weights of the various parts.

In the live animal it is difficult to measure the capacity of any part of the stomach except the reticulo-rumen. In excised parts there is the problem of abnormal distention and "over-filling." The reticulo-rumen is normally never completely filled with liquid and solids since it contains appreciable amounts of gas. In addition, it is restricted in shape by its own tissue as well as by the organs or tissue against which it rests. The volume of the excised stomach may also be different as a result of relaxation of muscles and ligaments. Presumably, the best measure of "physiological fill" should be a measurement of stomach contents of a "normally" fed animal. Some of the published data on relative size of stomach compartments are tabulated in Table 2-1.

The water fill and wet stomach contents give somewhat comparable data, but both differ from the wet stomach tissue method, particularly in estimating the relative amount of the reticulo-rumen. The data also show that the omasum of the sheep is relatively smaller than that of cattle and that the abomasum is relatively larger. If the reticulo-rumen is subdivided, the data on adult sheep show the following relative percentages of wet stomach tissue: reticulum, 11%; rumen, 62%; omasum, 5% and abomasum, 22-23%. Comparable values for cattle are approximately 5-7%, 50-55%, 26-30% and 13-14%, respectively.

The weight of stomach contents for animals of comparable size is quite variable, as might be anticipated, and will be influenced primarily by type of diet and condition of the animal. Data in the literature indicate that reticulo-rumen contents might be expected to vary between 10-20% of body weight. Stomach contents will normally increase as the amount of roughage in the ration increases (see Ch. 10); as an animal gets fat, stomach contents will usually decrease (as a % of body weight).

Table 2-1. Relative size of the ruminant stomach compartments as determined with different techniques.[a]

| Method | Animal | Age | Percent found in | | |
			reticulo-rumen	omasum	abomasum
Water fill	cattle	adult	86-88	6-7	6-8
	sheep	adult	85-87	2-3	11-12
Wet stomach contents	cattle	adult	81-87	10-14	3-5
	sheep	adult	88-93	2	5-10
Wet stomach tissue	cattle	adult	56-60	26-30	13
	sheep	adult	69-73	5-6	22-23

[a] Data cited by Warner and Flatt (1965)

Comparison of Bovine Stomach to Other Ruminants

The stomach of the sheep (and goat) is quite similar to that of cattle, although considerably smaller, having an average capacity of about 15 1. The dorsal sac of the rumen is a little longer than the ventral sac. The ventral sac is relatively larger and more of its volume extends to the right of the medial plane than in cattle. The caudo-ventral sac extends further back than that of the dorsal sac (Fig. 2-12). There are two longitudinal grooves on the right side which join at each end, thus enclosing a long, narrow and prominent area. The dorsal groove contains the right ruminal artery and the ventral one corresponds to the pillar. The left coronary grooves do not extend to the curvatures. There is no dorsal coronary groove on the right side, but the ventral one is very distinct and extends to the curvature (Sisson and Grossman, 1953).

The reticular cells are smaller in diameter and not as deep (Plate 2-1, 2-7). The papillae in the sheep rumen lack the pigmentation of bovines and are considerably smaller, particularly in the cranial and ventral sacs. They are usually somewhat tongue-like in shape. Although somewhat more dense in the ventral areas, the dorsal sac is papillated, not glabrous as in cattle. The lateral part of the reticulo-ruminal fold ends half an inch or more behind the cardia and the fold is relatively larger and more developed in sheep than in bovines. Its ventral part curves more

backward and less to the right than in cattle. The cranial sac is relatively smaller in sheep and does not extend as close to the abdominal floor. The omasum is much smaller than the reticulum, its capacity being only about 500 ml. It is oval and compressed laterally. The leaves are much less numerous than in cattle, with about 50 leaves the usual number. The sequence of leaves (in order of size) is: 1, 2, 1, 3, 1, 2, 4. The abomasum is relatively larger and longer than in cattle with a capacity about twice that of the reticulum (Sisson and Grossman, 1953; author's unpublished data).

The rumen of American deer (black-tailed, mule) is relatively much larger than that of cattle or sheep (as % of total stomach). The caudo-ventral blind sac is much shorter than that of sheep (Fig. 2-12) and there is a distinct dorsal coronary groove on the right side. The omasum and abomasum are relatively quite small as compared to domestic species. Reticular cells are small in diameter and very shallow (Plate 2-1), and rumen papillae tend to be dark brown and cylindrical in shape; although somewhat more dense in the cranial and ventral sacs. The papillae are relatively uniform in density throughout the rumen. Omasal leaves number about 50 and are in the sequence of 1, 2, 1, 3, 1, 2, 1, 4. In the abomasum, the spiral folds number about 12, but they tend to be more narrow and thicker than in sheep.

Pronghorn antelope have a rumen somewhat more similar to sheep than that of deer in relative shape and size. The caudo-ventral

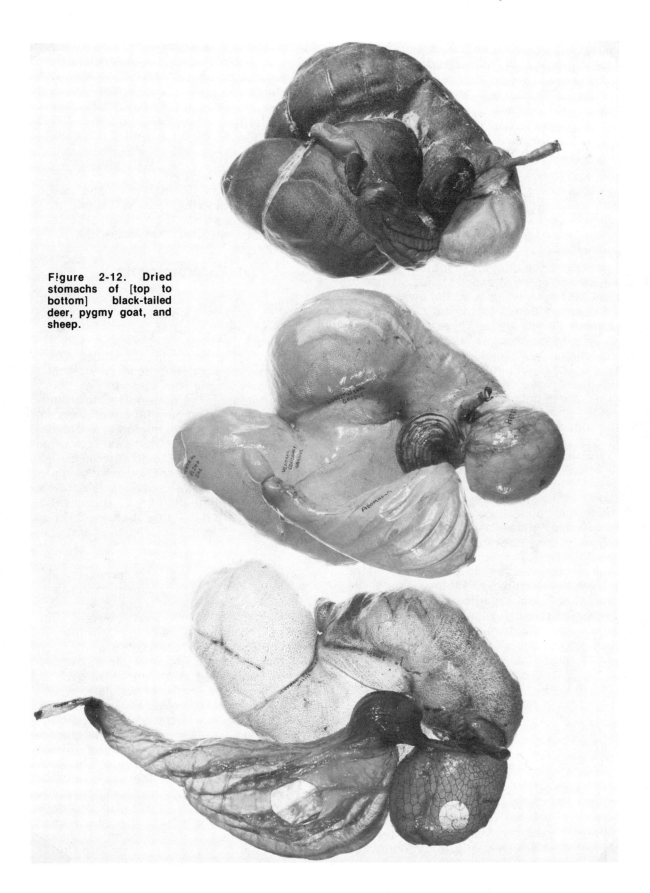

Figure 2-12. Dried stomachs of [top to bottom] black-tailed deer, pygmy goat, and sheep.

sac is of intermediate length and there is no well defined dorsal coronary groove on the right side. Reticular cells are about the same diameter as in sheep but are more shallow. Rumen epithelia are relatively uniform in density. The omasum is relatively large with about 50 leaves which are in the sequence of 1, 3, 1, 4, 1, 3, 1, 4, 1, 2, 3. The abomasum is also relatively large, especially as compared to deer.

Hofmann (1968) has a paper which is highly recommended for readers interested in comparative anatomy of wild ruminant species, African in this case. On the basis of his studies, Hofmann has divided ruminants into roughage or grass eaters, selective eaters, and transitional forms. His general description of the stomach characteristics of these different types is as follows:

Roughage Eaters (domestic cattle are an example). These animals have a large rumen which extends caudally into the pelvic inlet. The rumen is characterized by powerful pillars. The reticulum is relatively small, but has high thick-walled crests and deep cells with distinct subdivision into secondary and tertiary crests. Papillae show an uneven distribution with great variation in size and shape and generally with few in the dorsal sac. The omasum tends to be large, spherical in shape with numerous leaves of several orders. The leaves are thin and covered by short and usually conical papillae. The abomasum is relatively big and spacious.

Selective Eaters. These are animals which generally consume softer and juicy forage low in fiber. The rumen is smaller and usually does not extend much beyond the last lumbar vertebrae. Rumen pillars are small and weak, particularly so for the longitudinal pillar. The reticulum is relatively large and has extensive but shallow cells; secondary crests are frequently missing and tertiary crests are nearly always lacking. Rumen papillae show a regular distribution and are usually big, flat and tongue-shaped or somewhat reduced in size and number in the dorsal sac. The omasum is flat and kidney-shaped and relatively small or very small. It contains not more than a few leaves, often of only one order. The abomasum is relatively small.

Transitional Forms. These have been divided into (A) roughage eaters in wet environments — animals in which the stomach shows a reduced capacity with omasal leaves which are rather numerous and very thin, or (B) selective eaters in three subclasses: (1) those consuming hard, juicy leaves of desert plants; these animals tend to have relatively larger omasums and powerful rumen pillars; (2) animals showing seasonal intake of dry and fibrous forage; these show partial decrease in dorsal papillae; and (3) animals eating leaves and twigs; they tend to have big, soft, dense papillae in all parts of the rumen and a relatively large omasum.

Hofmann suggests that domestic cattle are typical of the roughage eaters and that sheep and goats should be classified in the transitional form described under B2.

Pseudoruminants

The camel, dromedary and new world camelids — llama, alpaca, guanaco, vicuna — are sometimes called pseudoruminants because their stomach is somewhat different than that of true ruminants. Presumably, their evolutionary development was similar to that of ruminants up to a point. Pseudoruminants are similar in many respects such as regurgitation of ingesta, having active stomach microbial fermentation, and stomach contractions somewhat related to ruminants. Minor differences are noted between the camel and the camelids.

The stomach of the camelids (Fig. 2-13, 14) has been studied by numerous investigators. Recent data have been published from Cornell University (Vallenas et al, 1971; Cummings et al, 1972). These papers indicate that the stomach of these animals is divided into three distinct compartments. The first compartment, frequently compared to the rumen, contains about 83% of the total volume. It is divided ventrally into cranial and caudal sacs by a pillar or transverse sulcus. In the ventral portions of both sacs there are areas containing oblong, raised, thin-walled sacculations (Fig. 2-15, 16). In areas not lined by sacculations, the lining is a stratified squamous epithelium. The second compartment, often compared to the reticulum, is small and contains glandular cells on its greater curvature. These animals have a ventricular groove (Fig. 2-14) which apparently serves the same function as the reticular groove in true ruminants. The third compartment is lined with glandular mucosa which is arranged in nonpermanent folds along the initial 1/5 and in permanent longitudinal pleats in the middle 3/5. In the initial 1/5 and terminal 1/5, tissue corresponds to true gastric gland tissue.

The function of the cells in the first compartment (previously called water cells) remains to be completely defined, but information indicates that these cells probably secrete both mucous and buffers (Cummings et al, 1972).

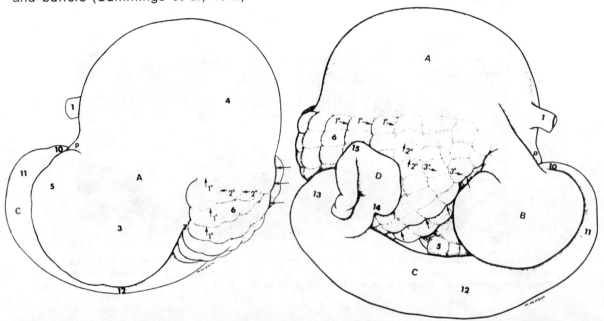

Figure 2-13. New-world camelid stomach. Left view. A, first compartment; C, third compartment; p, elliptical pouch of first compartment; 1, esophagus; 3, cranial sac; 4, caudal sac; 5, sacculated area in cranial sac; 6, sacculated area in caudal sac; 7, transverse sulcus; 10, tubular passage to third compartment; 11, initial one-fifth of third compartment; 12, middle three-fifths of third compartment; 1°, primary grooves; 2°, secondary grooves; arrows, attachment of greater omentum. Right view. B, second compartment; D, duodenal ampulla; 13, terminal one-fifth of third compartment; 14, pylorus; 15, duodenum; 3°, tertiary grooves. From Vallenas et al [1971].

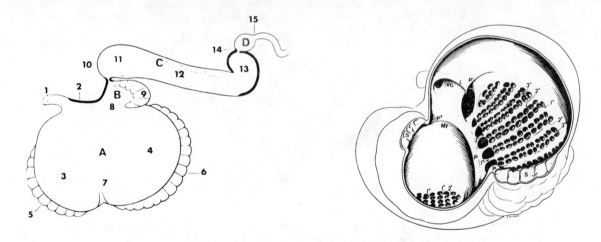

Figure 2-14. New world camelid stomach. Left. Diagrammatic representation of the llama and guanaco stomach. A, first compartment; B, second compartment; C, third compartment; D, duodenal ampulla; 1, esophagus; 2, ventricular groove; 3, cranial sac; 4, caudal sac; 5, sacculated area in cranial sac; 6, sacculated area in caudal sac; 7, transverse sulcus; 8, entrance to second compartment; 9, glandular cells of second compartment; 10, tubular passage to third compartment; 11, initial one-fifth of third compartment; 12, middle three-fifths of third compartment [lines represent mucosal pleats]; 13, terminal one-fifth of third compartment; 14, pylorus; 15, duodenum. Right. Llama stomach from the left with a portion of the left wall removed to allow visualization of the mucosal surface. E, entrance to second compartment; L, lip of ventricular groove; MF, mucosal folds in cranial sac; P, transverse pillar; P1, caudal limb of pillar; P2, cranial limb of pillar; S, glandular saccules; VG, ventricular groove; 1°, primary crests; 2°, secondary crests; 3°, tertiary crests. From Vallenas et al [1971].

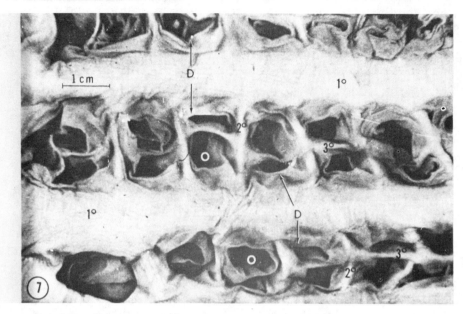

Figure 2-15. Camelid stomach. Portion of the sacculated area from the caudal sac of the first compartment of llama. D, mucosal diaphragms; O, saccular orifices; 1°, primary crests; 2°, secondary crests; 3°, tertiary crests. From Vallenas et al [1971].

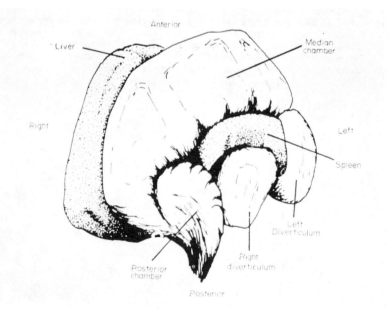

Figure 2-16. Drawing of the ventral view of the stomach of a foetal hippopotamus as positioned in the abdomen. From Arman and Field [1973].

Comparison of the Ruminant Stomach to that of Ruminant-like Animals

There are a number of animals exclusive of ruminants and pseudoruminants in which some pregastric fermentation occurs (Moir, 1965). The Gambian or Hamster rat [*Cricetoyms gambianus*] and the Golden Hamster [*Mesocricetus auratus*] have sacculated stomachs, one portion of which is nonglandular and inhabited with microorganisms. In other rodents some species of

Notomys, Neotoma, Peromyscus, Perognathus, Dipodomys and *Megachiroptera* have similar stomach structures. The three-toed tree sloth [*Bradypus tridatylus*] has a remarkably complex stomach which is believed to retain plant leaves for an extended period of time and is probably inhabited by microorganisms. In pigs and related genuses [*Suiformes*] the stomach varies "from the simple form of the domestic pig, through some greater subdivision in the peccaries, to the enormous stomach of the hippopotamus with its three compartments and anterior diverticula. The ruminant-like characteristics of this stomach are reinforced by the presence of an esophageal groove bypassing the anterior stomach, and by the lack of a cecum. Whether there is, in fact, ruminant-like digestion in the hippopotamus is not known at the present time, and remains a subject for investigation" (ibid).

A drawing of a fetal hippopotamus stomach is shown (Fig. 2-16, from Arman and Field, 1973). Volatile acid content indicates fermentative activity in the stomach and recent papers (Thurston and Grain, 1971; Thurston and Noirot-Timothee, 1973) identify two new genera and four species of holotrich ciliates and two new genera and three new species of ento-diniomorph ciliate protozoa from the hippopotamus stomach.

Body fats of the hippopotamus, kangaroo [*Macropus major*], wallaby [*Protemnodon eugenii*] and quokka [*Setonis brachyurus*] are similar to that of ruminants, indicating some pregastric fermentation. The fact that animals such as the euro [*Macropus robustus*] and wallaby can utilize ingested nitrogen and incorporate urea into bacterial and protozoal protein in the stomach clearly indicates active microbial fermentation (Lintern-Moore, 1973). Data also indicate that the langur monkey has a complex stomach in which fermentative activity resembles that of ruminants in many ways (Bauchop and Martucci, 1968).

The Intestinal Tract

Generally, the anatomy and physiological functioning of the intestinal tract of ruminants is believed to be similar to that of other mammalian species. However, a brief discussion of the arrangement of the intestines is probably in order at this point.

Beginning at the pylorus of the abomasum, the first part of the intestine (duodenum) passes dorsally and forward to the visceral surface of the liver, between the liver and rumen, where it is attached to the liver and rumen by the lesser omentum. Here it forms an S-shaped curve. The bile duct opens in the ventral part of the S-shaped curve and the pancreatic duct opens further back. The second part of the SI (jejunum) runs backward and then forward forming the iliac flexure. The remainder of the SI is arranged in numerous very close coils which lie chiefly in the space bounded medially by the right face of the ventral sac of the rumen, laterally and ventrally by the abdominal wall, dorsally by the large intestine, and cranially by the omasum and abomasum. A few coils may find their way behind the blind sacs of the rumen at the left side (Sisson and Grossman, 1953).

The terminal part of the ileum is straight and runs cranially between the cecum and colon and is attached to the cecum by the ileo-cecal fold. The cecum is a simple tubular structure with a blind end which points in the general direction of the pelvis. Ruminants, in general, have a relatively small ceca in comparison with other herbivores. There is no clear demarcation between the cecum and colon, but the site of the ileo-cecal valve is the acknowledged junction. The proximal colon is a comparatively wide tube which is looped on itself in double elliptical coils before it narrows to form the spiral colon which consists of tightly and regularly arranged centripetal (traveling toward the center) and centrifugal (receding from the center) coils. The number of centripetal coils is estimated to be: cattle, 1-2.5; sheep, 2-4; and goats, 2.5-3.5. The incidence of aberrant coiling is about 20% in sheep and 3% in cattle (Ash, 1969). The spiral colon is considered to end near the dorsal level of the colon and is continued by the distal colon which leads into the rectum. The distal colon gradually diminishes in caliber. The terminal part leaves the spiral mass, passes forward to the great mesenteric artery, and runs forward (cranial) to the terminal part of the duodenum. It inclines to the right in relation to the ventral surface of the right kidney, forms an S-shaped curve near the pelvic inlet and joins the rectum (Sisson and Grossman, 1953; Ash, 1969).

In sheep, Hecker and Grovum (1971) report that the large intestine of Merino ewes (ca. 40 kg) ranged in length from 360 to 550 cm, and the calculated surface area was 1,921 cm^2 (see Table 9-11 for area of individual sections). These authors also point out that grooves in the digesta indicating commencement of pellet formation were observed first ca. half-way along the centripetal colon while the first distinct pellets were present in the middle of the centrifugal colon.

Surgical Modifications of the Ruminant GIT

The development of various surgical techniques that allow the collection of data or improved observations of specific organs or tissues has been a great help in furthering our knowledge on physiology and function of living organisms. The ruminant animal is no exception to this general statement. Of the domestic animals, far more work of this type has been done on ruminants than on other species. A number of the techniques that have been used are mentioned briefly. Examples of fistulated or cannulated animals are shown in appropriate chapters.

Rumen Fistulation

A fistula is described as a tube or canal formed by an incomplete closure. Methods describing the construction of rumen fistulas have been in the literature for many years. Fluorens in 1833 is believed to be one of the first to describe such a procedure. Another early investigator was Colin in 1854. More recent techniques have been described by Schalk and Amadon (1928), Phillipson and Innes (1939), Dougherty (1955), Binns and James (1959), Perry and Macleod (1969) and McCann et al (1973).

The techniques vary somewhat in detail and type of hardware used, but all require an opening in the left side behind the ribs and below the lumbar area. An opening is made through the skin, fascia, muscle and peritoneum and the rumen is usually sutured to the opening, with the result that adhesions form between the body wall and the rumen wall. Various types of plugs are available, including hard plastic, flexible plastic or rubber, inflatable rubber or wooden. If the surgery is properly done and if the plug is a good fit, the animal will get by with no apparent discomfort, little, if any, soreness and only a slight amount of leakage around the cannula (Fig. 2-17).

Rumen fistulas have been a tremendous help to investigators studying rumen physiology and metabolism. One can observe rumen contractions and the ingestion of feed. Sampling of rumen contents is greatly simplified, and this aids the study of rumen microorganisms or rumen chemistry. Instruments can readily be placed in the rumen and reticulum to measure temperature, pH, gas pressure or other variables of interest. Saliva can be collected in the cardial area. With reasonable care, instrumentation or tubes can be inserted into the omasum and abomasum also. These examples are just a partial list of types of information that can be obtained more readily from animals with rumen fistulas than from intact animals. If all of the fistulated animals that have contributed to M.S. and Ph.D. dissertations were included as coauthors, there would be quite a long list indeed.

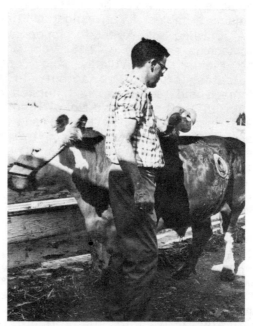

Figure 2-17. The author, shown with a fistulated steer and a dried stomach, lecturing to students on the complexity of the ruminant stomach.

Rumen Pouches

Small pouches have been used to study absorption through the rumen wall. Such pouches are constructed of normal rumen tissue and have an exteriorized opening so that samples can be obtained or material added (Tsuda, 1956; Foss and Black, 1972).

Esophageal Fistulas

The techniques of establishing and using esophageal-fistulated animals has been described by Torell (1954), Cook et al (1963) and Bishop and Froseth (1970) among others. In this technique, a fistula is established into the esophagus at a convenient location on the neck. Usually, a cannula of the appropriate size is placed in the opening. When in use the cannula is removed, thereby allowing saliva and ingested feed or water to pass through the fistula into a collection bag attached to the animal's neck (see Plate 4-1). Esophageal-fistulated animals take a large amount of care, but fistulated sheep, cattle and deer have been used successfully in studying grazing selectivity of plants, estimation of dry matter intake, and the collection of saliva.

Tracheal Cannulas

Colvin et al (1957) and Fujihara et al (1973) have published on techniques for establishing a tracheal cannula in cattle and goats, respectively. In this procedure the trachea is transected and the ends are exteriorized to the surface. With an appropriate arrangement of a face mask and with tubing attached to the anterior end of the transected trachea, rumen gas production can be measured separately from expired gases from the lung (see Ch. 16).

Salivary Cannulas

Cannulation of the parotid salivary glands was described by Denton (1957) and Hyden (1958) among others. Such cannulas have been used to study the effect of ingestion on secretion and salivary composition and, the effect of drugs and nerve stimuli on salivary production (see Ch. 5).

Omasal Cannulas

The omasum is a difficult organ on which to work, but cannulation techniques have been developed and used to a very limited extent to study digesta coming from the forestomachs (Bouchaert and Oyaert, 1954; Ash, 1962; Willes and Mendel, 1968; Willes, 1972).

Abomasal Cannulas

A variety of procedures have been published for use on sheep (Phillipson, 1952; Singleton, 1961), goats (Singleton, 1961) and cattle (Conner et al, 1957). In most of these, the cannulas have been designed as re-entrant cannulas. An exteriorized loop is inserted between the abomasum and the duodenum. Samples can then be taken and the digesta can otherwise follow its normal course. Some types (see Ch. 7) are designed primarily to allllow sampling of digesta coming from the abomasum.

Intestinal and Cecal Cannulas

Cannulas similar to the exteriorized (see Ch. 7) or re-entrant abomasal cannulas have been placed in various parts of the small intestine, thus allowing measurement of flow rates or sampling. Methods for intestinal cannulas have been reported by Hogan and Phillipson (1960), Goodall and Kay (1965), Ruckebush (1970) and Thivend and Poncet (1971) and for a cecal cannula, by MacRae et al (1973).

Preparations of Ruminant Stomachs for Educational Purposes

The use of appropriate models, visual aids, or samples in the classroom or for adult education is a convenient and valuable means of demonstration and teaching. Fresh specimens are quite useful, but those of some species may be difficult to obtain or desired ages may not be available. Furthermore, the normal shape is not always easy to visualize after fresh specimens have been partially dissected. Several papers have been published on preparation of the ruminant stomach, and these are discussed briefly.

Hix (1954) described a method for preparation of fetal stomachs of calves. In this procedure, the stomach is washed out and placed in 5% formalin solution for hardening. After several days it is washed and injected with paraffin wax (M.P. 50-57°C) preheated to 85-90°C. The stomach is then held under tap water to harden the wax which is forced into all compartments by manipulation. Air pockets are removed with a needle and paraffin injected to replace the air. The preparation is then dried thoroughly. External fat is then removed and a heavy coat of banana oil-cellulose acetate in acetone is applied as a preservative.

Scott (1960) described a technique in which the stomach is washed and trimmed and then placed in a 10% formalin solution for at least 72 hr. After thoroughly washing in running water for 12-24 hr, the stomach is placed in 45% v/v glycerin-water solution which contains crystal of thymol (2-3 g/l.) which act as a bacteriostat. The specimen is then dried and inflated with a continuous stream of air until dry. The specimen need not be coated with preservative, but a 12% solution of Saran 120 in methyl ethyl ketone is satisfactory for this.

Evans (1966) used a technique for fetal stomachs which involves injection with red latex (Ward's Natural Science Establishment) by tying a needle into the esophagus of a fresh fetus. Gentle steady pressure will fill the stomach. The esophagus is tied off and the fetus placed in a 10% formalin solution. This allows the latex to set while the fetus is floating in fluid with the result that stomach shape is more natural than with some other methods of preparation. The formalin treatment is extended to at least a week and the specimen is then macerated in HCl. This removes the stomach wall and leaves a cast corresponding to the internal structures. The cast must be stored in 2% formalin, otherwise it dries beyond recognition. An example is shown in the article by Warner and Flatt (1965, p 25).

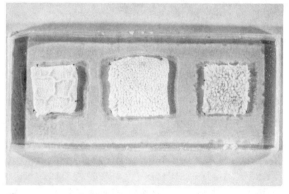

Figure 12-18. Sections of the ruminant stomach [reticulum, dorsal and cranial sac, respectively] mounted in transparent plastic.

Albright et al (1963) discuss several methods of preserving stomach specimens. In one case inflatable stomachs can be prepared as follows: soon after slaughter remove the adipose tissue from the surface. Wash out the stomach with water and rinse the rumen in Wickersheimer's fluid. To 10 l. of boiling water add the following: alum, 33 g; NaCl, 83 g; KNO_3, 40 g; K_2CO_3, 200 g; and As_2O_3, 33 g. Cool and filter, and to the solution obtained above add: glycerine (or propylene glycol), 4 l.; and methyl alcohol, 1 l. Submerge the digestive tract into the solution and stir daily for ca. one month. The odor will disappear when the rumen is, for all

practical purposes, tanned and completely dry. Add valves to the esophagus and duodenum ends so that it can be inflated with forced air or other gas. These authors (ibid) also discuss a method for preserving sections of the stomach mounted in plastic (see Fig. 2-18) and describe a periscope that can be constructed to view rumen activity.

Kitchell et al (1961) have published details of a method designed to produce a very durable specimen for class use. As with other methods, the stomach is cleaned of ingesta and inflated and the excess fat removed. The stomach is then immersed in 99% isoporpyl alcohol and partially filled with alcohol, being allowed to soak for about 2 wk. Following this the stomach is dried with air while suspended with cheese cloth. After it is dried fiber glass mats are applied as a covering material with the aid of resins. Several coats of resin are then applied to the specimen. Sprott and Smallwood (1974) have published details of a similar procedure.

Benevenga et al (1969) have published a procedure which is similar, in the preliminary stages, to that of Kitchell. It differs, however, in that the stomach is frozen after it is suspended and inflated. After 1-2 wk in the freezer, it is removed and drying is completed by blowing air through it.

Another method is one which has been used in the author's laboratory (Church, 1968). It has the advantage of being simple, yet adequate for most purposes. The fresh stomach is trimmed of excess fat, but care should be taken not to disturb connective tissue which is attached to the abomasum-rumen and the reticulum-cranial sac as the stomach is more difficult to dry in its normal shape. The stomach can be cleaned by filling with water, kneading and expelling the diluted digesta through the esophagus or pylorus, taking care not to exert too much pressure; failing that it can be opened and cleaned. Soaking in 70-80% ethanol is recommended to dehydrate the tissue and extract some of the lipids. Addition of an antioxident such as Ethoxyquin® at this point will probably help to prevent rancidity at a later date. In most cases, some alcohol should be poured into the inside cavities. Alcohol is preferred to formalin as the latter tends to result in a rubbery specimen. After soaking for 7-10 days, the stomach is suspended in cheese cloth in as natural a shape as can be devised and it is dried by passing air through it, taking care not to over inflate it as this will not allow a normal appearance. Any holes must be closed reasonably tight. In thicker and ventral parts of the stomach, pin holes will help to dry the tissue. Air pressure must be watched in the early stages as leakage through the tissue may change and the stomach may dry in a partially deflated position. Drying can be speeded up by directing a fan toward the specimen. Following drying, the stomach parts can be labeled with india ink and the stomach coated with some type of plastic resin or lacquer which will tend to increase durability. Holes can also be cut in various sections to allow one to see the internal structure. This method results in a light weight specimen which has no unpleasant odor and is reasonably resistant to handling. Examples from three species are shown in Fig. 2-12.

References Cited

Albright, J.L., C.L. Davis and T.H. Blosser. 1963. J. Dairy Sci. 46:1142.
Anderson, W.D. and A.F. Weber. 1969. J. Animal Sci. 28:379.
Arman, Pamela and C.R. Field. 1973. E. Afr. Wildl. J. 11:9.
Ash, R.W. 1962. J. Physiol. 164:4P (abstr).
Ash, R.W. 1969. Proc. Nutr. Soc. 28:110.
Bauchop, T. and R.W. Martucci. 1968. Science 161:698.
Becker, R.B., S.P. Marshall and P.T.D. Arnold. 1963. J. Dairy Sci. 46:835.
Benevenga, N.J., S.P. Schmidt and R.C. Laben. 1969. J. Dairy Sci. 52:1294.
Binns, W. and L.F. James. 1959. J. Amer. Vet. Med. Assoc. 135:603.
Bishop, J.P. and J.A. Froseth. 1970. Amer. J. Vet. Res. 31:1505.
Bouchaert, J.H. and W. Oyaert. 1954. Nature 174:1195.
Church, D.C. 1968. J. Animal Sci. 27:1525.
Colvin, H.W., J.D. Wheat, E.A. Rhode and J.M. Boda. 1957. J. Dairy Sci. 40:492.
Conner, H.G., A.D. McGilliard and C.F. Huffman. 1957. J. Animal Sci. 16:692.
Cook, C.W., J.T. Blake and J.W. Call. 1963. J. Animal Sci. 22:579.
Cummings, J.F., J.F. Munnell and A. Vallenas. 1972. J. Morphol. 137:71..
Denton, D.A. 1957. Quart. J. Expt. Physiol. 42:72.
Dougherty, R.W. 1955. Cornell Vet. 45:331.
Evans, H.E. 1966. Personal Communication. Cornell University.
Foss, D.C. and D.L. Black. 1972. J. Animal Sci. 34:999.
Fujihara, T., T. Furuhashi and I. Tasaki. 1973. J. Dairy Sci. 56:820.
Goodall, E.D. and R.N.B. Kay. 1965. J. Physiol. 176:12.
Habel, R.E. 1964. Guide to the Dissection of Domestic Ruminants. Edwards Bro. Inc., Ann Arbor, Michigan.
Hecker, J.F. and W.L. Grovum. 1971. Aust. J. Biol. Sci. 24:365.
Hix, E.L. 1954. J. Animal Sci. 13:49.
Hofmann, R.R. 1968. In: Comparative Nutrition of Wild Animals, pp 179-194. Academic Press Inc., London.
Hogan, J.P. and A.T. Phillipson. 1960. Br. J. Nutr. 14:147.
Hyden, S. 1958. Biol. Abstr. 35:4528.
Hyden, S. 1965. Cornell Vet. 55:419.
Kitchell, R.L., J. Trunbull, R.A. Nordine and S.C. Edgell. 1961. J. Amer. Vet. Med. Assoc. 138:329.
Lambert, P.S. 1958. Vet. J. 104:302.
Lavker, R., W. Chalupa and P. Opliger. 1969. J. Dairy Sci. 52:266.
Lintern-Moore, S. 1973. Comp. Biochem. Physiol. 44A:75.
MacRae, J.C., C.S.W. Reid, D.W. Dellow and R.S. Wyburn. 1973. Res. Vet. Sci. 14:78.
McCann, C.P., R.J. McLaren, R.L. DeLay and J.K. Matsushima. 1973. Proc. West. Sec. Amer. Soc. An. Sci. 24:377.
Moir, R.J. 1965. In: Physiology of Digestion in the Ruminant. p 1. Butterworths Pub. Co.
Perry, F.G. and G.K. Macleod. 1969. J. Dairy Sci. 52:264.
Phillipson, A.T. 1952. J. Physiol. 116:84.
Phillipson, A.T. and J.R.M. Innes. 1939. Quart. J. Expt. Physiol. 29:333.
Ruckebush, Y. 1970. Ann. Rech. Veter. 1:265.
Schalk, A.F. and R.S. Amadon. 1928. N. Dak. Agr. Expt. Sta. Bul. 216.
Scott, H. 1960. Unpublished data. Ohio State University.
Sellers, A.F. and C.E. Stevens. 1966. Physiol. Rev. 46:634.
Singleton, A.G. 1961. J. Physiol. 155:134.
Sisson, S. and J.D. Grossman. 1953. The Anatomy of the Domestic Animals. 4th ed. W.B. Saunders Co.
Sprott, L.R. and J.E. Smallwood. 1974. Southwest. Vet. 27 (no. 1).
Stevens, C.E. and B.K. Stettler. 1966. Amer. J. Physiol. 210:365.
Thivend, P. and C. Poncet. 1971. Ann. Biol. Anim. Bioch. Biophys. 11:275.
Thurston, J.P. and J. Grain. 1971. J. Protozool. 18:133.
Thurston, J.P. and C. Noirot-Timothee. 1973. J. Protozool. 20:562.
Torell, D.T. 1954. J. Animal Sci. 13:878.
Tsuda, T. 1956. Tohoku J. Agr. Res. 7:231.
Vallenas, A., J.F. Cummings and J.F. Munnell. 1971. J. Morphol. 134:399.
Warner, E.D. 1958. Amer. J. Anat. 102:33.
Warner, R.G. and W.P. Flatt. 1965. In: Physiology of Digestion in the Ruminant. Butterworths Pub. Co.
Willes, R.F. 1972. J. Dairy Sci. 55:1188.
Willes, R.F. and V.E. Mendel. 1968. Amer. J. Vet. Res. 25:1302.

CHAPTER 3 — GROWTH AND DEVELOPMENT OF THE RUMINANT STOMACH

Fetal Development

There have been sufficient studies of the fetal development of the ruminant stomach to be able to characterize generally the changes which occur (see Warner and Flatt, 1965, for a review). These studies show that the stomach develops from a long spindle-shaped dilation of the primitive gut which gives rise to the concurrent but differential development of the various stomach compartments. In the case of bovine embryos, Warner (1958) found the stomach to be apparent at 28 days (9.5 mm embryos). By 36 days (14.7 mm), epithelial changes indicated development of adult stomach regions. These developed rapidly until about 56 days when definitive pouches could be observed. Becker and Marshall (1951) found that the rumen was the largest compartment early in fetal life, but the abomasum generally weighed more by ca. 5 mo. of fetal age and, at birth, the abomasum represented about 47% of total stomach weight. The honeycomb structure of the reticulum developed between 72 and 100 days; the omasum was relatively large in early fetal life, but did not continue to increase in size as rapidly in later stages.

In sheep, compartmentization of the stomach may be distinguished in embryos measuring only 9 mm; by 20-24 days the reticulo-rumen and abomasum are distinguishable and the omasum by 43 days (Warner and Flatt, 1965). As late as 100 days the epithelial surface is smooth and no papillae visible, although they develop to some extent by birth (Wardrop, 1961), and are of the stratified squamous epithelia typical of the forestomach. Some folding of the epithelia of the reticulum can be seen by 70 days and the outline of the reticular ribs is clear at 100 days; the honeycomb structure is well developed at birth. The leaf structure of the omasum is apparent by 70 days (Wardrop, 1961).

Wallace (1948) studied fetal development of stomachs from lambs which were from ewes bred for 56, 84, 112 or 140 days. At 56 days, the rumen represented about 45% of stomach weight; its relative weight declined to 26% at 140 days. Comparable data for other stomach parts were: reticulum, 14-10%; omasum, 24-8%; and abomasum, 17-56%.

Fetal development of the stomach might be expected to be relatively uniform within a species since the intra-uterine environment is, presumably, rather constant. Available data are not sufficient to demonstrate any effect of breed, size, plane of nutrition or general health of dam on development of the fetal stomach. No doubt some developmental changes may be modified by environmental influences on the dam, but they are probably minor in extent.

Postnatal Development of the Stomach

An appreciable volume of data are available on various aspects of postnatal development of the ruminant stomach. The data, in general, indicate that differential development continues for some period of time, being modified by such factors as species differences, diet, and nutritional stress. Wallace (1948) suggested that the organs develop more or less in the order of their functional importance and that, at any one age, the organs most affected by nutritional stress are those which are growing at their maximum rate.

Position in the Abdomen

Benzie and Phillipson (1957) have studied stomach development of kids, lambs and calves using radiographic techniques (X-ray). Some of their findings are as follows: at birth the rumen and reticulum are small in comparison to the abomasum in all three species, but these organs develop relatively more rapidly after birth. The abomasum (goat) in the first few hours after birth is seen to be a saccular organ situated immediately behind the diaphragm and with its long axis running dorso-ventrally. The disposition in the calf is the same. The rumen and reticulum at this stage are still small structures. Although the reticulum, owing to its movements, may exhibit variations in size, it does not occupy as much space as in older animals. During the first 3 wk of life the abomasum of the goat retains its position and on viewing the organ when full in the dorso-ventral plane, it is seen to be situated on the left side of the body extending from the diaphragm to the caudal third of the abdomen. The pyloric antrum is to the right of the midline where it turns dorsally to lead to the pylorus and duodenum. During the second and third wk of life the reticulum enlarges and the body of the abomasum moves caudally away from the diaphragm. Its final position, however, is not attained until the animal is eating large quantities of solid food. The abomasum increases in size at a much slower rate than the rumen; it is found entirely on the right side of the body and in the epigastric region of the abdominal cavity. The area occupied by the abomasum, when viewed in either the lateral or dorso-ventral positions, varies with the degree of filling. Its posterior part has no fixed limits. The pylorus itself occupies a position that cannot change very much and most of the changes in position of the abomasum occur in the body (as opposed to the pylorus). Further information on development of the goat's stomach has been described by Tamate (1956).

Tamate and co-workers (1962) have studied the stomach development of dairy calves fed in a normal manner (milk, concentrate, hay). Observations indicated that a rapid development occurred in the reticulo-rumen as early as 4 wk of age. At 8 wk it occupied the entire left half of the abdominal cavity, except for a small space filled by the anterior part of the body of the abomasum, and extended considerably into the right half. Caudally, the extremities of the rumen extended to a point opposite the 5th lumbar vertebra or the pelvic inlet. Ventrally, the bottom of the ventral sac of the rumen reached the floor of the abdominal cavity at 12 wk of age. The reticulum expanded primarily in a posterior (caudal) direction. No extensive development of the omasum was observed. The relatively small abomasum was located between the abdominal floor and the ventral sac of the rumen, extending caudally to the 3rd lumbar vertebra at 8 wk of age, but only to the 2nd vertebra at 12 wk of age. It became confined for the most part to the right half of the abdominal cavity to accommodate the extension of the rumen.

Normal Developmental Changes

The differential development of the compartments of the stomach of cattle and sheep has been investigated by a number of authors. Data from several sources on bovines [Bos tarus] have been compiled by Warner and Flatt (1965) and are shown in Table 3-1. Data on some other ruminant species are shown in Table 3-2.

Table 3-1. Percentage of bovine stomach tissue contributed by each compartment.[a]

	Age in weeks						
	0	4	8	12	16	20-26	34-38
Reticulo-rumen	38	52	60	64	67	64	64
Omasum	13	12	13	14	18	22	25
Abomasum	49	36	27	22	15	14	11

[a] Includes data from Becker and Arnold (1952); Godfrey (1961); Tamate et al (1962); and Warner et al (1956).

The information presented in Tables 3-1 and 3-2 indicates a rapid increase in size of the reticulum and rumen as soon as the animal starts to ingest dry feed. The abomasum gradually regresses in relative size, although not in absolute size, and the

Table 3-2. Changes in the ruminant stomach with age.

Animal	Age	Percentage in the various stomach compartments			
		Reticulum	Rumen	Omasum	Abomasum
		Tissue Weight			
		Reticulo-rumen			
Domestic buffalo[a]	3 wk	59		7	34
	6 wk	65		8	27
	9 wk	69		14	16
	12 wk	68		14	17
	15 wk	69		15	15
Sheep[b]	9 days	8	24	8	60
	7 days	7-8	22-23	5-6	64-65
	14 days	6-8	28-29	4-5	58-60
	20-21 days	9-10	45-46	5-6	39-40
	28-30 days	11-12	44-51	5-6	32-39
	40-42 days	10-11	57-60	4-5	26-29
	56-57 days	10-11	64-66	5-6	18-20
	62-63 days	11	60-62	5-6	22-23
	Adult	11	62	5	22
Deer[c]	0 days	6	23	6	65
	14 days	8	31	6	55
	1 month	8	53	4	35
	2 months	9	62	6	23
	3 months	8	71	4	17
	4 months	7	77	5	11
	Adult	6	74	8	12

Animal	Age	Volume	
		Reticulo-rumen	Omasum-abomasum
Goats[d]	1-2 days	15-27	73-85
	7-10 days	21-45	55-79
	13-16 days	19-68	32-81
	15 days	37-56	44-63
	32-38 days	36-56	44-64
	37-40 days (grass diet)	81-95	5-19
	50-68 days (grass diet)	71-95	5-29
	53-72 days (milk diet)	33-68	32-67

[a] Data from Singh et al (1973); fed milk for 3 wk, then 1:1 concentrate and hay.
[b] Includes data from Church et al (1962); Palsson and Verges (1952) Wallace (1948), Walker and Walker (1961); and Wardrop and Coombe (1960).
[c] Data from Short (1964).
[d] Data from Tamate (1957).

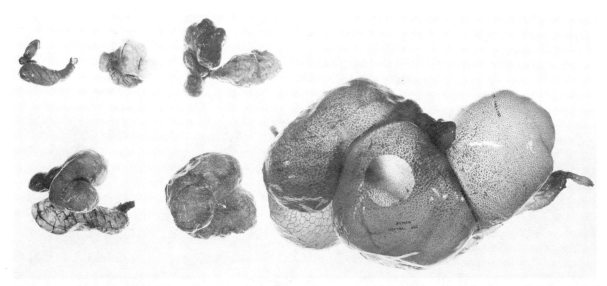

Figure 3-1. Change in size of the ovine stomach with age. Top row: at birth, 2 wk, and 4 wk of age. Bottom row: 6 wk, 8 wk, and stomach from a fat lamb of unknown age.

omasum develops slowly, taking longer to reach relative mature size than the reticulum or rumen. The reticulo-rumen of calves has made its most rapid relative growth prior to 8 wk of age, and the relative mature size probably is attained by 12 wk, although Godfrey (1961) and Blaxter et al (1952) indicate that relative mature size may not be attained by 12 wk or from 6-9 mo., respectively. Variances of this type are related partially to different feeding regimens (see later section).

The omasum is still increasing in relative size up to 36-38 wk in cattle, and the abomasum is still regressing. With respect to lambs, the data show that the reticulum has reached its relative mature size by 30 days. Rumen growth is quite marked between 7 and 30 days and it is of mature relative size by 8 wk of age. The omasum is still undersized at 8 or 9 wk, although the abomasum is of relative mature size. Fig. 3-1 illustrates the changes in size of the stomach in sheep, Fig. 3-2 shows the relative changes with age in one experiment (Oh et al, 1972) and changes with age in deer are illustrated in Fig. 3-3.

Only limited information on stomach development is available on species other than sheep and cattle. Information on goats is not directly comparable, but indicates that stomach development is relatively complete at 7-9 wk. Domestic buffalo apparently are comparable to cattle, but it would seem that, in deer, the stomach development takes

somewhat longer, the limited information indicating relative mature size of the rumen at 3-4 mo. and the abomasum at 4 mo., somewhat later than for sheep or goats. Information on these different species indicates a positive relationship between the length of gestation period and time required for stomach development. There is probably also a correlation between development and length of the normal nursing period.

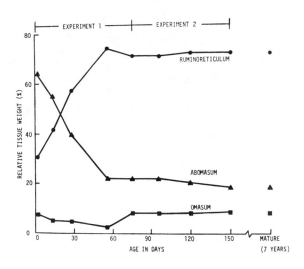

Figure 3-2. Relative changes in wet tissue weights of the stomach of lambs. From Oh et al [1972].

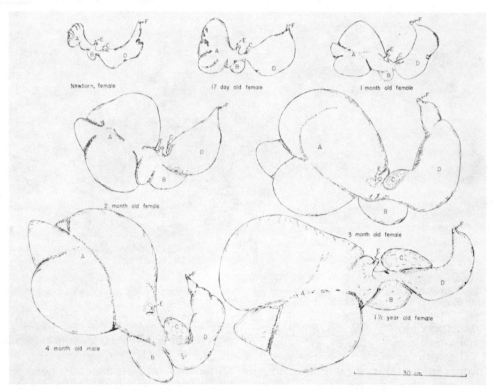

Figure 3-3. Diagrammatic representation of sequential development of deer [white-tail] stomach. A, rumen; B, reticulum; C, omasum; D, abomasum; E, esophagus; F, duodenum. From Short [1964].

Stomach Capacity

Data cited by Warner and Flatt (1965) indicate that the stomach contents in adult cattle are distributed 81-87% in the reticulo-rumen, 10-14% in the omasum and 3-5% in the abomasum. Comparable figures for sheep are 88-93%, 2% and 5-10%, respectively (weight basis). Chandler et al (1964) found that the stomach contents of 15-wk-old calves were distributed 86, 7 and 7%, respectively in the stomach compartments, figures which agree well with those for adults. Kesler et al (1951) observed rumen contents in 16-wk-old calves on a liquid diet to be about 10% of live wt, somewhat less than for most adults. Recent data on 10-13-wk-old calves on various types of roughage diets (Hodgson, 1973) showed that 79-92% of the wet digesta was recovered from the reticulo-rumen, 3.4-11.3% from the omasum, and 1.9-10.6% from the abomasum. As a % of body wt, the reticulo-rumen contents ranged from 13.8 to 25.6%. With respect to the bovine omasum, one report indicates an increase in volume of 60 fold between 10 and 150 days of age (Becker et al, 1963).

With lambs, Walker and Walker (1961) found reticulo-rumen contents to increase from 191 g at 21 days of age to 1,408 g at 77 days of age. When expressed as a % of live wt, mean values for reticulo-rumen contents were: 21 days, 2.5; 28 days, 3.9; 35 days, 4.6; 42 days, 8.6; and 77 days, 15.9. Wardrop and Coombe (1961) observed that the volume of the abomasum showed little change with age in grazing lambs. The volume of the rumen contents increased with age and the rate of this increase was most marked from 3 wk of age onwards. The volume of the rumen contents, relative to both live wt and volume of the abomasum contents, was constant from 8 wk of age onwards. Data reported by Church et al (1962) showed a rumen volume of 325 ml in 2-wk-old lambs, 969 ml at 4 wk, and 1,461 ml at 40 days of age; volume of rumen measurements was found to be highly correlated to rumen wet tissue wt (r = .97).

Relative Capacity of the Total GIT

In the adult sheep, the length of the intestines, when stripped out of the omentum, is approximately as follows:

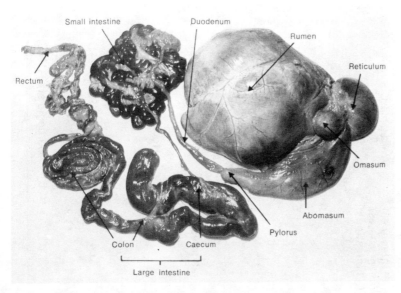

Figure 3-4. The stomach and intestines of the sheep. Courtesy of C.S.I.R.O.

small intestine, 24 m (75-85 ft); cecum, 0.5 m (1.7 ft); and for the colon and rectum, 8-9 m (28-30 ft). Comparable values (Sisson and Grossman, 1953) given for cattle are: small intestine, 40 m (130 ft), cecum, 0.75 m (2.5 ft); and the colon, 10-11 m (35 ft).

The stomach and intestines of the sheep are illustrated in an excellent photograph in Fig. 3-4 which gives some perspective on comparative size; tabular data illustrating relative differences between species or during growth are shown in Table 3-3.

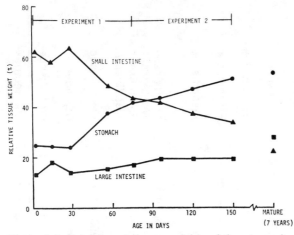

Figure 3-5. Relative wet tissue weights of the stomach [circles], small intestine [triangles] and large intestine [squares] of lambs from two experiments. Data from Oh et al [1972].

In the adult sheep, the intestines account for ca. 50% of the wt of the stomach and intestines. This represents a decrease from about 78% in day-old lambs (Wardrop and Coombe, 1960). Changes observed in one experiment (Oh et al, 1972) are illustrated graphically in Fig. 3-5. Although fewer values are available for cattle, data in Table 3-3 indicate that the intestine decreases from 70% to about 33-35% in adult animals. The only direct comparison between species (done by same people and at same time) known to the author is that made by Longhurst and Douglas (1953) between deer and sheep. It was of a very limited nature. These values, however, indicate that the reticulo-rumen of the deer is relatively larger than that of sheep, which in turn, is slightly smaller than that of cattle. On the basis of % of body weight, however, the reticulo-rumen of most deer species is smaller than that of domestic ruminants (Prins and Geelen, 1971).

Factors Affecting Stomach Development

Normal development of the stomach is an orderly process, presumably mediated by the endocrine glands. At a given age and weight and when an animal is on a typical diet, the approximate relative development of the stomach compartments can be predicted with reasonable accuracy. In addition to species differences, age, and weight (affected by the environment), there are a number of factors which may influence stomach development. These are discussed in succeeding paragraphs.

It has been demonstrated by a number of investigators that restriction of young ruminants to a liquid diet of milk or milk replacer will delay development of the forestomach. The reticulo-rumens of such animals will usually be smaller than normal for their age, with thinner walls, have less capacity, and will lack the normal development and coloration of papillae usually found in these compartments (Warner et al, 1956; Loe et al, 1959; Niedermeier et al,

Table 3-3. Relative capacity of the gastro-intestinal tract.

Animal	Basis of estimate	Percent of (in) the GIT							Author
		Reticulum	Rumen	Omasum	Abomasum	Small intestine	Cecum	Large intestine	
Deer, 67 lb wt	Volume	1.1	57.8	0.5	1.4	26.2	2.3	10.8	Longhurst & Douglas (1953)
Sheep, 77 lb wt	Volume	2.8	47.8	1.2	6.0	28.3	4.0	10.0	"
Sheep, 1 wk of age	Fresh tissue	7.5		17.0		60.7		14.7	Large (1964)
4 wk of age	Fresh tissue	16.9		11.1		60.9		11.1	"
8 wk of age	Fresh tissue	24.8		8.9		53.0		13.3	"
16 wk of age	Fresh tissue	31.9		11.4		38.7		18.0	"
Sheep, 4 wk of age	Fresh tissue	3.0	14.3	1.4	9.0	72.5 (all intestines)			Wardrop & Coombe (1960)
8 wk of age	Fresh tissue	3.6	21.5	1.5	6.0	67.4 (all intestines)			"
adult	Fresh tissue	5.5	28.4	3.9	11.2	50.9 (all intestines)			Rogerson (1958)
adult	Dry digesta	5.2	52.4	8.9	2.8	9.3	6.4	14.9	"
Fat lambs	Fresh tissue	30.2		3.6	6.9	34.3		25.0	Randall (1974)
	Wet digesta	67.3		2.3	5.6	11.7		13.1	"
	Dry digesta	73.4		2.8	5.0	7.2		11.6	"
Pygmy goats, 30 lb wt	Dry tissue	4.8	44.0	4.7	6.5	27.1	1.6	11.3	Wilson (1958)
Saanen goat, adult	Fresh tissue	40.0		1.7	5.7	30.2	8.0	14.4	Hamada (1973)
Calves, liquid diet	Fresh tissue	14.5		13.5		54.6		17.4	Kesler et al (1951)
Calves, 12 wk of age	Fresh tissue	19.0		11.4	11.4	69.5 (all intestines)			Tamate et al (1962)
Calves, 10-13 wk of age fed chopped grass	Fresh tissue	31		7	7	39		16	Hodgson (1973)
	Wet digesta	77		3	3	8		9*	"
fed pelleted grass	Fresh tissue	28		9	8	39		16	"
	Wet digesta	63		4	8	13		12*	"
Steers, 250-400 kg	Fresh tissue	36.4		13.9	12.0	14.8	3.4	5.8	Tulloh (1966)
Cows, adult	Dry digesta	66.8		4.8	4.3	20.8		13.2	"
Cows, adult	Fresh tissue	42.8		15.9	7.3	25.3	1.6	10.8	Carnegie et al (1960)

*Data exclude contents of the rectum.

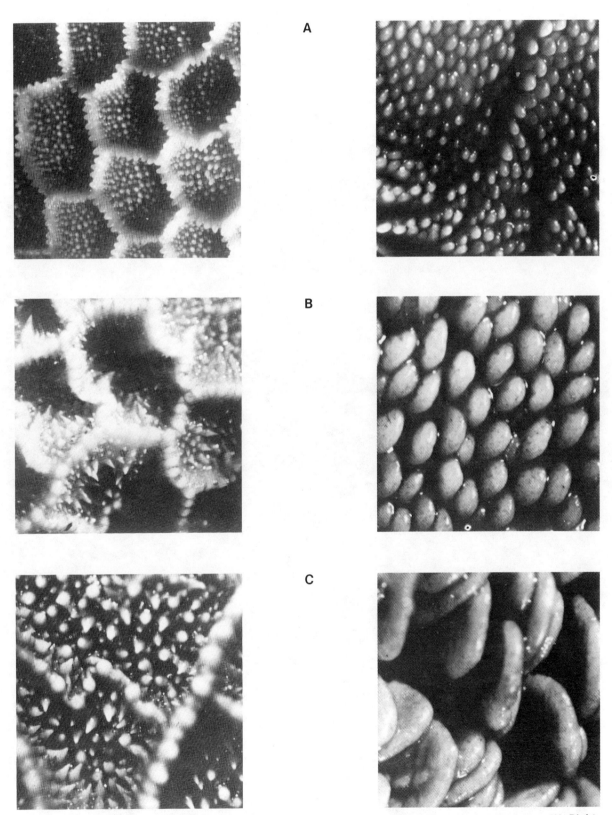

Plate 3-1. Left. Reticular epithelia of lambs [A] at birth, [B] 20 days of age, and [C] 91 days of age. Mag. ca. 3X. Right. Rumen dorsal sac epithelia of lambs at the same ages. Mag. ca. 7X. From Wardrop [1961].

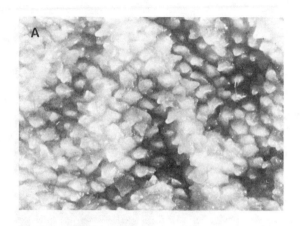

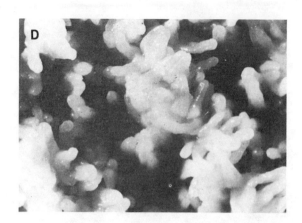

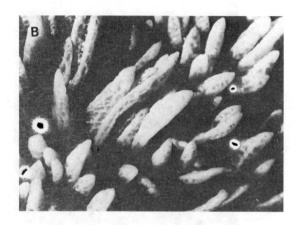

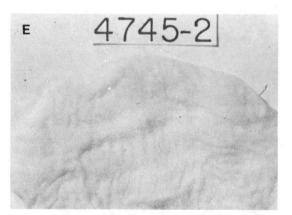

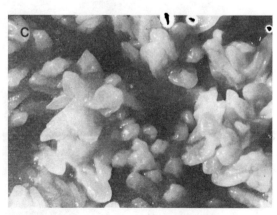

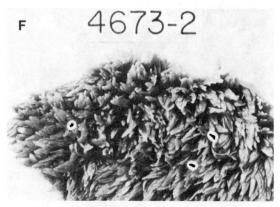

Plate 3-2. Effect of diet on rumen papillae growth: [A] 8-wk-old calf fed milk via nipple; [B] 8-wk-old calf fed milk, hay, and grain; [C] 8-wk-old calf fed milk + 16.1 kg of VFA containing 70% acetate and 30% propionate; [D] 8-wk-old calf fed milk + 6.7 kg Na butyrate and 1,120 sponges; [E] 12-wk-old calf fed milk; [F] 12-wk-old calf fed milk, hay and grain. From Tamate et al [1962]. Courtesy of A.D. McGilliard, Iowa State Univ.

1959; Smith, 1961; Tamate et al, 1962; Stobo et al, 1966; Omori et al, 1968; Singh and Yadava, 1971; Oh et al, 1972; Roy et al, 1973). Data reported by Harrison et al (1960), in fact, demonstrated that rumen papillae will regress in size and number when an animal is changed from a grain-hay ration back to a milk diet. Other reports, for that matter, indicate that some regression in rumen papillae occurs after birth and probably continues until consumption of roughage begins. In calves surgically modified to bypass the forestomach, the rumen may continue to increase in capacity but it has thin walls, atrophied pillars and no papillae (Stewart et al, 1966). Examples of normal changes with age in reticular and ruminal epithelia are shown in Plate 3-1.

Roy et al (1973) have recently demonstrated that calves can be maintained for some time (219-270 days of age) on liquid diets while growing at very acceptable rates. These cattle (av. wt 336 kg at slaughter) had relatively little rumen development as indicated by % of the total GIT; reticulo-rumen, 20.1; omasum, 3.4; abomasum, 7.7; intestines, 68.8. In grazing beef calves suckling their dams, it has been shown that relatively little rumen development occurred by 9 wk of age (Stewart, 1971), as indicated by rumen weight, papillary development, and rumen contents.

Ample evidence is available from experimental studies (see previous paragraphs) to demonstrate that ingestion of roughage is stimulatory to development of the reticulo-rumen in terms of weight and thickness of the tissues and the development of normal papillae. Concentrates may, however, result in greater stimulation than will roughage of papillary development in early life (Harrison et al, 1960; Stobo et al, 1966; Peron, 1970).

At least part of the stimulus for development of papillae is the presence in the rumen of organic acids, particularly the volatile acids (VFA) normally found in the adult — acetic, butyric, propionic and valeric. That part of the stimulus is due to acids was shown by Flatt and coworkers (1958). In these experiments rumen papillary development was relatively normal when salts of the VFA were introduced into a rumen-fistulated milk-fed calf. Plastic sponges, providing inert bulk, were ineffective. Results of a similar nature have been obtained by other workers (Sander et al, 1959; Smith, 1961; Gilliland et al, 1962; Tamate et al, 1962; and

Rickard and Ternouth, 1965). Candau (1971) has also shown that ammonia is stimulatory to papillae development.

The development of normal adult color of rumen papillae (bovine) does not occur in milk-fed calves. Presumably, the dark pigmentation of adult papillae results from feeding roughages, but the origin of the pigment is not clear although ingestion of both iron (Hamada et al, 1970) and soil (Healy and Wilson, 1971) have been implicated.

In addition to the effect of roughage on the rumen, it has been suggested that feeding roughage results in a longer small and large intestine in cattle and that greater volumes of gastric juice may be secreted (Krosota, 1968).

The effect of underfeeding on changes in the GIT has been studied in one laboratory recently (Carnegie et al, 1969). Results indicated weights of the abomasum and small intestine were less, but weights of the omasum, cecum and colon-rectum were not appreciably altered by moderate underfeeding.

Surgical Removal or Alteration of the Stomach

It was reported some years ago (Trautmann, 1933) that partial removal of the reticulo-rumen and omasum was followed by regeneration of the tissues. More recently, a number of papers have reported techniques and results where different portions of the stomach have been removed or when the reticulo-rumen and omasum have been bypassed surgically. Those dealing with surgical removal include Sauer and Brisson (1961), Lupien et al (1962), Williams et al (1966) and Hamada (1973). Those concerned with surgical modifications include: omasal-abomasal cannulation, Kameoka and Morimoto (1962); forestomach bypass surgery (esophageal or reticulo-abomasal anastomosis), Ruckebusch and Marquet (1962), Ruckebusch et al (1966), Stewart et al (1966), and Huber et al (1969); removal of omasal leaves, Bell and Mewborn (1968) and Hamada (1973). These various procedures have been devised in order to isolate or remove the rumen and, thus, treat the young ruminant animal as a monogastric species, or to facilitate collection of digesta between parts of the stomach.

In animals with either the forestomach

removed or bypassed, voluntary food intake is reduced. Animals tend to eat more slowly, chew food more thoroughly, and usually prefer finely chopped or ground feed. Total food intake is reduced. While these animals may show a tendency to want to eat normal fibrous feeds, which may stimulate the rumination reflex (Lupien et al, 1962; Ruckebusch and Marquet, 1965), this is apt to cause severe discomfort (Stewart et al, 1966). Digestibility of fiber tends to be depressed in operated animals (Hamada, 1973).

Survival past 2-3 months has been relatively rare. In those which have survived for several months, the cecum tends to be enlarged considerably (Hamada, 1973).

In sheep, removal of omasal leaves (Bell and Mewborn, 1968) was noted to result in lower fiber digestibility (40%) as compared to controls (44%). With a goat on a highly digestible milk replacer type of ration (Hamada, 1973), there was little apparent effect of the surgery. Bone particles (from fish meal in the diet) did accumulate in the reticulum.

Conclusions

Fetal development of the ruminant stomach is relatively rapid, with the various compartments being distinguishable by 43 days in sheep and 56 days in cattle. The epithelial surface develops more slowly with no papillae present at 100 days in sheep. Postnatal development of the stomach is related to size and/or age, and diet. A liquid diet delays development of the reticulo-rumen both in terms of tissue thickness and weight and in papillary development. Normal development results in rapid growth of the reticulo-rumen after the young animal starts to ingest solid feed. Inert roughage will stimulate development of growth as evidenced by an increase in tissue thickness, but the presence of fermentable materials which yield the volatile fatty acids and ammonia appears to be a necessary factor for papillary maturation. Relative mature size of the stomach is reached in about 8 wk in sheep and goats, 3-4 mo. in deer, and 5-6 mo. in cattle. As the stomach develops, it represents an increasing percentage of the total GIT.

References Cited

Becker, R.B. and S.P. Marshall. 1951. J. Dairy Sci. 34:329.
Becker, R.B. and P.T.D. Arnold. 1952. Proc. Assoc. S. African Workers. 49:78.
Becker, R.B., S.P. Marshall and P.T.D. Arnold. 1963. J. Dairy Sci. 46:835.
Bell, M.C. and W.B. Mewborn. 1968. J. Animal Sci. 27:1160 (abstr).
Benzie, David and A.T. Phillipson. 1957. The Alimentary Tract of the Ruminant. Oliver and Boyd Pub. Co.
Blaxter, K.L., M.K. Hutcheson, J.M. Robertson and A.L. Wilson. 1952. Br. J. Nutr. 6:i.
Candau, M. 1971. Ann. Biol. Anim. Bioch. Biophys. 11:284.
Carnegie, A.B., N.M. Tulloh and R.M. Seebeck. 1969. Aust. J. Agr. Sci. 20:405.
Chandler, P.T., E.M. Kesler and R.D. McCarthy. 1964. J. Animal Sci. 23:870.
Church, D.C., G.L. Jessup and Ralph Bogart. 1962. Amer. J. Vet. Res. 23:220.
Flatt, W.P., R.G. Warner and J.K. Loosli. 1958. J. Dairy Sci. 41:1593.
Gilliland, R.L., L.J. Busch and J.D. Friend. 1962. J. Dairy Sci. 45:1211.
Godfrey, N.W. 1961. J. Agri. Sci. 57:173.
Hamada, T. 1973. J. Dairy Sci. 56:473.
Hamada, T., S. Maeda and K. Kameoka. 1970. J. Dairy Sci. 53:588.
Harrison, H.N., R.G. Warner, E.G. Sander and J.K. Loosli. 1960. J. Dairy Sci. 43:1301.
Healy, W.B. and G.F. Wilson. 1971. N.Z. J. Agri. Res. 14:122.
Hodgson, J. 1973. Animal Prod. 17:129.
Huber, T.L., J. Kittrell and M. Adsit. 1969. J. Animal Sci. 28:34.
Kameoka, K. and H. Morimoto. 1962. Japanese Bul. Nat. Inst. Agr. Series G, 21:175.
Kesler, E.M., M. Ronning and C.B. Knodt. 1951. J. Animal Sci. 10:969.
Krasota, V.F. 1968. Nutr. Abstr. Rev. 38:1343.
Large, R.V. 1964. Animal Prod. 6:169.

Loe, W.C., O.T. Stallcup and H.W. Colvin. 1959. J. Dairy Sci. 42:395.
Longhurt, W.M. and J.R. Douglas. 1953. Trans. N. Amer. Wildlife Conf. 18:168.
Lupien, P.J., F. Sauer and G.V. Hatina. 1962. J. Dairy Sci. 45:210.
Niedermeier, R.P., N.N. Allen and R.W. Bray. 1955. J. Dairy Sci. 38:622.
Oh, J.H., I.D. Hume and D.T. Torrell. 1972. J. Animal Sci. 35:450.
Omori, S. et al. 1968. Japanese Bul. Nat. Inst. Animal Indust. 18:61.
Palsson, H. and J.B. Verges. 1952. J. Agr. Sci. 42:1.
Peron, N. 1971. Revista Cubana de Ciencia Agr. 5:195.
Prins, R.A. and M.J.H. Geelen. 1971. J. Wildl. Mgmt. 35:673.
Randall, R.P. 1974. Ph.D. Thesis, Oregon State Univ., Corvallis.
Rickard, M.D. and J.F. Ternouth. 1965. J. Agr. Sci. 65:371.
Rogerson, A. 1958. Br. J. Nutr. 12:164.
Roy, J.H.B., I.J.F. Stobo, P. Ganderton, and S.M. Shotton. 1973. Animal Prod. 16:215.
Ruckebusch, Y. and J.P. Laplace, J.P. Perret and Y. Doare. 1966. C.R. Soc. Biol. 160:2334.
Ruckebusch, Y. and J.P. Marquet. 1965. C.R. Soc. Biol. 159:394.
Sander, E.G., R.G. Warner, H.N. Harrison and J.K. Loosli. 1959. J. Dairy Sci. 42:1600.
Sauer, F. and G.J. Brisson. 1961. Amer. J. Vet. Res. 22:990.
Short, H.L. 1964. J. Wildl. Mgmt. 28:445.
Singh, M. and I.S. Yadava. 1971. Ind. J. Animal Sci. 41:922.
Singh, M., I.S. Yadava and A.R. Rao. 1973. J. Agr. Sci. 81:55.
Sisson, S. and J.D. Grossman. 1953. The Anatomy of the Domestic Animals. 4th ed. W.B. Saunders Co.
Smith, R.H. 1961. J. Agr. Sci. 56:105.
Stewart, A.M. 1971. Rhod. J. Agr. Res. 9:53.
Stewart, W.E., G.E. Henning and J.H. Nicolai. 1966. J. Dairy Sci. 49:1543.
Stobo, I.J.F., J.H.B. Roy and J.H. Gaston. 1966. Br. J. Nutr. 20:171.
Tamate, H. 1956. Tohoku J. Agr. Res. 7:209.
Tamate, H. 1957. Tohoku J. Agr. Res. 8:65.
Tamate, H., A.D. McGilliard, N.L. Jacobson and R. Getty. 1962. J. Dairy Sci. 45:408.
Trautmann, A. 1933. Cited by Hungate, R.E. 1966. The Rumen and Its Microbes. Academic Press.
Tulloh, N.M. 1966. N.Z. J. Agr. Res. 9:999.
Walker, D.M. and G.J. Walker. 1961. J. Agr. Sci. 57:271.
Wallace, L.R. 1948. J. Agr. Sci. 38:93, 243, 367.
Wardrop, I.D. 1961. J. Agr. Sci. 57:335.
Wardrop, I.D. and J.B. Coombe. 1960. J. Agr. Sci. 54:140.
Wardrop, I.D. and J.B. Coombe. 1961. Aust. J. Agr. Res. 12:661.
Warner, E.D. 1958. Amer. J. Anat. 102:33.
Warner, R.G. and W.P. Flatt. 1965. In: Physiology of Digestion in the Ruminant. Butterworths Pub. Co.
Warner, R.G., W.P. Flatt and J.K. Loosli. 1956. J. Agr. Food Chem. 4:788.
Williams, E.I., D.E. Williams, D.D. Goetsch and P.O. Firth. 1966. Amer. J. Vet. Res. 27:1777.
Wilson, P.N. 1958. J. Agr. Sci. 51:4.

CHAPTER 4 — INGESTION AND MASTICATION OF FEED

The ingestion of food by ruminants under pasture or range conditions often occupies a third or more of their time, thus it is an important aspect of digestive physiology. Many different environmental and physiological factors affect the rate of eating or the amount of food that may be consumed. Unfortunately, quantitative data on some of these are not as prevalent as might be wished. A number of these factors are discussed in this chapter. Those more specifically concerned with appetite and its control are discussed in the second volume of this series.

Prehension

The term **prehension** means the seizing and conveying of food to the mouth. In ruminant species the lips, teeth and tongue are the principal prehensile organs. However, their relative importance varies with the species of animal, its age and the type of food being eaten.

One peculiarity of ruminant animals is that they do not have upper incisor teeth. Rather, the upper incisors are replaced with a tough dental pad (Fig. 4-2), which provides a surface against which the lower incisors can put pressure. Although the elephant is probably an exception, no other herbivorous species suffer the handicap of not having upper incisors.

In bovines, the chief prehensil organ is the tongue. The tongue, a long mobile organ, is used to pull grass or other herbage into the mouth where it can be clipped off with the incisor teeth and dental pad. If the herbage is long and coarse, it is pulled into the mouth by the tongue and is partially pulled and partially bitten off. Near the tip of the tongue (Fig. 4-1), there are a number of filiform papillae which are stiff and project in a caudal direction. These papillae aid in collecting small particles of food; they are also useful in normal grooming of the hair coat.

The lips, which are relatively immobile in bovines, become more important as prehensile organs when the animal is cropping lush, young grass or when eating food of relatively small particle size such as grains, meals, pellets and so forth. Sheep and numerous other species have an upper lip, often partially cleft, which is much more mobile than that of bovines. This type of a lip permits very close grazing, although the incisor teeth and tongue are considered to be the principal prehensile structures. The tongue is not protruded as much in grazing as it is in cattle. This type of prehensile lip, which is facilitated by the manner in which the tongue is used, allows many species to be very selective when consuming grass, mixed herbage, browse or forbs.

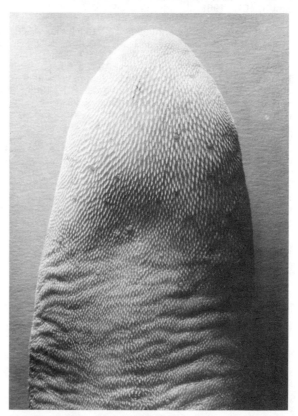

Figure 4-1. The tip of a bovine tongue showing the filliform papillae. These papillae project caudally and aid in prehension.

Mastication

Mastication or chewing is the mechanical reduction of food to a smaller particle size. In non-herbivorous animals, mastication is accomplished primarily by movements of the

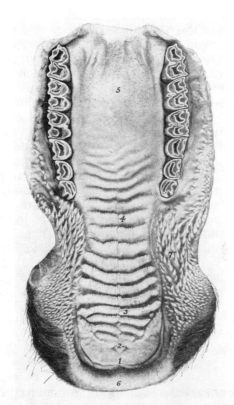

Figure 4-2. The hard [upper] palate of the bovine. 1, dental pad or plate; 2, placed on papilla incisiva with lines to orifices of ductus incisivi; 3, ridge of palate; 4, raphe of palate; 5, smooth part of palate showing orifices of palatine glands; 6, upper lip; 7, conical papillae of cheek. From Sisson and Grossman [1953]. Courtesy of Saunders Pub. Co.

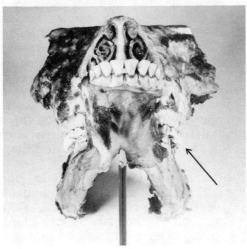

Figure 4-3. Partially disected head of the bovine. The arrow points to the molar teeth with the object of showing the difference in width between the upper and lower jaws. The result being that the animal cannot chew on both sides of the jaw at the same time.

mandible in a vertical plane. In herbivores, well-developed lateral movements greatly facilitate the grinding action which is required to reduce fibrous plant material to a size or shape that may be swallowed. In addition, the upper jaw is wider than the lower jaw making it possible for the animal to use the molars on only one side at a time (see Fig. 4-3). Due to the lateral movements of the jaw, the molar teeth develop a chisel-shaped grinding surface. The sharp edge of the lower molar teeth is innermost, whereas that of the upper teeth is outermost. At times, these edges may become sharp enough to damage the tongue or cheek, respectively. In addition, the teeth are composed of layers varying in hardness and resistance to wear, resulting in the development of a rough surface which greatly facilitates grinding of fibrous material. Furthermore, the grinding surfaces of the molars are in different planes, thus increasing efficiency of mastication. In cattle, the permanent incisor teeth appear between 1-1.5 and 4 yr of age and the permanent molars from ca. 6 mo. to 4 yr of age (Sisson and Grossman, 1953).

Even though ruminants are well equipped to thoroughly masticate fibrous food material, it is not their custom to do so while ingesting food. As a general rule, only enough chewing occurs to mix the food with saliva and to form a bolus of suitable size and consistency so that it may be swallowed. As noted by Hungate (1966), Camper in 1803 stated, "Most of these (wild) animals, fearful of their enemies have little time to devote to feeding; in consequence they consume suitable forage as quickly as possible; they hide or rest like domestic animals, and ruminate at their ease the food which has already undergone a little alteration or digestion." This observation, although recorded some 170 years ago, is probably as logical an explanation as any regarding the mastication habits of ruminants.

Although ruminants do eat hurriedly, the fibrous nature of their normal rations requires that a considerable amount of time and energy be expended during either ingestion or rumination. Fuller (1928) noted that dairy cows made an average of 94 jaw movements/min when eating grain and silage and 78/min when eating hay. He calculated that a dairy cow makes ca. 4,700 jaw movements daily while eating grain and silage and 10,530 while eating hay. In addition, there were ca. 26,400 jaw movements during rumination, or a total of ca. 42,000/day. Gill et al (1966) have studied the eating habits of cows given hay or fresh herbage. These authors reported that their cows made about 5,000 to 10,000 jaw movements/day during ingestion, the number being influenced by the amount and type of forage fed. Estimates of the number of chews while eating can be derived from published data if we apply "typical" values for number of chews/min (74/min for hay; 94/min for grain). In one case values are: long hay, 18-24 lb/day, 17,310; straw, 8-10 lb/day, 14,800 (Freer et al, 1962). In another experiment, when cows were consuming ca. 20 lb of feed/day, estimates are: long hay, 19,350; dried grass, 22,190, and concentrates, 5,170 (Freer and Campling, 1965). In the case of sheep fed alfalfa hay, oats or fresh grass (Popescu and Florescu, 1959), the number of jaw movements during eating works out to be about 9,000 for oats to 43,000 for alfalfa hay. When the number of jaw movements made during rumination are added (ca. 40,000), the total/day would be from 50,000-80,000 (Gordon, 1958).

For dairy cows the mean particle size of swallowed hay or forage varied from 1.6-1.2 mm (Gill et al, 1966). Food swallowed the first few minutes of eating contained particles of a larger average size than those at any other time during the meal, although the frequency of jaw movements did not vary appreciably during a meal. Increasing the amount of hay given to the cows by 50% or giving a different hay did not cause any significant alteration in the average size of particles of swallowed hay. With a diet of herbage, the average particle size of swallowed food was larger than that of hay (easier to swallow?) and there were slightly more jaw movements/min.

In studies with young calves, Hodgson (1971) observed that they spent 2.3-2.4 hr/day eating pelleted diets as opposed to 4.8 hr/day for hay. Food dry matter was consumed at a rate of 14-17 g/min for pellets and 4.2 g/min for hay.

The effectiveness of mastication on releasing soluble nutrients from ingested feed has been investigated by a number of laboratories. For example, Bailey and Balch (1961) studied the effect of chewing on hay by allowing a cow with a rumen fistula to eat normally vs. administration of the hay through the fistula. Digestibility of the dry matter of the hay and % of dry matter in the reticulo-rumen contents were not changed by "fistula feeding," but the amount of dry matter in the reticulo-rumen was increased. In addition, the amount of time spent ruminating increased approximately from 30 to 44% of the day when hay was placed directly in the rumen. In a subsequent paper (Bailey, 1962), samples of swallowed and unswallowed grass were placed in nylon bags in the rumen of a fistulated cow. In this case digestion of dry matter, protein and ash in the swallowed grass during the first hour was considerably greater than in the unswallowed samples and differences were still evident after 13 hr. Hogan (1965) and Doyle (1967) have also presented data obtained from fresh grass or clover boluses from sheep, indicating that more of the plant nitrogen was readily extractable from swallowed samples than from unswallowed grass or clover.

The Food Bolus

As observed by Schalk and Amadon (1928), the bolus is projected into the stomach with considerable force and is deposited in the anterior rumen or the **antrium ventriculi** (reticulo-rumen fold area). The rapid movement of a bolus is, presumably, made possible by the presence of striated muscle in the ruminant esophagus, a type of muscle not normally found in the esophagus of most other mammals. The ruminant esophagus is also characterized by a cardial sphincter (near juncture of esophagus and reticulum), a pharyngo-esophageal sphincter near the pharynx and, apparently, a diaphragmatic sphincter where the esophagus passes through the diaphragm (Dougherty and Habel, 1955). These structures are, presumably, of more importance in the regurgitation phase of rumination and/or eructation than in normal deglutition (swallowing).

The form, weight and consistency of the bolus varies considerably, depending upon the type of food being ingested. Forage material, such as cured hay, is formed into a firm, oblong mass with rounded extremities and will hold its shape even after extensive handling. Cured hay boli have a low moisture content and will float in water although their weight increases rapidly after arrival within the rumen. Boli of concentrates are much heavier, as would be expected. Ground feed forms a bolus which is doughy in consistency and quite often is dry in its central portion, when eating is rapid. The weight of forage boli tends to be smallest when eating first begins; it increases to a peak weight by the time 1/3 to 2/3 of the meal has been consumed, and declines somewhat by the end of ingestion (Gill et al, 1966). These authors found that the average wet weight of forage boli ingested by dairy cows was about 140-160 g. The initial weights were 80 to 100 g, a value similar to that reported by Schalk and Amadon (1928). Schalk and Amadon reported that wet weights for hay were 85 g, for whole corn 81 g, and for whole oats 140 g. Gill et al (1966) found that dry weights (more accurately measured) were between 12 and 28 g, with mean values about 22-24 g. The difference between the wet and dry weights would represent moisture added from saliva during mastication.

Eating Behavior

Only a relatively few papers are available on the effect of different variables on chewing (or eating) rate or other parameters of eating behavior. On the basis of observations by many different people, it must be assumed that palatability of a feedstuff or a ration (however it may be measured) is a factor along with hunger in the modification of normal chewing rates. Palatability and taste might be expected to be influenced by such physical and chemical parameters as the hardness of seeds or pellets; those very hard objects being masticated at a slower rate. Other factors that are apparently involved would include quantity of feed, particle size, presence of objectional objects such as thorns, burrs or rocks, the doughiness and dustiness of grains and meals, texture, chemical taste sensations, the moisture content, and the presence of coarse, fibrous plant tissues which require a great deal of mastication to reduce in size. Some papers on this general subject are discussed in subsequent paragraphs. However, the reader should keep in mind that quantitative data on many of these factors have not been published.

Dry or Harvested Feeds

The effect of hunger on eating rate was clearly demonstrated by Schalk and Amadon (1928). After being off feed for 24 hr, a mature cow ingested 30 boli of green alfalfa during the first 5 min of eating, but only 19 boli during the succeeding 5 min. Freer et al (1962) observed that the eating rate of dairy cows was increased when cows were restricted to less than 4½ hr/day, and markedly increased by restriction to 2 hr. Results of one experiment (Freer and Campling, 1965) clearly show the effect of restricting feeding time on eating rate: restricted feeding, dried ground grass, 4.5 min/kg; long dried grass, 8.1 min/kg; ad libitum feeding, dried ground grass, 10.7 min/kg and dried long grass, 18.2 min/kg. Data from this experiment station (Balch, 1971) also clearly indicate that a reduction in eating caused by restriction in time to eat resulted in an increase in rumination time, so that the total time spent eating and ruminating was about constant for a given roughage.

The effect of physical form of feed on eating rate is partly exemplified by differences in consumption of concentrates and roughage. For example, Schalk and Amadon (1928) reported that whole corn boli were swallowed at a rate of 1 1/3/min; ground feed at 3 1/4/min and whole oats at 2 1/3/min. Bailey (1959), using dairy cows, found the eating rate to be markedly affected by physical form. Mean rates (g/min) were: long hay, 70; dried grass, 83; silage, 248; fresh grass, 282; and a pelleted ration, 357. With concentrates, information at hand indicates that cows generally eat faster as the amount is increased and cubes are eaten faster than meal, although there may be considerable differences between cows (Jones et al, 1966; Stoddard, 1969).

Most experiments clearly indicate that feeds requiring considerable chewing are usually eaten (swallowed) at a slower rate than less fibrous feeds (Tables 4-1, 2), although Putnam et al (1967) observed in one experiment that the response of cattle varied when given a choice of ground or pelleted high-roughage (89%) and low-roughage (25%) rations. For the low-roughage, rate of consumption was least for the pelleted form (40 vs. 12 min/kg consumed) while for the high-roughage, the pelleted form was consumed at about the same rate as the ground form (16 vs. 19 min/kg). Results of Ilan et al (1973) with moderate-roughage diets are probably more typical. They found that young cattle on a medium-roughage (40%) diet spent 26% more time eating and 5% more time drinking as well as 19% more time ruminating than those on a low- roughage (18%) ration.

Table 4-1. Eating and ruminating time of cows given diets of single feedstuffs.[a]

Feedstuff	Time range observed*		
	Eating	Ruminating	Total
Oat straw	41-58	94-133	145-191
Medium quality hay	20-40	63-87	103-109
Good quality hay	27-31	55-74	87-105
Grass silage	31-58	60-83	99-120
Dried grass	8-18	33-39	44-53
Concentrates, pelleted	4-10	(0-25)**	(4-29)**
Finely ground oat straw	11-24	(0-20)**	(11-31)**
Finely ground hay	13	(0-6)**	(13-19)**
Finely ground dried grass	5-12	(0-11)**	(5-18)**

[a] Data from Balch (1971) * min/kg dry matter consumed ** Higher values in the ranges shown in () show the extent of irregular chewing with finely ground diets.

Generally, with forage, grinding, chopping or pelleting will usually increase rate of consumption (Campling and Freer, 1966). Addition of urea or concentrates to straw diets — which speeds up rumen digestion — has also been shown to increase eating rates (Freer et al, 1962) when cows were fed in meals, reflecting less material in the reticulo-rumen and, thus, hunger. It is doubtful that the same reaction would be seen in cows fed ad libitum because the stomach would probably not empty out to the same degree. With respect to physical nature of the feed, the main factors seem to be those which affect the amount of chewing required to reduce particle size and to mix saliva with the food in order that a satisfactory bolus may be formed for swallowing.

Gill et al (1966) observed that eating rates varied with the type of roughage supplied to

Table 4-2. Eating and ruminating time of cows given different mixed diets.[a]

Diet	Time range or mean*		
	Eating	Ruminating	Total
Oat straw + urea	23-40	67-79	98-117
Finely ground oat straw + urea	15-18	0-22	15-37
Hay + concentrates:			
67%**	19	47	66
44%	18	42	60
31%**	15	37	52
17% Hay in diet	11	24	35
8%	21	19	40
7%	16	20	36
0%	10	0	10
Barley straw + concentrates:			
60%**	18	44	62
40%** Straw in diet	17	36	53
20%**	16	20	36
0%	21	0	21

[a] From Balch (1971) * min/kg dry matter consumed ** pelleted; hay or straw was coarsely chopped.

cows, but jaw movements generally were within the range of 70-80/min and cows usually took about 15-18 min to eat a kg of hay. Gill et al also noted a considerable individual variation between cows; however, mean values for animals consuming hay were between 2.6 and 2.9 boli swallowed/min. They did not observe a decline in eating rate during the meal, although this has been reported for both silage and low-quality hay by Suzuki et al (1969).

Feeding habits for cows fed silages indicate that rate of eating was highest during the first 5-10 min and then gradually declined. The highest rate of eating occurred at the evening meal (fed 2X daily), but the rate declined at much the same speed for each meal when cows received from 2-5 meals daily. When given a large meal of silage, three stages of eating were observed: fast, moderate decreasing to slow, but this change was not noted with hay. The authors (Suzuki et al, 1969) suggested the initial high rate was partly psychological, the cows being influenced by a large amount of silage in view. Silage dry matter was consumed at about twice the rate of hay dry matter when restricted amounts were given. In addition to quality of feed, individuality of the cows and stage of reproduction were obvious factors. Pregnant cows ate longer and slower than lactating cows. When given a choice between silage and hay (Webb et al, 1963), dairy cows tend to spend more time eating silage than hay (4 vs 2¼ hr) and most of the time is during the daylight hours (74% between 0600 and 1800). Frequency in this case averaged 18 visits to the feeders, with visits during the day being of longer duration. Campling (1966) has studied the frequency of eating in heifers, pregnant females and lactating cows (pairs of twins). When heifers were fed hay, the number of daily periods ranged from 7 to 14 with a mean of 11. In pregnant animals, eating periods ranged from 9 to 20 with a mean of 12, and in lactating cows the range was from 8 to 16 with a mean of 12.

The stage of the reproductive cycle also has an effect on eating patterns as observed by Putnam and Bond (1971). Their data indicating that less time is spent at the feeder during estrus even though the diurnal pattern was not changed. No differences were observed in feeding patterns or daily time at the feeder during early and mid-gestation, but less time was spent at the feeder immediately before and after calving,

and lactating cows were seen to be more uniform in eating patterns than nonlactating cows.

Data on the feeding behavior of sheep are considerably less extensive than those on cattle, although more information is available on rumination (see section on rumination, Ch. 6). In older work, Popescu and Florescu (1959) fed alfalfa hay, oats or fresh grass to sheep. Average eating times were about 6.25, 1.75 and 4 hr when consuming 1,553,797 and 6,840 g of feed. The number of mastications/min were 116, 86 and 141 while eating and 72, 89 and 55 when ruminating. More recent information on sheep which were fed silage has been presented by Dulphy (1971, 1972) and Dulphy and Demarquilly (1972). Their studies show that daily time spent eating was shorter for sheep fed silage than for green forage or hay prepared from the original herbage. The length of silage meals was shorter and their number higher. The eating rate of sheep on silage was variable in that silage was eaten less rapidly than hay in one trial and at the same rate in another. When animals received silage without transition from hay, dry matter intake progressively decreased for 4 days. When fed hay again, dry matter intake immediately increased as well as the length of the meal. Further data showed that fine chopping before ensiling increased feed intake, daily time spent eating and number of meals. Chopping after ensiling also increased intake and the number of meals increased slightly although rate of eating decreased. Other work on consumption of haylage produced from alfalfa or vetch cut at different stages (Peterson et al, 1974; Fig. 4-4) indicated that stage of maturity and type of preservation (haylage or hay) had no appreciable effect on numbers of meals (9-11 meals/day on average), or 7.1 for vetch and 12.1 for alfalfa. Meal size was not statistically affected by forage species (102.9 g for vetch vs. 95.8 for alfalfa) or maturity. Haylage-fed sheep ate smaller meals than those on hay. Vetch-fed sheep spent 20% more time at the feeder (325 min) than those fed alfalfa (272 min). The authors noted a high correlation (0.91) between bulk density of the forage and rate of dry matter consumption.

Feeding behavior of sheep on complete diets (20% chopped hay, 80% concentrate) has been studied in a limited way (Chase and Wangsness, 1973). Average meal size was 135 g; other parameters noted were:

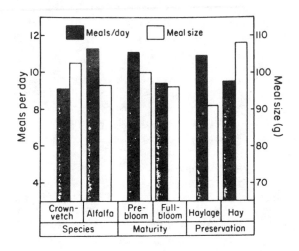

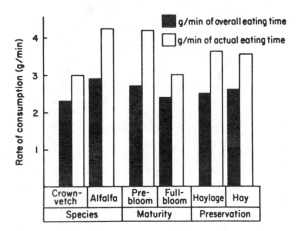

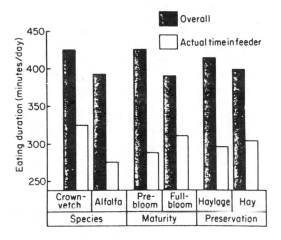

Figure 4-4. [Top] The effect of forage species, maturity and preservation on numbers of meals and meal size. [Middle] The effect of forage species, maturity and preservation on rate of dry matter consumption [g/min]. [Bottom] The effect of forage species, maturity and preservation on total overall and actual eating duration. From Peterson et al [1974].

duration of meals, 12.6 min; eating rate, 11.7 g/min. Their data indicated that, with increasing meal size, the sheep apparently adjusted both eating rate and meal duration, although eating rate increased less with large meals than the duration of eating.

Rapid alteration of the amount of light has an effect on ewes (Ruckebusch and Laplace, 1968). Based on 12 hr of light from 0900 to 2100, then 24 hr of either light or dark increased the number of meals and rumination periods, and light increased the proportion of time spent in feeding, but not the amount of feed consumed.

Kennan and McManus (1970) have studied eating habits of wethers restricted for 4 wk periods sufficient to cause substantial losses in weight. The sheep were then fed alfalfa which was chopped, pelleted or pelleted with wheat. Results indicated that feed intake increased slowly for 4 wk after the restriction period. After short-term deprivation of food (24 to 72 hr), sheep that ate 8.5 meals/day under normal conditions then consumed 11.8 meals after 24 hr or 7.0 meals after 72 hr of fasting (Peterson et al, 1972).

Feedlot Behavior

Putnam and Davis (1963) have used photoelectric cells and recorders to study feeding habits of steers fed ground or pelleted rations varying in roughage content. About ¾ of the time spent at the feeder was between 0600 and 1800, although the steers fed at intervals throughout the night. Pelleting reduced time spent at the feeder by about 30%. Average number of feeding periods ranged from 9 to 14/day. In another experiment (Putnam et al, 1967), they found that steers spent 112-127 min/day at feeders, with no difference in time from October to February. Further studies of this type (Chase et al, 1971) with steers have shown that the greatest concentration of eating activity occurred during two periods, peaking at 0600 and 1630 with smaller peaks at 0930 and 1430.

Hoffman and Self (1973) found that total daily eating time of steers averaged about 143 min/day and was unaffected by season of the year, but varied greatly during the day. In summer, greatest activity occurred in late afternoon (1500-1800) and early evening (1800-2100) with a smaller peak near sunrise (0600-0900). In winter, greatest activity occurred in the late afternoon (1500-1800). Water consumption and time spent drinking

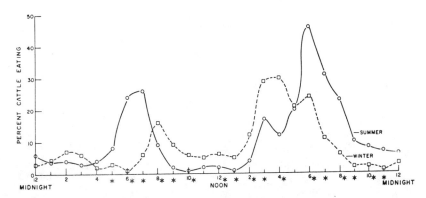

Figure 4-5. Seasonal influence on diurnal eating activity of yearling steers in the feedlot. An asterisk [*] indicates a significant [P<.001] difference between seasons. From Ray and Roubicek [1971].

were greater during the summer than winter. Further information on effect of seasonal patterns on food and water consumption in a hot climate have been presented by Ray and Roubicek (1971) as illustrated in Fig. 4-5, 6. Note that the summer feeding pattern in the morning peaked at an earlier time and that there was less feeding during the afternoon hours, the major peak of the day being about 1800 as opposed to a broader peak during the winter between 1500 and 1600 hr. Water consumption patterns indicate that a higher percentage of steers were drinking during the hot periods of the day in the summer.

Confinement Feeding of Cows

Mature lactating beef cows fed under confinement have been shown, in one study, to spend about 170 min/day eating during the day and 29 min at night but the time spent was related to level of intake as percentage of the day utilized by eating was 22.1, 12.9 and 7.1 for cows fed at a level of 2.5, 2.0 and 1.5% of body weight, respectively (Schake and Riggs, 1969). Similar data have been reported by Rugh and Wilson (1971). When fed at a level of 115 or 85% of NRC recommendations, the cows spent 1.92 or 1.74 hr eating, respectively. Mastication frequency of the 115% cows was greater (a combined count of eating and ruminating). When fed 2X daily in equal amounts, cows tended to eat faster at the evening meal, but eating rate does not appear to be affected by changing the interval between meals from 12 hr to 6 hr (Suzuki et al, 1969).

Suckling Behavior

Recent data on suckling behavior of young animals are not very plentiful. Newborn calves are said to suckle about 6X daily (Walker, 1950). Cartwright and Carpenter (1961) observed that little nocturnal nursing occurred. Average nursing frequency and duration were said to be 4.2 times and 38.0 min for Herefords and 3.5 times and 28.7 min for Brahman-Hereford cross calves. Walker (1962) indicates that the majority of calves suckled 3-5X/day and observed that Hereford-Angus heifers suckled their calves more frequently but for shorter times than Angus heifers. The most regular suckling time was near daybreak, and intervals between sucklings tended to increase as the season advanced. When beef calves were allowed to nurse only 2X daily, average time spent for morning and evening nursings was 14.8 and 15.3 min, respectively (Schake and Riggs, 1970). In calves with an initial age of 76 days, observations by Rugh and Wilson (1971) indicated they nursed on average 6.14X/day and spent 1.19 hr/24 in this activity. With artificially raised calves, Hafez and Lineweaver (1968) found that Holstein calves took from 0.9-2.2 min to consume 700 ml of milk. Other data on nursing behavior of calves are given by Stephens (1974).

Munro (1955) reported that young lambs may suckle as frequently as once hourly up to the age of 14 days; there was a gradual reduction in the time the ewe allowed the lamb to suck and a sudden shortening of this period occurred at ca. 14 days. More recent data on naturally raised lambs (Ewbank, 1967) indicate that the duration of nursing in wk-old lambs was about 40 sec, but this decreased to ca. 14 sec by 8 wk of age. Data were not obtained over a complete 24-hr period, but observations indicated that single lambs suckled 13-15X/day at 1 wk of age, decreasing to ca. 8X/day at 6 wk. Twins

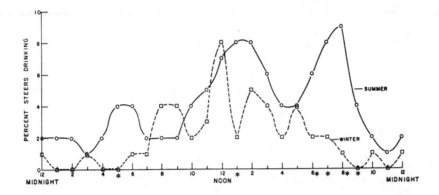

Figure 4-6. Seasonal influence on diurnal drinking activity of yearling steers in the feedlot. An asterisk [*] indicates a significant [P <.001] difference between seasons. From Ray and Roubicek [1971].

suckled at much more frequent intervals up to the 4th wk of life. Studies of suckling behavior in artificially raised lambs (Stephens and Baldwin, 1971) indicate that wk-old lambs tend to nurse 6X daily for a total time of 17.5 min. This decreased to 4X and 10 min, respectively, by the time they were 6 wk of age. When in groups, lambs tended to nurse at intervals of ca. 80 min and the group spent about 21 min/period.

Miscellaneous

In studies with sheep on purified diets, Purser and Moir (1966) observed that eating rate was highly correlated with rumen volume when animals were fed 1X daily. Further studies of this type have been carried out with fattening lambs on a high-roughage pelleted diet (Randall, 1974). When eating rate was expressed in terms of an eating rate index (g food consumed/$BW^{0.75}$) or in terms of food consumed in 30 or 60 min, high correlations were observed between eating rate and parameters such as daily gain, feed efficiency, rumen contents and abomasum weight.

Grazing Behavior

The grazing patterns of ruminant animals may be modified by a number of factors. Animal factors — age, physiological status and nutritional needs; plant factors — herbage yield, palatability, plant height and

so on; and environmental factors — rainfall, temperature, humidity, etc., all very likely combine to have some effect on any particular set of parameters. Thus, the reader should keep in mind that data obtained in one particular set of circumstances may not be applicable in all others.

Animals with esophageal or rumen fistulas have been used extensively by many different laboratories to sample herbage. Although esophageal-fistulated animals (see Plate 4-1) require considerable care; they are very useful in studying the qualitative nature of grazed material. The technique has been used successfully with sheep and cattle (Weir and Torell, 1959; Cook et al, 1963; Ridley et al, 1963; Wallace and Henham, 1970; many other papers) and also with deer (Veteto et al, 1972).

Data available from fistulated animals clearly demonstrate that sheep, which are selective eaters, choose parts of the plant which are of higher quality (and more digestible) than cattle when both species have access to the same herbage. When ingested material is compared to the forage that is available to the animal, studies show that both sheep and cattle (Table 4-1) select a diet which is higher in crude protein and P and lower in fiber. Esophageal samples, however, tend to be higher in ash, particularly P (from saliva) and may be variable in other chemical components (Langlands, 1966; Little, 1972; Scales et al, 1972). In rumen samples when the organ is not evacuated, data indicate that fewer forbes

Table 4-3. Chemical composition of hand sampled and esophageal-fistula samples and comparison of sheep and cattle samples.

Forage	Chemical component, %						Reference
	CP	ADF	Cellulose	Lignin	Ash	P	
Dairy cows							
Bermuda grass							
hand-clipped	16.9	35.6		6.3	6.9		Guthrie et al,
esophageal	20.3	32.0		4.8	15.4		1968
Esophageal samples, same range area							
Sheep	12.3		21.8	13.1	12.4	.38	Cook et al,
Cattle	8.9		27.0	12.5	10.6	.29	1963

and more grasses are apt to be found than were in the diet (Rice et al, 1971).

The grazing habits of domestic ruminants have been investigated in a number of environmental situations. One of the more extensive reports is that of Wagnon (1963), which is based on data from the foothills of California.

Observations from many different areas indicate that beef or dairy cows may spend from ca. 25 to as much as 58% of their time grazing. This time will be influenced by the availability of forage. Wagnon (1963) noted that the higher value (58%) occurred when cows are grazing short, new grass. Most of the papers indicate that grazing during the summer season would average about 40% of a 24 hr period (Johnstone-Wallace and Kennedy, 1944; Castle et al, 1950; Hancock, 1950; Hardison et al, 1956; Furr and Nelson, 1961; Walker, 1962; Lucci et al, 1972a, b). Wagnon's data indicate that supplemental feeding reduced the grazing time from 56 to 44% of the time during winter months.

While grazing, cattle tend to average over 50 bites/min (Hardison et al, 1956; Larsen, 1963), although this rate is apt to be higher on young grass and bites/min are apt to be much slower (25 or less) by the end of a grazing period (Hancock, 1950; Larsen, 1963).

Stobbs (1973) has studied bite size in Jersey cows with esophageal fistulas and with electronic apparatus to count the number of bites (Fig. 4-7). Data were obtained on a variety of tropical grasses. Some of his information on variation in bite size of individual animals grazing three species is shown in Table 4-4. Results of

these studies indicate that bite size varies appreciably between individual animals. Stobbs feels that a high density of leaf and a low stem content are the main factors affecting bite size. These plant factors may be affected, in turn, by amount of regrowth, time after plants were cut or grazed, N fertilization and growth regulators. Stobbs does not give data on wet weight of bites, but the mean bite size (mg of organic matter) ranged from a low of 70 to a high of 590. Stobbs goes on to say that cows may show a rate of biting in excess of 4,000/hr for short periods, but rarely exceed 36,000/day.

Table 4-4. Variation in mean bite size (g organic matter/bite) of three Jersey cows grazing three pasture species.[a]

Animal #	Plant species			Mean
	Siratro	Setaria	Pangola	
1	0.24	0.38	0.30	0.31
2	0.19	0.34	0.33	0.29
3	0.29	0.24	0.39	0.31
Mean	0.24	0.32	0.34	0.30

[a]From Stobbs (1973)

Studies with sheep (Arnold, 1960, 1964) indicate that a decrease in pasture availability results in increased grazing time and increased rate of eating until herbage becomes quite scarce. Allden and Wittaker (1970) have shown that the size of a bite increases almost linearly with increasing tiller length of herbage and that the number of bites decreases proportionately so that

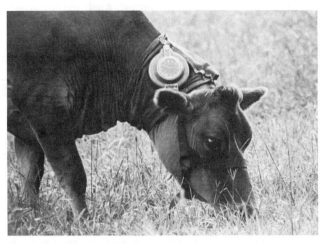

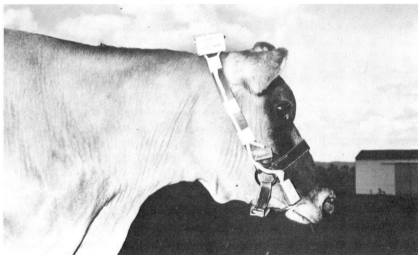

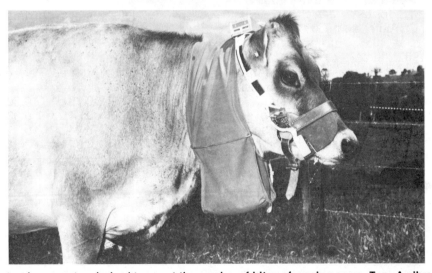

Figure 4-7. Electronic apparatus devised to count the number of bites of grazing cows. Top, A vibracorder attached to a cow for recording grazing time and periodicity of grazing. Middle, equipment for automatically recording jaw movements of cattle. Bottom, the same equipment plus an esophageal collection bag, allowing data to be collected on number of bites and amount consumed. Photos courtesy of T.H. Stobbs, CSIRO, The Cunningham Laboratory, Qld, Australia.

rate of intake is relatively stable (see Fig. 4-8). These authors calculated that the size of the bite ranged from 25 mg of dry matter at a tiller length of 3.7 cm to 420 mg of dry matter at a tiller length of 36.7 cm. The bites/min ranged from 73 at a tiller length of 5 cm to 18/min at a tiller length of 36.7 cm.

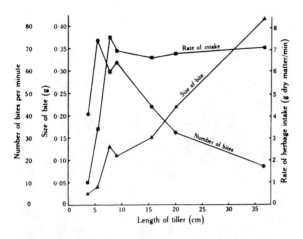

Figure 4-8. Relation between length of tiller and rate of herbage intake, rate of biting, and size of bite. From Allden and Whittaker [1970].

Although ruminants may graze at all hours during the day or night, they tend to be relatively regular and cyclical in their habits. Wagnon (1963) found that the peak periods of grazing for beef cattle occurred from daybreak up to 6 hr later, and from late afternoon until darkness or later. Most of the night feeding was done around midnight, the least from 0200 to daybreak. Night feeding accounted for about 25% of the total in summer months and about 32% when getting supplemental feed. Sheppard et al (1957) found that daily patterns of high grazing activity occurred at about 0400-0800 and 1600-2000, with medium activity at 1000-1200. On a variety of pastures the peak activity was between 1600-2000 with medium activity at 1000-1200. Hancock (1950) reported that 40% of grazing occurred at night by dairy cows in New Zealand, and Hardison et al (1956) found that dairy cows grazed about equal amounts between a.m.-p.m. milkings. Minimal grazing occurred between 2000 and 0300. Hancock (1950) also found that the rate of grazing (bites/min) was similar during light and dark feedings. Lucci et al (1972) observed that periods of more intense grazing were after the afternoon milking until darkness (1630-1830), immediately after the morning milking (0700-0900),

between 2100 and 2300, at 1200 and 0230.

The time spent grazing, as indicated earlier, may be modified by a great number of factors. Of these nutrient needs is a critical one and a number of reports indicate that lactating animals spend more time grazing than those with a lesser demand (Hardison et al, 1956; Bumbry, 1959; Arnold and Dudzinski, 1967; Lucci et al, 1972a). For example, deer frequently graze very little during daylight hours (Montgomery, 1963), yet it is very common in the summer time to see does with young fawns grazing and browsing during the middle of the day.

High daytime temperatures have been shown to increase the time spent grazing at night (Harker et al, 1954; Hardison et al, 1956; Wilson, 1961). Although Larkin (1954) found that high temperatures resulted in a reduction in total as well as daytime grazing in tropical areas of Queensland, Australia. Moonlight nights may also encourage more grazing at night when nutrient demand is greater.

Lofgreen et al (1957) have reported data on grazing behavior of cattle and sheep (see Fig. 4-9) on alfalfa and trefoil-orchard grass pasture and on consumption of soilage. Their data indicate that grazing times increased as forage became less available. The distribution of grazing time for sheep was similar to that of cattle, although sheep tended towards more cyclical patterns, with more time spent in the hours from 2000-2400 and less during the early afternoon hours. Perhaps hot weather may have been partially responsible for this species difference. With unherded sheep in mountain summer range, Bowns (1971) found that sheep spent 67-80% of daylight hours grazing, the time increasing as the season progressed and forage became more scarce. This time was generally divided into a period of grazing activity in the morning and another in the afternoon separated by a period of rest during the middle of the day. The afternoon period was longer and feeding appeared to be more intensive. These sheep generally watered early in the morning, either during or following the morning grazing period. When salt was taken, it generally followed watering in the morning.

In the studies with sheep fed fresh forage (Dulphy, 1971), data indicated that sheep consumed 9.8 meals/day and spent 26-42 min/meal. Earlier work (Tribe, 1950) showed that pregnant ewes carrying twins grazed

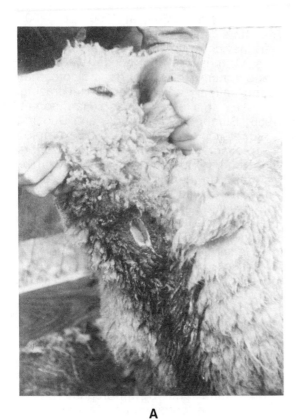

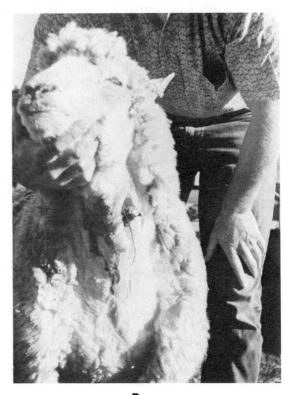

A

B

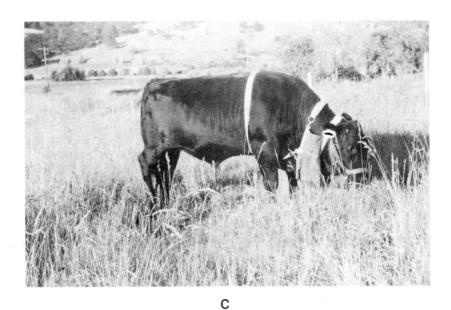

C

Plate 4-1. Esophageal fistulas. A, sheep with an open esophageal fistula; B, an animal with a cannula in place to allow normal passage of ingesta through the esophagus; C, a steer with a collection bag attached [with cannula removed]. Courtesy of T.E. Bedell, Oregon State University.

about 1 hr longer than those carrying singles. It was also observed that grazing by a hungry animal tends to increase the grazing time of other well-fed sheep in the same flock, however there could well be a difference in intake resulting from a difference in rate of eating or in size of bite. Arnold (1966) has also studied the effect of sight on grazing habits of sheep by using blinders. He found that the diet composition differed from controls in some pasture situations, although preference ranking of forage was unaltered.

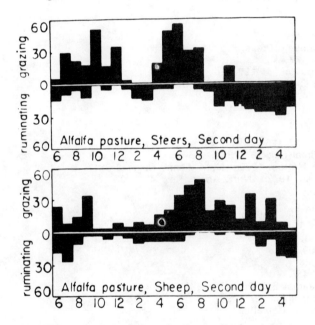

Figure 4-9. Grazing and ruminating patterns of steers and sheep on alfalfa pasture. From Lofgreen et al [1957].

Conclusions

Ruminant species differ in the use of their prehensile organs depending upon the nature of feed being consumed, but those with mobile lips can be very selective. Cattle, at least, masticate ingested feed only enough to form a bolus of suitable size to swallow it easily. The number of jaw movements during mastication would appear to be on the order of 15,000 to 20,000 in cattle and 10,000 to 45,000 in sheep with approximately an additional 25,000 and 40,000 during rumination in cattle and sheep, respectively. The total daily mastications would, therefore, be on the order of 35,000-85,000 for sheep and 40,000-45,000 for cattle. Mastication appears to increase the solubility of some nutrients. The rate of mastication varies with hunger and nature of the feed.

The grazing behavior of ruminants is cyclical in nature with major activity during early morning and evening hours and intermittent activity at other times, probably being affected by temperature as well as other environmental and physiological factors. Grazing habits appear to be similar in sheep and cattle. Data indicate that a reduction in available forage increases grazing time. In the dry lot feeding is also intermittent, but a majority occurs during daylight hours.

References Cited

Allden, W.C. and I.A. McD. Wittaker. 1970. Aust. J. Agr. Res. 21:755.
Arnold, G.W. 1960. Aust. J. Agric. Res. 2:1034.
Arnold, G.W. 1964. In: Grazing in Terrestrial and Marine Environments. Blackwell Scientific Publications, Adlard & Son Ltd., Dorking, England.
Arnold, G.W. 1966. Aust. J. Agr. Res. 17:521.
Arnold, G.W. and M.L. Dudzinski. 1967. Aust. J. Agr. Res. 18:349.
Bailey, C.B. 1959. Proc. Nutr. Soc. 18:1.
Bailey, C.B. 1962. Can. J. Animal Sci. 42:49.
Bailey, C.B. and C.C. Balch. 1961. Br. J. Nutr. 12:183.
Balch, C.C. 1971. Br. J. Nutr. 26:383.
Bowns, J.E. 1971. J. Range Mgmt. 24:105.
Bumbry, P.J. 1959. N.Z.J. Agr. Res. 2:797.
Campling, R.C. and M. Freer. 1966. Br. J. Nutr. 20:229.
Cartwright, T.C. and J.A. Carpenter. 1961. J. Animal Sci. 20:904 (abstr).
Castle, M.E., A.S. Foot and R.J. Halley. 1950. J. Dairy Res. 17:215.
Chase, L.E., A.H. Rakes, A.C. Linnerud and J.D. Pettyjohn. 1971. J. Dairy Sci. 54:1835.
Chase L.E. and P.J. Wangsness. 1973. J. Animal Sci. 37:340 (abstr).
Cook, C.W., J.T. Blake and J.W. Call. 1963. J. Animal Sci. 22:579.

Dougherty, R.W. and R.E. Hable. 1955. Cornell Vet. 45:459.
Doyle, J.J. 1967. Aust. J. Expt. Agr. Animal Husb. 7:318.
Dulphy, J.P. 1971. Ann. Biol. Anim. Bioch. Biophys. 11:289.
Dulphy, J.P. 1972. Ann. Zootech. 21:429.
Dulphy, J.P. and C. Demarquilly. 1972. Ann. Zootech. 21:443.
Ewband, R. 1967. Animal Behav. 15:251.
Freer, M. and R.C. Campling. 1965. Br. J. Nutr. 19:195.
Freer, M., R.C. Campling and C.C. Balch. 1962. Br. J. Nutr. 16:279.
Fuller, J.M. 1928. N. Hamp. Agr. Expt. Sta. Tech. Bul. 35.
Furr, R.D. and A.B. Nelson. 1961. J. Animal Sci. 20:959 (abstr).
Gill, J., R.C. Campling and D.R. Westgarth. 1966. Br. J. Nutr. 20:13.
Gordon, J.G. 1958. J. Agr. Sci. 50:34.
Guthrie, L.D., G.H. Rollins and G.E. Hawkins. 1968. J. Dairy Sci. 51:710.
Hafez, E.S.E. and J.A. Lineweaver. 1968. Z. Tierpsychol. 25:187.
Hancock, J. 1950. Empire J. Expt. Agr. 18:249.
Hardison, W.S., H.L. Fisher, G.C. Graf and N.R. Thompson. 1956. J. Dairy Sci. 39:1735.
Harker, W.H., J.I. Taylor and D.H.L. Rollinson. 1954. J. Agr. Sci. 44:193.
Hodgson, J. 1971. Animal Prod. 13:15.
Hoffman, M.P. and H.L. Self. 1973. J. Animal Sci. 37:1438.
Hogan, J.P. 1965. Aust. J. Agr. Res. 16:855.
Hungate, R.E. 1966. The Rumen and Its Microbes. Academic Press.
Ilan, D., D. Levy and Z. Holzer. 1973. Animal Prod. 17:147.
Johnstone-Wallace, D.B. and K. Kennedy. 1944. J. Agri. Sci. 34:190.
Jones, C.G., K.D. Maddever, D.L. Court and M. Phillips. 1966. Animal Prod. 8:48.
Keenen, D.M. and W.R. McManus. 1970. J. Agr. Sci. 74:477.
Langlands, J.P. 1966. Animal Prod. 8:253.
Larkin, R.M. 1954. Queensland J. Agr. Sci. 11:115.
Larsen, H.J. 1963. J. Animal Sci. 22:1134 (abstr).
Little, D.A. 1972. Aust. J. Expt. Agr. and Animal Husb. 12:126.
Lofgreen, G.P., J.H. Meyer and J.L. Hull. 1957. J. Animal Sci. 16:773.
Lucci, C. de S., H.J. Sartini, F.L. Pires and J.C.A. de Mattos. 1972a. Nutr. Abstr. Rev. 42:731.
Lucci, C. de S., H.J. Sartini, J.P. Sobral and O. Rehfeld. 1972b. Nutr. Abstr. Rev. 42:730.
Montgomery, G.G. 1963. J. Wildl. Mgmt. 27:422.
Munro, J. 1955. Agr. Progress 50:129.
Peterson, A.D., B.R. Baumgardt and T.A. Long. 1974. J. Animal Sci. 38:172.
Peterson, A.D., L.E. Chase and B.R. Baumgardt. 1972. J. Animal Sci. 35:192 (abstr).
Popescu, F. and S. Forsecu. 1959. Nutr. Abstr. Rev. 30:106.
Purser, D.B. and R.J. Moir. 1966. J. Animal Sci. 25:509.
Putnam, P.A. and J. Bond. 1971. J. Animal Sci. 33:1086.
Putnam, P.A. and R.E. Davis. 1963. J. Animal Sci. 22:437.
Putnam, P.A., R. Lehmann and R.E. Davis. 1967. J. Animal Sci. 26:647.
Putnam, P.A., R. Lehmann and W. Luber. 1968. J. Animal Sci. 27:1494.
Randall, R.P. 1974. Ph.D. Thesis, Oregon State University, Corvallis.
Ray, D.E. and C.B. Roubicek. 1971. J. Animal Sci. 33:72.
Rice, R.W., D.R. Cundy and R.R. Weyerts. 1971. J. Range Mgmt. 24:121.
Ridley, J.R., A.L. Lesperance, E.H. Jensen and V.R. Bohman. 1963. J. Dairy Sci. 46:128.
Ruckebusch, Y. and J.P. Laplace. 1968. Nutr. Abstr. Rev. 38:558.
Rugh, M.C. and L.L. Wilson. 1971. J. Animal Sci. 32:727.
Scales, G.H., C.L. Streeter and A.H. Denham. 1972. Proc. West. Sec. Amer. Soc. Animal Sci. 23:192.
Schake, L.M. and J.K. Riggs. 1969. J. Animal Sci. 28:568.
Schake, L.M. and J.K. Riggs. 1970. J. Animal Sci. 31:414.
Schalk, A.F. and R.S. Amadon. 1928. N. Dak. Agr. Expt. Sta. Bul. 216.
Sheppard, A.J., R.E. Blaser and C.M. Kincaid. 1957. J. Animal Sci. 16:681.
Sisson, S. and J.D. Grossman. 1953. The Anatomy of the Domestic Animals. 4th ed. W.B. Saunders Co.
Stephens, D.B. 1974. Animal Prod. 18:23.
Stephens, D.B. and B.A. Baldwin. 1971. Res. Vet. Sci. 12:219.
Stobbs, T.H. 1973. Aust. J. Agr. Res. 24:809; 821.
Stoddard, G.E. 1969. J. Dairy Sci. 52:844.
Suzuki, S., H. Fujita and Y. Shinde. 1969. Animal Prod. 11:29.
Tribe, D.E. 1950. Nature 166:74.
Veteto, G., C.E. Davis, R. Hart and R.M. Robinson. 1972. J. Wildl. Mgmt. 36:906.
Wagnon, K.A. 1963. Calif. Agr. Expt. Sta. Bul. 799.
Walker, D.E. 1962. N.Z. J. Agr. Res. 5:331.
Walker, D.M. 1950. Bul. Animal Behav. 8:5.
Wallace, J.D. and A.H. Henham. 1970. J. Animal Sci. 30:605.
Webb, F.M., V.F. Colenbrander, T.H. Blosser and D.E. Waldern. 1963. J. Dairy Sci. 46:1433.
Weir, W.C. and D. Torell. 1959. J. Animal Sci. 18:641.
Wilson, P.N. 1961. J. Agr. Sci. 56:351.

CHAPTER 5 — SALIVARY PRODUCTION AND FUNCTION

It has been well documented that sheep, cattle and buffalo secrete large volumes of alkaline and well-buffered saliva in the normal course of feed ingestion and rumination. Presumably, all other ruminant animals produce comparable saliva in terms of amounts and quality, but data on other species are rare or nonexistant.

The chief salivary glands and their distribution in sheep have been described by Kay (1960a) and more recently in buffalo by Venkatakrishnan and Mariappa (1969). In the sheep there are five sets of paired glands and three unpaired glands. The paired glands (located bilaterally on each side of the head) are: the parotid, which extends from the base of the ear to the posterior end of the mandible; the submaxillary, found at the base of the maxilla and mandible; the inferior molar, found in the cheek; the ventral sublingual, underneath the tongue; and the buccal, also found in the cheek. The unpaired glands include the palatine, in the hard and soft palate; the pharyngeal, near the pharnyx; and the labial, in the corners of the mouth (see Fig. 5-1).

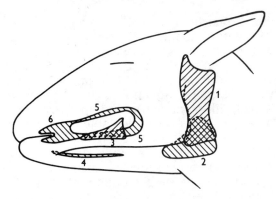

Figure 5-1. The main paired salivary glands of the sheep. 1, parotid; 2, submaxillary; 3, inferior molar; 4, sublingual; 5, buccal; 6, labial. The pharyngeal and palatine glands are not shown. From Kay [1960a].

Saliva is generally produced by glands classified as serous (thin, watery saliva containing protein but no mucin); mucus (thick, slimy saliva which contains the glycoprotein, mucin); and mixed (combination of both). A more complete description of the salivary glands of the sheep is given in Table 5-1 and Fig. 5-1 from Kay's paper (ibid). As shown in the table the parotid and inferior molar glands produce serous saliva; the palatine, buccal and pharyngeal produce mucus saliva, and the submaxillary, sublingual and labial produce mixed saliva.

Nasolabial Glands

Nasolabial glands are small glands situated in the dermis of the muzzle skin of ruminant species such as cattle and buffalo (Mackie and Nisbet, 1959). The watery secretion of the glands keeps the muzzle moist. Both buffalo and cattle are known to make deliberate efforts to mix this secretion with their food. They frequently thrust their muzzles into the feed and, during rumination, run their tongues into the nostril and over the muzzle, thus bringing the secretion into the mouth (Majeed et al, 1970). The moisture on the muzzle may play a very small part in evaporative cooling; cessation of secretions occurs during many illnesses and a dry, hot muzzle is often used as evidence of disease. The rate of secretion in an adult cow is said to be 80 mg/20 cm^2/5 min, a rate which is increased threefold when food of high palatability is given (Toutain et al, 1973). Majeed et al (1970) have characterized the chemical properties of nasolabial secretions and found them to be similar to saliva. They also noted relatively high levels of amylase and, since the levels in buffalo were not correlated to blood levels, suggested that these glands may be the source of amylase sometimes reported to be present in ruminant saliva.

Functions of Saliva

There are a number of salivary functions in ruminants that have been confirmed by experimental data. These are discussed in subsequent paragraphs, not necessarily in the order of importance.

As an Aid in Mastication and Swallowing

Except in the case of lush vegetation, the ruminants' feed is often dry, and that of

Table 5-1. Summary of characteristics of the salivary glands of sheep.

Glands	Mean weight	Weight relative to parotids (%)	Cell type	Factors governing rate of flow	Estimated saliva volume (l./24 hr)	Saliva type
Both parotid	23.5	100	Serous	Continuous flow when denervated. Respond to stimulation of mouth, esphagus and reticulo-rumen	3-8	Fluid and isotonic. Strongly buffered with HCO_3 and HPO_4
Both inferior molar	5.9	25	Serous	Continuous flow when denervated. Responds to stimulation of mouth, esophagus and reticulo-rumen	0.7-2.0	Fluid and isotonic or nearly so. Strongly buffered with HCO_3 and HPO_4
Palatine, buccal and pharyngeal	20.7	88	Mucus	Very slow continuous flow when not stimulated. Respond to stimulation of mouth, esophagus and reticulo-rumen	2-6	Very mucus and isotonic or nearly so. Strongly buffered with HCO_3 and HPO_4
Both submaxillary	18.2	77	Mixed	No flow when denervated. Strongly stimulated by feeding. Little or no response to stimulation of esophagus or reticulo-rumen	0.4-0.8	Variably mucus and hypotonic. Weakly buffered
Both sublingual	1.3	6	Mixed	Continuous flow when not stimulated. Moderately stimulated from esophagus; other reflexes not studied	0.1 (?)	Very mucus and hypotonic. Weakly buffered
Labial	10.9	46	Mixed	Little or no flow when not stimulated. Little or no response to stimulation of esophagus and reticulo-rumen; other reflexes not studied.	?	Very mucus and hypotonic. Weakly buffered

domestic ruminants may frequently be of a powdery nature that would be extremely difficult to ingest, if not for the moistening effect of saliva. A bolus collected in the cardial area may contain saliva equivalent to several times the weight of the dry feed ingested. In addition, the location of mucus-secreting glands — buccal, palatine, and pharyngeal — is such that a bolus may be easily coated with mucus, thus making it easier to swallow.

Enzymic Activity of Saliva

The saliva of many mammals contains salivary amylase, although this does not appear to be the case in ruminants (see previous section on nasolabial glands). However, domestic ruminants are known to produce an enzyme that Ramsey et al (1960) and Ramsey (1962) identify as a group of pregastric esterases and which Grosskopf (1965) calls salivary lipase. Data from several different laboratories (Ramsey and Young, 1961; Wise et al, 1968; Gooden, 1973; Hamilton and Raven, 1973) indicate that this enzyme(s) preferentially acts on short-chain triglycerides, i.e., those containing butyric acid or other similar fatty acids. Hydrolysis of long-chain triglycerides is much slower and less complete. Activity is considerably less than that of pancreatic lipase (Gooden, 1973) and there is little activity remaining at a pH of 2.5 (Siewert and Otterby, 1970) or in the small intestine (Siewert and Otterby, 1971; Gooden and Lascelles, 1973).

Other Properties

The large quantity of Na and K salts secreted in saliva appears to function primarily as buffers against the acids produced during fermentation in the rumen. Mucin, urea, P, Mg and Cl are present in relatively high concentration in saliva and probably supply readily available nutrients to rumen microorganisms. Last, and probably not least, some data indicate that the anti-frothing properties of saliva are an important factor in prevention of bloat in ruminants (see Ch. 17).

Chemistry of Saliva

The chemical composition of saliva from individual glands and mixed saliva from all glands have been studied by a number of investigators. An example of the composition that might be expected from data collected by McDougall (1948) and that by Kay (1960a) is shown in Table 5-2.

Table 5-2. Composition of saliva

Gland	Nature of secretion	Ion content							
		Na$^+$	K$^+$	Ca^{++}	Mg^{++}	P	Cl$^-$	HCO$_3^-$	HPO$_4^=$
		mg% [a]							
Mixed	from mouth	370-462	16-46	1.6-3.0	0.6-1.0	37-72		25-43	
Parotid	fistula	352-447	12-45	0.1-2.0	0.4-1.1	19-129		19-238	
		meq/l. [b]							
Parotid	from anesthetized sheep	182-189	5				9-16	91-99	71-79
Inferior molar	from anesthetized sheep	175	7-10				7-12	97-110	44-51
Palatine	from anesthetized sheep	179	4				25	109	25
Submaxillary	from anesthetized sheep	3-66	15-51				2-9	1-9	14-175
Sublingual	from anesthetized sheep	16-47	6-25				16-40	8-18	0.3-2.0
Labial	from anesthetized sheep	29-47	3-9				34	2-4	2-10

[a] From McDougall (1948)

[b] From Kay (1960a); Kay's values represent collections from resting or stimulated glands.

Denton (1957) found that the electrolyte concentration of parotid saliva was considerably higher than that of plasma and thus considered saliva as being hypertonic to plasma. However, Kay (1960a) has shown that osmotic pressure of mixed saliva, as measured by freezing point, is isotonic to plasma. Consequently, the salivary glands, as a whole, are required to do no osmotic work. Kay (1960a) feels that this is one explanation of the ability of the salivary glands to produce such copious quantities of saliva.

McDougall (1948) found the dry matter content of mixed and parotid saliva to be 1.0-1.4% and 1.1-1.4%, respectively. The ash content was 0.7-0.9 and 0.8-1.1%; and the pH varied from 8.4-8.7 and 7.7-8.2 for mixed and parotid saliva, respectively. Turner and Hodgetts (1955) have shown that the buffering capacity of parotid saliva is relatively greater on the acid side than at basic pH's (see Fig. 5-2).

The nitrogen content of saliva is variable as are the other constituents but is usually on the order of 0.1-0.2% (McDougall, 1948; Lyttleton, 1960; of which 60-80% is urea nitrogen. Salivary protein comes primarily from the mucus-producing glands and is made up of glycoproteins. Sialic acid (N-acetylneuraminic acid) is found in large quantities. N-acetyl glactosamine and hexosamine are also found in appreciable amounts (Lyttleton, 1960; Nisigawa and Pigman, 1960). Other data on chemistry of saliva from goats (Komi and Snyder, 1963) and buffalo (Das et al, 1966; Setia et al, 1971) are available.

Amount of Secretion

Salivary production in domestic ruminants has been studied in a number of different laboratories. Data are not always easy to compare, however, since saliva has been collected in a number of different ways. Cannulation of the parotid duct has been used most frequently, but this obviously ignores all of the saliva that is produced by other glands and, most frequently, the cannulation has been done on only one gland. Cardial collections made in rumen-fistulated animals have been used in recent years. Collections have also been made on esophageal-fistulated animals. Carbachol has been administered at times to stimulate salivary flow. Consequently, the range in estimates of salivary production have usually been obtained over a limited time period and results extrapolated to a 24 hr basis; thus any errors may be magnified appreciably. Tomas (1973) has recently published details of a technique for cannulation of both parotid glands, a method which allows return of saliva to the animal. This procedure has been used over a period of several months. It is one which should give a reliable estimate under more nearly normal physiological conditions.

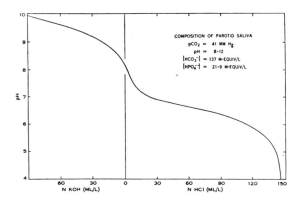

Figure 5-2. An illustration of the buffering capacity of parotid saliva. Note that between pH 7 and 6 a large amount of HCl is required to lower the pH. From Turner and Hodgetts [1955].

Some of the published estimates of total salivary production/day for sheep include: Hyden (1958), 6-12 l.; Kay (1960a), 6-16 l.; McManus (1961), 7.8 l.; Sasaki and Umezu (1962), 1-24 l.; and Somers (1957), 5 l. For cattle some of the published data include: Bailey (1959), 74-110 l., exclusive of rumination in dairy cows; Bailey (1961), 98-190 l.; Mendel and Boda (1961), 100 l.; Meyer et al (1964), 117-183 kg; Putnam et al (1966), 33-54 l. in 350 kg steers; and Yarns et al (1965), 25-51 l. in steers. It is obvious that a great deal of variation occurs between animals and between different experiments. However, we might conclude that sheep probably secrete 6-10 l./day and mature cattle 150 ± l./day. If, however, parotid saliva accounts for 40-50% of the total saliva as suggested by data of Kay (1960a) and Tribe and Peel (1963), then these estimates may be low as Tomas (1973) found that sheep produced 3-10 l. of parotid saliva, and Benavides and Rodriquez (1971) found that young bulls produced 24-37 l. of parotid saliva.

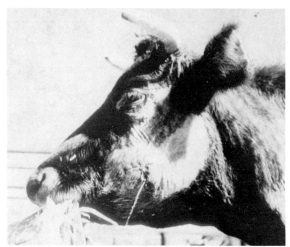

Figure 5-3. An illustration of the flow of parotid saliva during mastication in a cow with a parotid cannula. Courtesy of D.A. Denton, U. of Melbourne.

Variables Affecting the Quality or Quantity of Saliva

The range in output of saliva can be partially accounted for by the fact that saliva production is greater when eating than when not eating (resting); also, the physical nature and moisture content of feed being consumed have quite a bearing on salivary production. Presumably, palatability of a ration as affected by physical nature and taste would be an important factor. Data published by Bailey (1959) illustrate the effect of different feeds (cardial collections):

Feed	Salivary production g/g food	ml/min	Eating rate, g food/min
Pelleted ration	0.68	243	357
Fresh grass	0.94	266	283
Silage	1.13	280	248
Dried grass	3.25	270	83
Hay	3.63	254	70

Balch (1958) has published data on salivary secretion similar to that published by Bailey. He collected boli from cows eating hay, concentrates in meal and pelleted form, flaked corn, beets, and grass and determined the amount of saliva added to the ingested feed. Mean values (lb) for saliva added per 10 lb of ingested food were: hay, 50.2; concentrates as meal, 13.0; concentrates as pellets, 10.1; flaked corn, 13.7; beets, 5.0; and grass, 9.3. His data show a ten-fold difference in salivary secretion as affected either by the nature of the ingested food or by different feeds. There were also appreciable individual differences. For example, with the cows eating hay, the range in saliva added/10 lb of ingested hay was from 43.0 to 56.9 lb. Subsequent research by Bailey (1966) indicated that rate of swallowing could be used to calculate salivary production. Consumption of grass resulted in a rate of secretion of 73 ml/min and hay of 58 ml/min. The rate of swallowing of boli was 1.81 for grass and 1.60/min for hay. Further data of this type (Hawkins and Autrey, 1968) indicate a low correlation between parotid saliva production and crude fiber when alfalfa hay was fed, but a good correlation between dry matter and saliva volume when Bermudagrass hay was fed. When cattle were fed rations varying from 20-100% hay (Emery et al, 1960), it was observed that the pH and ash content of saliva increased as the hay content increased. Salivary N tended to decrease as the percentage of hay in the ration increased, but hexosamines were higher in the high-grain rations.

In studies with sheep, Warner and Stacy (1968) calculated that total salivary production amounted to ca. 0.7-0.8 l./hr while the animals were eating chopped roughage. During resting periods, production was ca. 0.2-0.3 l./hr. If it is assumed that production is about the same during eating and rumination and that these activities occupy about 16 hr/day, then total daily production would be ca. 14 l./day. Other papers indicating qualitative or quantitative changes in saliva as affected by ration or additions to the rumen include those of Meyer et al (1964), Boda et al (1965), Oltjen et al (1965), Yarns et al (1965), Hawkins and Little (1968), Benavides and Rodriguez (1971) and Obara et al (1972b).

McManus (1962) studied the effect on rumen contents of diverting saliva through an esophageal fistula or allowing it to enter the rumen. When saliva was diverted through the fistula, rumen pH consistently fell lower and the volatile fatty acids rose to higher concentrations than when saliva entered the rumen.

Wilson (1964) found that sectioning the parotid ducts and nerves decreased the intake of an alfalfa chaff diet by 42% and an alfalfa hay diet by 35%, but it had no effect on diets of straw or ground alfalfa hay. The rate of passage through the GIT was decreased as was cellulose digestion. Water intake was not changed. Secretion of residual saliva increased. In two sheep there was little change in rumen volatile acids, pH, or ammonia N.

Numerous experiments have been done on ruminants with cannulated parotid glands. Denton (1957) found that the rate of secretion increased during eating and rumination, but decreased during starvation or water depletion. Stewart and Dougherty (1958) reported similar data and found that rumen dry matter content influenced secretion rate of parotid saliva. After watering or administration of water via a rumen fistula, the flow of parotid saliva decreased (parotid saliva production tends to be inversely related to water intake). Bailey and Balch (1961) observed that chewing on the operated side of the mouth (side with a parotid cannula) was the most effective stimulus to saliva secretion. When chewing occurred on the opposite side, the rate of secretion was raised little or not at all above that found during periods of rest, indicating that mastication adjacent to the parotid gland was required for stimulation of secretions. The rates of secretion found at the end of each period of rest increased from about 5 ml/min immediately after eating to about 20 ml/min immediately before the next eating period. This pattern of gradual increase throughout the period between meals was also observed during rumination when mastication occurred on the operated side of the mouth. The rate of flow from one parotid gland averaged 20, 25, and 10 ml/min during eating, rumination, and rest, respectively, for a daily output of about 23 l. Bruggemann et al (1966) reported that parotid secretion rates of sheep during the rumination rose to about 3½ times the resting rate. Average daily output for one gland was (ml/min): semi-purified diet, 0.9; pelleted hay and concentrates, 1.8; and hay, 2.9-4.1. Fig. 5-4 shows data from Lawlor et al (1966) indicating how saliva production may vary from time to time during the day. These authors estimated daily production of parotid saliva to be 2.7, 5.4, and 11.5 l. for semi-purified diets, hay-concentrate, and hay rations, respectively.

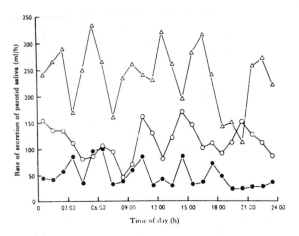

Figure 5-4. Diurnal variation in secretion of parotid saliva in sheep fed a semipurified diet; ●—●; a roughage-concentrate diet, o—o ; and hay, △—△ . From Lawlor et al [1966].

Denton (1956, 1957) has demonstrated that a Na-deficient diet has a marked effect on the Na and K content of parotid saliva, and he further demonstrated that a salivary fistula was an easy way to produce Na deficiency if the secreted saliva was not returned to the sheep either orally or intraruminally. In his sheep, Denton found that the Na-K concentration was about 180 and 10 meq/l. with a normal diet, and that adequate replacement of Na had little effect. If Na replacement was not allowed, the animal became grossly depleted, saliva volume decreased from about 3 to 1 l./day, and the Na concentration fell from 180 to 60 meq/l. and K concentration rose to approximately 120 meq/l. Total P in the saliva rose, but the total amount secreted per day was unchanged. The increased desire for Na by fistulated sheep was shown by the consumption of NaCl. In one case a sheep with a fistula licked 5-15 g/day off a salt block whereas prior to the operation it usually licked off only 0.5-2 g/day. Other effects on the animal when saliva is not returned have been noted by Obara et al (1972a). Data on parotid secretion during Na deficiency have been reported by Bailey and Balch (1961), Denton (1958), Dobson et al (1960), Kay (1960a), and Setia et al (1971).

Somers (1961) found that dietary urea intake or urea infusions via the rumen resulted in a marked increase in urea content of saliva and blood and that there was a good correlation between the two. Further data of this type (Alieva and Alieva, 1969) show that feeding NPN compounds resulted in increased urea in blood, saliva and urine. When cannulated parotid ducts were blocked, there were increases in blood urea, saliva in the non-cannulated gland, rumen ammonia and urinary urea. These changes became progressive. When NPN was removed from the diet, one sheep gradually recovered and one sheep died when NPN was not removed from the diet. Oltjen et al (1969) found that placement of large amounts of urea in the rumen of cattle caused a reduction in salivary flow to 20% of the base value when ruminal ammonia was high and symptoms of urea toxicity were evident. Rozybakiev (1967) has shown that Mn (1.6 mg/kg BW) increased parotid saliva production in sheep along with an increase in salivary urea and a lesser fall in Cl.

After carrying out intravenous infusions of P in sheep, Clark et al (1973) have concluded that the salivary glands probably have a major role in regulating P balance, at least during short intervals of time.

Reflex Control of Salivary Stimulation

Hungate (1966) has summarized briefly some of the information available on innervation of the salivary glands. Only brief mention will be made here of a few pertinent papers. Data reported by Comline and Kay (1955), Ash and Kay (1959), Kay and Phillipson (1959) and Phillipson and Mangan (1959) show that stretching the terminal esophagus, cardia, reticulo-rumen fold, or reticulo-omasal orifice caused large increases in parotid secretion. Whereas, light tactile stimulation of these areas and of the walls of the reticulum and cranial pillar had little effect on parotid flow. Inflation of the rumen in anesthetized sheep or calves to pressures below 20 mm Hg increased the flow of parotid and residual saliva up to 10 fold, but progressively inhibited secretion as pressure was increased. Inflation of the esophagus alone stimulated parotid secretion; when only the rumen was inflated, secretion was inhibited. Inflation of the abomasum was slightly inhibitory in some experiments. Inflation of the rumen produced approximately a 5 fold increase in the mucoprotein concentration of submaxillary saliva without materially altering the concentration of other components.

Boda et al (1965) and Yarns et al (1965) have reported that ruminal infusions of volatile fatty acids, HCl and water have little effect on salivary flow, although Ash and Kay (1959) noted a transitory effect on parotid secretion and Obara et al (1972b) found that both butyric and propionic acid infusion decreased parotid flow.

Development of Salivary Secretion in Young Ruminants

Wilson (1963), Wilson and Tribe (1961), Tribe and Peel (1963) and Kay (1960b) have studied the development of the salivary glands in lambs and kids. They have demonstrated that parotid glands develop more slowly in lambs on milk diets than when grazing. Glands of grazing, milk and hay, or milk-fed lambs were immature before 4 wk of age. Grazing lambs reached adult flow rates at 7-10 wk of age. Rate of flow was significantly correlated to fresh weight of the rumen, but not to body weight. In adults, residual saliva (all except the parotid) comprised about 41% of the total saliva but in lambs only 26%. Salivary composition varied with secretion rate and less with age. Cl concentration fell with age (Kay). In one experiment (Wilson, 1963) lambs were fed on wood shavings and milk; milk; milk and hay; or a synthetic diet containing starch, fortified whole milk powder and sodium bicarbonate. Data showed that lambs receiving the hay and milk or the synthetic diet secreted significantly less saliva than those receiving the milk or milk and shavings diets. In a different experiment comparisons were made between lambs that were 63 days of age which had grazed with their mothers, and lambs that were grazed until 63 days of age but were then confined to a milk diet for a further 70 days. Salivary production from the parotids of the grazing lambs was significantly greater than the secretion by lambs returned to the milk diet. It was concluded that the parotid glands developed in response to the mechanical stimulation of food (mouth, esophagus, stomach?) and that there was a regression of gland development when this stimulation was removed.

Sasaki (1969) has also shown that a marked increase occurs in salivary production with age in calves, parotid secretion/g tissue increasing 7 fold between 1-13 wk in calves fed milk, hay and grain, but very little increase in calves fed milk only. Mixed saliva also increased in MHG animals. Salivary Na (mixed saliva) was slightly higher in calves fed MHG and K was slightly lower, but no effect of age was demonstrated. Bicarbonate increased with age and Cl fell to adult levels by 6 wk in calves fed MHG and 9 wk in milk-fed calves.

Conclusions

Saliva is produced in copious amounts by 5 sets of paired glands and 3 unpaired glands, with the parotid glands apparently accounting for 40-50% of total production. Evidence indicates that sheep likely produce 6-10 l./day or more and adult dairy cows 150 l. or more. Saliva serves as an aid in forming and swallowing a bolus of food and as an important buffering agent in the rumen. A limited amount of lipase activity is present; some amylase activity may be derived from secretions of the nasolabial glands found in the dermis of the muzzle of some species. Saliva also provides some nourishment for rumen microbes from mucin, urea, and minerals, particularly P and Mg in addition to Na, K and Cl.

Production of saliva — both in quantity and quality — varies with eating, rumination and resting. Water content and physical nature of the food affect total production, and other dietary factors such as Na or urea may influence the composition of saliva. In the young animal, salivary glands develop in close coordination with rumen function.

References Cited

Alieva, A.A. and Z.M. Alieva. 1969. Nutr. Abstr. Rev. 39:428.
Ash, R.W. and R.N.B. Kay. 1959. J. Physiol. 149:43.
Bailey, C.B. 1959. Proc. Nutr. Soc. 18:1.
Bailey, C.B. 1961. Br. J. Nutr. 15:443.
Bailey, C.B. 1966. Animal Prod. 8:325.
Bailey, C.B. and C.C. Balch. 1961. Br. J. Nutr. 15:383.
Balch, C.C. 1958. Br. J. Nutr. 12:330.
Benavides, M.C. and J. Rodriguez. 1971. Revista Cubana de Ciencia Agr. 5:31.
Boda, J.M., P.G. McDonald and J.J. Walker. 1965. J. Physiol. 177:323.
Bruggemann, J., K. Walser-Karst and D. Giesecke. 1966. Nutr. Abstr. Rev. 36:734.
Clark, R.D. et al. 1973. Aust. J. Agr. Res. 24:913.
Comline, R.S. and R.N.B. Kay. 1955. J. Physiol. 129:55.
Das, S.C., J.S. Rawat and A. Roy. 1966. Indian Vet. J. 43:792.
Denton, D.A. 1956. J. Physiol. 131:516.
Denton, D.A. 1957. Quart. J. Expt. Physiol. 43:72.
Denton, D.A. 1958. J. Physiol. 140:129.
Dobson, A., R.N.B. Kay and I. McDonald. 1960. Res. Vet. Sci. 1:103.
Emery, R.S., C.K. Smith, R.M. Grimes, C.P. Joffman and D.W. Duncan. 1960. J. Dairy Sci. 43:76.
Gooden, J.M. 1973. Aust. J. Biol. Sci. 26:1189.
Gooden, J.M. and A.K. Lascelles. 1973. Aust. J. Biol. Sci. 26:625.
Grosskopf, J.F.W. 1965. Onderstepoort J. Vet. Res. 32:153.
Hamilton, R.K. and A.M. Raven. 1973. J. Sci. Food Agr. 24:257.
Hawkins, G.E. and K.M. Autrey. 1968. J. Dairy Sci. 51:627 (abstr).
Hawkins, G.E. and J.A. Little. 1968. J. Dairy Sci. 51:1817.
Hungate, R.E. 1966. The Rumen and Its Microbes. Academic Press, Inc.
Hyden, S. 1958. Biol. Abstr. 35:4528.
Kay, R.N.B. 1960a. J. Physiol. 150:515.
Kay, R.N.B. 1960b. J. Physiol. 150:538.
Kay, R.N.B. and A.T. Phillipson. 1959. Proc. Royal Soc. Med. 52:374.
Komi, N. and W.H. Snyder. 1963. Amer. J. Physiol. 204:1055.
Lawlor, M.J., D. Giesecke and K. Walser-Karst. 1966. Br. J. Nutr. 20:373.
Lyttleton, J.W. 1960. N.Z. J. Agr. Res. 3:63.
Mackie, A.M. and A.M. Nisbet. 1959. J. Agr. Sci. 52:376.
Majeed, M.A., I.H. Zaidi and A. Ilahi. 1970. Res. Vet. Sci. 11:407.
McDougall, E.I. 1948. Biochem. J. 43:99.
McManus, W.R. 1961. Nature. 192:1161.
McManus, W.R. 1962. Aust. J. Agr. Res. 12:907.
Mendel, V.E. and J.M. Boda. 1961. J. Dairy Sci. 44:1881.
Meyer, R.M., E.E. Bartley, J.L. Morrill and W.E. Stewart. 1964. J. Dairy Sci. 47:1339.
Nisigawa, K. and W. Pigman. 1960. Biochem. J. 75:293.
Obara, Y., et al. 1972a. Nutr. Abstr. Rev. 42:1360.
Obara, Y., S. Watanabe, Y. Sasaki and T. Tsuda. 1972b. Tohoku J. Agr. Res. 23:132.
Oltjen, R.R., P.A. Putnam and R.E. Davis. 1965. J. Animal Sci. 24:1126.
Oltjen, R.R., P.A. Putnam and E.E. Williams. 1969. J. Animal Sci. 29:830.
Phillipson, A.T. and J.L. Mangan. 1959. N.Z. J. Agr. Res. 2:990.
Putnam, P.A., R. Lehmann and R.E. Davis. 1966. J. Animal Sci. 25:817.
Ramsey, H.A. 1962. J. Dairy Sci. 45:1479.
Ramsey, H.A., J.W. Young and G.H. Wise. 1960. J. Dairy Sci. 43:1076.
Ramsey, H.A. and J.W. Young. 1961. J. Dairy Sci. 44:2227.
Rozybakiev, M.A. 1967. Nutr. Abstr. Rev. 37:752.
Sasaki, Y. 1969. Nutr. Abstr. Rev. 39:1140.
Sasaki, Y. and M. Umezu. 1962. Tohoku J. Agr. Res. 13:211.
Setia, M.S., J.S. Rawat and A. Roy. 1971. Indian J. Animal Sci. 41:525.
Siewert, K.L. and D.E. Otterby. 1970. J. Dairy Sci. 53:571.
Siewert, K.L. and D.E. Otterby. 1971. J. Dairy Sci. 54:258.
Somers, M. 1957. Aust. Vet. J. 33:297.
Somers, M. 1961. Aust. J. Exp. Biol. Med. Sci. 39:133; 145.
Stewart, W.E. and R.W. Dougherty. 1958. J. Animal Sci. 17:1220 (abstr).
Tomas, F.M. 1973. Quart. J. Expt. Physiol. 58:131.
Toutain, P.L., L. Bueno and J.P. Mangol. 1973. Extrait des Cahiers de Med. Vet. 42:41.
Tribe, D.E. and L. Peel. 1963. Aust. J. Agr. Res. 14:330.
Turner, A.W. and V.E. Hodgetts. 1955. Aust. J. Agr. Res. 6:124.
Venkatakrishnan, A. and D. Mariappa. 1969. Indian Vet. J. 46:768.
Warner, A.C.I. and B.D. Stacy. 1968. Br. J. Nutr. 22:389.
Wilson, A.D. 1963. Aust. J. Agr. Res. 14:226.
Wilson, A.D. 1964. Br. J. Nutr. 18:163.
Wilson, A.D. and D.E. Tribe. 1961. Aust. J. Agr. Res. 12:1126.
Wise, G.H., P.G. Miller, G.W. Anderson and J.C. Jones. 1968. J. Dairy Sci. 51:737.
Yarns, D.A., P.A. Putnam and E.C. Leffel. 1965. J. Animal Sci. 24:173; 805.

CHAPTER 6 — MOTILITY OF THE GASTRO-INTESTINAL TRACT

The stomach of the ruminant animal with its movement of ingesta in and out of compartments is a very complex physiological mechanism as compared to the simple stomach of monogastric species. Ingesta transport becomes more complicated because of the reticular groove, the act of rumination that is interspersed between intermittent periods of eating, the need to dispose of large volumes of gas produced by microbial fermentation, and the fact that most solid food is delayed for varying periods of time in the reticulo-rumen and the omasum. Modern recording apparatus and surgical procedures developed in recent times have made it possible to collect data which have helped to more clearly understand this complex series of events, but much still remains to be learned.

Reticular [esophageal] Groove

This structure, as described in Ch. 2, begins at the cardia and extends to the reticulo-omasal orifice. It is essentially a continuation of the esophagus as a groove or tube which bypasses the reticulo-rumen when contracted into a tube. The early workers in the field of ruminant physiology thought that the reticular groove served to bypass all ingested fluids or that the groove might be involved in regurgitation. However, the latter theory was disproved by partially suturing the lips of the groove without any effect on regurgitation.

Observations of groove functions in fistulated animals by authors such as Schalk and Amadon (1928), Wise and Anderson (1939), radiophotographic studies by Watson (1944) and Benzie and Phillipson (1957) as well as research from many other laboratories have demonstrated that the reticular groove functions primarily in the young suckling ruminant to bypass milk from the esophagus to the omasum (Phillipson, 1970). Closure of the groove may be accomplished by initiation of the suckling reflex and is apparently not affected by temperature or gross composition of the liquids, although solids in suspension may provide sufficient stimulus to initiate closure (Kay, 1972). The typical posture assumed while drinking is not, apparently, required for reflex closure (Watson, 1944). Experiments generally indicate that milk passes into the abomasum if the animal is accustomed to taking milk in the manner in which the fluid is given. If, in contrast, milk or water are given in a manner in which the animal normally quenches its thirst with water, the fluid passes mainly into the reticulo-rumen (Wise and Anderson, 1939; Watson, 1944).

In recent studies, Ruckebusch and Kay (1971a) observed that the reticular groove contracts with two distinct movements; first, by shortening, the right and left lips become firmly opposed allowing direct passage of 30-40% of the volume of liquid towards the abomasum. Then, the closure of the groove can be complete if the lips are inverted, mainly the right lip. In this case, 75-90% of the ingested liquid is recovered in the abomasum. The direct passage of liquid during suckling in the adult sheep is accompanied by momentary and immediate inhibition of reticulo-ruminal contractions. These authors also demonstrated that increased excitability provoked by showing a nipple bottle was sufficient in a trained subject to double or triple the volume of liquid collected in the abomasum after administration into the lower esophagus. Ørskov et al (1970) demonstrated that complete closure of the groove took place in lambs trained to drink small meals from a trough, similar to those drinking from a nipple bottle. Teasing with a bottle beyond their reach also caused groove closure; if not teased, the groove did not close; if they could discriminate between teasing and normal routine, the groove frequently did not close (determined by presence of barium passing into the reticulo-rumen or abomasum). Lawlor et al (1971) have used similar techniques (barium and X-ray) to study groove closure in lambs fed milk replacers either individually or in groups (see Fig. 6-1).

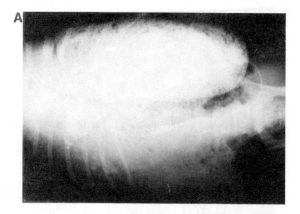

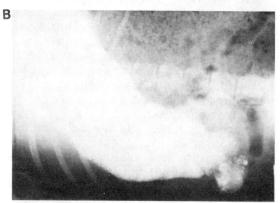

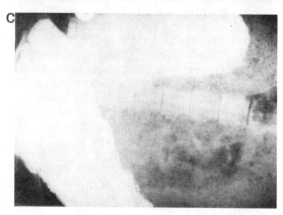

Figure 6-1. Radiographs showing location of barium sulfate in the stomachs of lambs. The barium was offered as a suspension with a milk replacer from either a teat-bottle or a bulk dispenser. In [A] it is located in the rumen, [B] shows it in the abomasum and in [C] it is present in the rumen and abomasum. The radiographs were taken with the lambs held on their backs. From Lawlor et al [1971].

In one experiment, the milk replacer consistently entered the abomasum in 7 of 10 individually-fed lambs and in 12 of 22 group-fed lambs. Similar values for a second experiment were 22 of 24 and 34 of 50 respectively. They found that poor sucking, low milk consumption and entry of milk into

the rumen resulted in very poor performance by the lambs which demonstrated a non-specific unthriftiness similar to 'tail enders' often observed in flocks.

Older observations have indicated that calves are more apt to have milk in the reticulo-rumen than are lambs, and that bucket-fed animals are apt to have more milk or gruel in the rumen than nipple-fed animals. Apparently the neural stimulation from drinking is not adequate to stimulate complete closure of the reticular groove when drinking from a bucket in relatively large amounts, although as indicated previously, small meals from a trough may pass into the abomasum. However, a keen appetite for milk is stimulatory, regardless of age or various environmental factors (Watson, 1944).

Closure of the reticular groove can also be stimulated by certain salts (Phillipson, 1970). Cu and Na salts are reported to be at least partially effective in sheep. In cattle, Na salts are apparently more effective than Cu. Glucose has also been reported to be an effective stimulant (Riek, 1954; Comline and Titchen, 1961). Reticular stretch or distension inhibits reflex closure of the groove in decerebrate animals (Sellers and Titchen, 1959) and sectioning of the vagus nerve completely abolishes the groove reflex (Duncan, 1953). Although the response diminishes with age, animals continued on nipple feeding may have a functioning groove into their adult years.

Movements of the Reticulo-Rumen

The orderly and synchronized movements of the reticulum and rumen aid in mixing newly ingested food with that already in the stomach, in regurgitation and eructation of gas and in moving food into the omasum. Consequently, an understanding of the normal activity is required for a complete appreciation of stomach function. The basic movements of the stomach were described rather completely in the 1920's by Schalk and Amadon and by Wester in Germany and by other authors using more sophisticated equipment in recent years. The reader is referred to reviews by Clark (1956), Reid (1963), Sellers and Stevens (1966), and Phillipson (1970).

The organization of the stomach movements is not as easily determined visually as might be imagined. As Schalk and Amadon (1928) relate, "Visual inspection of the rumen in an empty state reveals the cavity of the viscus in almost constant movement. The various muscular pillars of the rumen are advancing and retreating with a consequent alteration in size of the various subdivisions of the cavity. The relationship of these contractions is not at all evident upon preliminary visual inspection."

Research investigations on the motor activity of the reticulo-rumen generally indicate that most of the activity can be divided into (1) primary contractions, sometimes referred to as the mixing cycle, and (2) secondary contractions, sometimes called eructation contractions. However, there is not complete agreement on cyclical activity of the reticulo-rumen due to the fact that observations and measurements have been made by a variety of methods in different laboratories and on different species (see Sellers and Stevens, 1966). Also, it has been shown that motor activity may be influenced by eating, rumination, bloat, trauma and by deprivation of food or water with the result that a wide variety of motor activity may occur; some of which may represent complete cycles and others which may represent abbreviated cycles (Phillipson, 1970).

Primary Contractions

When reticulo-rumen activity resumes after a period of rest or inhibition, recordings of pressure in the different compartments indicate that contractions are first initiated by the reticulum, thus it is the point at which the normal cycle begins. As pointed out by Sellers and Stevens (1966) there is general agreement on the following activity:

a. An initial sharp contraction of the reticulum and the reticulo-ruminal foid during which the reticulum contracts to about ½ of its resting size.

b. A second (and the most powerful) contraction of the reticulum after which the wave of contraction passes caudally over the rumen, resulting in a lifting of the cranial sac due to contraction of the cranial pillars, contraction of the caudal and dorsal coronary pillars and compression of the dorsal sac of the rumen resulting, partially, from contraction of the longitudinal pillars.

c. The wave of contraction continues over the caudodorsal blind sac, ventral coronary pillar, ventral sac and caudoventral blind sac with some displacement ventrally of the cranial pillar.

It should be pointed out that these events result in a gradual wave of contraction followed by a wave of relaxation. As a matter of fact, some sacs may be dilating while others are contracting. For example, when the dorsal sacs are contracting in the primary cycle, the ventral sacs and the reticulum are dilating. Some of these various stages of contraction can be seen in the X-rays presented by Benzie and Phillipson (1957). Sketches of some of these are shown in Fig. 6-2.

The best diagrammatic illustrations of cyclical contractions of the sheep's stomach are those of Phillipson (1939) shown in Fig. 6-3. This figure illustrates the cyclical activity resulting in a flow of ingesta from the reticulum to the cranial sac, from the cranial sac into the dorsal sac; from the dorsal sac back through the cranial sac to the reticulum or into the ventral sac; from the ventral to the caudoventral blind sac and finally, from the caudoventral blind sac back into the ventral, dorsal and cranial sacs and into the reticulum. Thus, the contractions result in a circulation of semisolid digesta and fluids within the reticulo-rumen. This sequence of events requires 30 to 50 sec to complete when the animal is resting (neither eating or ruminating).

Secondary Contractions

Those contractions occurring in the rumen which involve only part of the organ are referred to as secondary. They may or may not occur after a primary contraction. These contractions generally involve the dorsal coronary pillar, contraction of the caudodorsal blind sac and dorsal sac and relaxation of the caudoventral blind sac. The longitudinal and cranial pillars are also probably involved (Reid and Cornwall, 1959). At times only the dorsal sac is involved. Secondary contractions require about 30 sec to complete in cattle (Schalk and Amadon, 1928; Phillipson, 1970) and are usually, although not always, associated with eructation (Dziuk and McCauley, 1965). When evaluating rumen contractions with electromyography (electrical activity in muscles), Ruckebusch and Tomov (1973) demonstrated that secondary contractions originated in the ventral blind sac, either independently or immediately following a primary contraction.

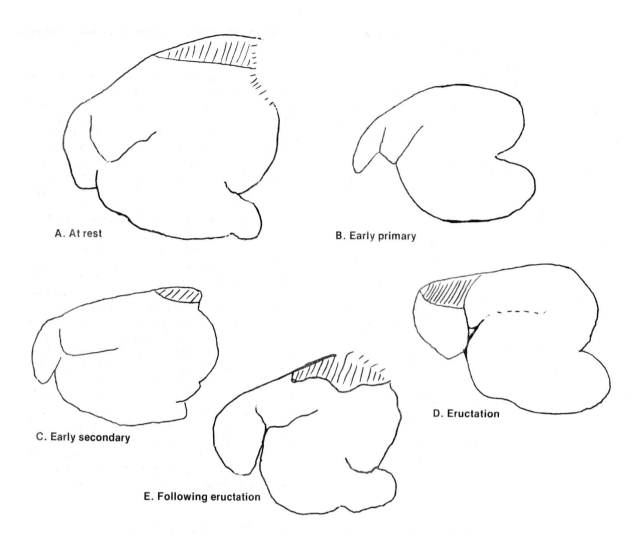

A. At rest

B. Early primary

C. Early secondary

D. Eructation

E. Following eructation

Figure 6-2. Diagrams from X-rays of ruminant stomachs. Diagrams A and B are typical of the reticulum at rest and the initial stages of a primary cycle, respectively. Diagrams C, D, and E are various stages of a secondary contraction. Disregard differences in size of the diagrams. A, stomach of a 37 day old goat at rest; B, the reticulum is contracted, the cranial pillar is contracting, and the caudoventral sac is dilated; C, the reticulum is at rest, the dorsal sac is relaxed, and the caudoventral sac is contracting; D, picture taken immediately after C showing the dilation of the reticulum with gas forced into the cardial area, contraction of the dorsal sacs, the dilation of the caudoventral sac; E, stage following that in D showing relaxation of the dorsal and ventral sacs but still some contraction of the cranial pillar and reticulo-ruminal fold. From Benzie and Phillipson [1957].

The wave of contraction was seen to pass in a circular manner to the dorsal blind sac, dorsal sac and ventral sac and back to the ventral blind, with eructation occurring at the end of contraction of the dorsal sac. The time required to complete a cycle was related to the strength of contraction of the ventral blind sac. For further details, see the section on eructation.

Variations in Motility Patterns

As noted previously, a number of varia-

tions have been reported in the accepted pattern of reticulo-rumen motility (Stevens and Sellers, 1966). Some of the variations may be due to different methods used, but there are, obviously, many different factors which affect stomach motility in the ruminant animal. Some of these are discussed in subsequent paragraphs.

Normal variations

Schalk and Amadon (1928) observed that there was a rather constant 1:2 rhythm between the primary and secondary contractions in the cows that they examined.

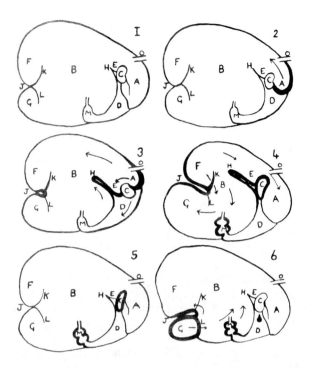

Figure 6-3. Cyclical activity of the ruminant stomach and the flow of digesta within. From Phillipson [1939].

However, Williams (1955) found that a 1:1 rhythm occurred a majority of the time (74% of 400 animals); a 2:1 rhythm occurred in 16% of the cows, whereas a 1:2 rhythm was found in 10%, only (palpation and auscultation). He found appreciable variation in animals in the same herd and on the same diet, part of which might be accounted for by variation in time of sampling after eating.

Phillipson and Reid (1960) reported that four major patterns of contractions occurred in the rumen of cattle as measured with pressure-sensitive recordings. These were (R = reticulum; D = dorsal sac; V = ventral sac): (1) R, D; (2) R, D, V; (3) R, D, D, V; and (4) R, D, V, D, V. They stated that these patterns accounted for 90% of the changes observed in four cows (see Table 6-1). In a more recent paper, Dziuk and McCauley (1965) recorded pressure changes in the reticulum (R), dorsal sac (D), caudodorsal blind sac (CDB), and the ventral sac (V) of cows during rest. The usual contractions, labeled as primary ($_p$) or secondary ($_s$) were as follows: (1) R, D_p, CDB_p, V_p; (2) R, D_p, CDB_s, D_s, V_s; and (3) R, D_p, CDB_p, V_p, CDB_s, D_s, V_s. The comparison of these two reports would indicate that patterns 2, 3 and 4 of Phillipson and Reid are probably the same type of pattern as 1, 2, and 3,

respectively, of Dziuk and McCauley.

Ruckebusch and Kay (1971b) have recently described 6 types of reticulo-ruminal motor activity in bovines. The first 4 are the same as those of Phillipson and Reid (1960). The other 2 were: R, D, CVB, D, V: and R, D, V, CVB, D, V. They did not distinguish between dorsal and caudodorsal blind sac contractions. These authors pointed out that contraction of the dorsal blind and dorsal sacs can occur independently of one another, but the blind sac always contracted before eructation and its contraction is associated with contraction of the ventral blind sac. Activity of the ruminal pillars did not always parallel contraction of the dorsal sac. Movements of the reticular groove and the atrium followed each reticular contraction. Data of a similar type on sheep have been presented by Ohga et al (1965; see Table 6-1).

Data on time intervals in stomach contractions are available from many different publications. Much of this data was obtained from rumen-fistulated animals. For example, Morillo and De Alba (1960) found the mean rate of rumen contractions in pregnant lactating cows to be 25.9 seconds/cycle. This was not affected by breed, but varied with different rumen activities, being 22.7, 26.4 and 28.7 sec/cycle during eating, ruminating and resting, respectively. The rate also varied with rumen fill and varied with different pastures.

When radio telemetry methods were used (Mooney et al, 1971) on intact animals that were fistulated at a later date, it was shown that fistulated animals had slower contractions during rest although not during feeding or ruminating. Rumen pressures were also greater in intact animals while feeding. Some of their data are shown in Table 6-2. When using similar procedures with intact dairy cows fed hay and grain, Dracy et al (1972) found the average duration of contraction cycles to be 37.3, 43.8 and 56.5 seconds while eating, resting and ruminating, respectively.

Reid and Cornwall (1959) observed in sheep a complete disappearance for long periods of the ventral phase of the primary cycle during resting periods (see Fig. 6-7). Balch (1955) and Dziuk and McCauley (1965) have also reported the absence of rumen motility during periods of apparent sleep in cattle, sheep and goats. Ruckebusch and Bueno (1972) note that the motility of the

Table 6-1. Incidence (%) of pressure waves in the rumen of cows and sheep.

Activity	a*					b**		
	D[c]	DV	DSV	DVSV	Others	Primary (DV)	Modified primary (D)	Secondary (SV)
					Cows[d]			
Feeding	1	27	5	56	11	55	4	41
Resting	10	35	25	22	8	41	25	34
Ruminating	22	28	37	6	7	25	43	32
					Sheep[e]			
Feeding	0	45	1	46	8	65	1	34
Resting	2	48	4	39	7	64	4	32
Ruminating	4	48	13	30	6	57	12	31

*Total patterns analyazed under (a) = 5998;   **The analyses under (b) excludes the group "others" under (a).

[c]D, primary wave in dorsal sac; V, pressure in ventral sac; S, secondary wave in dorsal sac, which at its peak usually coincides with a sharp spike of pressure in the anterior and ventral sacs of the rumen and which accompanies eructation. Those under (a) represent the sequences of these changes and the incidence of which about 10% cannot be classified into the 4 main categories listed. Those under (b) indicate the incidence of primary waves (DV), modified primary in which the ventral sac shows no pressure change (D), and secondary waves (SV).

[d] From Phillipson and Reid (1960);   [e]From Ohga et al (1965) as modified by Phillipson (1970).

Table 6-2. Effect of rumen fistulation on frequency and amplitude of reticular contractions.[a]

Treatment	contractions per min	amplitude, mm Hg
Resting		
Intact	1.2	18.2
Fistul.	1.4	5.9
Feeding		
Intact	2.0	22.1**
Fistul.	2.0	9.4
Ruminating		
Intact	1.1	10.4
Fistul.	1.1	10.9

[a]Data from Mooney et al (1971). **Statistically greater than 9.4.

forestomach is considerably slower during sleep or paradoxical sleep, generally with the cycles having a greater duration than 60 seconds, and a number of different papers show rumen contractions to occur at a slower rate when animals are lying as opposed to standing.

Species comparisons

Phillipson (1939) and Reid and Cornwall (1959) have studied motility of the sheep's stomach using pressure-sensitive recorders, and Dziuk et al (1963), Dziuk and McCauley (1965), Dziuk (1965), and Bhattacharyya and Mullick (1965), respectively, have studied motility in the white-tailed deer; cattle, sheep and goats; the American bison and the Asian buffalo. Consequently, a relatively large amount of data on ruminant species is available.

Comparisons of reticular contractions indicate that the reticular contractions of cattle and bison are essentially two separate pressure waves, whereas in sheep, goats and white-tailed deer, the reticular contraction is more of a biphasic contraction. Work from Dziuk's laboratory indicates that the motility patterns of cattle and bison are similar, but that those of sheep and goats are somewhat less variable. Secondary contractions of the caudodorsal blind sac occurred with each secondary cycle, and the secondary cycles also included a secondary contraction of the ventral rumen in the goat and usually in the sheep. In all three species, the primary caudodorsal blind sac contraction began after the dorsal sac contraction and peaked later. In the cow, the secondary contraction of the caudodorsal blind sac began before dorsal sac contraction. However, in goats and sheep these contractions were simultaneous. During rumination in sheep, the modified primary wave (Table 6-1) occurred less frequently than in cattle (Phillipson, 1970). The rates of primary to secondary contractions were similar for the cow, bison, sheep and goat. Although the deer showed a higher frequency of cycles (about 2/min) and a higher ratio of primary to secondary contractions, the number of secondary contractions were about the same as in cattle. In the buffalo, Bhattacharyya and Mullick (1965) found that the numbers of total, primary and secondary contractions were less than in cattle; the interval between primary contractions being longer, although the interval between secondary contractions was similar to that of cattle. Examples of differences observed in five different species when the stomach was at rest (neither eating or ruminating) are shown in Fig. 6-4, 5, 6.

Effect of Eating

Schalk and Amadon (1928) and Balch et al (1951) have reported that ingestion of food results in an increased rate of rumen motility in cattle, with the latter noting that the rate increased from 60 to 105 cycles/hr from a resting state to feeding. Reid and Cornwall (1959) have reported similar observations on sheep (Fig. 6-7) and Dziuk et al (1963) found that deer increased resting motility from about 120 to about 170 cycles/hr when eating corn. Consumption of hay resulted in rates of contraction about the same as when ruminating (slightly above the resting rate). Figs. 6-6, 7 illustrate differences in rate when bison and sheep, respectively, are resting, eating and ruminating. Limited data (Mahipaul and Mishra, 1971) indicate that eating increased stomach contractions of cattle about 1.5X as compared to 2X or more in buffalo. Reid (1963) found that motility in the feeding sheep was characterized by a high frequency of contractions — as many as 3/min; a ratio of primary to secondary contractions of about 1:1; a high level of tonic activity with strong rumen contractions with the contractions of the ventral sacs being prolonged and polyphasic; and a change after about 30 min to a different form of primary and secondary sequences of the ventral sacs more typical of contractions during rest. During feeding, the ventral

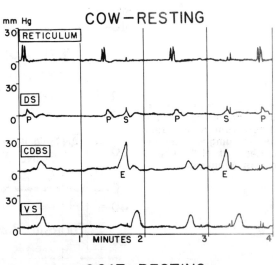

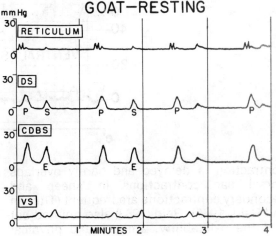

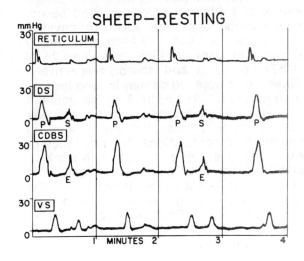

Figure 6-4. Pressure recordings in the reticulo-rumen of a cow, sheep and goat during rest [neither eating or ruminating]. Primary [P] and secondary [S] contractions are identified as are eructations [E]. Courtesy of H.E. Dziuk, Univ. of Minnesota.

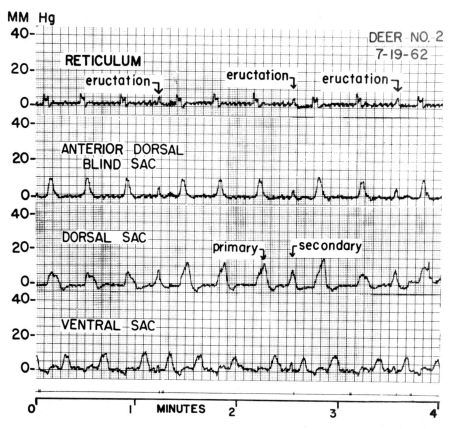

Figure 6-5. Typical pressure events recorded in the reticulo-rumen of deer when standing and resting. Courtesy of H.E. Dziuk, Univ. of Minnesota.

contraction is delayed and barely overlaps dorsal sac contractions in sheep and secondary contractions are frequent (Titchen and Reid, 1965). Reid (1963) also pointed out that the palatability, amount and physical form of the ration had marked effects on the nature and duration of primary and secondary contractions. The effect of physical form of the feed has also been observed by Colvin and Daniels (1965) and Pharr et al (1967) on cattle and sheep, respectively. When cattle were fed oat hay in long form or ground through 1/4 or 3/32 in. hammermill screens, the finest grind resulted in a slower rate of contractions, but no change in amplitude of contractions. The amplitude of rumen contractions took from 2 to 6 wk to stabilize after animals were changed from one diet to another, a change from the 3/32-in. hay to long hay taking the longest time. With sheep (Pharr et al), grinding the hay also resulted in reduced amplitude of rumen contractions.

Effect of rumination and eructation

One of the primary differences in reticulo-rumen motility between rumination and that of the resting phase or eating is the occurrence of an extrareticular contraction (or triphasic) that occurs prior to the usual biphasic contraction (see Fig. 6-6, 8, 9). This extrareticular contraction has been demonstrated and observed by many individuals and occurs a few seconds prior to the usual reticular contraction. Dziuk and McCauley (1965) point out that, in sheep and goats, the first phase of the biphasic contraction following regurgitation and, to a lesser extent, the second reticular pressure change were either of a very low amplitude or were absent (see Fig. 6-8).

Dziuk et al (1963) have noted that some regurgitation contractions in deer occur out of phase with respect to the usual biphasic reticular contraction (see Fig. 6-9). Reid and Cornwall (1959) reported similar events in cattle, although they occurred with lower frequency than in deer. Dziuk and McCauley (1965) also found that pressure changes associated with secondary ventral sac contractions extended into the subsequent reticulo-rumen cycle during rumination, with the terminal phases occurring during the regurgitation contraction of the reticulum in sheep, goats and cattle. This change was not related to the length of cycle as it was sometimes found in both short and long cycles.

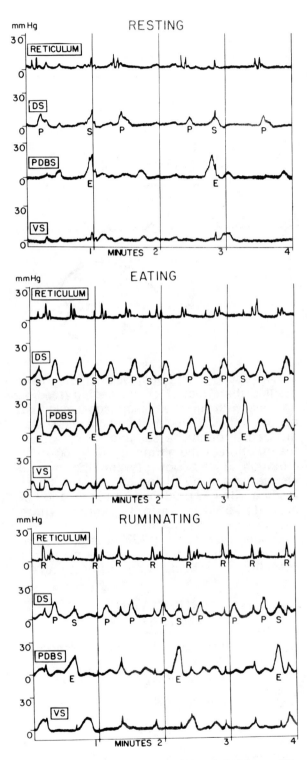

Figure 6-6. Reticulo-ruminal activity of the bison while resting, eating and ruminating. Note the increased activity during eating, contractions occurring at 2-3X the rate while eating as while resting. Contractions during rumination are also accelerated, and the extra-reticular contraction associated with regurgitation is quite evident in the lower recording. Courtesy of H. E. Dziuk, Univ. of Minnesota.

Eructation in deer (Dziuk et al, 1963) has been observed to occur during secondary rumen contractions; however, in cattle, goats, and sheep, eructation may occur, at times, during primary contractions. In goats, it has frequently been observed during rumination that two secondary contractions took place with eructation occurring during each contraction (Dziuk and McCauley, 1965). Eructation or secondary contractions will be more frequent when gas formation is rapid; i.e., 30 min-2 hr after a meal and, also, usually after a period of rumination.

Effect of Fasting and Water Deprivation

Reid (1963) has made extensive studies on the effect of diet and fasting on motility of the sheep's stomach. In sheep fasted 18-24 hr, he found the motility to be characterized by: (1) a low frequency of coordinated sequences with only 1 to 0.3 contractions/min; (2) a low proportion of secondary contractions — as few as 1 to every 5 primary contractions; (3) a low level of tonic activity; (4) short, simple, relatively weak rumen contractions in which ventral sacs may not contract during primary sequences; and (5) the emergence of a characteristic form of both primary and secondary sequences. Nesic (1961) has also shown that fasting for 6 days resulted in weak contractions at about half the normal rate for sheep and information on cattle (Attebery and Johnson, 1969) shows a marked decrease in amplitude of contractions as well as frequency.

Miscellaneous Factors

Many different physiological abnormalities or diseases will cause alteration or cessation of normal stomach motility cycles (see Ch. 17 for some examples). One example of this type of alteration in reticular contractions is shown in Fig. 6-10 (Holtenius et al, 1971b). In this case the cow developed traumatic peritonitis (hardware disease) caused by a nail piercing the reticulum and irritating other tissues. Presumably, the resulting pain altered the normal reflex in an attempt to reduce further damage.

The function of hormones in stomach motility of ruminant animals has not been clearly defined. One recent paper (Ruckebusch, 1971) demonstrates that pentagastrin, a synthetic peptide similar to gastrin, caused contractions of the reticulo-rumen to cease ca. 20 sec after administration I.V.

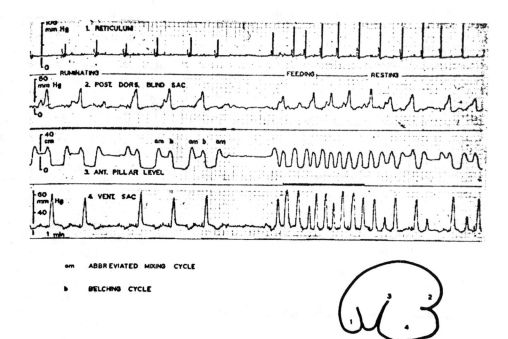

Figure 6-7. Recordings illustrating the activities of the reticulo-rumen during rumination, feeding and rest in sheep. From Reid and Cornwall [1959].

With respect to ambient temperature, Attebery and Johnson (1969) exposed cows to temperatures up to 38°C for up to 5 days. This resulted in a decrease in the amplitude of rumen contractions and a trend toward less frequent contractions. Exposure to this temperature for 1 or 2 days had little effect, however. Fasting resulted in slow, weak contractions.

When deprived of water, Schalk and Amadon (1928) observed that the resting period was prolonged as the rumen dehydrated and that the contractions were weak; the contents of the rumen formed a doughy mass of ingesta that was subject to little mixing by rumen contractions.

Mahipaul and Mishra (1971) have studied diurnal, seasonal and age effects on rumen motility in cattle and buffaloes. In cattle, rumen motility was higher in summer than in winter (diets varied with season) in animals over 1 yr of age. The rate of contractions gradually increased with age and was greater in adult males than in females. Contractions were slower in buffalo than in cattle, ranging from 12-15/10 min (vs. 16-18/10 min in cattle). Motility was higher in winter than in summer and higher in females than in males and increased with age in buffalo as it did in cattle. Drinking also caused an increase in rate of contractions, although this is not evident in data of Dracey et al (1972) with cattle.

Ruckebusch and Laplace (1967) have studied the effect of sham feeding (feeding animals with an open esophageal cannula) on motility. If regurgitated digesta was diverted through the cannula, this reduced the duration of the normal cycle by 50-75%, although it did not prevent the normal peristaltic activity of the esophagus. Sham feeding with hay produced an acceleration of motility of the reticulo-rumen which depended on mastication.

Schalk and Amadon (1928) pointed out that closure of the reticular groove caused a cessation of reticular and rumen contrac-

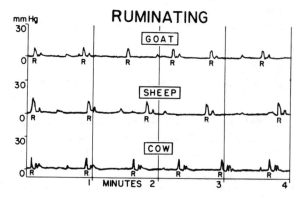

Figure 6-8. Pressure recordings in the reticulum of the goat, sheep and cow during rumination [R]. Note in cattle, that the normal reticular contraction tends to e more biphasic than in the goat or sheep. Courtesy of H.E. Dziuk, U. of Minnesota.

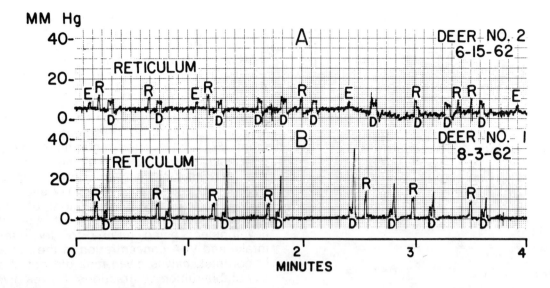

Figure 6-9. Pressure recordings in the reticulum of two deer [A & B], indicating regurgitation [R] occurring out-of-phase with respect to the reticulo-rumen cycle as indicated by the positions of reticular doublets [D] in deer A on the right side of the chart. E = eructation. Courtesy of H.E. Dziuk, Univ. of Minnesota.

tions. Recent data (Kay and Ruckebusch, 1971) confirm this indicating that suckling either milk or water causes reticular contractions to become more frequent, but weak, or to cease altogether. After the fluid passes into the abomasum, reticular contractions slow down. Rumen and omasal motility are more fully inhibited than the reticulum by sucking.

Development of Motility in Young Ruminants

Relatively little information is available on young animals. Schalk and Amadon (1928) demonstrated that the reticulo-rumen contractions in calves were low in frequency although of a typical cyclic nature. Other observations indicate that motility develops in conjunction with intake of solid food, but the movements may be imperceptible with methods such as palpation and auscultation (Mahipaul and Mishra, 1971). Using fluoro-scopic methods, Benzie and Phillipson (1957) reported that movements of the reticulum and rumen occurred in young suckling animals, even though these organs contained no solid food. Regular cyclic contraction set in when solid food was eaten. Dziuk and Sellers (1955) indicated that

spontaneous rumen contraction was more regular and stronger in roughage-fed calves than in milk-fed animals. Asai and Sasaki (1970), using fluoroscopic methods in young calves, state that at 2 wk of age a feeble movement of the bottom of the reticulum

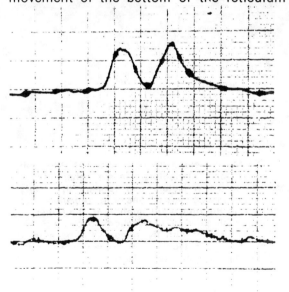

Figure 6-10. Reticular presure patterns of [top] normal cow and [bottom] cow with spontaneous traumatic peritonitis, caused by tissue damage from a nail in the reticulum. Note the prolonged second contraction. From Holtenius et al [1971b].

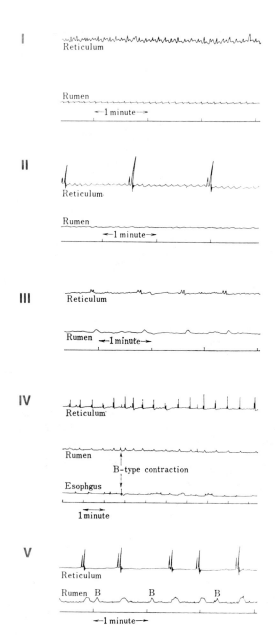

Asai (1973) has studied rumen movements in more detail using rumen-fistulated calves and pressure-sensitive recorders in calves from 2 to 10 wk of age which were fed a variety of different diets — milk; milk, hay and grain; milk + sponges; milk + VFA; or milk + sponges + VFA. As a result of these studies, reticular and rumen motility was arbitrarily divided into five stages of development (Fig. 6-11). These graphs show the progressive development from no motility to well defined reticular and rumen contractions. In calves allowed milk, hay and grain ad libitum, eructation contractions of grade V were recorded at 3-10 wk of age, the development being related to dry matter intake and VFA concentration in the rumen. In contrast, calves given milk did not show any stable rumen contractions. Calves given milk + sponges reached grade IV at 7-9 wk, and those given milk + VFA reached grade IV-V at 10 wk of age. The combination of milk, sponges and VFA allowed development to grade V at 3-5 wk of age. Typical eructation contractions were seen by 5-6 wk of age in calves fed normally.

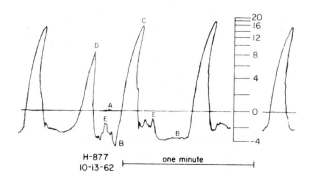

Figure 6-12. Rumen gas pressure of fasting steer fed on long oat hay. A, atmospheric pressure; B, resting rumen pressure; C, primary rumen contraction; D, eructation contraction; E, deflection caused by movement of the steer. Scale is graduated in cm of water. From Colvin and Daniels [1965].

Figure 6-11. Developmental motility of the calf stomach. I, only respiratory pressure changes are recorded in the reticulum and rumen; II, clearly identifiable biphasic contractions of the reticulum, but no change in the rumen; III, motility in the rumen is now seen with primary contractions occurring; IV, further development with the rumen showing eructation contractions [B type]; V, the rumen now shows well defined primary and secondary contractions. From Asai [1973].

was observed; a feeble movement of the reticulum followed by a slow movement of the rumen at 3 wk, and active biphasic contraction of the reticulum and strong contractions of the rumen occurred at 6 wk of age.

Rumen Pressures

Data from many different sources are available on rumen pressure changes, particularly where studies with bloat have been the prime interest (see Ch. 17). However, the pattern of pressure changes, when free gas pressure is recorded, is quite different than that of pressure curves that

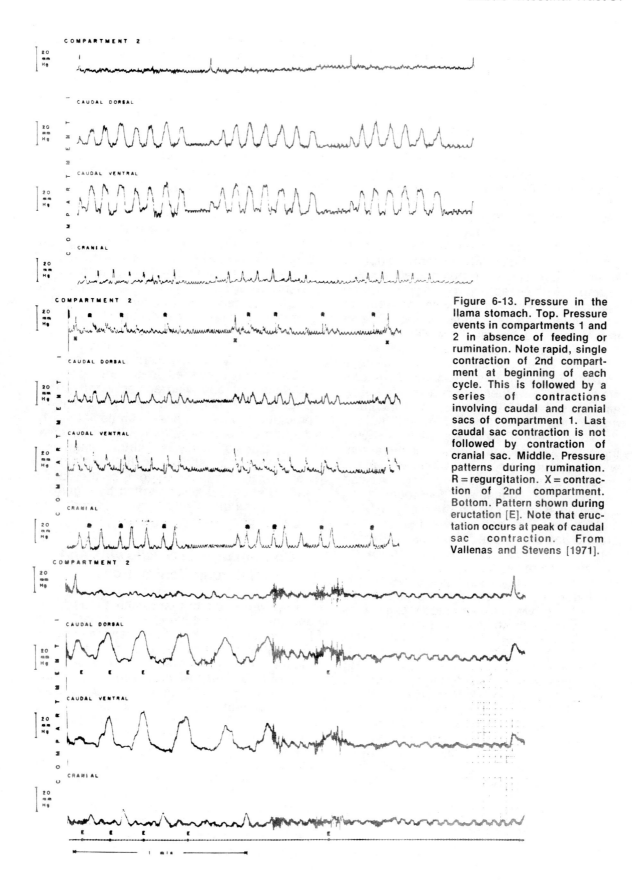

Figure 6-13. Pressure in the llama stomach. Top. Pressure events in compartments 1 and 2 in absence of feeding or rumination. Note rapid, single contraction of 2nd compartment at beginning of each cycle. This is followed by a series of contractions involving caudal and cranial sacs of compartment 1. Last caudal sac contraction is not followed by contraction of cranial sac. Middle. Pressure patterns during rumination. R = regurgitation. X = contraction of 2nd compartment. Bottom. Pattern shown during eructation [E]. Note that eructation occurs at peak of caudal sac contraction. From Vallenas and Stevens [1971].

have been shown in other graphs earlier in this chapter where pressure was recorded by sensors immersed in the fluids. One example of the pressure waves to be expected is shown in Fig. 6-12 from Colvin and Daniels (1965). This illustrates one fact long known, that gas pressure, when the rumen is at rest, is subatmospheric, but it increases in a sharp spike when either primary or secondary contractions occur. Phillipson and Reid (1960) noted that rumen pressures encountered in sheep on normal rations ranged from -5 to -15 mm of water during the resting phase to as high as 70+ during active contraction. Other relatively recent data on this subject provide confirmation of earlier studies at many different stations. For example, with sheep, Pharr et al (1967) found that rumen pressures to 14 cm of water in animals fed long hay; pressure was reduced in animals fed ground hay. Resting pressures were nearly always subatmospheric. Alderson et al (1972) noted that average (maximum) rumen gas pressures were 12.9 cm of water in wethers fed coarse alfalfa hay as opposed to 16.2 for those fed medium-ground hay (not typical of most studies). Data on cattle (Colvin and Daniels, 1965) indicate average maximum pressures (cm water) ranging from 7.3 when fed finely ground hay to 17.2 when fed long hay, and Attebery and Johnson (1969) found peak rumen pressures to be on the order of 14-15 cm of water in dairy cows fed coarsely ground hay and grain. When fasted (rumen contents removed and replaced with water), pressures were ca. 4-5 cm of water. In deer, Dziuk et al (1963) found pressures in the caudodorsal blind sac to be as high as 65 mm of Hg in two deer, although mean values were from 29 to 40 mm of Hg.

In intact animals (radio telemetry methods), pressures observed in steers, presumably in the fluid, were 10.4 mm Hg while ruminating to 18.2 during rest and 22.1 while feeding (Table 6-2, Mooney et al, 1971). By contrast, fluid pressures seen in the reticulum (peak at second spike of biphasic contraction) of intact cows are much higher, average values being 143 mm Hg while resting, 147 while eating, 167 while drinking, and 32-53 while ruminating (Dracy et al, 1972).

Stomach Motility in Camelids

As pointed out in Ch. 2, the stomach anatomy of camels and camelids is quite different than that of true ruminants. Recently, Vallenas and Stevens (1971) have made detailed studies of motility in llamas and guanacos and a brief condensation of their findings is presented here. The reader may wish to refer to illustrations on anatomy in Ch. 2 (Fig. 2-13, 14, 15).

Results of these studies (see Fig. 6-13) show that the first two compartments undergo cyclic motility. Like the reticulum of ruminants, the second compartment contractions are rapid and lead the cycle of contractions. First compartment contractions are multiple, often having 6-8 contractions before the next contraction of compartment 2. The glandular pouches were usually everted early in this cycle. The duration noted was 1.8/min at rest. This increased to a rate of ca. 4/min in the cranial sac while feeding, and then decreased to ca. 1.4/min during rumination. The amplitude of contractions also increased during feeding.

Eructation occurred near the peak of caudaldorsal and ventral sac contractions (Fig. 6-13). It occurred 3-4X/cycle. Usually, eructation was followed immediately by deglutition, but the latter could be observed at any stage of the cycle. During rumination, the cranial sac showed extra contractions not preceded by contractions of the caudal sac. These were accompanied by regurgitation. A single cycle could include 3-4 regurgitations.

Coordination of Swallowing and Reticular Contractions

In view of the fact that rumen contractions are highly coordinated and that such phenomena as regurgitation and eructation are highly coordinated, it is of interest to look at some graphs showing the relationship of swallowing (deglutition) and reticular contractions. As examples, figures from three different publications are shown (Fig. 6-14, 15, 16). Timing of swallowing in rumination is relatively obvious in these figures. For example in Fig. 6-15, 16 on the esophageal traces, the first spike of rumination presumably represents swallowing of the rumination bolus and the others represent the events of rumination that follow (see later section); thus, the bolus is swallowed prior to the extra-reticular contraction that occurs in rumination. When

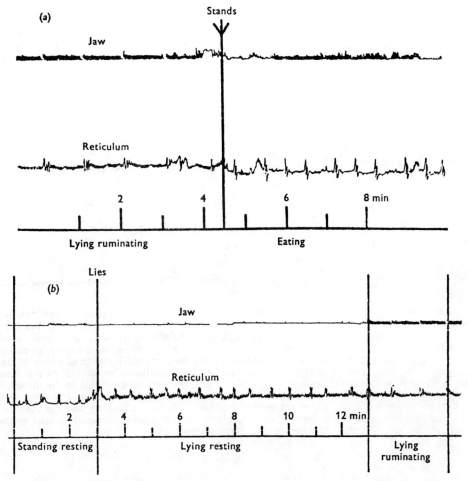

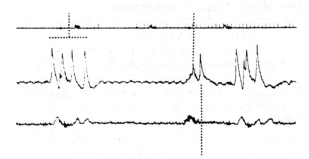

Figure 6-14. A recording which shows the coordination of jaw movements with reticular activity during rumination and eating. From Balch [1971].

Figure 6-15. Recordings from the reticulum and the esophagus in a normal cow during rumination. At top, time marker in seconds; middle, the esophagus tracing; bottom, reticulum tracing. From Holtenius et al [1971a].

eating, the timing is less clear and graphs showing this relationship are not as adequate as might be desired, but they do tend to show that the bolus is swallowed slightly before the normal biphasic contraction of the reticulum.

Movement of Ingested Boli

As noted in Ch. 4, ingested boli are deposited in the cardial area of the reticulo-rumen. Schalk and Amadon (1928) point out that one bolus, or sometimes several, may accumulate before the reticulum contracts. The reticular and cranial sac contractions rapidly move the bolus posteriorly in the rumen, depending upon the specific gravity of the particles in the bolus. Observations reported by Schalk and Amadon in cattle

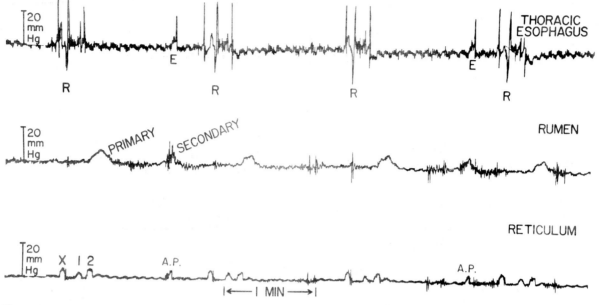

Figure 6-16. A graph showing three complete cycles of reticulo-ruminal contractions during rumination. The double reticular contraction, 1 and 2, and a primary and secondary rumen contraction are labeled for the first cycle. The extra-reticular contraction associated with regurgitation [X] is also labeled. The esophageal pressure changes during regurgitation are labeled [R] and consist of a small positive pressure wave, followed by the negative deflection due to inspiration against a closed glottis and then, immediately, the large positive deflection due to antiperistaltic esophageal contraction. Regurgitation is usually soon followed by deglutition [unlabeled] of the fluid expressed from the bolus at the beginning of mastication. A wave of deglutition, carrying the bolus to the rumen, is also seen on the esophageal trace at the end of each cycle of rumination and just before the next regurgitation. Note the close integration of the rumination and reticulo-ruminal cycles. Eructation [E] is also labeled, and the associated increase in pressure due to abdominal press can be seen on the reticular trace [A.P.] and also superimposed on the secondary wave of rumen contraction. Courtesy of Stevens and Sellers [1968].

indicated that light weight boli of forage move back into the dorsal sacs, whereas boli of high specific gravity, which disintegrate rapidly, may not move past the cranial sac. As the reticulum dilates in conjunction with contractions of the blind sacs and the ventral sac, the rush of ingesta back towards the reticulum will carry many of these particles into the reticulum. Unfortunately, observations of this type on other species are available only as X-rays. Benzie and Phillipson (1957) show a few pictures on sheep indicating that appreciable amounts of boli from barium-cereal ingesta reached the dorsal and ventral sacs, and that such boli disintegrate rapidly.

Rumination

This phenomenon of "chewing the cud" or rechewing rumen contents ingested at some earlier time is one of the features most characteristic of ruminant animals. Briefly, rumination involves regurgitation of ingesta from the reticulo-rumen, swallowing of regurgitated liquids, remastication of the solids accompanied by re-insalivation and reswallowing of the bolus.

The Mechanics of Rumination

As pointed out earlier in this chapter, the regurgitation phase of rumination is associated with an extrareticular contraction that precedes the usual biphasic contraction by a short time (see Fig. 6-6 to 6-9, 6-15, 16). This contraction results in a marked increase in fluid pressures in the cardial area (Bell, 1958; Dracy et al, 1972). Accompanying the reticular contraction, in most cases, is an inspiratory effort of greater volume than usual. This results in a sharp contraction of the diaphragm and a negative pressure in the trachea which has been observed to occur in animals with a cannulated trachea (Webster and Cresswell, 1957), thus indicating that the glottis does not have to be closed to create the negative pressure. Webster and Cresswell (1957) suggest that the walls of the esophagus are normally collapsed but, at the moment of regurgitation, the cardia and posterior portion of the esophagus dilate, producing a ballooning of the walls of the esophagus. Since this is accompanied by a negative pressure in the thoracic cavity and an increased pressure of fluids in the cardia, it could easily account for the aspiration of reticular contents into the esophagus. Sucking sounds associated with these events are easily heard in fistulated animals and Schalk and Amadon (1928) pointed out that a strong flow of reticular contents can be detected by the hand. Aspiration of reticular contents into the esophagus is facilitated by the fact that ingesta in the reticulum is more fluid in nature (and of lower dry matter content) than that found in the cranial or dorsal sacs of the rumen. Phillipson (1970) points out that regurgitation can occur when the reticulum has been immobilized by administration of atropine, thus contraction is apparently not an essential part of regurgitation.

Movement of digesta being regurgitated from the distal portion of the esophagus to the mouth is apparently accomplished by a wave of antiperistaltic contraction which has been timed at ca. 107-112 cm/sec in calves and 42-54 cm/sec in sheep in one case (Winship et al, 1964), 107 cm/sec in cows (Stevens and Sellers, 1960) and 182 cm/sec in sheep in another experiment (Dougherty et al, 1971). This rapid movement is apparently possible due to the fact that esophageal muscle in ruminants is striated, and thus capable of rapid contractions (Stevens and Sellers, 1960; Winship et al, 1964). Rapid contraction would also be facilitated by the physical nature of the regurgitated material, which is a semifluid or slurry rather than a descrete bolus. In contrast, normal swallowing is much slower, i.e., 25 cm/sec (Winship et al, 1964; Dougherty et al, 1971). In sheep, liquid from the rumination bolus is swallowed at a rate of 35 cm/sec and the bolus, after remastication, at a rate of 21 cm/sec (Dougherty et al, 1971).

Rousseau (1971) concludes that opening of the cardia during regurgitation and its closure at the end of swallowing depend upon action of the same, but quantitatively different, esophageal muscle layers.

When regurgitated material reaches the mouth, the excess liquids are swallowed and soon appear as a spurt of liquid at the exposed cardia (Schalk and Amadon, 1928). Remastication, re-insalivation and swallowing of the bolus follow. Refer to some of the graphs shown, particularly Fig. 6-15, 16, 17.

Mastication and Fate of the Rumination Bolus

During the remastication that occurs while ruminating, the bolus is re-insalivated; however, salivary secretion is of a different nature than that which occurs during eating. According to Bailey and Balch (1961) the parotid glands may secrete more saliva during rumination than during eating. However, Kay's (1960) data indicate that the mucogenic glands do not secrete much during rumination.

The solids regurgitated during rumination are remasticated in a more deliberate manner than is usual on initial ingestion of dry feed, although perhaps at a faster rate than may occur during grazing. Fuller (1928) found that cows made 94 chews/min when eating grain and silage, 74/min when eating hay, but only 55/min when ruminating. Johnstone-Wallace (1953) recorded 42 chews/min in ruminating beef cattle, and Hardison et al (1956) observed 64/min in lactating dairy cows as opposed to 58 bites/min in the latter when grazing. The number of jaw movements calculated from data of Freer et al (1962) and Freer and Campling (1965) are as shown: cows fed 8-10 lb of straw/day, ca. 26,500; cows fed 18-24 lb of hay, ca. 34,400. In cows fed ca. 20 lb of hay, dried grass or concentrates: hay, 50,100; dried grass, 36,100; and concentrates, ca. 11,000.

In the case of sheep, Gordon (1958) found that one sheep chewed at a rate of 75/min when ruminating as compared to about 100/min when eating. Data of Gordon's show that the average bolus was in the mouth from 49-54 sec and that the average number of chews/bolus was about 70 compared to 54-58 chews/bolus reported by Pearce (1965a). The interval between, ranging from 7-12 sec is utilized to swallow the bolus, regurgitate and swallow the excess liquids. Burger (1967) has investigated rumination patterns in a variety of ruminant species in zoological gardens and observed 20-70 chews/bolus.

Data on the number of jaw movements in sheep are rather scarce. Gordon (1958) noted 38,000-39,000 chews, and Pearce (1965a) observed 6,300-36,700, depending upon the type of ration; most were on the order of 30,000 chews/day. If we assume that a sheep makes about 70 chews/bolus, then we can calculate from some of Gordon's data (1961) that sheep fed 640 g of concentrates and 400 g of chopped hay made about 31,500 chews/day. Krzywanek (1968) observed 44,000 jaw movements during rumination in sheep fed hay and 23,000 when on pasture.

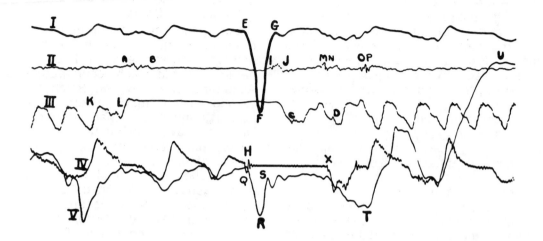

Figure 6-17. Tracings of regurgitation and related events in a steer with a rumen fistula. I: Intra-tracheal pressure. F, the negative pressure associated with regurgitation. Note at G that there is no particular rise of intratracheal pressure following the negative pressure. II: Movements of boluses in the cervical part of the esophagus. AB, the swallowing of the remasticated bolus. IJ, the regurgitated bolus passing up. MN and OP, the swallowing of fluid squeezed out of the bolus in the mouth. III: Jaw movements, which cease at L and begin again at C. IV: Nasal pressure. The glottis is closed from H to X. There appears to be a slight lag in the closure of the glottis, producing the dip just below H. V: Changes in abdominal girth. An enlargement is indicated at R. This is synchronous with F. At U the rumen contraction which always follows regurgitation is under way. Time intervals of 1 sec. From Downie [1954].

Fig. 6-18 illustrates the pattern of jaw movements in sheep during idling, eating, ruminating and while fasting.

The bolus, when swallowed, returns to the cardial area. One might suspect that it might be regurgitated again, since a rather brief interval elapses between swallowing and regurgitation of the next batch. However, this apparently does not occur to any extent due to the fact that the regurgitation contraction of the reticulum probably suffices to move the bolus back into the cranial sac. Direct observations (Schalk and Amadon, 1928) indicate that the reswallowed bolus is moved into the cranial or dorsal sac of the rumen if specific gravity or particle size is not conducive to passage into the omasum via the reticular-omasal orifice. Even in the case of this alternative, some time would be required for distintegration of the bolus and settling of the particles of higher specific gravity.

into many periods with intervals of feeding, drinking and rest interspersed. Since ruminant animals generally spend ⅔ to ¾ of their eating time in daylight hours (see Ch. 4), on any kind of a typical feeding schedule

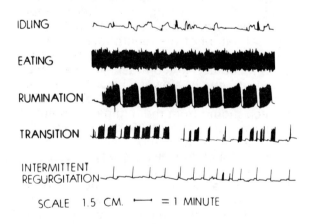

Figure 6-18. Typical jaw motion patterns. Transition patterns were recorded during the first part of a fasting period, and represent intermediates between the normal rumination and the intermittent regurgitation seen during fasting. From Welch and Smith [1968].

Time Spent Ruminating

Time spent ruminating is generally divided

they spend more time ruminating at night than during daylight hours (see Fig. 4-8; 6-19). This has been known by livestock people for many, many years and has been confirmed in a number of cases with experimental evidence where rumination periods have been observed around the clock or where records have been made of jaw movements (for example with sheep, Krzywanek, 1968; Welch and Smith, 1968; Gordon and McAllister, 1970; and cattle, Freer et al, 1962).

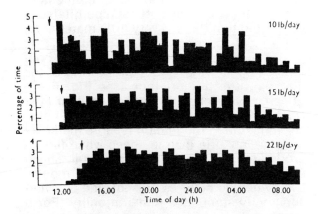

Figure 6-19. Mean percentage of the total time spent ruminating daily by four cows which occurred in each 30 min period of the day, at each of three levels of intake of hay; the arrows show the mean times at which eating ceased. From Freer et al [1962].

Data on sheep (Gordon, 1958, 1961) indicate that there may be many periods of rumination when animals were fed concentrate and hay. These periods may range from ca. 30 sec to 2 hr, but half or more were shorter than 30 min (Gordon, 1958). When fed 1X daily, sheep had from 9 to 18 rumination periods/day; when fed frequently, the number ranged from 12 to 35; mean values were on the order of 14 for those fed 1X and ca. 18 for those fed frequently. The number of boli regurgitated/period was also variable, mean values being 25 for frequent feeding and 31 for 1X feeding. Other studies with sheep (Pearce and Moir, 1963; Pearce, 1965; Weston and Hogan, 1967; Welch and Smith, 1968, 1969a, b) indicate that sheep will spend about 8-9 hr/day in rumination, the amount being affected by a number of different variables (see later section).

Studies with confined cattle indicate fewer rumination periods than with the sheep of Gordon's study. Schalk and Amadon (1928) present data which are quite variable, but which would average ca. 30 ruminating periods/day for cattle on dry feed. With dairy cows on a variety of different roughages and with different amounts of feed, Freer et al (1962) observed from 11 to 21 periods/day, Freer and Campling (1965) observed from 8 to 17 in cows fed hay or dried grass, and Campling (1966) found mean values to be 15, 16 and 16 in heifers, pregnant cows and lactating cows, respectively, fed roughage or roughage and concentrates. In these latter experiments, reticular contractions were measured. Assuming that each contraction produced a bolus (double or triple reticular contractions counted as one contraction), Freer et al (1962) observed mean values during rumination of 448/day in cows fed ca. 10 lb of straw and 686 in cows fed 22 lb of hay; Freer and Campling (1965) observed 635 in cows fed 21 lb of hay, 438 in those fed 29 lb of dried grass, and 109 in those fed 20 lb of concentrates. Schake and Riggs (1969, 1970) have observed beef cows and calves while in confinement. They noted that the cows spent an average of 197 min during the day and 259 min at night in rumination and the calves spent ca. 120 min during the day and ca. 180 min at night. Data from several sources indicate that cattle may spend from 35 to 80 min of ruminating time/kg of roughage consumed.

In the case of grazing cattle, average rumination times reported by Castle et al (1950) were 5.6 hr, with 9-13 periods/day. Hardison et al (1956) reported average time spent ruminating at about 7-8 hr, Johnstone-Wallace and Kennedy (1944) gave average values of 7 hr, and Wagnon (1963) reported a range from 6 to 10 hr, depending upon the availability and maturity of forage. Thus, we might expect cattle to spend 6 to 10 hr/day in rumination activity.

Stimulation of Rumination

Habel (1956) has demonstrated that the rumen is innervated primarily by the dorsal trunk of the vagus nerve and Duncan (1953) showed that sectioning the vagus nerve completely inhibited rumination. Bell and Lawn (1955, 1957) and Clark (1953) have investigated centers in the brain which control rumination with results indicating that a subcortical area anterior to the pituitary is the site of control. Kay (1959) demonstrated that rumination could be stimulated by injection of adrenalin. Factors which result in distension of the lower GIT and which inhibit rumen motility would, presumably, inhibit rumination.

Leek (1969) has studied nerve receptors in the rumen and notes that those designated as mechanoreceptors are located mainly in the medial walls of the reticulum and the cranial sac, the reticular groove, the reticulo-ruminal fold, the dorsal and ventral sacs and the omasal canal. The receptors in the reticulum and the rumen appeared to be deep in the muscle layers, but those in the reticular groove were more superficial.

All of the factors stimulating or inhibiting rumination have not been clearly defined. However, Schalk and Amadon (1928) demonstrated some time ago that tactile stimulation of reticular and ruminal epithelium proved to be a powerful stimulus and was most effective when applied to the cranial wall of the reticulum. The response became progressively weaker from this point to the caudal region of the rumen. The pressure exerted by a recording balloon, the hand, or handfuls of hay was also effective. When the rumen was packed with hay, rumination began within a few minutes. Sawdust and shavings stimulated regurgitation, but the taste was apparently so undesirable that further rumination was inhibited for an extended period. Feeding only grain or finely ground hay resulted in a cessation of rumination. These observations indicated rather clearly that rumination was initiated, at least partially, as a result of tactile stimulation of the epithelia from roughage in the reticulo-rumen. However, change from a pattern of eating to rumination is rather gradual. Pearce (1965a) points out that the lag period following ingestion of feed occurs during a time when tactile stimulation should be maximal, thus indicating that chemical receptors may be a factor which would reflect changes in rumen contents as digestion proceeds.

Rumination may also be stimulated by milking or suckling young. Andersson et al (1958) found that reflex rumination occurred within 2-3 sec after milking began and independently of the time since the last contraction of the reticulum. The reflex was apparently initiated by receptors in the part of the udder which was innervated by lumbar nerves.

Other Factors Influencing Rumination

As noted previously feeding grain only, or finely ground roughages, will result in cessation of rumination or in pseudo rumination (Balch, 1952; Gordon, 1958; Freer and Campling, 1965; Welch and Smith, 1970, 1971; Balch, 1971). In pseudo rumination, the time spent ruminating is greatly reduced in total and for each bolus. When this occurs, there does not appear to be an adequate stimulus to the rumen epithelia or the amount of coarse material regurgitated is so limited that there is very little material for the animal to chew. Pseudo rumination is characterized by regurgitation, a brief interval of chewing, and reswallowing of the material after a short time (see Fig. 6-18). Sheep may be observed smacking their lips. Ruckebusch et al (1970) point out that bolus chewing during rumination is more markedly reduced in cattle than in sheep when fed on ground roughage and that chewing in sheep may occur without a bolus in the mouth. Even when no bolus is present, the chewing apparently stimulates rumen motility. For a given particle size in ground material, we might expect cattle to react more, as their stomach is larger, particle size of digesta is larger, and what is a fine grind for cattle might well be a medium grind for sheep.

It might be noted that regurgitation in ruminants is somewhat similar to vomiting. In ruminants, vomiting occurs only infrequently, although data (Dougherty et al, 1965) definitely show that ruminants can be induced to vomit by administration of drugs. Other data show that electrical stimulation of certain brain centers will cause vomiting (Bell, 1961), and toxins of one kind or another may induce vomiting.

The urge to ruminate must be rather strong as evidenced by the research of Lupien et al (1962), Ruckebusch and Marquet (1965) and Ruckebusch et al (1966). In these cases the forestomach and rumen, respectively, were surgically removed, yet the animals still regurgitated ingesta.

Pearce (1965a, b, c) has studied a number of factors influencing the normal pattern of rumination. When sheep were fed once daily, the pattern of rumination was characterized by a period of inactivity (lag period) after eating, followed by a period of increasing intensity of rumination, leading to a maximum intensity in the early hours of the morning, then a period of reduced activity up to the next feeding time. A high level of roughage feeding was associated with a shortened lag period, while a low level of feeding resulted in a prolonged lag period and a highly skewed distribution. The pattern retained its general characteristics despite changes in the chemical and physical composition of the ration and despite variation in the method of administration of the ration. When fed ad libitum, rumination tended to be distributed without apparent order over the whole day. The lag period was progressively shortened when increasing proportions of a ration of oat and alfalfa chaff were administered via rumen fistulas. The effect was much reduced when high protein sheep cubes were added to the chaff. The removal of rumen contents after voluntary feeding and then their immediate return to the rumen tended to cause an early commencement of rumination. When the rumen contents were "pasteurized" before return, however, rumination did not occur for an extended period of time. When the rumen contents were replaced with buffer solutions plus roughage, variable rumination responses occurred; in one instance apparently uninhibited rumination resulted. No consistent effect of pH on rumination was found when rumen contents were replaced with buffered mixtures at pH values ranging from about 5.1 to 6.95. However, rumination tended to be irregular at the lower pH levels. The addition of sodium carbonate to the rumen to prevent a fall in pH after feeding had no apparent effect; neither did the infusion of volatile fatty acids or urea solutions into the rumen. Removal of part of the saliva by aspiration during eating, or adding previously aspirated saliva had no effect, nor did the manual mixing of rumen contents. After teasing with food, one sheep did not recommence rumination for several hours, another showed practically no reaction and the remaining two showed intermediate responses.

Balch (1971) points out that data obtained from his laboratory indicate that the amount of chewing — both during eating and rumination — gives an index of the fibrous nature of roughages. Studies at this station and at others indicate that the rate of eating roughage is faster with small amounts, but the rumination time/unit of roughage consumed is longer (Freer et al, 1962; Freer and Campling; 1965; Welch and Smith, 1969b). Frequency of feeding has a slight effect in increasing rumination (Gordon, 1961) and, of course, amount of feed, particularly roughages has a marked effect (Balch, 1971; Welch and Smith, 1969b) as does the physical nature of the feed (Balch, 1971; Welch and Smith, 1971; Voskuil and Metz, 1973) and quality of the forage (Balch, 1971; Welch and Smith, 1969a). Welch et al (1970) have also presented data indicating that there are breed differences in dairy cattle; in their case Guernsey cows averaged less rumination time than Holstein or Jersey cows.

Arnold (1960) found that rumination time of sheep was significantly reduced as pasture availability declined, and Lofgreen et al (1957) noted that the ratio of eating time: ruminating time decreased in cattle grazing on small plots whereas that of sheep did not. They attributed the decreased ratio to the reduced selectivity of cattle resulting in an intake of forage of lower digestibility and higher fiber content.

Gordon (1965) has studied rumination behavior of sheep restricted from water for 4-5 days. No important change occurred during the first day or two. However, by the 4th day of deprivation, chewing time decreased by 39%, 34% fewer boli were regurgitated and food intake fell by 46%. When sheep were fasted for 56 to 72 hr (Welch and Smith, 1968), a rapid decline occurred in rumination time and rumination ceased after 36 hr of fasting by animals that were initially fed chopped grass hay. When the sheep were refed, rumination time was back to normal by the second day.

Rumination in Young Animals

As indicated in a previous section (Development of Motility), rumination in young ruminants is closely related to the consumption of solid feedstuffs that enter the reticulo-rumen. Asai (1973) has researched this subject in some detail with calves fed different diets. In this study, rumination was recorded even before the normal rumen or reticulo-rumen contractions were detected. The data indicated that rumination occurred at 2-3 wk of age in calves fed milk, hay and grain or milk + VFA. Rumination was delayed in calves fed milk (seen at 4-10 wk of age). Asai points out (Fig.

6-20) that regurgitation sometimes occurs without a follow-up of the usual biphasic reticular contraction. In older work, Swanson and Harris (1958) studied rumination in young dairy calves. Rumination had begun in 18 of 26 calves in the first 2 wk, and in 25 by the 4th wk. Rumination time increased rapidly to an average of nearly 5 hr/day at 6-8 wk of age when calves were consuming about 0.5 kg of hay. Rumination was initiated before any appreciable amount of hay was consumed. These results are similar to those reported by Schalk and Amadon (1928) and Flatt et al (1959). Tamate et al (1962) also noted that VFA stimulated calves to ruminate at about 1 wk of age. In young (3-4 wk of age) calves fed through an abomasal fistula, Ruckebusch and Candau (1969) found that rumination was not suppressed even though there was no solid food in the rumen. Infusion of VFA into the rumen over a 5-6 hr period, in amounts equivalent to that produced from normal fermentation of forage, inhibited rumination for several hr. Plastic material in the rumen stimulated rumination. In older calves (Hodgson, 1971a, b), it appears that they chew somewhat faster than adults during rumination (80-85 chews/min when given hay); chews/bolus increased as the roughage in the diet increased, ranging from 36-67 when given pellets or baled grass in one experiment and from 51 to 71 in a second experiment. The time spent ruminating increased rapidly for 2-3 wk after weaning until the calves were eating 1-1.5 kg of dry matter/day; after that changes in ruminating time were small. Calves on pelleted diets ruminated < 3 hr/day as compared to > 7 for those receiving hay, and some of them on the pelleted diet were never seen to ruminate. Baccari et al (1970) note that there was a negative correlation in Zebu calves between age at the start of rumination and weight gain at weaning, suggesting that weaning weight was greater when rumination starts earlier.

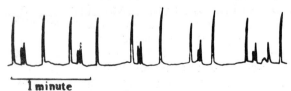

Figure 6-20. Pressure changes in the reticulum of the young calf showing that regurgitation [longest spikes] sometimes occurs without a follow up of the usual biphasic reticular contraction. From Asai [1973].

Studies with hand-raised lambs (Stephens and Baldwin, 1971) indicate that 3 of 9 lambs had started to ruminate by the end of 1 wk of age. During the second wk, 7 of the lambs ruminated and by the beginning of the third week all lambs were ruminating. There was a gradual increase in ruminating time (Fig. 6-21).

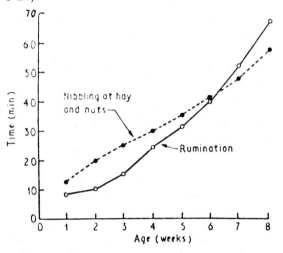

Figure 6-21. The amount of time spent in ruminating or nibbling at solid food during a 6 hr period. Graph is based on pooled data from 9 lambs observed over a period of 8 wk. From Stephens and Baldwin [1971].

Value of Rumination to the Animal

The actual value of the rumination process to the animal remains in doubt due to a lack of scientific evidence, although two papers shed some light on the subject. In one study (Pearce and Moir, 1963), sheep were fed a chopped roughage ration on which rumination was either allowed to occur normally or was restricted by means of a muzzle; they also fed a finely ground ration with either normal rumination allowed or with the addition of polyethylene flakes to stimulate rumination. Their data showed that grinding resulted in a shorter retention time in the GIT and a lower digestibility of dry matter, organic matter, and crude fiber. The effect of muzzling was to markedly increase retention time which was associated with a higher digestibility of dry matter, organic matter, and crude fiber (this would result in a reduction in intake, however). The addition of polyethylene flakes to the ground ration tended to further decrease retention time, compared to ground hay, and reduced digestibility. Jean-Balin et al (1972) have carried out experiments in which rumination was suppressed by administration of morphine; repeated injections prevented rumination for periods from 24 hr to 10 days. Treated sheep fed long hay usually showed some reduction of feed intake. Elimination of stained feed particles was prolonged in all sheep. Digestibility of cellulose was increased in 10 of 12 trials; the increase was greatest on pelleted diets and only slight on long hay. Retention of N was improved and most sheep maintained or even gained weight. The authors concluded that the chief effect of rumination is to accelerate emptying of the rumen, thus permitting greater feed intake.

From an evolutionary point of view, why did ruminants develop this complicated mechanism? The answer remains for future scientists to unravel, of course. However, the most logical answer seems to be that ruminants could eat rapidly during daylight hours and spend "leisure" time at night rechewing their fibrous diet at their convenience during a period when they are less apt to be attacked by predators than if they were actively feeding during the night hours.

There is little doubt that ruminants expend an appreciable amount of energy in the rumination process. For sheep, Graham (1964) has estimated the energy cost at 0.24 Kcal/hr/kg body weight over a range of diets. Thus, when comparing long and ground forage, we could estimate differences in energy expenditure. Assuming that other parameters do not change, Weston and Hogan (1967) calculate that reduction in rumination on ground hay might result in a 9% saving of metabolizable energy. Whether it requires more energy than would be required to chew food thoroughly when eating is open to question, but the soaking process undergone in the reticulo-rumen undoubtedly makes mastication more efficient for fibrous feeds. The rumination process no doubt, serves to maintain a more uniform amount of ingesta in the GIT during a 24-hr period, probably due largely to the rather continuous remastication. Remastication should aid in maintaining a more uniform population of rumen microorganisms and of microbial end products in the rumen of lower GIT, something akin to feeding at frequent intervals as opposed to 1X/day (see Ch. 16). In animals fed 1X/day, data show that following a period of rumination there is a surge of microbial growth and

an increase in the VFA concentration. Rumination should, then, contribute substantially to more efficient utilization of the heat increment resulting from microbial fermentation in the rumen and body tissues and, thus, to more efficient utilization of other nutrients. If, as suggested in the two papers reviewed, rumination reduces rumen turnover time of solid digesta and, thus, allows greater feed intake, this is obviously an advantage to animals consuming low quality feedstuffs.

Eructation

Eructation is the mechanism whereby the ruminant animal belches or gets rid of the large quantities of gas produced in the forestomach as a result of microbial fermentation. The average volume of gas produced in the reticulo-rumen of cattle may be expected to be on the order of 2 l./min for an adult animal; comparable values for sheep would be about 5 l./hr. During periods of peak gas production (30 min to 2 hr after feeding), gas production may increase tremendously. Colvin et al (1958) found that steers feeding on alfalfa green chop produced 12-27 l./min and 3-17 individual eructations/min occurred although most were within the range of 10-15. From 0.5 to 1.7 l. of gas were given off at each eructation (see Ch. 16 for further details). Consequently, the mechanism for getting rid of gas must be rather efficient to handle this volume. Weiss (1953) has reviewed some of the older literature on eructation; for other reviews see papers by Dougherty (1961, 1968) and Dougherty et al (1965).

The events of the eructation mechanism have been shown to be associated with secondary rumen contractions for the most part, although there are some species differences in this respect (see preceding sections). Dougherty and Habel (1955) and Dougherty and Meredith (1955) have used radiographic photography to study eructation and found that the biphasic contractions of the reticulum — the beginning phases of a normal primary cycle of contractions — cleared the cardial area of much of the ingesta. Although eructation usually does not occur until some period of time after the reticular contractions (perhaps 20-30 sec in cattle), the reticulo-ruminal fold and the cranial pillar remain in a contracted state acting as a dam restraining the ingesta from

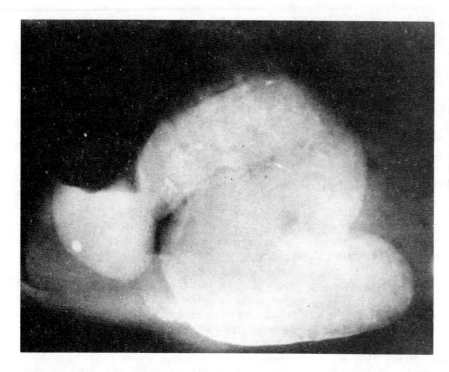

Figure 6-22. Lateral X-ray view of goat's stomach showing the reticulum dilated with gas in its upper part. The reticulo-ruminal fold has contracted and prevented the comparatively liquid contents of the cranial sac from entering the reticulum. Note that the caudoventral blind sac is dilated. From Benzie and Phillipson [1957, Plate 20].

filling the reticulum. Dilation of the reticulum, coinciding with contraction of the dorsal and caudodorsal blind sacs and relaxation of the caudoventral blind sac, allows rumen gas to be forced into the cardial area. Radiographs of sheep (Benzie and Phillipson, 1957; Fig. 6-22) indicate that the caudoventral sac is dilated, probably to provide room for ingesta forced out of the dorsal sacs.

During periods of high gas production, two or more secondary contractions may frequently occur in a normal complete cycle of contraction. Presumably, the cranial pillar must remain in a state of contraction when this occurs, but evidence is lacking on this subject. Ruckebusch and Tomov (1973) point out that sustained gaseous distension elicited numerous secondary contractions concurrent with a lower frequency of reticular contractions. Some of the secondary contractions were incomplete, but all began with contraction of the ventral blind sac and were associated with eructation.

Dougherty (1961) has described the remainder of the mechanism, indicating that the cardia and a zone of constriction about 2 in. anterior to it (diaphragmatic sphincter) than relax, admitting gas to the thoracic esophagus; this action is repeated rapidly, the cardia and diaphragmatic sphincter alternately closing and opening. When the

esophagus has filled with gas and the cardial and diaphragmatic sphincters closed, the pharyngo-esophageal sphincter relaxes and the gas is forced out of the esophagus into the nasopharynx. Just prior to this expulsion the nasopharyngeal sphincter closes. The glottis remains open and the lips are closed during eructation with the result that a considerable part of the eructated gas enters and penetrates deeply into the respiratory passages (trachea and lungs).

In cows equipped with face masks and tracheal cannulas (see Fig. 16-8), Dougherty and Cook (1962) found that 3-7X as much gas was expelled through the trachea as through the face mask (i.e., gas which would normally go into the lungs). Hornicke et al (cited by Dougherty et al, 1965) found that 0.5-33% of eructed gas escaped by mouth or nose, the remainder being respired from the trachea. Gas production in alpacas appears to be comparable to cattle, but data (Dougherty and Vallenas, 1968) indicate relatively more goes into the trachea.

Hill (cited by Dougherty et al, 1965), Stevens and Sellers (1960) and Dougherty et al (1971) have studied the speed of eructation and find that gas travels up the esophagus at a speed of 160, 227 and 200 cm/sec, respectively. Multiple eructations (see previous section) may occur during one secondary contraction of the rumen.

As the reader may know, eructation is a silent process in ruminants as contrasted to belching in (some) humans. This, no doubt, is a protective mechanism which would help these animals avoid predators during quiet periods of rumination while at rest.

Stimulation of Eructation

Cole et al (1945), Weiss (1953) and others have shown that inflation of the rumen with gas stimulates the eructation reflex. The work of Stevens and Sellers (1959) and Iggo (1951) indicates that tension (stretch) receptors in the cardial area have a stimulatory action on eructation. When using decerebrate sheep, Dougherty et al (1958) determined that eructation was inhibited when an area around the cardia was covered with ingesta, water, foam or mineral oil. With the decerebrate animal on its back and with a well-filled rumen, eructation was completely inhibited even with elevated rumen pressures; with an empty rumen, eructation was as efficient as in a standing position. Nickols (1951) and Weiss (1953) have shown that over filling of the rumen with liquids will inhibit eructation. Ruckebusch and Tomov (1973) find that chemical stimulation of the rumen by fatty acids (pH 5.5-5.9) increased the ratio of secondary to primary contractions of the rumen to a variable extent, depending on their initial rate (for further detail see Ch. 17). Dougherty's work indicates that, in sheep, the area around the cardial is kept free of ingesta by strong contractions of the reticulo-ruminal fold and the cranial pillar whereas in cattle, which have a less well developed fold, the cranial pillar may assume the major role in clearing the cardia.

The research cited indicates that neural receptors in the cardial area inhibit eructation when the presence of ingesta, foam, or liquids is detected. In view of the fact that a large proportion of eructated gases is disposed of via the lungs, this is an understandable protective device, since foreign bodies in the lungs may easily lead to pneumonia or other undesirable reactions.

Comparison of the eructation and rumination mechanisms indicates that they are stimulated in different ways. Eructation is stimulated by gas pressure in the rumen, whereas rumination is stimulated by tactile and chemical means and can be experimentally produced by administering insulin to decrease blood sugar (Augusto and Vallenas, 1956; Bowen, 1962). Although both involve passage of material up the esophagus, the pressure waves associated with eructation are faster than those associated with rumination. Regurgitation occurs in association with an extrareticular contraction, while eructation is associated, for the most part, with secondary rumen contractions. Eructation is inhibited if the cardial area is not evacuated of solids or fluids, whereas regurgitation requires that the cardia be below fluid level.

Omasal Motility

In a review paper, Sellers and Stevens (1966) point out that the anatomical location of the omasum has made it a difficult organ to study. Nevertheless, a fair amount of information is available (see Bost, 1970), although the information is rather incomplete with respect to known functions. Information on digesta passage is presented in Ch. 7 and that on absorption in Ch. 9.

With respect to motility, the sequence of contractions is the neck (which connects with the reticulum), the omasal canal and the body of the organ. Omasal contractions are relatively slow and prolonged (see Fig. 6-23, 24), when compared to rumen contraction, and there is said to be considerable variability between animals (cattle) although contractions in sheep and goats are said to be more regular. Until recently, no evidence has been presented to show contractions of the leaves (Sellers and Stevens, 1966), although Phillipson (1939) observed with radiographic studies that the whole organ undergoes considerable changes in position and shape during a normal contractile cycle. Some of the papers giving data on omasal motility are reviewed in subsequent paragraphs.

Balch et al (1951) studied movements of the omasal orifice in relation to contractions of the reticulum, cranial pillar of the rumen, the omasum, and abomasum by means of small, lightly inflated balloons. During resting, eating, rumination, lying, drinking and while the cow was being milked, the R-O orifice functioned in a constant pattern. For the greater part of the reticulo-ruminal cycle of contraction, the orifice was loosely open but following the last reticular contraction, the orifice closed strongly. The last reticular contraction was accompanied by a marked fall in pressure in the neck of the omasum, followed by a marked rise of pressure in the omasum which coincided with the closure of the orifice. The transfer of digesta from the reticulum and cranial rumen sac most likely occurred at the time of the last reticular contraction, coinciding with the fall in pressure in the omasum. The authors stated that it is probable that the passage of digesta from the reticulo-rumen is relatively continuous throughout the day and is largely controlled by the valve-like action of the omasum.

Borgatti and Matscher (1956) also noted that contraction of the omasal orifice was always associated with reticular contractions and that the contractions were biphasic but of much longer duration, lasting 25-35 sec. They observed that swallowing was associated with monophasic contractions of the esophageal groove and the omasal orifice; however, these contractions were absent if swallowing occurred during the refractory period after a reticular contraction.

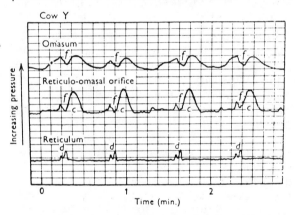

Figure 6-23. Pressure changes in the reticulum, reticulo-omasal orifice, and the omasum of a cow at rest. The double contraction of the reticulum [d], the sudden fall in pressure in the omasum and reticulo-omasal orifice [f], and the powerful contraction of the orifice [c] are shown. From Balch et al [1951].

Stevens et al (1960) found that pressure recordings made between the leaves of the omasal body and in the omasal canal were quite different in character (see Fig. 6-23) with the body contractions being of much greater amplitude than those from other parts of the stomach (30-40 mm of Hg). The body contractions were also of longer duration than the canal contractions, sometimes overlapping into the next ruminal cycle. Another difference was that the canal contractions occurred with each reticular cycle whereas the body contractions did not always occur, at times being absent for 2-5 cycles. These authors proposed that canal contractions force the more fluid components of the ingesta from the canal between the leaves of the omasal body and that the contraction of the omasal body forced ingesta out of the intra-leaf space into the abomasum. The greatest flow of ingesta from the reticulum appeared to occur directly following the canal contractions. Backflow of large volumes of ingesta from the omasum to the reticulum was occasionally noted and seemed to occur when the omasal body contracted during closure of the omasal-abomasal orifice.

In suckling animals, Kay and Ruckebusch (1971) note that the act of suckling inhibits action of the omasum and that filling of the abomasum also inhibits its action. Other data from this laboratory (Ruckebusch and Kay, 1971) show pressure patterns similar to those of Balch et al (1951); recordings from the omasal canal showed two peaks, the first accompanying the first phase of reticular contraction and the second following the second phase. The body of the omasum gave rise to a rhythmic pattern of pressure change which was much slower than the reticulo-ruminal cycle. Tactile stimulation of the reticulum and its orifices accelerated the omasal cycles as well as reticulo-ruminal cycles and sudden distension of a balloon in the omasum or introduction of fluid into the abomasum often resulted in a marked reduction in rate of contraction.

Laplace (1970) indicates that omasal motility shows an association between food intake and omasal filling and between rumination and omasal emptying and this author concludes that the omasum plays a regulating role in transit of ingesta and in rumination behavior. Bueno and Ruckebusch (1974), using sheep with surgically placed balloons and/or strain gauges, observed two patterns of contraction. One, confined to the oral and middle thirds of the organ, originated at the omasal groove and proceeded to the right and then left surfaces and ceased at the onset of reticular contraction. The other was limited to the third of the organ near the abomasum. In this part, the contractions were prolonged regardless of the reticular contraction. The characteristic cyclic motility of the omasum (Fig. 6-24) was slightly reduced in sheep fasted for 48 hr. Water restriction resulted in prolonged irregular contractions which were reestablished to normal by drinking. Motility was affected by normal activity. During feeding, the contractions of the omasal body increased in frequency in parallel with those of the reticulum. Cycles/min observed in two sheep were: 1.02-1.05 during rest; 1.40-1.60 while eating, and 1.-6-1.09 while ruminating. These authors point out that rumination periods usually finish with two or three long intervals between contractions and, subsequently, by prolonged contractions of the omasal body.

Pressure waves from the reticulo-omasal orifice indicated it always dilated strongly during the second phase of reticular contraction and also during the extra-reticular contraction associated with regurgitation. Alternating opening and closing movements were seen at a frequency of 5-7/min. Contractions of the omasal leaves were also demonstrated, these being independent of contractions of the omasal body and which occurred at 2-3/min. These contractions passed from the free border to the base and traveled in an aboral (away from the mouth) direction. It was also shown that local application of fatty acids increased the frequency of leaf contraction.

Other papers presenting data on omasal motility include those of Ohga et al (1965), Newhook and Titchen (1972) and Zieba (1972).

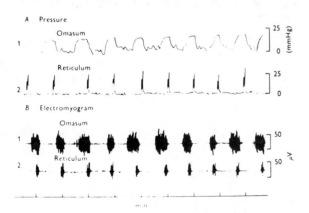

Figure 6-24. Motility of the omasum and the reticulum. A, pressure changes recorded in a sheep at rest from one small balloon inserted midway along the greater curvature of the omasum [1] and another between the muscular layers of the ventral pole of the reticulum [2]. B, electromyograms recorded from electrodes situated in close proximity to the balloons. From Bueno and Ruckebusch [1974].

Abomasal Motility

In terms of normal motility, the abomasum has largely been ignored, although an appreciable amount of information is available on factors affecting flow through it (see Ch. 7). Generally, the contractions of the abomasum resemble those seen in the simple stomach. The fundus is usually quiet, but the body shows numerous peristaltic waves. The phyloric part shows peristaltic waves and, at times, several may be traveling simultaneously. Based on fluoroscopic studies of animals consuming meals with barium, Phillipson (1970) states that activity of the walls of the filled abomasum is confined mainly to the pyloric antrum. Strong waves of contraction can be seen to pass over this part of the stomach but the main body remains relatively inactive. In young lambs, strong contractions of the body of the stomach can occasionally be seen before a meal when they are hungry, while the reticulum lifts the part of the abomasum immediately adjacent to it when it contracts. Electromyographic studies (Ruckebusch and Kay, 1971) show that electrical activity consists of a rhythmic discharge which was much more frequent than the cycles of the forestomach.

Abomasum activity is influenced by the contents of the duodenum and can be inhibited by the introduction of a number of substances into the duodenum, such as fat emulsions and weak acid solutions (see Ch. 7 for further detail).

Intestinal Motility

Studies of intestinal motility have also been rare in ruminants although a considerable amount of information is available on passage of digesta. Electromyographic studies (Dardillat and Ruckebusch, 1973; Ruckebusch and Bueno, 1973) have identified three types of waves of contraction — dispersed, propulsive (peristalsis) and segmental — at the gastroduodenal junction. It was suggested that the difference between propulsive waves and segmental seems to lie mainly in the speed at which the contraction wave moves down the intestine. Segmental contractions, which normally occurred every 40 min, decreased in frequency during digestion of milk, although not during fasting. When calves were weaned onto hay, segmental contractions increased by >30%. In older calves the number and velocity of contractions in the lower small intestine were reduced.

In the cecum, fluoroscopic studies of lambs (Phillipson, 1970) show peristaltic and antiperistaltic movements which originate at the ileocecal junction and pass to the apex of the organ and return. Periods of quiescence, slow movement and of great activity have been observed; in the high activity period, 6-15 movements have been noted in a 10 min period. Berehoiu (cited by Ash, 1969) described a total contraction of the cecum which forces cecal contents into the sigmoid colon. Successive contractions at 12-20 min intervals occurred until the cecum was almost empty. Svendsen and Kristensen (1970) have observed cecal activity in Jersey cows with cecal fistula. When fed hay, contractions occurred at the rate of 13.6/min; this decreased to 8.2/min when cows were fed grain. With rams (Svendsen, 1972) it observed that an 0.1 mM solution of VFA increased cecal motility; 1.0 mM slightly and 10 mM solutions strongly inhibited motility.

Summary

Stomach motility, as we have seen, is a result of a complex, highly organized system that mixes ingested feed, provides for rumination and eructation, provides for bypassing the reticulo-rumen when milk is ingested, and moves ingesta into and through the omasum and abomasum.

The basic movements of the reticulo-rumen, called primary contractions, are designed to circulate ingesta in the organ and result from coordinated contractions and dilations of the various pillars and sacs. Secondary contractions are primarily involved in eructation of rumen gas; a substantial variety of motility patterns may occur that have been related to species differences, ingestion of feed, eructation, rumination, fasting and water deprivation.

Rumination provides an opportunity for the animal to rechew hastily ingested feed, although its value to the domestic animal is difficult to calculate. Animals may commonly spend about a third of their time in rumination depending upon the nature of the diet. Rumination appears to be stimulated by the presence of coarse material in the stomach, but there is evidence which certainly indicates that rumen chemistry is a factor. Eructation, on the other hand, is stimulated by pressure of gas in the stomach and is a necessary adjunct to a system that depends on pregastric fermentation by microorganisms.

Data on the omasum indicates that it contracts in coordination with reticulo-rumen cycles, although in a slower, more deliberate manner. Abomasal contractions appear to be similar to those of the monogastric stomach as do those of the small intestine. Sheep and cattle apparently have well coordinated contractions allowing ingesta to be moved into and out of the cecum.

References Cited

Alderson, N.E., G.E. Mitchell, C.O. Little and J.L. Call. 1972. J. Animal Sci. 35:102.
Andersson, B., R. Kitchell and N. Persson. 1958. Acta. Physiol. Scand. 44:92.
Arnold, G.W. 1960. Aust. J. Agr. Res. 2:1034.
Asai, T. 1973. Jap. J. Vet. Sci. 35:239.
Asai, T. and Y. Sasaki. 1970. Tohoku Agr. Exp. Sta. Bul. 40:209.
Ash, R.W. 1969. Proc. Nutr. Soc. 28:110.
Attebery, J.T. and H.D. Johnson. 1969. J. Animal Sci. 29:734.
Augusto, G. and P. Vallenas. 1956. Amer. J. Vet. Res. 17:79.
Baccari, F., M.R.G. Kuchembuck and H.M. Barros. 1970. Arq. Exc. Vet. 22:119.
Bailey, C.B. and C.C. Balch. 1961. Br. J. Nutr. 15:371.
Balch, C.C. 1952. Br. J. Nutr. 6:366.
Balch, C.C. 1955. Nature 175:940.

Balch, C.C. 1971. Br. J. Nutr. 26:383.
Balch, C.C., A. Kelly and G. Heim. 1951. Br. J. Nutr. 5:207.
Bell, F.R. 1958. J. Physiol. 142:503.
Bell, F.R. 1961. In: Digestive Physiology and Nutrition of the Ruminant, Butterworths.
Bell, F.R. and A.M. Lawn. 1955. J. Physiol. 128:577.
Bell, F.R. and A.M. Lawn. 1957. Br. J. Animal Behavior 5:125.
Benzie, D. and A.T. Phillipson. 1957. The Alimentary Tract of the Ruminant. Oliver and Boyd. Pub. Co.
Bhattachrayya, N.K. and D.N. Mullick. 1965. Indian J. Exp. Biol. 3:255.
Borgatti, G. and R. Matscher. 1956. Nutr. Abstr. Rev. 27:414.
Bost, J. 1970. In: Physiology of Digestion and Metabolism in the Ruminant. Oriel Press, Newcastle upon Tyne, England.
Bowen, J.M. 1962. Amer. J. Vet. Res. 23:948.
Bueno, L. and Y. Ruckebusch. 1974. J. Physiol. 238:295.
Burger, M. 1967. Nutr. Abstr. Rev. 37:751.
Campling, R.C. 1966. Br. J. Nutr. 20:25.
Castle, M.E., A.S. Foot and R.J. Halley. 1950. J. Dairy Res. 17:215.
Clark, C.H. 1953. Amer. J. Vet. Res. 14:376.
Clark, R. 1956. J. So. African Vet. Med. Assoc. 27:79.
Cole, H.M. et. al. 1945. J. Animal Sci. 4:183.
Colvin, H.W., P.T. Cupps and H.H. Cole. 1958. J. Dairy Sci. 41:1565.
Colvin, H.W. and L.B. Daniels. 1965. J. Dairy Sci. 48:934.
Comline, R.S. and D.A. Titchen. 1961. In: Digestive Physiology and Nutrition of the Ruminant. Butterworths.
Dardillat, C. and Y. Ruckebusch. 1973. Ann. Rech. Veter. 4:31.
Dougherty, R.W. 1961. In: Digestive Physiology and Nutrition of the Ruminant. Butterworths.
Dougherty, R.W. 1968. Ann. N.Y. Academy Sci. 150:22.
Dougherty, R.W. and H.M. Cook. 1962. Amer. J. Vet. Res. 23:997.
Dougherty, R.W. and R.E. Habel. 1955. Cornell Vet. 45:459.
Dougherty, R.W. and C.D. Meredith. 1955. Amer. J. Vet. Res. 16:96.
Dougherty, R.W. and A. Vallenas. 1968. Cornell Vet. 58:3.
Dougherty, R.W., R.E. Habel and H.E. Bond. 1958. Amer. J. Vet. Res. 19:115.
Dougherty, R.W., J. Hill, H.M. Cook and J.L. Riley. 1971. Amer. J. Vet. Res. 32:1247.
Dougherty, R.W., C.H. Mullenax and M.J. Allison. 1965. In: Physiology of Digestion in the Ruminant. Butterworths.
Downie, H.G. 1954. Amer. J. Vet. Res. 15:217.
Dracy, A.E., A.J. Kurtenback, D.E. Sander and L.F. Bush. 1972. J. Dairy Sci. 55:1156.
Duncan, D.L. 1953. J. Physiol. 119:157.
Dziuk, H.E. 1965. Amer. J. Physiol. 208:343.
Dziuk, H.E., B.A. Fashingbauer and J.M. Idstrom. 1963. Amer. J. Vet. Res. 24:772.
Dziuk, H.E. and E.H. McCauley. 1965. Amer. J. Physiol. 209:324.
Dziuk, H.E. and A.F. Sellers. 1955. Amer. J. Vet. Res. 16:411.
Flatt, W.O., R.G. Warner and J.K. Loosli. 1959. Cornell U. Agr. Exp. Sta. Memoir #361.
Freer, M. and R.C. Campling. 1965. Br. J. Nutr. 19:195.
Freer, M., R.C. Campling and C.C. Balch. 1962. Br. J. Nutr. 16:279.
Fuller, J.M. 1928. N. Hamp. Agr. Expt. Sta. Tech. Bul. 35.
Gordon, J.G. 1958. J. Agr. Sci. 50:34.
Gordon, J.G. 1961. Animal Behav. 9:16.
Gordon, J.G. 1965. J. Agr. Sci. 64:31.
Gordon, J.G. and I.K. McAllister. 1970. J. Agr. Sci. 74:291.
Graham, N. McC. 1964. Aust. J. Agr. Res. 15:384.
Habel, R.E. 1956. Cornell Vet. 46:555.
Hardison, W.A., H.L. Fisher, G.C. Graf and N.R. Thompson. 1956. J. Dairy Sci. 39:1735.
Hodgson, J. 1971a. Animal Prod. 13:15.
Hodgson, J. 1971b. Animal Prod. 13:25.
Holtenius, P., S.O. Jacobsson and G. Jonson. 1971a. Acta Vet. Scand. 12:313.
Holtenius, P., S.O. Jacobsson and G. Jonson. 1971b. Acta Vet. Scand. 12:325.
Iggo, A. 1951. J. Physiol. 115:74.
Jean-Blain, C., R. Boivin and J. Bost. 1972. Nutr. Abstr. Rev. 42:512.
Johnstone-Wallace, D.B. 1953. J. Roy. Agr. Soc. England. 114:11.
Johnstone-Wallace, D.B., and K. Kennedy. 1944. J. Agr. Sci. 34:190.
Kay, R.N.B. 1959. Nature 183:552.
Kay, R.N.B. 1960. J. Physiol. 150:515.
Kay, R.N.B. 1972. Rowett Institute. Personal Communication.
Kay, R.N.B. and Y. Ruckebusch. 1971. Br. J. Nutr. 26:301.
Krzywanek, H. 1968. Nutr. Abstr. Rev. 38:462.
Laplace, J.P. 1970. Physiol. Behav. 5:61.
Lawlor, M.J., S.P. Hopkins and J.K. Kealy. 1971. Br. J. Nutr. 26:439.
Leek, B.F. 1969. J. Physiol. 202:585.
Lofgreen, G.P., J.H. Meyer and J.L. Hull. 1957. J. Animal Sci. 16:773.
Lupien, P.J., F. Sauer and G.V. Hatina. 1962. J. Dairy Sci. 45:210.
Mahipaul, S.K. and B. Mishra. 1971. J. Res. Punjab Agr. Univ. 8:125.
Mooney, G.A., H.D. Radloff and J.J. Cupal. 1971. Proc. West. Sec. Amer. Soc. Animal Sci. 22:255.

Morillo, F.J. and J. DeAlba. 1960. Cornell Vet. 50:66.
Nesic, P. 1961. Nutr. Abstr. Rev. 31:113.
Newhook, J.C. and D.A. Tichen. 1972. J. Physiol. 222:407.
Nickols, R.E. 1951. Amer. J. Vet. Res. 12:199.
Ohga, A., Y. Ota and Y. Nakazato. 1965. Jap. J. Vet. Sci. 27:153.
Ørskov, E.R., D. Benzie and R.N.B. Kay. 1970. Br. J. Nutr. 24:785.
Pearce, G.R. 1965a. Aust. J. Agr. Res. 16:635.
Pearce, G.R. 1965b. Aust. J. Agr. Res. 16:649.
Pearce, G.R. 1965c. Aust. J. Agr. Res. 16:837.
Pearce, G.R. and R.J. Moir. 1963. Aust. J. Agr. Res. 16:635.
Pharr, L.D., H.W. Colvin and P.R. Noland. 1967. J. Animal Sci. 26:414.
Phillipson, A.T. 1939. Quart. J. Exp. Physiol. 29:395.
Phillipson, A.T. 1970. In: Dukes' Physiology of Domestic Animals. 8th ed. Comstock Publ. Associates, Ithaca, N.Y.
Phillipson, A.T. and C.S.W. Reid. 1960. Proc. Nutr. Soc. 19:XXVII (abstr).
Reid, C.S.W. 1963. Proc. N.A. Soc. Animal Prod. 23:169.
Reid, C.S.W. and J.B. Cornwall. 1959. Proc. N.Z. Soc. Animal Prod. 19:23.
Riek, R.F. 1954. Aust. Vet. J. 30:29.
Rousseau, J.P. 1971. Ann. Biol. Anim. Bioch. Biophys. 11:283.
Ruckebusch, Y. 1971. Separatum Experientia 27:1185.
Ruckebusch, Y. and L. Bueno. 1972. Ann. Rech. Veter. 3:399.
Ruckebusch, Y. and L. Bueno. 1973. Br. J. Nutr. 30:401.
Ruckebusch, Y. and M. Candau. 1969. Nutr. Abstr. Rev. 39:1140.
Ruckebusch, Y., J. Fargeas and J.P. Dumas. 1970. Revue Med. Vet. 121:345.
Ruckebusch, Y. and R.N.B. Kay. 1971a. Ann. Biol. Anim. Bioch. Biophys. 11:282.
Ruckebusch, Y. and R.N.B. Kay. 1971b. Ann. Rech. Vet. 2:99.
Ruckebusch, Y. and J.P. Laplace. 1967. C.R. Soc. Biol. 161:1581.
Ruckebusch, Y., J.P. Laplace, J.P. Perret and Y. Doare. 1966. C.R. Soc. Biol. 160:2334.
Ruckebusch, Y. and J.P. Marquet. 1965. C.R. Soc. Biol. 159:394.
Ruckebusch, Y. and T. Tomov. 1973. J. Physiol. 235:447.
Schake, L.M. and J.K. Riggs. 1969. J. Animal Sci. 28:568.
Schake, L.M. and J.K. Riggs. 1970. J. Animal Sci. 31:414.
Schalk, A.F. and F.S. Amadon. 1928. N. Dakota Agr. Exp. Sta. Bul. 216.
Sellers, A.F. and C.E. Stevens. 1966. Physiol. Rev. 46:634.
Sellers, A.F. and D.A. Titchen. 1959. Nature 184:645.
Stephens, D.B. and B.A. Baldwin. 1971. Res. Vet. Sci. 12:219.
Stevens, C.E. and A.F. Sellers. 1959. Amer. J. Vet. Res. 20:461.
Stevens, C.E. and A.F. Sellers. 1960. Amer. J. Physiol. 199:598.
Stevens, C.E. and A.F. Sellers. 1968. Handbook of Physiology, Section 6, Alimentary Canal. Amer. Physiol. Soc., Washington, D.C.
Stevens, C.E., A.F. Sellers and F.A. Spurrell. 1960. Amer. J. Physiol. 198:449.
Svendsen, P. 1972. Nord. Vet. 24:393.
Svendsen, P. and B. Kristensen. 1970. Nord. Vet. 22:578.
Swanson, E.W. and J.D. Harris. 1958. J. Dairy Sci. 41:1768.
Tamate, H., A.D. McGilliard, N.L. Jacobson and R. Getty. 1962. J. Dairy Sci. 45:4-8.
Titchen, D.A. and C.S.W. Reid. 1965. In: Physiology of Digestion in the Ruminant. Butterworths, Washington, D.C.
Vallenas, A.P. and C.E. Stevens. 1971. Amer. J. Physiol. 220:275.
Voskuil, G.C.J. and J.H.M. Metz. 1973. Neth. J. Agr. Sci. 21:256.
Wagnon, K.A. 1963. Calif. Agr. Expt. Sta. Bul. 799.
Watson, R.H. 1944. Bul. Comm. Sci. Ind. Res. Austral. 180.
Webster, W.M. and E. Cresswell. 1957. Vet Rec. 69:527.
Weiss, K.E. 1953. Onderstepoort J. Vet. Res. 26:251.
Welch, J.G. and A.M. Smith. 1968. J. Animal Sci. 27:1734.
Welch, J.G. and A.M. Smith. 1969a. J. Animal Sci. 28:813.
Welch, J.G. and A.M. Smith. 1969b. J. Animal Sci. 28:827.
Welch, J.G. and A.M. Smith. 1970. J. Dairy Sci. 53:797.
Welch, J.G. and A.M. Smith. 1971. J. Animal Sci. 33:1118.
Welch, J.G., A.M. Smith and K.S. Gibson. 1970. J. Dairy Sci. 53:89.
Weston, R.H. and J.P. Hogan. 1967. Aust. J. Agr. Res. 18:789.
Williams, E.I. 1955. Vet. Rec. 67:907.
Winship, D.H., F.F. Zboralski, W.N. Weber and K.H. Soergel. 1964. Amer. J. Physiol. 207:1189.
Wise, G.H. and G.W. Anderson. 1939. J. Dairy Sci. 22:697.
Zieba, D. 1972. Weterynaria 27:67.

CHAPTER 7 — PASSAGE OF DIGESTA THROUGH THE GASTRO-INTESTINAL TRACT

Experimental work on the passage of food through the ruminant GIT is not new. Balch (1961) cites work by two Germans, Colin in 1886 and Wester in 1926 on this topic, and Hungate (1966) cites work by Wildt in 1874. There has been quite a bit of recent work on this topic beginning about 1950. For reviews on the subject, the reader is referred to Hyden (1961), Balch and Campling (1965), Phillipson and Ash (1965), Hungate (1966; pp 209-223), Ash (1969) and Bost (1970).

When studying the passage of digesta, it is usually necessary to use markers or cannulas through which the flow can be measured in some manner. A wide variety of markers has been used including internal ones (natural feed components) such as lignin, chromogens (plant pigments), iron and silica. The use of such compounds, which are presumed to not be absorbed to any extent, allows the calculation of change in concentration of nutrients or water as ingesta progresses through the gut. For example, if the concentration of lignin/unit of dry sample obtained from the rumen is less than that from the omasum, it implies that ingesta has disappeared in the rumen. Such analyses can be carried out on the basis of fluid samples by which estimates can be made of absorption or secretion of fluid into the GIT, or on dried samples from which partial digestion can be estimated.

External markers such as chromic oxide, labeled chromic oxide, a Cr-EDTA complex, a gold-resin complex, cerium or cesium, various dyes, stained feed particles, polyethylene particles or other plastics, and polyethylene glycol have been used at different times in different laboratories. The plastics and dyes have been used primarily to determine the rate of passage or the time required for complete excretion of a single meal. Chromic oxide and other metals have been used for this purpose as well as to detect changes in concentration of nutrients passing through the gut, and polyethylene glycol has been used to estimate fluid changes in the gut.

These reference substances vary widely in physical and chemical characteristics. They may be solids, soluble in the fluids of the GIT, or be component parts of the food or complexed to it. As Hyden (1961) notes, the different types of markers will pass through a section of the GIT at different rates and the usefulness of different types is restricted to the study of particles with similar physical characteristics. This is especially true with regard to passage out of the rumen and through the omasum.

Passage of Digesta From the Rumen

The importance of the relatively large amount of fluids (with digesta in solution or suspension) passing into and out of the rumen (and other parts of the GIT) is aptly stated by Phillipson and Ash (1965):

"It needs little thought to appreciate that the maintenance of an adequate flow of liquid through the stomach and intestines is essential in order to transport the solid matter of the digesta, so that account has to be taken of the quantities of water added by the alimentary glands to the digesta and of the quantities absorbed. The propulsive movements of the stomach and gut, although constituting the motive force for the movement of digesta, are influenced by the volume of material present inside them or in other parts of the canal. An appreciation of the mechanisms concerned with the flow of digesta has to consider both aspects."

After ingested food reaches the reticulum, contractions of the reticulum, reticulo-ruminal fold and the cranial sac very effectively move coarse, fibrous ingesta into the dorsal sac of the rumen where it may remain for some time. Following a meal of hay, examination of a fistulated bovine will reveal a rather tightly packed mass in the upper part of the dorsal sac. Thereafter, contractions of the various sacs tend to move some of the ingesta in somewhat of a circular fashion, particularly the more fluid portions. The contents of the reticulo-rumen are more fluid (lower dry matter content) towards the ventral and cranial parts. Each contraction of the rumen will force liquid into the upper part of the dorsal sac with the result that the ingesta is periodically bathed by the rumen fluids. It appears likely that the material in the ventral sac, which is more fluid and contains finer particles, is either soon regurgitated or passed on into the omasum. An example of stratification of ingesta possible in the reticulo-rumen is shown in Fig. 7-1 (Sisson and Grossman, 1953).

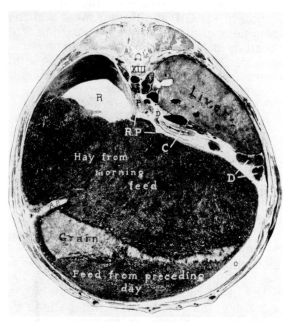

Figure 7-1. Stratification of ingesta in the reticulo-rumen. Picture of a cross section through the last thoracic vertebra. This animal was well fed the evening before embalming; the following morning a feed of cracked corn, followed by all the hay she desired, then embalmed, frozen, and sectioned. From Sisson and Grossman [1953]. Courtesy of Saunders Pub. Co.

Fluid Exchange in the Reticulo-Rumen

The net exchange of fluid in the reticulo-rumen is rather large and would be expected to have a substantial effect on passage of solids from the stomach. Quantitative estimates of salivary production (Ch. 5)

indicate that 6+ l. of saliva enters the reticulo-rumen in the sheep and >100 l. in adult cows. There are also indications that water may be secreted through the walls of the rumen, but quantitative estimates of this fraction are uncertain. Estimates of passage of digesta from the reticulo-rumen have been published by a number of authors. However, the animals used, rations fed and methods employed have varied appreciably with the result that the range in estimated flow is rather wide.

When using disappearance of polyethylene glycol (PEG) as a basis of estimation, Hydén (1961) calculated that about 7 l./24 hr passed from the rumen of sheep fed twice daily on hay or hay and meal. This is equivalent to ca. 300 ml/hr or a flow rate of ca. 6.4% of estimated rumen fluid volume/hr, or a turnover rate of a little more than once per day. In the case of a hay-fed cow (530 kg body wt) the mean rumen fluid volume was 50 l. and the flow was 150-170 l./24 hr. During the period of daylight, the flow rate was approximately 13-15% of fluid volume/hr and somewhat less at night. In the case of fasted sheep, flow rate declined to ca. 2% of fluid volume/hr after 40-50 hr.

Corbett et al (1959) studied flow rate in cattle fed pellets impregnated with chromic oxide and PEG in addition to a daily ration of grass hay. Average flow rate was ca. 18% of fluid volume/hr, a value equivalent to a turnover rate of ca. 4.2 times/day. Tulloh et al (1965), using PEG, estimated flow rates to be 6-15 l./hr in grazing cattle (twins), or 20-33%/hr. The flow rate for milking cows was 30-50% higher than for the dry twin. In other studies with cattle, Poutiainen (1968) calculated that rumen fluid outflow amounted to ca. 2.5-9 l./hr in adult cows, as feed intake increased from 3-14 kg/day. Volume was affected by amount of dry matter consumed and physical nature of the feed. With most diets, flow was faster by day than at night. With Hereford steers (weight not given), Mangan and Wright (1968) calculated a loss of marker (PEG or lithium sulfate) from the rumen to be from 4.6 to 7.9%/hr, values equivalent to a flow rate ranging from 2.8 l. to 4.2 l./hr.

Sutherland et al (1962) devised apparatus to circulate rumen contents with a pump via a rumen fistula in order to keep rumen contents well mixed. With this apparatus they found that the decrease in concentration of PEG was linear within 30 min after introduction into the rumen. In the case of sheep weighing 55 kg and fed 1 kg of finely ground pellets in two meals/day and drinking 2-3 l. of water daily, they found outflow from the rumen to be about 6 kg, or 250 g/hr, a somewhat lower value than reported by Hydén. Ulyatt (1964) estimated the flow rates from sheep grazing a variety of pastures with the aid of PEG. From his data he calculated that 650-900 ml/hr passed out of the rumen, values equivalent to 20-24% of estimated rumen volume. Turnover time would thus be 4-5 hr.

Hogan (1964) studied flow from the reticulo-rumen of sheep by reference to radiochromium complexed with EDTA which was slowly infused into the rumen. When fed a variety of diets, estimated rate of low varied from 5.8-18.0 l./day. For most diets the flow varied from 8-14 l./day for dry diets and green fodders. With adult sheep given dry feed 1X daily, Mangan and Wright (1968) estimated loss of markers from the rumen to be in the range of 4.9-6.9%/hr, or on a volume basis, 320 to 360 ml/hr.

Engelhardt (1963, 1964) has investigated secretion of water into the rumen and flow out of the rumen by using tritiated water and PEG, respectively, in goats. He calculated that about 40 l. of water passed through the rumen wall in each direction, averaging 55 ml/cm^2/hr (in vitro estimate), although estimates were quite variable. Passage of fluids out of the rumen via the omasum averaged 390 ml/hr for a turnover time of about 10 hr. The addition of urea or ammonia to the rumen, resulting in rumen osmotic pressure values comparable to blood, reduced flow of water into the rumen. Ternouth (1967) has also shown that substantial amounts of water may pass into the rumen through the wall. His data indicate a flow into the rumen after feeding whether the ingesta is hyper-osmolar or hypo-osmolar with respect to serum, with maximum inflow occurring 6-7 hr after feeding.

There is some question as to the route taken by ingested water. Schalk and Amadon (1928) state that during water deprivation (or refusal of water) the reticulo-rumen contents provide water to other tissues. When water is given to the thirsty animal, the rumen and reticular cavities are the first to be flooded by the fresh supply and a rapid transfer of liquids could be detected (by the hand) from the reticulum to the omasum (ibid). This movement of fluid was said to occur

independently of the reticulo-rumen motility and these authors found that an aspiratory action was exerted upon the contents of the ventral part of the reticulum. Wise and Anderson (1939) found that water, consumed from an open pail by calves, frequently flowed from the cardia into the rumen in amounts almost equal to the quantity consumed, indicating that most of it was delayed, at least for a time, in the rumen. Nanda and Singh (1941) state that small amounts of water flowed directly into the abomasum when given to sheep held off food and water for several days. However, Watson (1944) found, when using X-ray techniques, that 90-100% of ingested water passed into the reticulo-rumen of sheep which had been deprived of food and water for a period of time. He further stated that liquids passing through the reticulo-omasal orifice generally do not pass between the omasal leaves. Phillipson and Ash (1965) quote results from a thesis by Briggs regarding water passage from the rumen. When a sheep with an omasal cannula drank water, gushes (18-100 ml) of cool fluid flowed from the omasum during or immediately after drinking. This indicates a differential flow stimulated by drinking which represents a different pattern of flow than that normally observed from the omasum (see subsequent section). Presumably, a substantial amount of freshly drunk water must enter the reticulo-rumen since drinking cold water results in a marked reduction in the rumen temperature (Cunningham et al, 1964). The relative osmolality of the rumen and blood may be a modifying factor and, perhaps, accounts for some of the variance in the reports cited.

Passage of Solids From the Reticulo-Rumen

The passage of solids from the reticulo-rumen appears to be more complicated than that of fluids. A number of physical characteristics influences passage as well as the rapidity and extent of digestion which occurs in the rumen. Probably the best estimates can be made on indigestible (or undigested) material, but this may not be a good estimate of the outflow of digestible nutrients, which probably would be intermediate between the pattern of fluids and solids.

The rapidity with which markers such as chromic oxide and monastral blue (a dye) may pass down the tract was demonstrated by Lambourne (1957). A sheep grazing on forage was dosed with chromic oxide 1.5 hr and with monastral blue 0.5 hr before being slaughtered. Observations and analysis of gut contents indicated that some of the monastral blue had progressed as far as the omasum and the chromic oxide two-thirds of the length of the small intestine. Fibrous materials such as stained hay do not, however, appear to move as rapidly as this. In the case of goats, Castle (1956) found that 11-15 hr were required for the appearance of stained hay to appear in the feces, and Stielau (1967) observed particles in sheep feces as early as 10 hr after consumption. With cows, Balch (1950) found that stained hay appeared in the feces 12-24 hr after feeding, depending upon the physical nature of the hay. O'Dell et al (1963) reported similar results with minimal times varying from 12 to about 20 hr. Murray et al (1962) used a circulating pump to mix rumen contents in sheep. With this technique they reported that outflow of finely ground digesta reached a maximum 1-2.5 hr after feeding and showed a second peak in the period 7-10 hr after feeding.

These various experiments, although differing in many respects, indicate that some ingested feed passes very rapidly out of the reticulo-rumen, through the omasum, and on down the GIT. The physical nature of the feed appears to be a most important factor controlling the rapidity with which it leaves the rumen. Schalk and Amadon (1928) felt that specific gravity of the solid ingesta was the determining factor as regards the route to be followed from the cardia to the reticulo-omasal orifice. Other factors that are known to influence the passage of ingesta from the rumen include the particle size, the rapidity or ease with which the food is digested and the level of feed intake. These are discussed more fully in later sections.

Time Spent in the Reticulo-Rumen

The amount of time the average feed particle spends in the rumen is difficult to determine because of the uncertainty of how long it may stay in the omasum. Piana (1952) has provided some information on this by studying retention time in sheep which had

their rumens surgically removed. The first appearance of marker (fuchsin) was 6 hr after feeding chopped oats; the maximum amount was on the second and third days and the final appearance was on the 6th day. Particle size of excreted particles increased from the first to the 5th day. With normal sheep, the first traces of dye were found after 22 hr; the maximum excretion was on the second and third days and the final appearance was after 19 days. Thus, these data indicate that the rumen causes a delay of some 16 hr in initial appearance of the marker, but has little effect on time of maximum excretion as maximal levels occurred on the second and third days in both cases. Final excretion was delayed considerably in intact animals. Retention time in the omasum would be a maximum of 6 days minus 6 hr and maximum time in the rumen would be 19 days minus 6 days, or 13 days.

Balch and Campling (1965) cite a number of examples of their data with dairy cows indicating that the mean retention time in the reticulo-rumen and omasum is on the order of 60-80 hr depending upon the nature of the diet. Feedstuffs, such as straws, which are resistant to digestion, may be excreted in the feces over a very long period of time; in some cases for 10 days after the feed was consumed. Hungate (1966, pp 224-225, 242) has tabulated data from a number of sources and has calculated rumen turnover time. For cattle, the times ranged from 1.3 to 3.7 days, with most values being on the order of 2.1-2.7 days, or about 50-60 hr. For sheep the calculated times are less, ranging from 0.8-2.2 days, with most values being slightly over one day.

In research with sheep, Ingalls et al (1966) fed various forages and the sheep were killed either 6 or 12 hr after a meal or following a 12 hr period of ad libitum access to feed. Passage from the rumen was expressed as retention time and calculated by dividing the amount of the constituent in the rumen by the daily intake of the constituent. Legumes had a lower retention time than grasses. The values for dry matter being (days): alfalfa, 0.62; trefoil, 0.68; timothy, 0.84; and canary grass, 0.94 (means of 6 and 12 hr samples). For the four different forages, retention time of dry matter averaged 0.83 days for the 6 hr time and 0.71 days for the 12 hr time. In vitro data from other sources clearly show that legumes are attacked more rapidly in the rumen than grasses; consequently, we would anticipate more rapid turnover. The 12 hr values, of course, should show a lower retention time than the 6 hr times but, if expressed on a rate basis, the 6 hr values would probably be much higher.

Minson (1966) has calculated retention times for a variety of forages when fed at hourly intervals to sheep by removing rumen contents about 30 min after the last feeding. Data indicated that organic matter was retained for 10-25 hr and N for 12-61 hr. Increasing the level of intake reduced the retention time for both constituents. Weston (1968) found mean retention times (sheep) to be 36.3 hr for straw and 10.8 for alfalfa. In the case of the straw, he calculated that 17.7 hr were required to degrade straw to a size that

could readily pass out of the rumen, and that 16.6 hr were spent in "residence" in the rumen and omasum as small particles.

Relatively recent data on sheep (Hogan and Weston, 1971; Weston and Hogan, 1971), which were given ^{51}Cr-EDTA, indicate that passage out of the rumen is affected markedly by level of feeding (Table 7-1). Data from these papers indicate that flow from the rumen was higher for a second cutting than for a first cutting (not shown in table) and also between different clovers harvested at early or late maturity. Although the time the marker stayed in the rumen was not drastically different between treatments (clovers or harvests), increasing the feeding level with straw resulted in a more rapid turnover.

Table 7-1. Effect of different treatments on flow from the rumen and abomasum and on rumen volume and marker residence time.

	Treatment		
	Alkali-treated straw[a]		
	Level of feeding		
Item	High	Medium	Low
Organic matter intake, g/day	723	444	310
Flow from rumen, l./day	10.4	7.3	5.1
l./100 g OM intake	1.44	1.64	1.65
Rumen volume, l.	4.2	4.0	3.0
Marker residence time, hr	10.0	14.0	14.7
Flow from the abomasum, l./day	12.7	8.1	5.7

| | Clover Studies[b] | | | |
| | Early Maturity | | Late Maturity | |
	Sub. cl.[c]	Bers. cl.[c]	Sub. cl.	Bers. cl.
Organic matter intake, g/day	1095	960	689	925
Flow from the rumen, l./day	11.4	12.8	11.6	14.6
l./100 g OM intake	1.04	1.33	1.68	1.58
Rumen volume, l.	5.46	4.66	3.86	4.41
Marker residence time in rumen, hr	9.2	11.1	11.9	11.8
Flow from the abomasum, l./day	20.3	23.3	15.1	16.6
Ratio of flow from abomasum to flow from rumen	1.78	1.82	1.30	1.13

[a] Data from Hogan and Weston (1971)
[b] Data from Weston and Hogan (1971)
[c] Subterranean and Berseem clovers

It would be expected that the passage of solids out of the reticulo-rumen would be markedly affected by contraction of the reticulo-omasal orifice. While this has not been shown experimentally, Bueno (1972) has shown that fluid flow can be increased by 2.2 to 2.7X by keeping the orifice open with a cannula.

It is interesting to note the difference in rumen retention time between sheep and cattle. Speculation as to the reason would indicate several possibilities: (1) that sheep chew their food more thoroughly than cattle; however, the particle size resulting from mastication may not be smaller in relation to the size of the reticulo-omasal orifice; (2) that the greater selectivity of sheep when ingesting feed may result in more digestible diets; (3) that rumen metabolism of the sheep is more rapid or (4) that digesta may be held for less time in the omasum since the omasum in cattle contains a greater relative amount of stomach contents and many more leaves than in sheep. As a general rule, as the rate of passage increases digestibility is somewhat reduced. However, the turnover rate in the rumen (and other segments of the GIT) is of importance in that it has a controlling action on the amount of forage that can and will be ingested. An increased intake of feed and the more rapid passage associated with it will usually more than compensate for a slight reduction in digestibility insofar as resulting in an increase in metabolites to the tissues and greater productivity of the animal.

Passage of Digesta From the Omasum

Data on passage of digesta from the omasum are relatively limited, although several reports are available. In order to obtain such data without compounding errors with abomasal secretions, it is necessary to get at the omasum by direct fistulation (Bost, 1957; Willes and Mendel, 1968) or to establish cannulas or re-entrant cannulas between the omasum and abomasum. This procedure is difficult because of the large opening between these two organs. Papers describing this type of technique include those of Kameoka and Morimoto (1959), Oyaert and Bouchaert (1961), Ash (1962a), and Bost (1964).

Bost (1970) points out that many experimenters have questioned how ingesta could enter the deep interlaminar spaces of the omasum, as it is often thought that the omasal canal is nearly horizontal. In addition, he points out that this is a misconception as anatomical studies and radiographic pictures have definitely shown that the omasal canal is nearly vertical (see Fig. 2-6), thus the ingesta flowing into the omasal atrium will flood the free edge of the laminae. It should also be mentioned, as illustrated in Ch. 2, that the ingesta present between the leaves of the omasum is much more uniform in size and of much smaller particle size than in the rumen, resembling dehydrated cakes of fine fibrous material. Information currently available is not sufficient to explain how this occurs. Some writers suggest that only the small particles coming from the rumen enter the intralaminar spaces, but evidence to support or refute this theory is lacking.

Ash (1962a) describes the flow of material from the omasum as being of three types: (1) oozes and trickles of a few ml of fluid devoid of solid matter and often occurring about the time of a reticular contraction; (2) gushes of 10-20 ml containing appreciable amounts of finely divided plant material and occurring at irregular intervals but between cycles of reticular contractions; or (3) the slow extrusion and "washing through" of lumps of relatively solid food. Oyaert and Bouchaert (1961) have used omasal cannulas along with the marker, PEG. They found that fluid was always expelled from the omasal cannula shortly after contractions of the reticulum. When PEG was given through a rumen fistula it took about 35-40 min for the concentration of PEG leaving the omasum to become equal to that in the rumen and thereafter the concentration leaving the omasum was higher (indicating water absorption). During 8-hr collection periods when material collected from the omasum was not returned to the abomasum, mean hourly volume ranged in 4 sheep from 380-691 ml and in 3 of them volume was greatest in the 8-hr period from 1600 to midnight. The pH of omasal fluid was consistently higher than that of rumen fluid, and the concentration of Na, K and ammonia was always lower (absorption). In acute experiments with anesthetized sheep, a considerable amount of water was shown to be absorbed from diluted rumen fluid and from several test solutions and there was absorption even from a hypertonic solution of 0.3 M concentration. Ash (1962b) found, when omasal fluid was not put into the abomasum, that the overall rate of flow from the omasum was usually high (max. 810 ml/hr) and, although continuous, random fluctuations in the volumes were observed between successive 5-10 min periods. Returning food to the abomasum approximately halved the rate of flow and tended to induce alternating periods of high and low flow from the omasum. The introduction into the rumen of 2.5-4.1 l. of the more fluid rumen fraction (5% DM) from donor sheep caused a pronounced increase in flow from the omasum within 5-12 min and the response lasted at least 2 hr. The rapid introduction of 300-400 ml of omasal fluid into the abomasum temporarily abolished the response and simultaneously reduced the force and frequency of the reticular contractions. Data demonstrated a direct relationship between flow rates and daily food and water consumption, but diets of chopped hay or dried grass produced greater flows than a diet of grass meal fed as pellets when given in equal amounts. The range of flow from sheep on all three diets when eating 750-1,100 g/day was 1,072-2,075 ml/6 hr. The effects of eating on the flow were variable but an increase usually occurred within 30 min on restricted diets, reaching a peak in 1-3 hr. Rumination had no apparent effect on the flow rate.

Kameoka and Morimoto (1959) carried out a number of experiments with Japanese goats 18 mo. to 3 yr of age which weighed 21-30 kg. When fed a variety of rations, their data indicated that flow rates were usually within the range of 150-200 ml/hr, a value which is probably equivalent to 350-400 ml/hr in sheep weighing 40-50 kg.

Benavides et al (1972) have reported using omasal-abomasal and abomasal-duodenal re-entrant cannulas in a young bull. Feed intake was very low (1.19 kg DM on the first day) and progressively decreased, so it is unlikely that flow rates given even approximate physiologically normal values.

Passage of Digesta From the Abomasum

The measurement of food passage out of the abomasum and into the duodenum can be accomplished by several means. In animals with a cannula such as that in the upper part of Fig. 7-2, it is commonly done in conjunction with a marker of some type. When the cannula is exteriorized (re-entrant cannula) such as that shown in Fig. 7-3, it can be provided with a valve for sampling contents in conjunction with a marker. In one

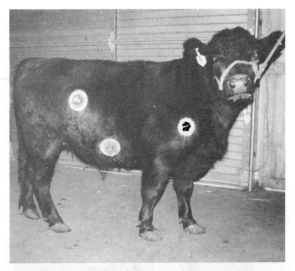

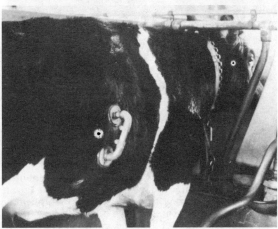

Figure 7-2. Upper. Steer with abomasal [lower] and intestinal cannulas. This type of cannula allows samples to be taken readily yet does not greatly interfer with digesta passage. Picture courtesy of C.O. Little, U. of Kentucky. Lower. A cow with a re-entrant cannula. This type may tend to restrict digesta passage, but is more useful for arriving at quantitative estimates of digesta passage.

instance, a re-entrant cannula containing an electromagnetic meter was used to measure flow rates (Ridges and Singleton, 1962). More recently, apparatus has been developed for automatically measuring flow and sampling digesta from re-entrant cannulas (Axford et al, 1971; Corse and Sutton, 1971; Thivend and Poncet, 1971; Weller et al, 1971) as illustrated in Fig. 7-4. Jones and Poulsen (1974) have used solutions of Na chromate (^{51}Cr) injected directly through the abdominal wall into the abomasum and quantitated passage rate by counting externally with a scintillation detector. Almost all of the published research with re-entrant cannulas to date has been done with sheep, goats or

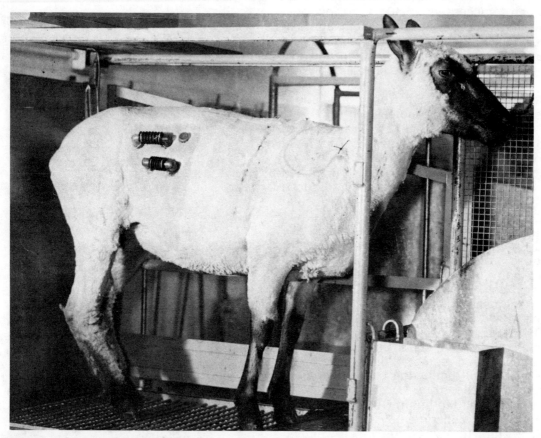

Figure 7-3. A sheep with multiple cannulas. The lower re-entrant cannula in the flank is an abomasal-duodenal cannula, in which the flow from the abomasum enters caudally and passes into the duodenum from the cranial entry. The upper cannula is a duodenal re-entrant cannula which is placed caudal to the common bile duct with flow in a caudal direction. Note the round "Thomas-type" cannula placed in front of the upper cannula; this is opposite the common bile duct and is used for collection of bile and pancreatic juices. Note the catheter on the shoulders. It goes from the thoracic lymph duct to the jugular vein and is used for studying flow of lymph, fat absorption, etc. Courtesy of F.A. Harrison, ARC, Institute of Animal Physiology, Babraham, Cambridge.

calves. Apparatus and techniques which allow continuous measurement no doubt provide more physiologically normal data than when flow is interrupted (see later section) as sampling and return of digesta alter flow rates. Some of these automated devices have been used continuously for several weeks, indicating that they must be working well.

From a historical point of view, Phillipson (1948) was the first to use abomasal-duodenal cannulas. In recent years this type of technique has been very popular and quite a number of publications are available on studies utilizing this technique with ruminant animals. For example, some of the older papers dealing with sheep include

those of Phillipson et al (1949), Phillipson (1952), Harris and Phillipson (1962), Hogan and Phillipson (1960), Badawy and Mackie (1964), and Topps et al (1968). Data on goats are given by Ridges and Singleton (1962), and papers on calves include those of Ash (1964), Phillips and Dyck (1964) and Smith (1964). Numerous others of a later vintage are available.

Studies with Sheep and Goats

Harris and Phillipson (1962) found that wethers with abomasal-duodenal re-entrant cannulas performed in a comparable manner to control sheep with respect to water and feed consumption, weight changes or digestibility. They noted that regular

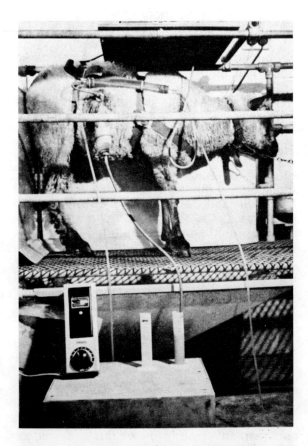

Figure 7-4. Apparatus designed to measure flow rates and sample digesta in sheep with re-entrant cannulas between the duodenum and abomasum. From Nicholson and Sutton [1969].

measurements of the flow of abomasal contents indicated an effect caused by feed ingestion and that rumination preceded an increased flow of abomasal contents (not noted with omasal studies). The average quantity of abomasal contents passed by four sheep was 398 ml/hr, and the use of chromic oxide in conjunction with the experiments indicated a recovery of 86-90%, so the flow rate was probably slightly less than might be expected. These sheep were fed on hay only. In an earlier experiment, Phillipson et al (1949) found that sheep weighing 41-68 kg and eating hay or hay and linseed meal had flow rates of 400-450 ml/hr. When the ration was changed to a 1:1 ratio of concentrate and hay, the 61-kg sheep had a flow rate of 272 ml/hr. Calculations, based on change in abomasal constituents as compared to rumen samples, indicated that abomasal juice accounted for 50-80% of abomasal contents. In another paper Hogan

and Phillipson (1960) found mean flow rate to be 360 ml/hr in sheep. Phillips and Dyck (1964) used sheep which were fed once daily. They noted that there was a monophasic diurnal flow pattern with the highest rates (400-500 ml on most rations) occurring just prior to and during feeding and the lowest rates (200-300 ml/hr) occurring 6-12 hr after feeding. There was a marked effect due to rations. However, passage was related to amount of food consumption and amount of fiber (or inversely to extent of digestible matter), averaging about 0.72-0.74 ml/g of food for high-fiber rations (75% oat straw) as compared to about 0.47-0.50 ml/g of low-fiber ration (16% straw). Topps et al (1968) found that duodenal flow rates were quite variable, observed values being 200-425 and 150-375 g/hr in sheep fed hay or concentrates, respectively. The minimal flow on the hay diet occurred from ca. 2000-2400 hr.

Harrison and Hill (1962) found that frequency of feeding had a marked effect on amount of digesta flowing from the abomasum. When sheep were fed once daily, the flow rate was ca. 270 ml/hr and increased to 785 ml/hr when fed the same ration three times daily and consuming about the same quantity of feed. In this case, collections averaging 7 hr in length may not have been representative of total daily flow. Thompson (1973) has also studied the effect of frequency of feeding. When sheep were given 900 g of a chopped straw and pelleted cereal ration and fed either 1X daily or hourly, he found flow rate into the abomasum to be considerably greater when fed hourly (av. of 8,113 and 9,156 ml/day on 2 different rations when fed hourly vs. 6,891 and 6,402 ml/day when fed 1X). Pickard (as cited by Thompson, ibid) observed a steady pattern of flow when sheep were fed 3X daily. This changed to a pattern in which up to 65% of the total daily flow occurred in the first 12 hr when the feeding regimen was changed to 1X daily. After the sheep became accustomed to the new regimen, the flow returned to a steady pattern. Pickard postulated that the rumen was emptied at a rapid rate shortly after feed was consumed in anticipation of further feeding and, when feed was not offered immediately, the rate of flow declined and the total daily digesta flow was not altered greatly by feeding.

In other studies, Thompson and Lamming (1972) found there was no consistent effect (2 sheep) when straw was given in long, chopped or ground form. Liebholz and Hartmann (1972) observed the flow of digesta to vary from 4.4 to 6.8 l./day when dry matter varied from 480-800 g/day; marked variation in flow was observed in their sheep (up to a 10-fold variation in 2-hr intervals). Other papers showing the effect of rations on flow rate into the duodenum include those of Weston and Hogan (1967, 1971) and Hogan and Weston (1971). Some of the data presented by these authors are shown in Table 7-1. The data show a marked effect of level of feeding and due to species and maturity of the forage fed to sheep.

Recent data of Ben-Ghedalia et al (1974) indicate a flow rate (0.05 m from pylorus) of 511 g/hr of which 24 g were dry matter. This was for sheep fed 2X daily on a ration with 400 g vetch hay and 600 g of concentrate.

In studies with goats, Ridges and Singleton (1962) used re-entrant cannulas equipped with an electromagnetic meter. They found flow rates to be in the range of 500-670 ml/hr.

Studies with Cattle

When working with young (2-5 wk of age) calves, Ash (1964) found that flow from the abomasum during fasting ranged from 75-218 ml/15 min. High rates occurred in the first 5-10 min when feed was given followed by a period of reduced flow. Peak flows occurred 30-60 min after a feed and again after 2-3 hr. In two calves flow 2.5 hr after a feed of 1,100 ml of milk was 1,432-1,520 ml, and in the third calf, 614-730 ml. The fat content of the milk did not appreciably affect flow rate in two of the calves, but did in the third one. Smith (1964) reported that milk was held up in the abomasum for about 0.8 hr before flowing into the duodenum in calves. Magnesium chloride reduced the retention time in the abomasum of either milk or glucose solutions. Casein had no effect, but wheat gluten caused a marked reduction in rate of emptying. No data on volume of flow were given, however. Mylrea (1966) reported that the flow from the abomasum in young calves (8-26 days of age) was about 200 ml/hr. After feeding, the flow rate increased to ca. 800 ml/hr with the maximum rate occurring in the first hour after feeding. The chyme at the site of the sample (pylorus) was thick, white and opaque before feeding, but it changed within a few minutes of feeding to a watery, greenish tinged, clear fluid with a few small fragments of milk clot. This type of chyme passed for 3-4 hr, then increasing amounts of milk clot appeared, changing by about 6 hr, to the type found before feeding.

Toullec and Mathieu (1973) have compared abomasal emptying in young calves given milk obtained early in the milking period vs. that obtained late in milking. They noted that stomach emptying was a little slower on milk from the early stage (81% passed out in 150 min vs. 64% from late-stage milk). Colvin et al (1969) found rate of passage of dry matter to be more rapid when calves were fed milk replacers containing soy flour vs whole milk, and Bell and Razig (1973) observed that glucose (3-10%) and lactose solutions (50-800 m. osmol/l.) inhibited abomasal emptying and acid production. NaCl and $NaHCO_3$ in concentrations hypotonic or isotonic with blood plasma stimulated abomasal emptying; hypertonic solutions inhibited emptying. Hypotonic solutions of KCl, $CaCl_2$, HCl and acetic acid also delayed emptying and high urea concentrations stimulated emptying.

In studies with cows, van't Klooster et al (1972) observed that flow of digesta was intermittent. Gushes varied between 100-500 ml and were separated by intervals of <1 to >15 min, but variation in hourly flow was not marked. Hourly flow rates averaged between 11.6 and 15.2 kg/hr for one cow and 8.3-9.5 for a second cow.

Passage of Digesta Through the Intestine

In the duodenum, Harrison and Hill (1962) have reported flow values in sheep. In one experiment on a single sheep, when abomasal flow was 312 ml/hr on 1X/day feeding, duodenal flow averaged 290 ml/hr. When fed 3X daily, abomasal flow averaged 885 ml/hr and duodenal flow 1,026 ml/hr. An average of three experiments for each method of feeding gave results of 273 ml and 785 ml/hr from the abomasum when fed once and three times; comparable values for duodenal flow were 263 and 864 ml/hr. When using sheep with abomasal-duodenal re-entrant cannulas and automatic sampling equipment, Nicholson and Sutton (1969) found that mean flow rates into the duodenum varied from 198 to 530 g/hr, the rates being affected by level of intake and make up of the ration (combinations of hay, dairy cubes and flaked corn). Badawy and Mackie

(1964) reported comparative values for flow from the upper and lower duodenum and the ileum of sheep fed grass, hay or hay and concentrates. Mean rates of flow of digesta in these three sites with grass were 73, 436 and 91 ml/hr, respectively. When hay was fed, the rates in the lower duodenum and ileum were 343 and 203 ml/hr, and with hay and concentrate, duodenal flow was 453 ml/hr. van't Klooster et al (1969) fed diets of different composition and amount to two sheep with re-entrant cannula in the distal duodenum. Mean flow rates ranged from 14 to 20 l./day. They noted appreciable differences between days and between sheep. Highest flow rate was before and during feeding in one sheep. In both sheep the rate tended to increase during the night, a change also observed by Topps et al (1968).

Hogan and Phillipson (1960) found a mean flow rate in the ileum of 180 ml/hr as compared to 360 ml/hr from the abomasum in sheep. Goodall and Kay (1965), using sheep with re-entrant cannulas in the terminal ileum, found flow in the terminal

45.

Grovum and Williams (1973) have used a combination of infusion of labeled Cr-EDTA and slaughter to estimate flow rates in sheep fed 400 or 1,200 g of chopped alfalfa hay. Calculated flow rates from the rumen, abomasum and small intestinal segments, each representing 20% of the total length, are shown in Table 7-2.

In sheep with multiple cannulas 0.05, 1, 3, 7, 15 and 25 m from the pylorus, Ben-Ghedalia et al (1974) found flow rates at these respective sites to be 511, 555, 433, 291, 205 and 181 g/hr; of this, water accounted for 487, 526, 408, 270, 187 and 162 g/hr.

In young calves (5-15 wk of age) Smith (1964) reported that the volume of flow from the ileum in ruminating calves was 5-10 fold that of milk-fed calves but gave no comparative data. Mylrea (1966, 1968) has investigated flow at various sites in the intestine of young calves and reported that flow rates at the duodenum were about 200 ml/hr; this increased to about 500 ml/hr after feeding.

Table 7-2. Flow rates of fluid along the GIT of sheep.[a]

Item	Rumen	Abomasum	Intestine, % of length				
			0-20	20-40	40-60	60-80	80-100
			ml/hr				
Fed 400 g/day	280	340	360	272	184	159	127
1,200 g/day	514	904	818	584	357	340	358

[a]Data from Grovum and Williams (1973)

ileum to be ca. 1.5 kg/day when the sheep were fed dried grass and ca. 2.7-2.9 kg/day when fed poor hay and concentrates or medium quality hay. Digesta flowed in discrete fractions of 20-30 ml in a series lasting 20-30 min, separated by intervals of 1-2 hr. There was no significant diurnal pattern nor any apparent effect of rumination. Dry matter of ileal effluent varied only from 6.9-8.8%, regardless of the diet. Topps et al (1968) have also used sheep with abomasal or duodenal or ileal re-entrant cannulas (different cannulas in different sheep). Mean flow rates (g/hr) when fed pelleted hay or concentrate were: abomasal, 407, 218; duodenal, 313, 200; and ileal, 190,

Data are also presented for other sites in the jejunum and the distal end of the ileum, at which point the flow was very irregular. Further studies with calves with duodenal re-entrant cannula (Ternouth and Buttle, 1973) indicated that volume of duodenal digesta increased from 5,505 to 7,709 ml/12 hr in calves from 7 to 63 days of age which consumed 3,392 to 4,930 ml of milk/day. When calves were given different types of milk replacers, duodenal digesta amounted to 6.06 to 6.22 l./12 hr. Minor differences in amount of flow were observed during the early hours after ingestion, being less with a milk replacer containing an overheated milk powder. Between 82 and 87% of the ingested fluids had passed from the abomasum in the first 6 hr after feeding (Ternouth et al, 1974).

Campling and Freer (1962) have studied the passage of rubber balls through the intestinal tract, when introduced into the abomasum. Depending on specific gravity, the minimum time found was 11 hr for cows fed dried grass. The rate of passage of particles varying in SG from 1.04-1.40 was indirectly related to density, mean values being 23-25 hr for SG of 1.02; 21-42 hr for 1.06; 32-46 hr for 1.12; and 41-61 hr for 1.21. For chromic oxide, King and Moore (1957) found average transit times of about 19 hr from the omasum until excreted by cattle. Mylrea (1966) has reported transit times for PEG in young milk-fed calves. He found that 92% of the PEG had been recovered in the 12 hr post-feeding period; the bulk of the PEG had reached the ileum by 8 hr. These data do not, however, include transit through the large intestine.

Coombe and Kay (1965) did not report rate of flow but did report that markers — discs of polyvinyl chloride, stained straw, or PEG — were retained for 2.2-4.5 hr in the small intestine of sheep, and for 10.2-26.5 hr in the large intestine. The retention times were inversely related to the dry matter intake of a particular ration. Shorter retention times were found on a hay diet than on an equal intake of more digestible dried grass (more undigested residue in the GIT). Weston (1968) calculated mean retention times in the abomasum and intestines to be 21.2 hr and 16.1 hr for straw and alfalfa, respectively, for sheep. This compares to a time of 12-14 hr for passage through the intestines of goats (Castle, 1956).

The intestine is capable of accommodating and propelling large volumes of digesta through it. Flow through the duodenum is essentially continuous while ileal flow is intermittent (Goodall and Kay, 1965) as noted earlier. Ash (1969) points out that flow through re-entrant cannula in the upper small intestine takes the form of gushes which occur in groups of about four which are separated by varying but usually short periods of quiesence. They may be followed by retrograde (backward) flow. When retrograde flow was expressed as a % of total aboral flow (away from the mouth), Singleton (1961) observed a range of 2-56% (mean 40%) in goats and 0-17% (mean 5%) in sheep. This data was obtained using an electromagnetic flowmeter in the cannula.

Digesta in the ileum flow in a steady stream toward the cecum; retrograde flow rarely occurs, although sometimes the contents remain stationary (Ash, 1969). Presumably, intermittent flow is associated with peristaltic contractions known to occur in the intestine (see Ch. 6).

Passage of Ingesta Through the GIT as a Whole

There have been numerous papers dealing with passage of food materials through the ruminant GIT as a whole. Some of these are reviewed briefly.

A good deal of the early work on food passage was done by C.C. Balch and associates. In one of his first papers (Balch, 1950), dairy cows were fed stained particles of long hay, ground hay and concentrates. Data from five experiments indicated that hay particles first appeared in the feces 12-24 hr after feeding. Excretion was characterized by a slow excretion of the first 10%, followed by a higher rate, typically resulting in passage of 80% within 70-90 hr. Seven-10 days usually elapsed before all particles were excreted. Ground hay, as a small addition to long hay, was excreted more rapidly than long hay, but completely ground hay rations were excreted over a longer period than long hay. Digestibility was not correlated to rate of passage.

Blaxter et al (1955) carried out experiments with sheep fed long roughage or as pellets made after the grass had been ground to a medium or fine degree of fineness. Three levels of feeding were used in the experiments. Results indicated that at each level of feeding, the fine-ground hay was excreted more rapidly than the medium-ground hay, which was, in turn, excreted more rapidly than the long hay. Increasing the amount of feed resulted in more rapid passage (a reduced rate of passage resulted in higher digestibility). In studies with adult sheep fed alfalfa hay, Stielau (1967) recovered stained hay as early as 10 hr, but other sheep took as long as 24 hr for first excretion. Neither amount or fineness of feed affected the time. The time for 5% of the marker to be excreted ranged from 19.5 to 40 hr, and 95% was excreted in 112-146 hr. Excretion time was greater as feed intake was reduced, but grinding had little effect.

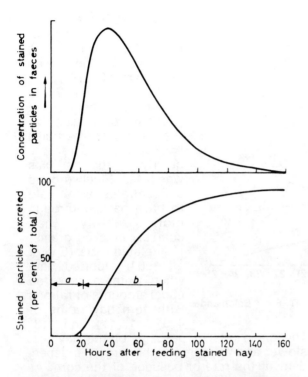

Figure 7-5. Time required for excretion of stained hay particles. From Balch [1961].

Campling and Freer (1966) found that the mean retention time of ground roughages was shorter than that for long roughages when equal and restricted amounts of each were fed to dairy cows. When offered ad libitum, there was little difference between mean retention time and the voluntary intake of long and ground dried grass was similar. O'Dell et al (1963) have reported similar results on retention time when comparing baled, ground or pelleted hay fed to dairy cows. Pelleted and ground hay was excreted more rapidly than baled hay. When the contents of the GIT were examined, the reticulo-rumens of cattle fed long hay had considerably more dry matter (9,305 g) than those fed ground hay (5,939 g) or pelleted hay (4,066 g) and the contents in the total GIT followed the same trend. Stained hay particles were excreted more rapidly by cattle fed pelleted hay (2.6% in 24 hr) than ground hay (1.8%) or long hay (1.0%). Other papers showing an effect of level of intake in cattle include those of Shellenberger and Kesler (1961) and Freer and Campling (1963). Miller et al (1974) have recently demonstrated that thyroid damage results in delayed excretion rates.

In the case of goats, Castle (1956) found that adult goats first excreted stained hay in 11-15 hr after feeding. Excretion reached a maximum at about 30 hr and was complete after 6-7 days. Mean retention time, when receiving rations of hay and concentrate, was ca. 38 hr (32-45 range). Retention time was not related to body weight, but to daily food intake, when expressed on the basis of metabolic size. In young goats (1-15 mo. of age) the rate of passage of hay increased up to weaning and remained relatively constant thereafter.

In studies with Asian buffalo fed roughage and protein meal, Ponnappa et al (1971) found that excretion time was somewhat longer for buffalo than cattle; 5%, 80.5% and mean values for buffalo and cattle, respectively were (hr): 32.3, 95.2; 91.2, 28.1, 79.7, 79.3. The cattle ate more, possibly accounting for some of the differences here.

Graphic examples of the excretion of a single dose of stained hay are shown in Fig. 7-5 and 7-6. These examples were taken from data published by Balch (1961) and Balch and Campling (1965). These examples indicate that a small quantity of food passes quickly out of the reticulo-rumen, however most of the digesta is retained for some period of time with the result that excretion is very gradual.

Figure 7-6, illustrating data from four cows, shows the marked effect of feeding level on retention time in the GIT. There was a considerable amount of difference between cows (E-H), but the trends were in the same direction in each case. Data obtained with ^{14}C-labeled hay are shown in Fig. 7-7 (Yadava et al, 1964) and illustrate another means of estimating retention time.

Lambourne (1957) has studied the excretion of sheep when on pasture. He found that markers appeared in the feces 5-8 hr after dosing and reached peak values about 10-18 hr after dosing. He found that, as quality of the forage decreased, peak marker levels occurred later and that high levels of intake (estimated) increased the rate of passage with the result that peak concentration of marker occurred at earlier times. Marker doses given at or near times of greatest feed intake were passed more rapidly than doses given after feeding. It seems likely that the markers may have been excreted more rapidly than would be typical for stained plant particles in studies with sheep.

A study of excretion of inert particles of

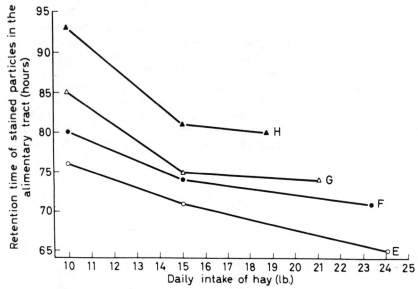

Figure 7-6. **Effect of level of feeding on retention time in the GIT. From Balch and Campling [1965].**

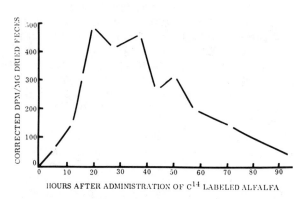

Figure 7-7. **Excretion of 14C from a single dose of 14C-labeled alfalfa hay. From Yadava et al [1964].**

various sizes has been reported by several authors. King and Moore (1957) used plastic particles ranging from 11-108 cm³/1,000 particles and varying in specific gravity from 0.92 to 1.24. A maximum passage rate occurred with particles ranging in size between 20-30 cm³/1,000 and SG of 1.18. Campling and Freer (1962) found that rubber particles with varying SG had the following retention times: SG 1.02, 78-119 hr; 106, 56-100 hr; 1.12, 55-90 hr; and 1.21, 59-103 hr. In another experiment, plastic particles 3.2, 4.0 or 4.8 mm in diameter were administered. Average retention times on a variety of rations were 80, 86 and 91 hr, respectively, for the three sizes. Derrickson

et al (1965) have also investigated passage of plastic particles, using particles having mean diameters of 4.76, 2.38, 1.19 or 0.60 mm. Within this range, the rate of passage decreased as the size of particles increased. Specific gravity of the particles was 1.425. Finely ground concentrates were said to have passed through more rapidly than coarsely cracked grains.

A related paper (Eng et al, 1964) reported data when wethers were fed equal amounts of rations with corn:hay ratios of 4:0, 3:1, 1:1 and 1:3. The mean rate of passage of the hay was slower and appeared to be largely independent of the rate of passage of the corn. As the amount of hay in the ration increased, the rate of hay excretion increased (similar to data from other papers). The passage rate of corn was at a maximum when no hay was fed and decreased as the level of hay in the ration increased.

Conclusions

Data on passage of digesta through the GIT are, for the most part, difficult to compare even within species because of the difference in experimental techniques, rations, ration preparation, the amount of feed given and other miscellaneous reasons. However, many of these experiments have provided useful physiological data that add to the knowledge on function of the ruminant digestive system. Some of the conclusions that might be drawn from these data include:

1. The passage rate of liquids is not necessarily the same as solids, particularly from the reticulo-rumen and the omasum. This is emphasized by the difference in passage time of markers of different types and the possibility that ingested water may travel a different route than rumen liquid.
2. Disappearance of solids from the rumen (and probably from the omasum) is influenced to a very great extent by

particle size, specific gravity, level and, probably, frequency of feeding as well as rapidity of digestion (which would reduce particle size and change specific gravity).

3. Passage through the intestines is influenced to some extent by specific gravity, but a major influence appears to be the amount of dry matter (and undigested fibrous material) present in these organs.

4. If the volume of liquid digesta increases in the abomasum or intestines, this has an inhibitory effect on passage from anterior organs.

5. Inadequate comparative data indicate that ovines have a much faster rumen turnover time than do bovines fed on similar rations, although direct comparative data are not available, and there is no direct evidence to explain the difference.

If the reader wishes to arrive at some estimated values for passage through the entire tract, the values given below might be a starting point for sheep.

Site	Possible values
Ingested feed	ca. 800 g/day = 33 g/hr
Saliva entering the rumen	6-10 l./day or 8 l./day = 330 ml/hr
Free water consumption	2-3 l./day or 2.5 l./day = 104 ml/hr
Fluid volume passing out of the rumen	350-900 ml/hr
Forestomach retention time of solids, mean value	25-40 hr
Fluid volume passing from the omasum	350-500 ml/hr
Fluid volume passing from the abomasum	300-650 ml/hr
Fluid volume passing from the duodenum	300-1,000 ml/hr
Fluid volume passing from the ileum	90-180 ml/hr
Weight of fecal matter	35 g/hr (includes water)

References Cited

Ash, R.W. 1962a. J. Physiol. 164:4P (abstr).
Ash, R.W. 1962b. J. Physiol. 164:24P (abstr).
Ash, R.W. 1964. J. Physiol. 172:435.
Ash, R.W. 1969. Proc. Nutr. Soc. 28:110.
Axford, R.F.E., R.A. Evans and N.W. Offer. 1971. Res. Vet. Sci. 12:128.
Badawy, A.M. and W.S. Mackie. 1964. Quart. J. Exp. Physiol. 49:346.
Balch, C.C. 1950. Br. J. Nutr. 4:361.
Balch, C.C. 1961. In: Digestive Physiology and Nutrition of the Ruminant. Butterworths, London.
Balch, C.C. and R.C. Campling. 1965. In: Physiology of Digestion in the Ruminant. Butterworths.
Bell, F.R. and S.A.D. Razig. 1973. J. Physiol. 228:499; 513.
Ben-Ghedalia, D., H. Tagari and A. Bondi. 1974. Br. J. Nutr. 31:125.
Benavides, M. et al. 1972. Revista Cubana de Ciencia Agr. 5:295.
Blaxter, K.L., N. McC. Graham and F.W. Wainman. 1955. Proc. Nutr. Soc. 14:iv (abstr).
Bost, J. 1957. J. Physiol., Paris, 49:56.
Bost, J. 1964. Ann. Nutr. Aliment. 18:73.
Bost, J. 1970. In: Physiology of Digestion and Metabolism in the Ruminant. Oriel Press, Newcastle upon Tyne, England.
Bueno, L. 1972. Ann. Rech. Veter. 3:83.
Campling, R.C. and M. Freer. 1962. Br. J. Nutr. 16:507.
Campling, R.C. and M. Freer. 1966. Br. J. Nutr. 20:229.
Castle, E.J. 1965. Br. J. Nutr. 10:15; 115; 338.
Colvin, B.M., R.A. Lowe and H.A. Ramsey. 1969. J. Dairy Sci. 52:687.
Coombe, J.B. and R.N.B. Kay. 1965. Br. J. Nutr. 19:325.
Corbett, J.L., J.F.D. Greenhalgh and E. Florence. 1959. Br. J. Nutr. 13:337.
Corse, D.A. and J.D. Sutton. 1971. Proc. Nutr. Soc. 30:18A (abstr).

Cunningham, M.D., F.A. Martz and C.P. Merilan. 1964. J. Dairy Sci. 47:382.
Derrickson, C.M., et al. 1965. J. Animal Sci. 24:879 (abstr).
Eng, K.S., M.E. Riewe, J.H. Craig and J.C. Smith. 1964. J. Animal Sci. 23:1129.
Engelhardt, W. 1963. Naturwissenchaften. 50:357.
Engelhardt, W. 1964. Plugers Arch. 278:141.
Freer, M. and R.C. Campling. 1963. Br. J. Nutr. 17:79.
Goodall, E.D. and R.N.B. Kay. 1965. J. Physiol. 176:12.
Grovum, W.L. and V.J. Williams. 1973. Br. J. Nutr. 29:13.
Harris, L.E. and A.T. Phillipson. 1962. Animal Prod. 4:97.
Harrison, F.A. and K.J. Hill. 1962. J. Physiol. 162:225.
Hogan, J.P. 1964. Aust. J. Agr. Res. 15:384.
Hogan, J.P. and A.T. Phillipson. 1960. Br. J. Nutr. 14:147.
Hogan, J.P. and R.H. Weston. 1971. Aust. J. Agr. Res. 22:951.
Hungate, R.E. 1966. The Rumen and Its Microbes. Academic Press, N.Y.
Hyden. S. 1961. In: Digestive Physiology and Nutrition of the Ruminant. Butterworths, London.
Ingalls, J.R., J.W. Thomas, M.G. Tesar and D.L. Carpenter. 1966. J. Animal Sci. 25:283.
Jones, B.E.V. and J.S.D. Poulsen. 1974. Nord. Vet. Med. 26:13.
Kameoka, K. and H. Morimoto. 1959. J. Dairy Sci. 42:1187.
King, K.W. and W.E.C. Moore. 1957. J. Dairy Sci. 40:528.
Lambourne, L.J. 1957. J. Agr. Sci. 48:273.
Liebholz, J. and P.E. Hartmann. 1972. Aust. J. Agr. Res. 23:1059.
Mangan, J.L. and P.C. Wright. 1968. Res. Vet. Sci. 9:366.
Miller, J.K. et al. 1974. J. Dairy Sci. 57:193.
Minson, D.J. 1966. Br. J. Nutr. 20:765.
Murray, M.G., R.S. Reid and T.M. Sutherland. 1962. J. Physiol. 164:26P (abstr).
Mylrea, P.J. 1966. Res. Vet. Sci. 7:333.
Mylrea, P.J. 1968. Res. Vet. Sci. 9:1.
Nanda, P.N. and G. Singh. 1941. Indian J. Vet. Sci. 11:16.
Nicholson, J.W.G. and J.D. Sutton. 1969. Br. J. Nutr. 23:585.
O'Dell, G.D., W.A. King, W.C. Cook and S.L. Moore. 1963. J. Dairy Sci. 46:38.
Oyaert, W. and J.H. Bouchaert. 1961. Res. Vet. Sci. 2:41.
Phillips, G.D. and G.W. Dyck. 1964. Can. J. Animal Sci. 44:220.
Phillipson, A.T. 1948. J. Physiol. 107:21P (abstr).
Phillipson, A.T. 1952. J. Physiol. 116:84.
Phillipson, A.T. and R.W. Ash. 1965. In: Physiology of Digestion in the Ruminant. Butterworths.
Phillipson, A.T., R. Green, R.S. Reed and L.E. Vowles. 1949. Br. J. Nutr. 3:iii (abstr).
Piana, C. 1952. Zootech. Vet. 7:445.
Ponnappa, C.G., M.N. Uddin and G.V. Raghavan. 1971. Indian J. Animal Sci. 41:1026.
Poutiainen, E. 1968. Ann. Agr. Fenn. 7: Suppl. 3, pp 1-66.
Ridges, A.P. and A.G. Singleton. 1962. J. Physiol. 161:1.
Schalk, A.F. and R.S. Amadon. 1928. N. Dak. Agr. Exp. Sta. Bul. 216.
Shellenberger, P.R. and E.M. Kesler. 1961. J. Animal Sci. 20:416.
Singleton, A.G. 1961. J. Physiol. 155:134.
Sisson, S. and J.D. Grossman. 1953. The Anatomy of the Domestic Animals. 4th ed. W.B. Saunders Co.,
    Philadelphia.
Smith, R.H. 1964. J. Physiol. 172:305.
Stielau, W.J. 1967. S. African J. Agr. Sci. 10:753.
Sutherland, T.M., W.C. Ellis, R.S. Reid and M.G. Murray. 1962. Br. J. Nutr. 16:603.
Ternouth, J.H. 1967. Res. Vet. Sci. 8:283.
Ternouth, J.H. and H.L. Buttle. 1973. Br. J. Nutr. 29:387.
Ternouth, J.H., J.H.B. Roy and R.C. Siddons. 1974. Br. J. Nutr. 31:13.
Thivend, P. and C. Poncet. 1971. Ann. Biol. Anim. Bioch. Biophys. 11:275.
Thompson, F. 1973. Br. J. Nutr. 30:87.
Thompson, F. and G.E. Lamming. 1972. Br. J. Nutr. 28:391.
Topps, J.H., R.N.B. Kay and E.D. Goodall. 1968. Br. J. Nutr. 22:261.
Toullec, R. and C.M. Mathieu. 1973. Ann. Rech. Veter. 4:13.
Tulloh, N.M., J.W. Hughes and R.P. Newth. 1965. N.Z. J. Agr. Res. 8:636.
Ulyatt, M.J. 1964. N.Z. J. Agr. Res. 7:713.
van't Klooster, A.T., A. Kemp, J.H. Geurink and P.A.M. Rogers. 1972. Neth. J. Agr. Sci. 20:314.
van't Klooster, A.T., P.A. Rogers and H.R. Sharma. 1969. Neth. J. Agr. Sci. 17:60.
Watson, R.H. 1944. CSIRO Bul. 180.
Weller, R.A., A.F. Pilgrim and F.V. Gray. 1971. Br. J. Nutr. 26:487.
Weston, R.H. 1968. Aust. J. Agr. Res. 19:261.
Weston, R.H. and J.P. Hogan. 1967. Aust. J. Agr. Res. 18:789.
Weston, R.H. and J.P. Hogan. 1971. Aust. J. Agr. Res. 22:139.
Willes, R.F. and V.E. Mendel. 1968. Amer. J. Vet. Res. 25:1302.
Wise, G.H. and G.W. Anderson. 1939. J. Dairy Sci. 22:697.
Yadava, I.S. et al. 1964. J. Dairy Sci. 47:1346.

CHAPTER 8 — EXCRETION AND DIGESTION

Fecal Excretion

Composition of Feces

Fecal material excreted by animals is comprised of undigested residues of food material; residues of gastric juices, bile, pancreatic and enteric juices; cellular debris from the mucosa of the gut; excretory products excreted into the lumen of the gut; and cellular debris and metabolites of microorganisms that grow in the large intestine with, most likely, some coming from the forestomach in the case of ruminants. The percentage of fecal material contributed by any one of these sources is difficult to determine in ruminants. Visek (1966) estimated that a 680 kg dairy cow might slough about 2,500 g of cells from the gut wall daily, based on data obtained with rats. This quantity represents ca. 500 g of digestible protein. Presumably, some of this cell debris would be digested and reabsorbed in the small gut, but that from the large gut would probably not be reabsorbed even if hydrolyzed by enteric enzymes or microorganisms. Some of the protein in the gut (endogenous origin) is, no doubt, derived from leakage of plasma proteins into the lumen (Fell et al, 1969).

Mitchell (1964) has reviewed some older publications on this topic and quotes several authors to the effect that fecal material from monogastric species is primarily a mass of bacterial cells. Virtanen (1966) theorized that practically all of the N of feces from cows fed purified diets is microbial protein. He based his estimate on the content of diaminopimelic acid (see Ch. 13) and estimated digestibility of rumen microorganisms. Some of this, no doubt, might be derived from cellular debris sloughed from the lining of the intestines.

Mason (1969) has made rather extensive efforts to fractionate fecal N into different sources — undigested (insoluble) dietary N; bacterial + endogenous N (intestinal cellular debris); water soluble N; and non-dietary fecal N. His calculations indicate that bacterial and intestinal cellular debris (that which could be centrifuged out) accounted for 70-81.1% of non-dietary fecal N. Further computations, based on diaminopimelic acid content of the different fractions, indicated that N from intestinal cell debris ranged from 0-32.5% of this fraction (bacterial and cell N); thus, his calculations indicate bacterial residues form the major source of fecal N. Data on other organic nutrients are lacking, however. Ørskov et al (1970) have carried out similar fecal fractionations. When sheep were fed 5-6.65 g of N/day, they recovered 0.38-1.07 g as insoluble and, presumably, undigestible N. N in suspension (bacterial and intestinal debris) amounted to 3.2-3.88 g/day, and water-soluble N amounted to 1.42-2.05 g/day.

Microscopic examinations of sheep feces (Mason, 1969) indicated bacterial residues in all samples, the residues tending to congregate on small dietary debris rather than on large fibers. Bacterial cells appeared to increase as the rations became more fibrous. No cells of animal origin could be identified in feces of sheep fed high-fiber rations. Dietary residues in the feces varied according to the nature of the ration fed. Straw, hay and grass residues were mainly composed of small amorphous pieces of lignified material together with pitted xylem vessels and xylem fibers. Concentrate rations contained undigested husks (barley) and much finer debris, but all feces showed marked degradation of dietary debris.

The color of feces is due to plant chromagens and to stercobilinogen produced by bacterial reduction of bile pigment. The odor is due to the presence of aromatic substances, primarily indole and skatole, which are derived from the deamination and decarboxylation of tryptophan in the large intestine. Compounds such as indole, skatole and phenol (derived from tyrosine) are absorbed to some extent by the blood. As such they are toxic, but are detoxified by conjugation with sulfuric acid or glucuronic acid in the liver and rendered nontoxic.

Relatively complete analyses of the feces of ruminant species are not as readily available in the literature, as one might think, although there are a great deal of data on digestibility in the literature. An example of some of the available data on feces from three ruminant species is shown in Table 8-1.

Table 8-1. Percentage composition of feces from different ruminant species (dry basis).

Constituent	Animal deer[a]	deer[a]	sheep[b]	sheep[c]	sheep[d]	calves[e]	steers[f]
	Feed source alfalfa hay	bitter-brush	pasture forage	alfalfa hay	alfalfa pellets	semi-synth. diet	alfalfa hay:conc., 1:1 ratio
Water content			50-69		54-64	80-82	76-79
Crude protein	16-17	11-12	10-16	11-25	9-10	37-58	13-19
Crude fat	3-4	8-9	7-10			34[h]	3-6
Crude fiber	39-40	30-32	21-29		41-49		32-44
Nitrogen-free-extract	28-29	43-44	26-36				28-46
Ash	11-13	6-7	8-11	15-25	16-19	13-21	4-8
Water extractives				8-16			
Alcohol-benzene ext.				7-13			
Hemicellulose				14-18[g]			
Cellulose				12-26	30-31		
Lignin				16-20			
Soluble carbohydrates						trace	
Undetermined				16-19			
Energy, Kcal/g			3.92-4.46		4.18-4.31		

[a] Dietz et al (1962)
[b] Schneider et al (1955)
[c] Jarrige (1965)
[d] Author's laboratory
[e] Blaxter and Wood (1951)
[f] Dowe et al (1955)
[g] Subdivided into xylans, 64.2%; arabans, 11.8%; hydrolyzable hexosans, 24.0%.
[h] Soap, 37-63%; other, 63-37%.

Data in the table show that a substantial part of feces from ruminants, consuming forage or forage-concentrate mixtures, is made up of the fibrous parts of the plant, primarily the cell wall components — lignin, cellulose, hemicellulose and NFE (which may be largely hemicellulose and lignin). The mineral elements (ash) may also make up a substantial percentage of the total.

Whether there is any real difference between species in the composition of dry matter excreted is questionable. The data shown do not allow a critical comparison because of the differences in analytical methods and in feedstuffs fed. There will usually be a difference in the water content of feces between sheep and cattle fed comparable rations. As a general rule, feces from sheep will run between 55 and 70% water and cattle from 70 to 85%, depending upon the diet. Those species which form fecal pellets are able to remove more water from feces, thus conserving it for other functions.

Amount and Frequency of Excretion

The amount of dry matter that will be excreted per day is affected by a number of variables, but the two most important factors are the amount of feed consumed and its digestibility. In the case of sheep grazing on grass, data published by Schneider et al (1955) indicate an excretion of ca. 200 g/day by sheep which weighed ca. 150 lb. Christian et al (1965) reported that organic matter excreted by stall-fed sheep given dried grass ranged from 50 to 185 g/day. Unpublished data from the author's laboratory show that dry matter excreted by lambs fed frozen chopped fescue ranged from 150 to 400 g/day, increasing as the quality of the forage decreased. The excretion of dry matter of 70-80 lb lambs fed alfalfa pellets averaged about 480 g/day, probably reflecting a more rapid passage of ingesta through the reticulo-rumen. Comparable values for lambs fed concentrate rations were on the order of 150 to 250 g/day.

The frequency of excretion in adult sheep has been reported in only one instance known to the author. In this experiment (Minson and Cowper, 1966), sheep were fed manually once daily or by a mechanical feeder every hour day and night. Neither frequency is, of course, typical of a free-feeding animal. Only graphical data were presented (Fig. 8-1), the graphs indicating some excretion every hour of the 24, ranging from a low of 3 g/hr (0800-1000) to 21 g/hr (2400-0200) for sheep fed 1X/day. For those fed every hour, fecal dry matter ranged from ca. 6 g/hr (1000-1200 and 2000-2400) to a high of about 17 g/hr (2400-0200). The fact that the sheep got up at least every hour to eat probably contributed to the frequent excretion since most ruminant animals will defecate after arising from a resting period. In other work, Blaxter et al (1956) have calculated fecal excretion curves based on periodic examinations of feces for stained particles. Calculated values are shown in Fig. 8-2. Their calculations indicate a substantial variation in fecal excretion of ground and pelleted forage, but relatively little when hay was fed long.

In the case of deer digestion data, Dietz et al (1962) reported that excretion ranged from a low of about 170 g/day for deer fed mountain mahogany (consumption 372 g) to a high of 540 g/day for deer fed alfalfa pellets (consumption 1,026 g/day). The deer averaged between 70 and 80 lb in live weight. No data were given on frequency of excretion. With confined mule deer, Smith (1964) observed 13-14 defecations/day. Thus, a comparison of deer and sheep excretion on similar diets would indicate comparable amounts of fecal excretion.

Available data on frequency of excretion in cattle have been collected primarily by making observations of grazing animals. Johnstone-Wallace and Kennedy (1944) reported that beef cows defecated an average of 12X/day

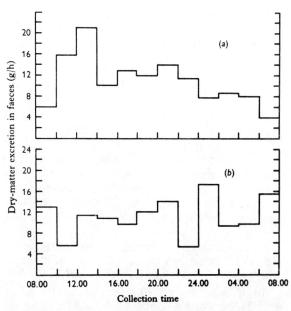

Figure 8-1. Diurnal variation in excretion of feces dry matter in sheep fed 912 g of air-dried alfalfa hay [a] once daily at 1000 or [b] 24X/day. Mean values for 6 sheep for 2 days. From Minson and Cowper [1966].

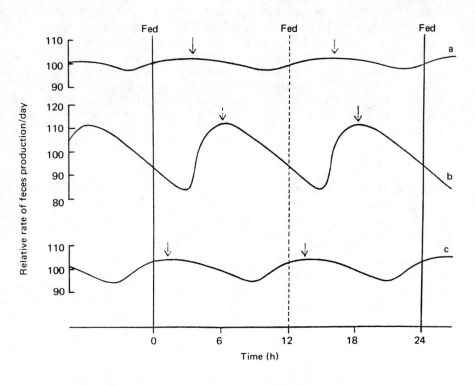

Figure 8-2. Estimated diurnal variation in fecal excretion by sheep. The graph shown was calculated from data obtained on excretion of stained particles of hay. The curves were derived from sheep fed 2X daily at 12 hr intervals. The sheep were fed [a] 1,200 g of long dried grass; [b] 1,500 g of finely ground and pelleted dried grass; and [c] 1,200 g of medium ground and pelleted dried grass. From Blaxter et al [1956].

when on summer pasture. Daily fecal weight was ca. 46 lb (wet), or 6.4 lb of dry matter. Wagnon (1963) also reported on average number of defecations at ca. 12X/day for beef cows on lightly grazed pasture. Grazing pastures closely reduced fecal output (less feed) to ca. 9½/day. A further decline on dry forage of closely grazed pastures to 4 defecations/day occurred. Supplementation during the winter had no effect on frequency, but dry cows averaged slightly less than lactating cows. Beef cows confined in dry lot and fed at different levels were observed to defecate an average of 6.4X/day, the frequency increasing as the level of feeding increased (Schake and Riggs, 1969). Suckling calves confined in the same facilities were observed to defecate an average of 4.9X/day (Schake and Riggs, 1970).

In the case of dairy cows, Castle et al (1950) reported a range of 7-15 defecations/day in the summer and fall months, with an average of 12, and Hardison et al (1956) observed an average of 15 defecations/day in the summer and fall.

With respect to the amount of feces voided/day, Dowe et al (1955) found the weight from steers to range from 6.3-20.6 lb wet or 1.7 to 4.7 lb dry. These values were for stall-fed animals. With cows on pasture, Lancaster et al (1953) reported values of 5.9-8.2 lb/day of fecal organic matter, and Hardison et al (1959) reported a range of 9-16 lb of dry matter/day for lactating cows.

Urinary Excretion

Chemical Nature of Urine

Urine represents the main route of excretion of nitrogenous and sulfurous metabolites of body tissues. In addition, urine is usually the principal route of excretion of some of the mineral elements, particularly Cl, K, and Na (see Ch. 19 of Vol. 2). Consequently, urine is, essentially, an aqueous solution of these various components with minor amounts of pigments and sloughed cells from the urogenital tract. Other urinary components, which are normally minor in quantity, include aromatic acids which are primarily glycine conjugates of benzoic and phenylacetic acids. These are excreted in much larger amounts by ruminants than by most other species (Martin, 1970). Phenylacetic acid in urine appears to be derived from rumen meta-

bolism of phenylalanine (Martin, 1973). In addition to these acids, sulfur-containing acids may be present in relatively large concentrations and ketones may be found at relatively high levels at times. Protein is found in the urine only infrequently (Weaver, 1970).

The color of urine is primarily due to urochrome, a metabolite of bile pigments complexed with a peptide (White et al, 1964). The specific gravity is usually on the order of 1.015-1.045 in sheep and goats and 1.030-1.045 for cattle (Dukes, 1955). The freezing point depression (osmotic pressure) is greater than for blood, thus indicating a concentration of solutes in urine. In regards to pH, it has been said in the past that urine is characteristically alkaline and that a basic reaction is characteristic of herbivorous animals due to the relatively large amounts of Na and K ions, especially K, found in vegetation. Relatively recent data from a number of different laboratories indicates, however, that urine pH of ruminants may be alkaline on dry forage, but is apt to be slightly acidic on many other diets. For example, Scott et al (1971) and Scott (1972) observed that calves or sheep generally excreted alkaline urine when fed on diets that were dried roughage or primarily roughage. When fed on concentrate diets of different types, the urine was acidic. In Norway, Hjelle (1969) observed that 92% of 1,248 urine samples from sheep were acidic, samples being obtained from sheep under different feeding regimens. Gasparini and Marangoni (1970) observed that fattening cattle had acidic urine, usually with a pH of ca. 6. Even on pasture, Weaver (1970) found that sheep excreted acidic urine for most of the year. Only during the months of May, June and July were mean urine pH values above 7.0. He suggests that normal urine values are within the range of pH 5-8, with most values being slightly acidic.

Relatively complete analyses of urine from ruminant species are not as available in the literature as for some other species, although data on many individual components can be obtained. Examples of some of the relatively recent data are shown in Table 8-2. The data clearly point out that urea is usually the principal nitrogen-containing compound present with lesser amounts of other components such as ammonia, allantoin, creatine and creatinine. The total or relative excretion of urea is primarily a function of N intake. For example, note the difference in the data from Topps (1966) in which sheep were fed a low protein (4%) diet vs an adequate level of protein (10%). On the low protein diet, ammonia accounted for slightly more urinary N than urea and other components such as allantoin, hippuric acid and creatinine represented substantial percentages of the total. However, when the crude protein was more nearly optimum, urea was by far the largest fraction present (71%). Urinary urea concentrations are, thus, a reflection of dietary intake of protein and resultant increased levels of plasma urea (Thornton and Wilson, 1972). The sheep, and possibly other ruminant species, responds to increased urinary urea with an increase in total urine production as it does not concentrate urine under these conditions (Rabinowitz and Gunther, 1972).

Differences in urinary composition between sheep and cattle are illustrated by the data of Nehring et al (1965) when the same rations were fed to both species. The data shown in Table 8-2, and that presented in the paper, indicate that sheep excreted less of the total N as urea and creatinine but more as ammonia and hippuric acid. Data summarized by Blaxter (1961) indicate that ruminants probably excrete much larger amounts of purine bases than do monogastric species. On fasting, the amount decreases markedly. This is, no doubt, a function of the high production in the rumen (McAllan and Smith, 1968) which results in high urinary excretion (Condon et al, 1970). There are, apparently, marked species differences between sheep and red deer in excretion of nucleic acids in urine (Razzaque and Topps, 1973).

Creatine excretion is generally thought to increase in cases of prolonged negative nitrogen balance, for example, in starvation, fever, hyperthyroidism or muscular atrophy;

Table 8-2. Composition of urine of ruminant animals.

Animal	Young lambs[a]	Sheep[b]	Sheep[b]	Sheep[c]	Cattle[c]	Calves[d]	Calves[e]
Conditions		roughage diet,	roughage diet,	mixed ration,		70-80 days	syn.
Item	4-5 kg wt	4% protein	10% protein	15% protein		of age	diet
Basis of measurement	mg/day	% of N	% of N	% of N		g/day	g/day
Nitrogenous constituents							
Ammonia	76	27.1	1.9	6.8	2.9		1.16
Amino acids	14						
Urea	1543	24.3	71.1	63.5	80.4		4.7
Allantoin	46	10.4	6.5	13.6	8.4		0.71
Uric acid	22	2.4	1.2	1.6	0.8		0.05
Purines	23						
Hippuric acid		17.2	6.5	10.2	4.1		
Creatine	45	1.9	1.0	0.9	0.7	1.9	0.22
Creatinine	52	13.7	4.8	3.4	0.7	2.6	0.38
Residual nitrogen	352	3.0	7.0				
Sulfurous constituents							
Inorganic	26						
Organic	32						
Reducing sugars	113						
Electrolytes							
Ca							0.02
Cl							11.3
K							17.0
Na							7.2
P							1.8

[a] Walker and Faichney (1964)
[b] Topps (1966)
[c] Nehring et al (1965)
[d] Woefel et al (1965)
[e] Blaxter and Wood (1951)

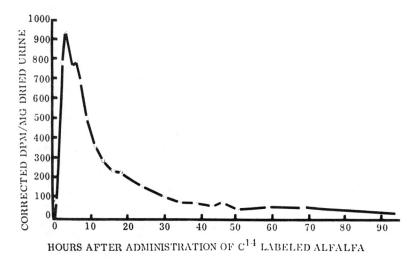

HOURS AFTER ADMINISTRATION OF C^{14} LABELED ALFALFA

Figure 8-3. Graph illustrating the excretion via urine of ^{14}C following the intra-ruminal administration of ^{14}C-labeled alfalfa hay. From Yadava et al [1964].

Urinary excretion of carbon is illustrated in Fig. 8-3. This curve showing excretion of ^{14}C would, presumably, be typical of that C which was fermented to one of the volatile fatty acids, absorbed by the GIT, and then excreted by the kidney as one of many possible C-containing compounds.

Abnormal Urine Constituents

Only traces of protein, amino acids, etc., are found in normal urine. The presence in quantity of proteins such as albumin and globulin is indicative of kidney disease in the adult animal. In the very young ruminant (and presumably other mammals), proteinuria is a normal thing. Pierce (1959) has shown that proteinuria occurred in calves given colostrum during the first 48 hr after birth, but not at older ages. When colostrum was replaced by boiled milk, proteinuria did not occur; the difference here being the lack of small protein molecules in the boiled milk. This reaction is related to the ability of the young mammal to absorb intact protein molecules of relatively small size during a short period of time following birth (see Ch. 9 for more detail). Pierce found, in one calf given 309 g of immune lactoglobulin, that 70 g appeared in the plasma of which 4.5 g were excreted in the urine. He further pointed out that proteins having molecular weights on the order of 30,000-35,000 pass through the kidney in a number of species.

Carbohydrates such as glucose or fructose may frequently be found in mammalian urine following the ingestion of a meal high in carbohydrates. In humans, normal levels may range from 10 to 20 mg% and in diabetic individuals as high as 12% glucose (White et al, 1964). In young ruminants small amounts may be found. For example, Walker and Faichney (1964) found 69-147 mg of reducing sugars were excreted per day by young lambs. In adult animals, however, the level of reducing sugars in urine would be expected to be negligible, since the kidney threshold is considerably higher than blood levels of glucose; i.e., the kidney is capable of returning the blood glucose which may pass

whereas creatinine (the anhydride of creatine) is usually related to body muscle mass (White et al, 1964), and is usually considered to be less influenced by diet. Data reported by Walker and Faichney (1964) on young lambs maintained on N-free diets for a few days indicated that creatine excretion was not greatly affected. Results reported by Topps (1966) and Nehring et al (1965) indicate, also, that creatinine excretion decreased markedly as crude protein intake increased, when expressed as a percentage of total N excreted via the urine. Topps stated that creatinine daily excretion showed little variation with the diet, results which have been confirmed by Kertz et al (1970). Only small quantities of sulfur (Table 8-2) are present in the urine of young lambs. Sulfur excretion is often proportional to the N:S ratio in body proteins. With respect to the mineral elements, urine composition of Cl, K, Na and P are markedly affected by dietary intake, although excretion is also regulated by absorption and excretion in the large gut. In ruminants, P is normally present in small amounts. Recent data of Scott (1972) indicate that sheep and calves fed a roughage diet did excrete an alkaline urine low in phosphate. However, when fed concentrate diets (80% barley), the urine was acid and contained large amounts of phosphate, of which a high proportion was present as phosphoric acid. The difference in excretion was not related to P intake. P is usually said to be present as the mono- or dibasic sodium salt.

through the glomeruli at these levels.

Ketones are commonly found in ruminant urine, especially in animals affected with starvation, ketosis, pregnancy toxemia and various other abnormal conditions. The kidney threshold for ketones is relatively low (see Ch. 25, Vol. 2), so these components might be expected to appear in urine of animals having only mild ketosis.

Porphyrins from the metabolism of the porphyrin nucleus of hemoglobin occur in small quantities in urine. Abnormal amounts may be present in cases of anemia, liver disease, anaplasmosis, and other diseases which result in a marked or rapid decrease in circulating erthyrocytes.

Amount and Frequency of Excretion

The amount of urine that will be excreted/day is, of course, extremely variable, being affected by the water intake, rate of respiration as affected by environmental and body temperature, intake of N and electrolytes, effect of hormones on the kidney, etc. In the case of sheep, normal excretion for an animal weighing 40-50 kg would be between 1 and 2 l./day. In the case of cattle, Dukes (1955) cites data indicating average excretion to be about 14 kg/day with a range of 9 to 23. Woefel et al (1965) found that calves weighing 70-90 kg excreted from 1-13 l./day, averaging about 3 l. when free water intake averaged 4.4 l./day.

Minson and Cowper (1966) reported that urinary excretion of sheep fed 1X daily ranged from a low of ca. 30 g/hr (0400-0900) to 100 g/hr (1600-1800); see Fig. 8-4. Lysov (1961) found that sheep with a bladder fistula excreted 10-15 ml/15 min when fasting and between 19-26 ml/15 min when fed. Rumination resulted in an increase, the peak being 45-60 min after commencement of rumination. Stacy and Brook (1964) noted that flow of urine in sheep before eating varied widely, from 0.3-4.0 ml/min. During eating the flow fell to 0.2 to 0.4 ml/min, but the specific gravity increased from ca. 1.01-1.03 to 1.03-1.08 after feeding. Na and K excretion also decreased after feeding as did pH, the pH being 6.9-8.4 before and 5.1-6.6 after feeding. Minson and Cowper (1966) also noted that SG was highest 4-6 hr after feeding and that N concentration reached a peak prior to feeding in lambs fed once daily. In those fed every hour, the peak N concentration occurred between 2000 and 2200 hr.

The frequency of excretion of urine by grazing cattle has been reported by a number of authors. Johnstone-Wallace and Kennedy (1944) observed that beef cows urinated an average of 9 times/day during the summer and fall months. Hardison et al (1956) reported 9.4 urinations for lactating dairy cows and Castle et al (1950) observed 9.8 urinations with a range of 5-14 during the summer months. Wagnon (1963) reported an average of 8.4 urinations (8-13) for beef cows on lightly grazed pasture as compared to 6.6 (5-11) for animals on closely grazed forage. On dry forage, cows urinated only 2 times/day. Beef cows fed in confinement have been observed to urinate 3.9X/day and suckling beef calves 4.9X/day (Schake and Riggs, 1969, 1970).

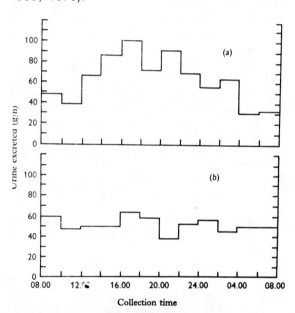

Figure 8-4. Diurnal variation in excretion of urine in sheep [a] given feed once at 1000 or [b] sheep fed 24X/day. From Minson and Cowper [1966].

Dermal Excretions

The importance of dermal excretions in ruminant species has yet to be determined. Some data are available on the amount of sweat produced (see Vol. 2, Ch. 18 on water requirements) and there are data on qualitative analyses (Dukes, 1955). The sweat glands, in addition to their cooling action, can apparently function to excrete salts such as Na, K and N. Species such as sheep produce appreciable amounts of oily secretions that maintain the water resistance of the wool. Mitchell (1964) points out that, in man, iron is excreted through the skin in appreciable amounts.

Digestion

Digestion is frequently defined as the preparation of food for absorption by the GIT. When used in reference to animals, the meaning implies that the action on food is limited to the act of eating, microbial digestion in the rumen or other parts of the stomach, gastric and enteric digestion occurring as a result of action by gastric, enteric and pancreatic enzymes, and digestion attributed to HCl in the stomach and bile from the liver. If digestive action were not restricted to the GIT, then changes such as those brought about by cooking and feed preparation could be included.

Many authors, particularly when writing about digestibility of feedstuffs, tend to use an implied definition meaning disappearance of food from the GIT. As such, this broad definition of digestion would include absorption as well as digestion. It is this general definition that will be used in discussion in this chapter, granted that it may not be a precise use of the term.

Reasons for Studying Digestibility

As indicated, evaluation of digestibility involves the determination of how much of an individual nutrient or feedstuff disappears in the GIT or, to put it another way, how

much material is not degraded and absorbed while passing through the animal. This is an important facet of nutrient utilization, since undigested residues and fecal excretions associated with digestion are the single biggest loss encountered in feed utilization, being somewhere on the order of 30-60% of the ingested feed for fibrous rations.

Digestion trials are carried out primarily for two principal purposes: to evaluate animal utilization of a particular nutrient, feedstuff, or ration and to quantitate the intake of digestible nutrients. In addition to the study of the effect of feed preparatory methods, feed additives, optimum combination of ration ingredients, other objectives might include study of the effect of age, species differences and so forth. Regardless of the specific objective, digestibility data, when used in conjunction with chemical analyses, have been used to a greater extent for nutritional research with domestic animals than any other type of data.

Methods Utilized

Conventional Methods. In conventional digestion studies animals are either confined in a crate or stall to facilitate collection of feces and/or urine or feces are collected with the aid of bags attached to the animal (see Fig. 8-5, 6, 7, 8). A uniform feed is supplied, the amount given is carefully weighed and samples obtained, feed refusals (orts) are weighed and sampled, and the feces are collected and sampled. It is normal practice to accustom an animal to the ration to be studied for a period of time to allow adaptation of the rumen microorganisms and to adjust feed intake to a stable level somewhat below maximum consumption. Feed intake is stabilized to reduce selectivity and because of a fluctuation in intake will result in a fluctuation in excretion. Excretion of fibrous fedstuffs may be delayed as much as 10 days; consequently, it is practically impossible to

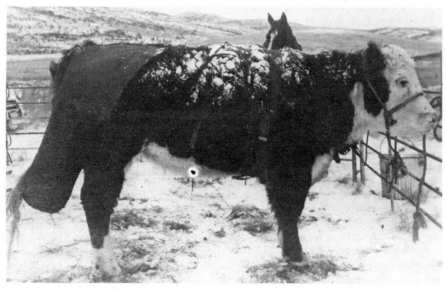

Figure 8-5. Steer with fecal collection bag of a type commonly used for complete collections. Courtesy of D.C. Clanton.

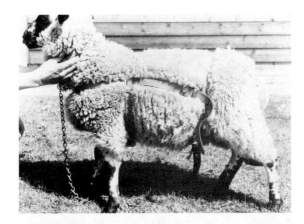

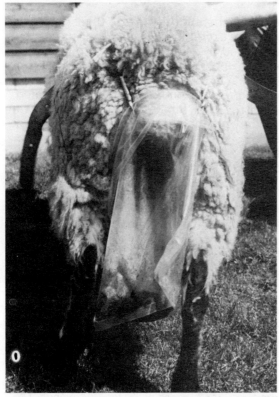

Figure 8-6. A sheep equipped with plastic collection bags, a type which is much easier to use as it is disposable. Courtesy of G. Fishwick, Glasgow University Veterinary School.

identify the excreta with consumptions on a given day. If feces are collected from 0900 on Monday for a 10-day period ending at 0900 on Thursday of the next week, it is hoped the feces are representative of the feed ingested during the 10-day period in which the feed carefully was weighed. If fluctuations in excretion occur, this is very likely not the case. In monogastric species such as swine or rats, some investigators follow the practice of giving dyes such as methylene blue or

carmine red at the beginning and end of a period and fecal collections are started when the animal passes the first dye and stopped when the second batch is passed.

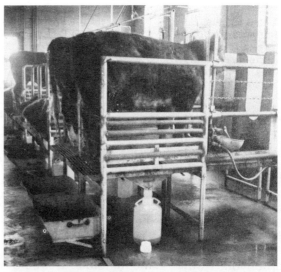

Figure 8-7. A metabolism crate used for collection of both feces and urine. Courtesy of J.P. Fontenot, V.P.I.

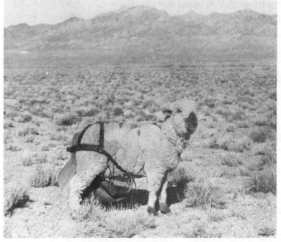

Figure 8-8. A sheep equipped for collection of both feces and urine while grazing on the range so that data can be collected for estimating metabolizable energy. Courtesy of L.E. Harris, Utah State University.

When the animal trial is complete, you now have data on the amount of feed consumed, the weight of wet feces excreted, and hopefully, representative samples of feed and feces. Chemical analyses of feed and feces then allow you to calculate the difference between the amount of a given nutrient consumed and the amount excreted. Data of this type, shown in Table 8-3, were obtained when lambs were fed alfalfa pellets.

Table 8-3.   Data obtained on digestibility of alfalfa pellets with sheep.

Item	Fresh weight	Nutrients						
		Dry matter	Crude protein	Crude fiber	Cellulose	Ash	Organic matter	Digestible energy
Feed analyses, %		91.9	13.0	25.5	22.2	11.3	88.7	4.325[a]
Nutrients consumed, g	5,800	5,329	659.4	1,395.2	1,501.7	600.7	4,728	23,047[b]
Fecal analyses, %		36.0	9.9	44.9	30.2	18.5	84.2	4.245[a]
Nutrients excreted, g	7,306	2,492	247.8	1,119.0	751.9	460.2	2,100	10,579[b]
Apparent absorption, g		2,837	411.6	276.2	749.8	140.5	2,628	12,468[b]
Apparent digestibility, %		53.2	62.4	19.8	49.9	23.4	55.6	54.1

[a] Expressed as Kcal/g
[b] Expressed as Kcal

As you will note in the table, the terms absorption and digestibility are preceded by the adjective, apparent. This term applies to any compound that is secreted or excreted through the wall of the gut into the large intestine and then as feces, particularly to nitrogenous compounds, lipids, some carbohydrates and some minerals. It would not apply to crude fiber or to cellulose since these fractions are foreign to animal tissue; therefore, when digestibility of cellulose or fiber is determined as described above, it is the true digestibility. The true digestibility of nutrients excreted into the gut must be determined by other means. For nitrogen, a common method is to place animals on a N-free diet or on diets with minimal amounts so that a regression line can be extrapolated back to zero intake and the nitrogen excretion can then be calculated; this allows the calculation of true digestibility of a test diet. In the case of minerals, isotopic techniques are usually required.

In many cases, it is desirable to evaluate

Table 8-4.   Data obtained on digestibility of an alfalfa pellet-seed screening mixture with sheep.

Item	Fresh weight	Nutrients						
		Dry matter	Crude protein	Crude fiber	Cellulose	Ash	Organic matter	Digestible energy
Feed Analyses								
Alfalfa pellets		91.9	13.0	25.5	22.2	11.3	88.7	4.325[a]
Seed screenings		90.0	13.2	11.8	12.2	5.4	94.5	4.381[a]
Nutrients Consumed, g								
Alfalfa pellets	5,250	4,824	629.5	1,263.0	1,359.0	543.8	4,280	20,863
Seed screenings	1,750	1,575	207.4	186.7	191.5	85.9	1,489	6,900
TOTAL	7,000	6,399	836.9	1,449.7	1,550.5	629.7	5,769	27,763
Fecal analyses, %		31.6	10.1	41.5	30.8	15.0	85.0	4.398[a]
Nutrients excreted, g	8,478	2,679	254.1	1,044.1	774.9	377.4	2,139	11,065
Apparent absorption, g		3,720	582.8	405.6	776.1	251.8	3,630	16,968
Apparent digestibility, %		58.1	69.6	28.0	50.1	40.0	62.9	60.1
Fecal excretion from								
alfalfa pellets, g[b]		2,258	236.7	1,012.9	680.8	416.5	1,900	9,576
remainder, g		421	17.4	31.2	94.1	-39.1	238	1,489
Absorbed from								
screenings, g		1,154	190.0	155.5	97.4		1,251	5,411
Apparent digestibility of								
seed screenings, %		73.3	91.6	83.3	50.9		84.0	78.4

[a] Expressed as Kcal/g; all others as Kcal
[b] Assumed that digestibility of alfalfa pellets the same as shown in Table 8-3.

Table 8-5. Digestibility of corn silage when fed with different feeds, dry basis.[a]

| Feedstuff | Digestibility, % | | | | | |
	OM	CP	Fat	Fiber	NFE	TDN
Alfalfa pellets	57	71	35	7	76	55
Steer finishing ration	77	73	81	49	83	78
Alfalfa + corn silage	68	73	80	44	77	69
Finishing ration + corn silage	70	69	82	47	78	72
Estimated digestibility of corn silage when fed with						
alfalfa pellets	80	75	96	80	79	86
finishing ration	61	62	82	45	68	67

[a] Data from Church (1969)

the digestibility of a feedstuff when fed in a mixture with one or more other feeds. An example would be protein supplements or grains — feedstuffs that would not normally comprise a complete ration. In this situation, it is necessary to determine digestibility by difference. An example of some of the data obtained and calculations required is shown in Tables 8-4 and 8-5. In the example, alfalfa pellets were fed with seed screenings. Digestibility of the alfalfa pellets was determined in a separate trial (Table 8-3). As Table 8-4 shows, a known amount of nutrients were fed and the fecal excretion determined. Then the coefficients of digestibility of alfalfa are used to calculate how much of the excreta should remain if the alfalfa pellets were digested to the same extent as when fed alone. The remainder of the excreta is attributed to the screenings, thus calculations for digestibility of the screenings can be made.

Determination of digestibility by difference presents problems where there is an **associative effect** between feeds. This term implies that the digestibility of two feeds may not be the same when fed together as when fed separately. In other words, there is a nonadditive effect. This is well illustrated in Table 8-4 by data on ash digestion. The digestibility of ash of alfalfa pellets fed alone was 23.4% and of the mixture, 40%. However, if the amount of ash consumed is multiplied by the coefficient for

alfalfa, we find that a -39.1 g of ash can be attributed to the screenings. In other words, the mixture improved the absorption of ash from alfalfa. The same situation probably applies to some of the other nutrients shown in the table. When alfalfa pellets and screenings were fed as a 50-50 mixture, the calculated digestibility of the screenings was (data not shown in table): dry matter, 71.9%; crude protein, 76.5%; and digestible energy, 71.6%; all values that were lower than when the screenings comprised only 25% of the total. An additional example of associative effect is shown in Table 8-5.

Indicator Methods. In order to carry out a digestion study as described, it is required that the animal be confined and fed a uniform diet. Obviously, there are many situations in which we might wish to have data under range or pasture conditions. The forage could be clipped and fed as soilage or stored and fed as frozen forage, but this restricts the natural selectivity of the animal. To overcome this problem the use of various inert reference materials has been studied by many investigators. Such reference materials are called indicators. Natural or internal indicators are those found in plant material and include materials such as lignin, silica, plant chromogens (pigments), and nitrogen. External (added material) indicators that have been used include such materials as chromic sesquioxide (Cr_2O_3), dyes, polyethylene glycol, and iron. For the benefit of those readers wishing more detail, Kotb and Luckey (1972) have prepared an extensive review on the use of markers in nutrition.

An ideal indicator should be insoluble in the GIT, be indigestible, pass through the tract at the same rate as ingested feed, have no undesirable pharmacological effect on the animal (such as diarrhea), and be suitable for chemical analyses. It is doubtful if any indicator would completely meet these specifications. For example, liquids and highly soluble nutrients will pass out of the rumen or be metabolized at a rapid rate whereas fibrous materials may persist in the rumen for days. Granular material would be expected to have a different passage curve than fibrous plant particles or liquid components. To overcome some of these problems, Cr_2O_3 has been complexed on plant fiber and administered in this manner with reasonably good results (Corbett et al, 1960), although some variation in excretion still remains due to irregular administration of the indicator. This is particularly true when short term collections are made (MacRae and Armstrong, 1969). Recovery is sometimes very low (Kiesling, et al, 1969). Cr_2O_3 complexed to paper (MacRae and Armstrong, 1969; Nelson and Green, 1969) or on beet pulp pellets (Yadava et al, 1973) has given good results.

With other external indicators, polyethylene glycol (PEG) has been a favorite in recent years for measuring fluid passage. However, Chandler et al (1966) demonstrated that administration of PEG for at least 7 days was required to achieve maximum concentration in the feces of calves and some diurnal variation was still encountered. Dosing 2X/day tends to give more uniform excretion of this marker (Hopson and McCroskey, 1972). Liquid parafin appears to be a promising marker for young calves (Volcani et al, 1973). Ellis and Huston (1967) have shown that rare earth markers, when absorbed on the feed, are valid markers for particulate digesta (indigestible residue), but not so for water-soluble or finely divided particles.

Internal indicators have generally met with less enthusiasm due to problems such as incomplete recovery (lignin, chromogens) or lack of sufficient indicator in dry forage (chromogens). Of the internal indicators, lignin has been used more than any other. Even though lignin is often said to be indigestible, there are ample data (see for example, Hogan and Weston, 1969; Porter and Singleton, 1971) to show that very substantial losses of lignin may occur in the ruminant GIT, probably most of it in the rumen.

The reader will probably have concluded that there are disadvantages to the use of the conventional as well as indicator methods. With conventional methods natural selectivity of the animal is greatly restricted or eliminated and consumption is nearly always less than for comparable unconfined animals, thus tending to result in lower digestibility values in the former and higher values in the latter case than would be expected in free-ranging animals. With the indicators, excretion may not be uniform, resulting in over or under recovery of the indicator, which, in turn, results in low or high estimates of digestibility, respectively. If we are dealing with an internal indicator under pasture or range conditions, there is the problem of adequately sampling the forage consumed. Fortunately, the use of esophageal-fistulated animals can largely overcome this problem. In actual practice there are a number of ways in which indicators may be used to advantage to collect data which might not otherwise be available. It is the author's opinion that somewhat inexact data are probably preferable to no data in many situations.

Different situations which are suited to indicator use are illustrated in succeeding paragraphs. Actual data from Johnson et al (1964) on indicator concentration are utilized in the illustrations. Cr_2O_3 was mixed and fed to sheep at a concentration of 0.242% of the dry matter and was present at a level of 0.510% of the fecal dry matter. Lignin represented 11.4% of the feed and 22.6% of fecal dry matter. Total intake of feed was about 1,500 g/day.

1. When feed intake is known and it is impossible or inconvenient to collect feces quantitatively. In this situation we could use lignin as an internal indicator or an external indicator such as Cr_2O_3 could be added to the feed or given via a capsule at regular intervals. "Grab" samples of feces are collected as they are voided or by collecting samples from the rectum at regular intervals throughout the trial. After analyses are

obtained on feed and feces for nutrients of interest and for the indicator, fecal output can be calculated as shown:

$$\text{Fecal output (g nutrient/day)} = \frac{\text{indicator consumed (g/day)}}{\text{indicator concentration in feces (g/g nutr.)}}$$

Substituting values from Johnson et al (Ibid) in the formula we have:

$$Cr_2O_3, \qquad \frac{3.63}{0.0051} = 712 \text{ g fecal dry matter/day}$$

$$\text{Lignin,} \qquad \frac{171.0}{0.226} = 757 \text{ g fecal dry matter/day}$$

If it is desired to calculate digestibility directly, it can be done using the formula below and substituting values for the appropriate nutrient (Schurch et al, 1952; Kane et al, 1953).

$$\text{Digestibility} = 100 - (100 \times \frac{\text{\% indicator in feed}}{\text{\% indicator in feces}} \times \frac{\text{\% nutrient in feces}}{\text{\% nutrient in feed}})$$

Substituting values from Johnson et al for crude protein in the formula and using Cr_2O_3 as the indicator, we have

$$\text{Digestibility} = 100 - (100 \times \frac{.242}{.510} \times \frac{12.65}{18.21}) = 67.1\%$$

2. When neither feed intake nor fecal output is known and a natural (internal) indicator can be used, digestibility can be calculated in the same manner as shown above. Substituting values from Johnson et al for crude protein and using lignin as the indicator, we have

$$\text{Digestibility} = 100 - (100 \times \frac{11.4}{22.6} \times \frac{12.65}{18.21}) = 65.0\%$$

In an example such as this one where we have analyses of the indicator on a dry basis, the formula can be abbreviated to calculate dry matter digestion as shown:

$$\text{\% dry matter digestion} = 100 - (100 \times \frac{\text{\% indicator in feed}}{\text{\% indicator in feces}})$$

3. When neither feed intake nor fecal output is known and an external indicator can be used, digestibility can be calculated as shown using an internal indicator and forage intake can then be calculated as shown (Kane et al, 1953):

$$\text{Nutrient consumption} = \frac{\text{total amount indicator consumed}}{\text{amount indicator in feces}} \times \frac{\text{amount nutrient in fecal sample}}{\text{\% nutrient indigestibility}}$$

Substituting values from Johnson et al, we have:

$$\text{Crude protein consumption} = (\frac{3.630}{0.0051} \times \frac{12.65}{35.0}) = 257 \text{ g/day}$$

In this example Cr_2O_3 was used as the indicator in feed and feces and nutrient indigestibility was derived by using lignin in the previous example, indicating how both internal and external indicators can be used together.

4. When fecal output is known, internal indicators can be used to calculate feed consumption. The only problem in this situation is to obtain a satisfactory sample of forage consumed in order to determine the concentration of the indicator in the forage.

It should be noted, when used as illustrated, that accuracy in estimating digestibility, fecal output, or nutrient consumption is only as good as the samples obtained and analytical methods utilized. Frequently, a considerable error may result due to non-uniform excretion of an indicator or difficulty in obtaining a representative forage sample. Nevertheless, a substantial amount of data has been obtained by using indicators that would otherwise not be available; much of it, particularly that showing seasonal trends, etc., should be adequate for the principal purposes even if a substantial error is present.

Indicator methods have also been used extensively to study changes in digesta that occur in the GIT and to estimate the extent of digestion that occurs in various segments (partial digestion).

In Vitro Rumen Digestion. In vitro, or artificial rumen, studies have been utilized extensively by investigators to evaluate utilization of feedstuffs as well as for studying rumen metabolism. There is a very substantial amount of literature on this subject. Some of the methods utilized to evaluate feedstuffs have been reviewed by Johnson (1966).

Although the procedures used may vary somewhat from laboratory to laboratory, the essential requirements include fermentation of rumen organisms with the test substrate (forage) in a buffered medium for a period of time usually ranging from 12-24 hr. The extent of fermentation of cellulose or dry matter is usually used to quantitate results. This technique requires a very small amount of test material and many forages can be evaluated in a relatively short time, as compared to the usual digestion trial. The possibilities for evaluating a new forage, particularly where the material is quite limited, are obvious. Correlation values between in vitro digestion of cellulose or dry

matter and in vivo digestion of dry matter or digestible energy may be expected to be 0.9 or better, thus permitting a rather good estimate of the digestibility of the test forage. McLeod and Minson (1972) point out that, on the average, in vitro data are better estimates of forage value than standard chemical analyses. A number of laboratories utilize this procedure to evaluate forage on a more or less routine basis.

Rumen Digestion. Digestion of feedstuffs occurring in the rumen, as distinct from that in the entire GIT, has also been utilized to evaluate feedstuffs. For individual feedstuffs this is usually accomplished by suspending the feed in a permeable bag of nondigestible material, such as nylon or dacron, in a rumen-fistulated animal. This technique, also called the nylon bag technique, has been studied extensively and shows more promise on feedstuffs high in starch than does the in vitro technique. Values obtained are suitable for relative comparisons, but correlations between nylon bag data and in vivo data are usually not sufficiently high enough to be useful (Scales et al, 1974).

Balance Trials. As related to nutritional research, a balance trial implies the quantitative measurement of the total intake and excretion of one or more nutrients. Data beyond those obtained for measurement of digestibility must be obtained for the organic nutrients since excretion may be via the urine, gases from the stomach or lungs, and via perspiration through the skin in some cases. Balance trials are commonly employed to evaluate nutritional utilization of the nutrients listed below:

Protein. Nitrogen retention is considered to be a much better method of evaluating protein utilization than apparent digestibility, especially for monogastric species. Since amino acids are not usually limiting in ruminant nutrition, this tends to reduce the value of nitrogen retention data, but it does provide additional information that aids in evaluating feedstuffs — such as calculation of the biological value of specific proteins or the effect of soluble carbohydrates on nitrogen retention.

Mineral nutrients. Balance studies have been quite useful in providing data used in establishing requirements of some of the major minerals, particularly Ca, Mg and P. Balance trials do not provide information on how such nutrients are utilized by body tissues, but the information on whether the animal is in a negative or positive state of retention is useful.

Energy. Nutrients that are oxidized to CO_2, water and/or other compounds require that the respiratory gases be measured if balance data are to be obtained. Of course, losses via feces and urine must be quantitated, too. Several methods are available to quantitate energy; these have been discussed elsewhere (Ch. 23, Vol. 2).

Factors Affecting Digestibility

There are numerous factors which have some influence on digestibility of feedstuffs or rations by ruminants. Some of these are discussed briefly:

1. Plane of nutrition (level of feeding). It was shown some years ago by Forbes et al (1928) and Mitchell et al (1932) that an increasing plane of nutrition results, usually, in a reduced digestibility of energy-supplying nutrients. More recent data of a similar nature have been published by Anderson et al (1959), Moe et al (1965), Reid et al (1966), Leaver et al (1969), Dijkstra (1972), and Tyrrell and Moe (1972).

True digestibility for the organic nutrients would normally be expected to decline as intake increases due to more rapid passage through the GIT. This results in less time for rumen or intestinal microorganisms to ferment the digesta or for digestive juices to act on it.

2. Amount of fiber and/or lignin in the feed. As a general rule, digestibility of feedstuffs decreases as the percentage of fiber increases. However, the lignin content is highly correlated with fiber content, so it is difficult to separate the effects. The physical and chemical masking effect of lignin apparently prevents the action of microbial cellulases on the fiber in this case. Minson (1971) has concluded that lignin has only a small effect on digestibility of soluble cell components in some grass species. He further concludes that the main factors controlling organic matter digestibility were the percentages of both hemicellulose and cellulose present and the extent to which they were lignified. Silicon was not a factor in digestibility of the celluloses. In an example cited by Blaxter (1962, p 188) digestible energy declined from 83% in first cutting ryegrass hay to 63% in the 4th cutting. At least part of this decline would be due to the increase in fiber and lignin.

3. Species differences. There have been a number of comparisons between the European breeds of cattle and sheep, but the results have been somewhat inconclusive. In a statistical study of published data, Cipalloni et al (1951) found that cattle generally digested dry roughages to a greater extent than sheep, whereas sheep were more efficient digesters of concentrates, particularly the ether extract fractions. Swift and Bratzler (1959) compiled data from a variety of experiment stations on 28 lots of forage and found that there were no significant differences between the two species in the digestibility of dry matter, crude protein or digestible energy. Alexander et al (1962) have also reported comparative results. Digestibility was quite similar on a variety of hays and silages, but they did find that sheep tended to digest grass hay of low quality or low protein content to a greater extent than cattle. Similar data of this type have recently been published by Schiemann et al (1971), results indicating that cattle digested crude fiber slightly better and that digestibility of protein by sheep was greater on high-protein diets.

Studies on rumen digestion by Hungate et al (1960) indicate that Zebu cattle had a more rapid fermentation rate than European breeds of cattle, results which were confirmed by Phillips (1961), who also found that Zebus digested ca. 3% more organic matter of low quality grass hay than Hereford steers. Ichhponani et al (1971) observed that Asian water buffalo digested cellulose in the rumen at a more rapid rate than Zebu cattle, the difference becoming more pronounced when the quality of feed was reduced. Pant et al (1963) ranked buffalo, sheep and goats in that order with respect to efficiency of rumen utilization, and Ponnappa et al (1971) found that buffalo digested more dry matter, crude protein, ether extract and cellulose than native cattle, the improvement being attributed to longer retention times in buffalo.

With red deer, Maloiy and Kay (1971) found that deer digested dry matter and cellulose a "little less well" than sheep, but there was no difference in crude protein when fed chopped or pelleted hays. Data on camelids (llama, Guanaco) indicate more efficient digestion of dry matter and fiber than sheep (Hintz et al, 1973), but apparently camels are less efficient in digesting dry matter but equal in digestion of crude protein of low quality grass hay as compared to Zebu steers (Maloiy, 1972).

4. Nutrient deficiencies. Many experiments indicate that a relative or absolute deficiency of protein will result in a marked reduction of digestible energy (and reduced feed intake). In ruminant species this is probably due, for the most part, to a depressing effect on microbial activity. Rumen digestion may also be depressed by deficiencies of Mg, P, and S of the macro minerals and by Fe, Co, Mn and Zn of the trace minerals (see Ch. 15). Other deficiencies, such as in the case of vitamin A, will have an effect due to the diarrhea which results.

5. Factors affecting appetite. Anything which will greatly modify intake can be expected to have an effect. This could include physical nature of the ration as well as the presence or absence of nutrients or appetite factors.

6. Frequency of feeding. Data presented by Gordon and Tribe (1952), Campbell and Merilan (1961) and Clark and Keener (1962) indicate that increasing the frequency of feeding tends to increase digestibility. Data presented by Gordon and Tribe (1952), Rakes et al (1961) and Graham (1967) indicate that

there is less heat loss and an improved N retention even though there may be little difference in digestibility. Other examples (Faichney, 1968; Hillier et al, 1968) show little or no apparent benefit of frequent feeding.

7. Feed preparation. There is a large volume of literature on this topic. The results, in general, indicate that grinding, rolling or flaking of grain may be expected to increase digestibility. Pelleting has been shown to have little effect for grains, and may result in a decreased digestibility of forages (more rapid passage) although the intake may increase markedly. Heating may improve some proteins, but too much heat can easily reduce digestibility. Steaming and cooking will usually improve the utilization of the carbohydrates in grains.

8. The associative effect of feedstuffs. This effect was illustrated previously and an additional and better example is shown in Table 8-5. Note how different the estimated digestion coefficients are when corn silage was fed with two different feedstuffs. When the feeds are fed together, part of the associative effect may be due to providing a more optimal combination of nutrients (if positive), or the digestibility of the basal ration may have been altered. For example, a

Table 8-6. Typical values for digestion coefficients by cattle.[a]

| Feedstuffs | Digestion coefficients | | | | | |
	Organic matter	Crude protein	Crude fiber	Nitrogen-free-extract	Ether extract	TDN
Straw, wheat	53	14	58	49	42	32
Hay						
Alfalfa	56	61	39	69	36	50
Mixed grass	54	23	62	50	28	44
Silage						
Alfalfa	60	67	52	61	60	14
Grass	71	60	78	70	55	16
Ryegrass, green	70	62	70	73	62	15
Grains						
Barley	81	70	6	88	63	78
Corn	87	75	19	91	87	80
Wheat	88	78	33	92	72	81

[a] Data from Schneider (1947) or NRC publications.

combination of alfalfa pellets and corn silage probably increases rumen retention time of the pellets, thus resulting in greater digestion of fiber from the pellets. Unfortunately, there is very little information in the literature to indicate how important this may be with a wide variety of different feedstuffs. The few illustrations available indicate that it may have a very substantial effect on digestibility in some specific situations. In comparing digestibility of alfalfa hay or beet pulp and the combination, Asplund and Harris (1971) found negative effects on ether extract and crude fiber but a positive effect on NFE and the observed value for N retention was lower than the calculated value.

9. Adaptation to ration changes. Unlike monogastric species, ruminants do not thrive on highly variable diets in which there is a marked change in the type of food consumed from day to day. A variable diet results in shifts in the rumen microbial population which require time to adjust to a different food source. One consequence of ration changes may be a lower digestibility than expected until this adaptation occurs. Data from a variety of sources indicate that animals need to be adjusted to ration changes for at least two to three weeks when conducting digestion trials in order to get a reasonably good estimate of digestibility. The extent of the change will, of course, determine the time required.

Amount of Various Nutrients Digested

The amount of a given nutrient in any particular feedstuff or ration that will be digested will be influenced by the variables listed previously as well as others not specifically listed. However, as a general estimate, the values listed in Table 8-6 would seem to be appropriate values for cattle.

Many people overlook the obvious biological fact that digestibility is subject to variation as a result of many different factors. Even within one animal or in identical twins, it may be difficult to confirm small differences. In addition, the difficulty in relating intake to excretion explains the conclusion that many factors have no effect on digestibility. Some of these would include such items as exercise, pregnancy, lactation, age and moderate changes in environmental temperature.

Even though digestibility is a biological variable, it has been and will continue to be a very useful criterion for evaluating feedstuffs, preparatory methods, seasonal differences in forages, nutrient intake by animals as well as numerous other objectives. This is so because digestion accounts for the single biggest loss in nutrient utilization by ruminant species.

References Cited

Alexander, R.A., J.F. Hentges, J.T. McCall and W.O. Ash. 1962. J. Animal Sci. 21:373.
Anderson, P.E., J.T. Reid, M.J. Anderson and J.W. Stroud. 1959. J. Animal Sci. 18:1299.
Asplund, J.M. and L.E. Harris. 1971. J. Animal Sci. 32:152.
Blaxter, K.L. 1961. In: Digestive Physiology and Nutrition of the Ruminant. Butterworths, London.
Blaxter, K.L. 1962. The Energy Metabolism of Ruminants. Hutchison Pub. Co., London.
Blaxter, K.L., N. McC. Graham and F.W. Wainman. 1956. Br. J. Nutr. 10:69.
Blaxter, K.L. and W.A. Wood. 1951. Br. J. Nutr. 5:11.
Campbell, J.R. and C.P. Merilan. 1961. J. Dairy Sci. 44:664.
Castle, M.E., A.S. Foot and R.J. Halley. 1950. J. Dairy Res. 17:215.
Chandler, P.T., E.M. Kesler and G.M. Jones. 1966. J. Animal Sci. 25:64.
Christian, K.R., V.J. Williams and A.H. Carter. 1965. N.Z. J. Agr. Res. 8:530.
Church, D.C. 1969. Oregon Agr. Expt. Sta. Sp. Rpt. 282.
Cipalloni, M.A., B.H. Schneider, H.L. Lucas and H.M. Pavlech. 1951. J. Animal Sci. 10:337.
Clark, B. and H.A. Keener. 1962. J. Dairy Sci. 45:1199.
Condon, R.J., G. Hall and E.E. Hatfield. 1970. J. Animal Sci. 31:1037.
Corbett, J.L., J.F.D. Greenhalgh, I. McDonald and E. Florence. 1960. Br. J. Nutr. 14:289.
Dietz, D.R., R.H. Udall, and L.E. Yeager. 1962. Colo. Game and Fish Dept. Tech. Pub. No. 14.
Dijkstra, N.D. 1972. Nutr. Abstr. Rev. 42:1589.
Dowe, T.W., J. Matsushima and V. Arthaud. 1955. J. Animal Sci. 14:340.
Dukes, H.H. 1955. The Physiology of Domestic Animals. 7th ed. Comstock Pub. Assoc., Ithaca, N.Y.
Ellis, W.C. and J.E. Huston. 1967. J. Nutr. 95:67.
Faichney. G.J. 1968. Aust. J. Agr. Res. 19:813.
Fell, B.F., E. Regoeczi, R.M. Campbell and W.S. Mackie. 1969. Quart. J. Expt. Physiol. 54:141.
Forbes, E.B., W.W. Braman and M. Kriss. 1928. J. Agr. Res. 37:253.
Gasparini, U. and S. Marangoni. 1970. Nutr. Abstr. Rev. 40:1443.
Gordon, J.G. and D.E. Tribe. 1952. Br. J. Nutr. 6:89.

Graham, N. McC. 1967. Aust. J. Agr. Res. 18:467.
Hardison, W.A., H.L. Fisher, G.C. Graf and N.R. Thompson. 1956. J. Dairy Sci. 39:1735.
Hardison, W.A., W.N. Linkous, R.W. Engel and G.C. Graf. 1959. J. Dairy Sci. 42:346.
Hillier, R.J., T.W. Perry, R.M. Peart and W.M. Beeson. 1968. J. Animal Sci. 27:227.
Hintz, H.F., H.F. Schryver and M. Halbert. 1973. Animal Prod. 16:303.
Hjelle, A. 1969. Acta Vet. Scand. 10:1.
Hogan, J.P. and R.H. Weston. 1969. Aust. J. Agr. Res. 20:347.
Hopson, D.E. and J.E. McCroskey. 1972. J. Animal Sci. 35:1054.
Hungate, R.E., G.D. Phillips, D.P. Hungate and A. MacGregor. 1960. J. Agr. Sci. 54:196.
Ichhponani, J.S., G.S. Makkar and G.S. Sidu. 1971. Indian Vet. J. 48:267.
Jarrige, R. 1965. Proc. IX International Grasslands Cong. Vol. 1, p 809.
Johnson, D.E., W.E. Dinusson and D.W. Bolin. 1964. J. Animal Sci. 23:499.
Johnson, R.R. 1966. J. Animal Sci. 27:855.
Johnstone-Wallace, D.B. and K. Kennedy. 1944. J. Agr. Sci. 34:190.
Kane, E.A., W.C. Jacobson, R.E. Ely and L.A. Moore. 1953. J. Dairy Sci. 36:637.
Kertz, A.F., L.R. Prewitt, A.G. Lane and J.R. Campbell. 1970. J. Animal Sci. 30:278.
Kiesling, H.E., H.A. Barry, A.B. Nelson and C.H. Herbel. 1969. J. Animal Sci. 29:361.
Kotb, A.R. and T.D. Luckey. 1972. Nutr. Abstr. Rev. 42:28.
Lancaster, R.J., M.R. Coup and J.C. Percival. 1953. N.Z. J. Sci. Tech. 35A:117.
Leaver, J.D., R.C. Campling and W. Holmes. 1969. Animal Prod. 11:11.
Lysov, F.F. 1961. Nutr. Abstr. Rev. 31:921.
MacRae, J.C. and D.G. Armstrong. 1969. Br. J. Nutr. 23:15.
Maloiy, G.M.O. 1972. Res. Vet. Sci. 13:476.
Maloiy, G.M.O. and R.N.B. Kay. 1971. Quart. J. Expt. Physiol. 56:257.
Martin, A.K. 1970. Br. J. Nutr. 24:943.
Martin, A.K. 1973. Br. J. Nutr. 30:251.
Mason, V.C. 1969. J. Agr. Sci. 73:99.
McAllan, A.B. and R.H. Smith. 1968. Proc. Nutr. Soc. 27:47A (abstr).
McLeod, M.N. and D.J. Minson. 1971. J. Br. Grassld. Soc. 26:251.
McLeod, M.N. and D.J. Minson. 1972. J. Br. Grassld. Soc. 27:23.
Minson, D.J. 1971. Aust. J. Agr. Res. 22:589.
Minson, D.J. and J.L. Cowper. 1966. Br. J. Nutr. 20:575.
Mitchell, H.H. 1964. Comparative Nutrition of Man and Domestic Animals. Vol. II. Academic Press.
Mitchell, et al. 1932. J. Agr. Res. 45:163.
Moe, P.W., J.T. Reid and H.F. Tyrrell. 1965. J. Dairy Sci. 48:1053.
Nehring, K., U. Zelck and R. Schiemann. 1965. Archiv. Tierernahrung. 15:45.
Nelson, A.B. and G.R. Green. 1969. J. Animal Sci. 29:365.
Ørskov, E.R., C. Fraser, V.C. Mason and S.O. Mann. 1970. Br. J. Nutr. 24:671.
Pant, H.C., M.D. Pandey, J.S. Rawat and A. Roy. 1963. Indian J. Dairy Sci. 16:29.
Phillips, G.D. 1961. Res. Vet. Sci. 2:202.
Pierce, A.E. 1959. J. Physiol. 148:469.
Ponnappa, C.G., M.D. Noor Uddin and G.V. Raghavan. 1971. Indian J. Animal Sci. 41:1026.
Porter, P. and A.G. Singleton. 1971. Br. J. Nutr. 26:3.
Rabinowitz, L. and R.A. Gunther. 1972. Amer. J. Physiol. 222:801.
Rakes, A.H., E.E. Lister and J.T. Reid. 1961. J. Nutr. 75:86.
Razzaque, M.A. and J.H. Topps. 1973. Proc. Nutr. Soc. 32:59A (abstr).
Reid, J.T., P.W. Moe and H.F. Tyrrell. 1966. J. Dairy Sci. 49:215.
Scales, G.H., C.L. Streeter, A.H. Denham and G.M. Ward. 1974. J. Animal Sci. 38:192.
Schake, L.M. and J.K. Riggs. 1969. J. Animal Sci. 28:568.
Schake, L.M. and J.K. Riggs. 1970. J. Animal Sci. 31:414.
Schiemann, R., W. Jentsch, H. Wittenburg and L. Hoffmann. 1971. Nutr. Abstr. Rev. 41:1054.
Schneider, B.H. 1947. Feeds of the World. W. Virginia Agr. Expt. Sta.
Schneider, B.H., B.K. Soni and W.E. Ham. 1955. Wash. Agr. Expt. Sta. Tech. Bul. 16.
Scott, D. 1972. Quart. J. Expt. Physiol. 57:379.
Scott, D., F.G. Whitelaw and M. Kay. 1971. Quart. J. Expt. Physiol. 56:18.
Schurch, A.F., E.W. Crampton, S.R. Haskell and L.E. Lloyd. 1952. J. Animal Sci. 11:261.
Smith, A.D. 1964. J. Wildl. Mgt. 28:435.
Stacy, B.D. and A.H. Brook. 1964. Aust. J. Agr. Res. 15:289.
Swift, R.W. and J.W. Bratzler (ed.). 1959. Pa. Agr. Expt. Bul. 651.
Thornton, R.F. and B.W. Wilson. 1972. Aust. J. Agr. Res. 23:727.
Topps, J.H. 1966. Proc. Nutr. Soc. 25:19.
Tyrrell, H.F. and P.W. Moe. 1972. J. Dairy Sci. 55:1106.
Virtanen, A.I. 1966. Science 153:1603.
Visek, W.J. 1966. Proc. Cornell Nutr. Conf. p 9.
Volcani, R., M. Ben-Yakov, D. Sklan and Z. Nitsan. 1973. J. Dairy Sci. 56:1107.
Wagnon, K.A. 1963. Calif. Agr. Expt. Sta. Bul. 799.
Walker, D.M. and G.J. Faichney. 1964. Br. J. Nutr. 18:201.
Weaver, A.D. 1970. Amer. J. Vet. Res. 32:5:813.
White, A., P. Handler and E.L. Smith. 1964. Principles of Biochemistry. McGraw-Hill Pub. Co.
Woelfel, C.G., et al. 1965. Connecticut Agr. Expt. Sta. Res. Rpt. 6.
Yadava, R.K., L.O. Gilmore and H.R. Conrad. 1973. J. Dairy Sci. 26:592.

CHAPTER 9 — PARTIAL DIGESTION AND ABSORPTION

The term **partial digestion** implies that the total digestion which occurs in the GIT can be subdivided into components that are digested in different parts of the tract. There has, in fact, been a considerable interest in this subject, particularly directed toward the reticulo-rumen in the earlier work and, more recently, to the intestinal tract. As in the case of studies on passage of feedstuffs through the tract, comparative data between species are inadequate, although data within species, especially sheep, are more complete.

In this chapter, as with some of the others, there is a question of what material to include or exclude. Since separate chapters dealing with rumen metabolism of the various nutrients are presented later, partial digestion data relating to the rumen will be primarily restricted to dry matter or major groups of nutrients, and that pertaining to specific nutrients will be presented in subsequent chapters. Likewise, data on absorption of the minerals are presented in Ch. 20 and 21 of Vol. 2 and will not be included here except for that on absorption by the forestomach.

Changes in Composition of Digesta Along the GIT

One method that has been used to estimate partial digestion in the GIT is to quantitatively collect digesta from the various parts of the GIT of slaughtered animals and to determine the chemical changes that have occurred. When used in conjunction with a marker such as lignin, PEG, or Cr_2O_3, such data allow the calculation of digestion or absorption in each segment of the GIT. Of course, saliva complicates the estimate for certain constituents in the rumen as do the digestive juices and sloughed cellular debris in the abomasum, duodenum and upper jejunum. Data of this type published by Rogerson (1958) are shown in Table 9-1 for sheep and data on dry matter content of the GIT in cattle (O'Dell et al, 1963) are shown for comparison. Other papers presenting information changes occurring in various parts of

the GIT include those of Boyne et al (1956), Badawy et al (1958a, b), Gray et al (1958), Weller et al (1962), and Mylrea (1966). An appreciable amount of information on specific nutrients is also available, especially in recent years from animals with multiple cannulas in the GIT. This will be mentioned and discussed in appropriate sections.

In regard to the data presented in Table 9-1, it is quite apparent that the dry matter content of various parts of the tract changes, reflecting secretion of the salivary or gastric fluids and absorption in the intestines (and probably the omasum). For comparative purposes it appears that cattle have an appreciably larger percentage of total digesta in the reticulo-rumen and omasum than do sheep and much less in the intestines.

The data shown in Table 9-1, when expressed on a dry matter basis, illustrate changes that might be expected to occur as some of the nutrients are digested and absorbed as digesta progresses through the GIT. For example, lignin is concentrated from the rumen to the omasum, indicating a loss of organic or inorganic nutrients. The decreasing concentration of lignin from the omasum (hay-fed sheep) to the abomasum and from the abomasum to the small intestine would indicate the production of large volumes of abomasal and intestinal juices. With respect to the intestines, a marked concentration of lignin occurs between the small intestine and the cecum, reflecting the large amount of absorption known to occur there. From the cecum through the colon only very slight changes occur, indicating a slight amount of absorption.

Partial Digestion in the GIT of Sheep or Goats

Robertson (1958) used data on composition from various sites in the GIT (similar to that in Table 9-1) and formulas similar to those used for indicator methods discussed in Ch. 8 to calculate the amount of digestion occurring in the rumen of sheep. From this data he calculated that ca. 40% of the dry

Table 9-1. Changes in composition of digesta in the gastrointestinal track of sheep or cattle.

					Sample site					
Ration fed and type of constituent	Ration	Rumen	Reticu- lum	Omasum	Abo- masum	S. int.	Cecum	Colon	Term. colon and rectum	Feces
Sheep [a]										
Hay, 600 g in 2 feeds										
Dry matter, %		10.1	11.5	18.8	15.5	9.8	13.5	14.6	25.8	
Dry matter, g		350.1	34.5	59.5	19.0	62.0	43.1	69.1	31.0	
Organ content, % of total		52.4	5.2	8.9	2.8	9.3	6.4	10.3	4.6	
Composition of digesta, %										
Lignin	11.33	19.73	15.49	23.78	18.52	12.38	20.86	21.18	21.04	22.16
Crude protein	6.90	8.46	10.32	9.33	12.25	17.96	8.38	8.19	8.58	7.76
Crude fiber	41.12	37.98	30.14	32.56	29.29	20.93	26.74	22.96	28.13	32.06
Energy (Kcal/g)	4.46	4.30	4.34	4.36	4.46	4.59	4.23	4.36	4.44	4.57
Soluble ash	5.34	7.21	4.89	4.87	4.15	10.36	8.33	6.92	5.13	4.47
Hay, 500 g and 300 g of cassava meal										
Dry matter, %		10.5	10.6	20.8	14.0	11.0	12.1	15.1	28.3	
Dry matter, g		321.4	26.8	37.0	12.5	44.9	42.6	42.9	53.5	
Organ content, % of total		55.3	4.6	6.4	2.1	7.7	7.3	7.4	9.2	
Composition of digesta, %										
Lignin	7.26	15.12	14.10	17.33	17.53	9.93	18.55	18.35	18.70	19.27
Crude protein	4.79	15.33	14.90	9.49	11.16	22.60	7.63	9.55	9.92	8.79
Crude fiber	26.56	29.35	29.51	33.69	29.70	19.46	28.42	26.84	29.08	31.47
Energy (Kcal/g)	4.27	4.40	4.36	4.48	4.43	4.54	4.26	4.31	4.40	4.44
Soluble ash	4.00	8.26	8.67	4.67	4.78	9.18	7.76	6.86	4.88	3.93
Dairy Cows [b]		Ret.-rum.				Up. Low.			L. int.	Total tract
Baled bermuda grass hay										
Dry matter, %		15.16		20.31	11.86	7.49 7.13	8.69		10.25	14.64
Dry matter, g		9,305		1,736	296	158 297	158		372	12,322
Organ content, % of total		75.5		14.1	2.4	1.3 2.4	1.3		3.0	
Ground bermuda grass hay										
Dry matter, %		14.61		20.88	11.56	8.72 7.43	10.61		10.95	14.56
Dry matter, g		5,939		1,617	224	168 202	146		276	8,572
Organ content, % of total		69.3		18.9	2.6	2.0 2.4	1.7		3.2	

[a] Data from Rogerson (1958)
[b] Data from O'Dell et al (1963)

matter was digested in the rumen of hay-fed sheep, ca. 50% when sheep were fed hay and cassava meal, and ca. 75% when fed 100% corn. His data indicate, for the hay and hay + cassava rations, that digestion and absorption of nutrients was almost complete by the time the cecum was reached.

Boyne et al (1956) studied the changes in composition of digesta in the GIT of sheep by killing the animals from 2-12 hr after feeding and isolating various segments of the GIT. The dry matter content of the reticulo-rumen as the percent of the total GIT was ca. 75% just after feeding and fell to ca. 60% in 12 hr. No calculations were given on partial digestion, however. In the papers by Gray et al (1958), sheep were fed on a mixture of wheat hay and wheat straw, or wheat hay or alfalfa hay. These authors estimated that 30, 40 and 50%, respectively, of the cellulose was digested in the rumen. Digestion of pentosans and other solids was similar to that of cellulose. For nitogenous material, they calculated that 100, 65 and 48% of dietary N reached the abomasum when sheep were fed the three rations. Data on cellulose (Gray, 1947) indicated that 70% of the digestible cellulose disappeared in the rumen, 17% in the cecum and 13% in the colon. Weller et al (1962) found that material entering the omasum was well digested in respect to plant N.

Badawy and co-workers (1958a, b) found that the reticulo-rumen contained ca. 74% of the contents of the GIT 4 hr after feeding. DM percentages were considerably higher in the omasum and the colon than in other parts of the tract, the omasum having the highest value. The highest concentration of ash on a DM basis was found in the abomasum, then the distal half of the small intestine, the proximal half, the cecum and colon and finally the omasum and the reticulo-rumen, in that order. The caloric values of the digesta were highest in those zones where dehydration was taking place, particularly in the omasum and, to a lesser extent, the cecum and colon.

Estimates of partial digestion have been reported by a number of other authors using methods such as marker flow from the reticulo-rumen, by emptying the reticulo-rumen and obtaining samples and with the aid of cannulas in various parts of the GIT. Some of these are reviewed briefly in subsequent paragraphs.

Oyaert and Bouchaert (1961) used sheep with omasal cannulas to determine the extent of rumen digestion when the sheep were fed 704 to 1,232 g of DM. Examination of omasal contents showed that 49-64% of total DM or from 52-75% of digestible DM disappeared in the forestomach, depending upon the diet fed. Kameoka and Morimoto (1959) have also used this technique with goats. When feeding a variety of diets, they found that 62-85% of the digestible organic matter disappeared by the time digesta has passed through the omasum. Apparent digestibility coefficients of crude protein in the forestomach varied widely and were positively related to dietary protein levels. The absorption of digestible protein ranged from -20 to 52%. In animals fed roughage alone, 62-73% of the digestible ether extract disappeared but in goats fed concentrates and hay, smaller amounts (-2.9 to 29%) were absorbed. Almost all of the digestible crude fiber (81-100%) was digested in the fore-stomach. Crude ash showed negative values (salivary secretion) except in one trial. Data from three of the trials conducted are shown in Table 9-2.

When using duodenal re-entrant cannulas, Ridges and Singleton (1962) estimated that, of the digestible constituents of the diet, 58% of the dry matter, 68% of the organic matter, 93% of the fiber, 11% of the crude protein and 81% of the soluble carbohydrates disappeared in the stomach and the remainder in the intestines. Hogan and Phillipson (1960) estimated that ca. 70% of the dry matter disappeared in the stomach and that ca. 25% of apparently digestible nitrogen was removed before digesta entered the duodenum. Phillips and Dyck (1964) fed sheep rations having low and high levels of starch supplemented with low and high levels of urea. Calculations indicated that appreciably more digestion of organic matter occurred in the intestines of sheep fed the low starch rations (30-35% vs 21-28% in the stomach). However, on the high starch diets, digestibility was considerably higher in the stomach (48-52%) as compared to the intestines (28-29%).

Cloete (1966) has studied partial digestion of dry matter using ruminal and intestinal cannulas in sheep fed grass pellets, cellulose or cellulose plus casein. On the cellulose diet, rumen function was affected but on the other two diets digestion was calculated to be 56 and 64% in the stomach for the pellets and casein diets, respectively,

Table 9-2. Estimated digestion in the forestomachs and the entire GIT of the goat.[a]

Ration	Site	Constituent, %					
		Organic matter	Crude protein	Ether extract	Crude fiber	NFE	Crude ash
Orchardgrass +	Forestomach	60.0	38.5	48.2	78.0	65.3	-25.9
red clover hay	Entire GIT	73.4	73.9	65.8	79.8	70.3	56.2
Hay and mixed	Forestomach	51.1	5.8	1.4	60.7	62.7	- 6.3
concentrates	Entire GIT	63.9	49.9	53.0	62.4	77.2	35.6
Hay and mixed	Forestomach	53.8	24.7	23.9	64.5	66.1	-18.7
concentrates (high starch)	Entire GIT	73.3	62.0	82.9	63.1	78.3	46.3

[a]From Kameoka and Morimoto (1959)

with 16 and 30% digestion in the small intestine and 28 and 6% in the large intestine, respectively. Data in Table 9-3 (Topps et al, 1968) illustrate that substantial digestion of dry matter and digestible energy may occur in the large intestine.

Information from some recent experiments on sheep fed a variety of diets is summarized in Table 9-4. When discussing partial digestion note that the relative amount which occurs in the stomach is dependent upon the type of diet, the amount of cereal grain in the diet, the kind of feed preparation used, and the nutrient of concern. These data clearly illustrate that the majority of the fibrous carbohydrates are digested in the fore-stomach, but, when pelleted feeds are fed, a very substantial amount may be degraded in the cecum or colon. Readily available carbohydrates are almost completely digested in the rumen, most papers indicating that 90-98% disappears there (Waldo, 1973). For readers who wish more information on it, this subject has been extensively reviewed by Armstrong and Beever (1969) and Waldo (1973). In addition to those references already cited, additional information on sheep may be found in papers by Tucker et al (1968), Ørskov et al (1969), Reed et al (1969), Vidal et al (1969), Holmes et al (1970) and Thivend and Vermorel (1971); and on goats, Porter and Singleton (1971).

Table 9-3. Partial digestion in the stomach and intestine of sheep fed hay or concentrates.[a]

Item	Percentage disappeared		
	Forestomach	Small intestine	Large intestine
Concentrate diet			
Digestible dry matter	69	17	14
Digestible energy	72	23	5
Hay diet			
Digestible dry matter	67	22	11
Digestible energy	81	7	12

[a]Topps et al (1968)

Regarding protein digestion in the stomach, it is apparent that some rations and experiments yield negative values. This is due, partly, to recycling of N via the saliva or through the rumen wall. For further discussion on this topic, refer to Ch. 13.

Data presented by Goodall and Kay (1965) on sheep with cannulas in the terminal ileum confirm the results of some other authors that very little digestion of cellulose occurs in the cecum or large intestine. However, Bazanova and Moiseev (1967) reported an experiment in which capsules containing filter paper were suspended via fistulas in the rumen and cecum of sheep. During the winter when the sheep were fed oats and hay, fiber digestion was generally more extensive in the cecum than in the rumen, although the data were variable and the difference was greater when fed mixed hay than alfalfa hay. In the summer when grazing grass, one sheep showed greater fiber digestion in the rumen, but the other was little changed. In the sheep that digested the greater amounts in the rumen, ciliate counts were higher. This experiment demonstrates that the microbial population in the cecum is apparently capable of hydrolyzing cellulose; presumably, the quality and physical nature of the diet might have a pronounced effect on the relative importance of cecal digestion.

In the case of starch, Tucker et al (1968) gave rations high in starch orally to sheep or via abomasal cannulas. Overall apparent digestibility of starch in four rations ranged from 88-94%; oral to abomasal (forestomach digestion) coefficients were between 64 and 80% and intestinal coefficients were 45-79% on rations containing 60-80% corn. Ørskov et al (1970) have studied starch fermentation in the cecum of sheep by infusing from 20-300 g/day. Infused starch in excess of 138 g appeared largely in the feces, indicating a limited but substantial capacity for starch fermentation. Infusions of starch increased N excretion from 5.8 to 9 g/day.

Partial Digestion Studies with Cattle

Experiments with cattle relating to partial digestion have been somewhat less extensive than those with sheep, partly because of the greater expense (and losses) when using animals with multiple cannulas in the GIT;

however, a number of papers of interest will be reviewed briefly. One of the first of these was by Hale et al (1947). When studying the disappearance of nutrients in the reticulo-rumen of alfalfa-fed steers, these authors estimated that loss of ingested nutrients from the rumen amounted to 48.4% of the dry matter, 59.6% of the crude protein, 43% of the cellulose and 83% of the other carbohydrates. Phillips et al (1960) calculated that when steers were fed on poor hay, rumen fermentation accounted for 50-70% of total dry matter digested. In the case of alfalfa hay-fed dairy cows, Yadava and Bartley (1964) based estimates of rumen digestion on disappearance from the rumen. They calculated that rumen fermentation accounted for the following amounts of total digestion: dry matter, 68.7%; fiber, 73.5%; NFE, 69.8%; crude protein, 65.4%; ether extract, 104.8%; and ash, 99%. Hinders and Owen (1968) have obtained similar data on steers fed alfalfa hay or dehydrated alfalfa pellets (see Table 9-5), using lignin ratio techniques. The values indicate that 90% of the digestible fiber disappeared in the rumen when alfalfa hay was fed as compared to <60% when dehydrated alfalfa pellets were fed. For NFE, 95 and 85%, respectively, disappeared in the rumen when hay and pellets were fed.

In examples where duodenal re-entrant cannulas were used, McGilliard et al (1957) estimated that forestomach digestion of organic matter accounted for 73, 58, 58 and 68% of the total when steers were fed rations varying from 100% corn to 100% alfalfa hay. Although no data were given, they did report that little or no fiber digestion occurred in the intestines. Putnam and Davis (1965) have obtained data on calves 4-14 mo. of age when fed a variety of feeds through an abomasal fistula. The data shown (Table 9-6) indicate that digestibility of dry matter and crude protein was less affected by abomasal feeding than was fiber. Calculated digestibility of the wood cellulose was 63% when fed orally and 29% when placed in the abomasum, a marked reduction, yet indicating very substantial digestion in the lower GIT. This paper differs from some papers by other authors who generally indicate little, if any, digestion of fiber from natural feedstuffs in the lower GIT of ruminants.

Other relatively recent research on partial digestion by bovines includes that of Dirksen et al (1972). In studies with cows with

Table 9-4. Partial Digestion of Different Nutrient Fractions of Various Rations with Sheep.

Ration, Site of digestion	Organic matter	N	CWC*	Digestibility, % Cellulose	Fiber Hemicellulose	RAC**	Energy	Reference
Sheep Fed Forages								
Alfalfa hay, chopped								Hogan and Weston (1967)
Stomach	64.6	24.1	86.8	89.8		82		
Intestine	35.4	75.9	13.2	10.2				
Alfalfa hay, pelleted								
Stomach	64.7	25.3	83.0	90.1		88		
Intestine	35.3	74.7	17.0	9.9				
Wheaten hay, chopped								
Stomach	67.2	-172	81.2	69.9		89		
Intestine	32.8	272	19.8	30.1				
Wheaten hay, pelleted								
Stomach	63.6	-119	67.6	76.5		91		
Intestine	36.4	219	33.4	23.5				
Forage oats, low-N fertilization								Hogan and Weston (1969)
Stomach	54.6	-7.8	88.8	95.6		95		
Forage oats, high-N fertilization								Weston and Hogan (1968)
Stomach	57.8	11.3	91.7	97.5		87		
Subterranean clover								
Stomach	65.0	7.2	91.9					
Berseem clover								
Stomach	61.5	20.6	93.0					
Alkali-treated straw, med. intake								Hogan and Weston (1971)
Stomach	55.6		91.9					
Dried, chopped ryegrass, early cut								Beever et al (1972) and Coelho Da Silva et al (1972b)
Stomach	64.4	-7.3		94.3	91.3		64.1	
Small intestine	29.4	97.4		2.7	0.8		31.7	
Cecum and colon	4.2	9.9		3.0	7.9		4.2	
Dried, pelleted ryegrass, early cut								
Stomach	56.2	-25.1		76.9	68.0		51.2	
Small intestine	33.7	114.8		6.0	8.8		39.2	
Cecum and colon	10.1	10.3		17.1	23.2		9.6	
Dried, chopped alfalfa								Thomson et al (1972) and Coelho Da Silva (1972a)
Stomach	47.3	-42.4		85.4	68.5		38.6	
Small intestine	29.4	107.8		-3.7	1.0		33.8	
Cecum and colon	23.3	34.6		18.3	30.5			

						Reference
Dried, pelleted alfalfa						MacRae and Armstrong (1969)
Stomach	33.6	− 35.0	63.3	55.2		23.3
Small intestine	42.1	111.0	9.2	3.7		51.1
Cecum and colon	24.3	24.0	27.5	41.1		25.6
Hay, chopped						
Stomach			91.0	95.3	81.8	67.1
Small intestine			0.2	3.4	18.2	21.2
Cecum and colon			8.8	1.3	0.0	11.7
Sheep fed diets containing cereal grains						
Hay 67, rolled barley 33						MacRae and Armstrong (1969)
Stomach			84.1	94.5	90.7	66.1
Small intestine			0.4	1.8	9.0	24.3
Cecum and colon			15.5	3.7	0.3	9.6
Hay 33, rolled barley 67						
Stomach			56.2	82.1	92.6	62.3
Small intestine			14.4	5.2	7.1	29.4
Cecum and colon			29.4	12.8	0.3	8.3
Hay 75, dairy cubes 25						Nicholson and Sutton (1969)
Stomach					89.2	70.0
Hay 20.5, dairy cubes 34.1, flaked corn, 45.4						
Stomach					96.2	68.3
Hay 18.9, dairy cubes 12.2, flaked corn, 69.1						
Stomach					94.5	62.3

*CWC = cell wall constituents
**RAC = readily available carbohydrates

Table 9-5.   Estimated digestibility in the rumen and intestines of steers fed alfalfa hay or alfalfa pellets.[a]

Feed, Site of digestion	Digestibility, %				
	NFE	Crude fiber	Acid det. fiber	Cellulose	Holo-cellulose
Long alfalfa hay					
Rumen	64.3	48.9	46.2	56.2	60.5
Intestines	3.4	4.0	5.1	-1.0	1.5
Pelleted alfalfa					
Rumen	57.7	25.9	25.7	25.4	30.1
Intestines	12.8	14.0	11.5	16.9	19.8

[a]From Hinders and Owen (1968)

Table 9-6.   Effect of feeding calves orally or via an abomasal cannula.[a]

Dry matter and ration fed	Age of calf, mo.	Method of feeding	Digestion coefficients, %		
			Dry matter	Crude protein	Acid detergent fiber
0.35 kg from milk	4	oral	78.1	78.2	52.1
+0.92 kg from ration	4.5	cannula	72.9	74.5	29.2
with 56.8% alfalfa		Diff.	-5.2	-3.7	-22.9
0.70 kg from milk	6	oral	81.5	87.0	49.2
+0.82 kg from alfalfa	8	cannula	71.5	74.4	28.6
		Diff.	-10.0	-12.6	-20.6
1.68 kg from ration containing 64% corn	11	oral	72.7	66.0	52.3
+0.29 kg from wood		cannula	70.2	69.3	37.6
cellulose	13	Diff.	-2.5	3.3	-14.7

[a]Putnam and Davis (1965)

duodenal cannulas, they found that 58-60% of digestible energy disappeared in the stomach when fed hay diets, 52-55% for those with more concentrates, and 20% for cows fed pellets. In the duodenum, 13-25% of α-linked glucose polymers (starch) remained, most on the concentrate rations. Watson et al (1972a, b) have used cows with re-entrant cannulas in the proximal duodenum and terminal ileum, and studied partial digestion in one cow when dry, pregnant and lactating, and a second cow when dry. Some of their data are shown in Table 9-7. These data indicate for energy that an increasing intake resulted in a reduction of digestibility in the stomach and a greater disappearance in the intestinal tract. The same trend is obvious, although more so, for N, showing that a negative amount of N disappeared from the rumen on two of the four examples. There was less difference for cellulose, although minor differences are noted and the α-linked glucose polymers were seen to be less digested in the rumen as intake increased or on a different ration. In studies where cellulose was infused into the abomasum of steers (Warner et al, 1972), mean digestion was 33%. Some digestion occurred in the ileum, but less than that in the large intestine. For sheep ca. 33% was digested when administered by this route.

Other data on cattle have dealt primarily with N (see Ch. 13) or starch utilization. Results indicate an appreciable difference in rumen although not in total GIT digestion, which is related to the source of cereal grain fed. Studies with barley as the major cereal component indicate that 92 to 99% disappeared in the rumen (Thivend and Journet, 1968; Topps et al, 1968). When corn was the major cereal grain, data from three laboratories indicate that appreciably larger amounts may pass into the duodenum, although total starch digestion is almost complete. Values cited range from 50-90% disappearance in the rumen, with means within the range of 67-76% (Karr et al, 1966; Thivend and Journet, 1970; Waldo et al, 1971). With sorghum grain, data from one experiment show a marked effect of processing methods (McNeill et al, 1971). The disappearance in the rumen was (%): ground, 42.0; reconstituted, 66.7; steam flaked, 83.4; and micronized, 43.0. In this experiment, total digestion was high (97-99.74%) and the authors calculated that post ruminal digestion accounted for 374 g (steam flaked) to 1159 g (micronized) of starch/day. In steers fed 100% hay, Jones and Ellis (1971) estimated that 120 g of starch passed from the reticulo-rumen/day; when the diet was 40% hay and 60% concentrate (mostly sorghum grain), 1,470 g of starch left the reticulo-rumen. The amounts from the two rations were calculated to account for 3.2 and 24.9%, respectively, of the digestible energy of the rations.

Table 9-7.   Partial digestion data on cows.[a]

| Item | Digestibility, % | | | |
| | Dried grass & rolled barley | | | Dried grass, flaked corn |
	Dry	Pregnant	Lactating	Lactating
Dry matter intake, kg/day	5.08	8.59	9.02	8.99
Disappearance of				
Digestible energy	73.2	73.7	72.2	74.8
Total GIT	66.7	64.5	58.4	53.4
Before duodenum*	17.4	19.1	33.0	34.7
In small intestine*	15.8	16.5	8.7	12.0
In cecum and colon*				
Digestible nitrogen				
Total GIT	72.6	75.6	71.3	71.2
Before duodenum*	40.8	20.7	-5.0	-15.5
In small intestine*	46.1	67.4	99.2	106.2
In cecum and colon*	13.1	11.9	5.8	9.3
Cellulose				
Total GIT	76.3	67.1		73.8
Before duodenum*	90.5	98.3		88.9
In small intestine*	-2.7	-2.7		3.9
In cecum and colon*	12.2	4.4		7.2
α-linked glucose polymers				
Total GIT	97.4	99.7		97.5
Before duodenum*	91.4	83.9		76.6
In small intestine*	9.0	12.4		16.1
In cecum and colon*	-0.5	3.7		7.3

[a]Data from Watson et al (1972a, b)
*Expressed as a % of total digestion

As pointed out in the introduction of this chapter, a substantial amount of information is available on partial digestion although it is sometimes difficult to compare experiments within or between species. In general, we can say that data indicate that substantial digestion occurs in the rumen for the organic nutrients, but the relative amount would seem to vary considerably from experiment to experiment. Many papers indicate that digestion of fibrous material in feedstuffs is essentially complete in the forestomach, although some papers indicate exceptions to this. Data also indicate that net absorption of ash in the forestomach is apt to be negative. About the only firm conclusion that can be made is that digestion is apt to be variable in various parts of the GIT; this, of course, is something that should be expected in a biological organism as complex as the ruminant animal.

Absorption from the Reticulo-Rumen and Omasum

For a long time it was considered unlikely that absorption could occur in the forestomach since these organs are characterized by a lining of cornified, stratified, squamous epithelial cells, a cell type not usually found covering absorptive surfaces. Barcroft et al (1944) pointed out that the epithelia of the forestomach differs from that of the skin, also cornified, stratified squamous epithelia, in that: the layer of cornified cells is thin, only 3-4 cells, probably due to the continued abrasion by rumen contents; the layer of granula cells, the *stratum granulosum,* is not a continuous layer; and there are no sebaceous glands, thus no greasy protection to assist in preventing passage of water, etc. In addition, these tissues are well supplied with blood.

The surface area of the forestomach is not particularly extensive. For example, in the dorsal parts of the rumen the papillae are small and sparse; papillae in the omasum are also small, although the leaves provide an appreciable surface area. It is of interest to note that rumen papillae are larger and more dense in the ventral and cranial sacs, areas that probably have the highest concentration of soluble nutrients. As a matter of fact, Aafjes (1967) has demonstrated that areas of the rumen wall with large numbers of papillae absorbed more volatile fatty acids than did areas with few papillae. It is also interesting to note that Sinclair et al (1958) found that the relative length of papillae in the ventral rumen sac of sheep was correlated ($r = 0.58$) to daily gain as was the pigmentation score of rumen epithelia ($r = 0.39$). This would suggest the possibility that productivity may be partially limited by absorptive surface in the rumen. Absorption of VFA is reduced in animals with rumen parakeratosis (see Ch. 17), which tends to reduce rate or efficiency of gain and to confirm this suggestion (Hinders and Owen, 1965).

Absorption from the stomach has been evaluated in a number of ways. One obvious method has been to determine changes in concentration of the compound being studied with or without the aid of a marker. A second method involves evacuating the rumen, adding a test solution and determining the change in concentration with time. Blocking the reticulo-omasal orifice to prevent outflow has been done as well as blocking of the esophagus to prevent inflow of saliva. For compounds that are absorbed in relatively large amounts or when radioactive labels are available in the compound of interest, absorption can be estimated by determining the difference in concentration of the test compound in portal blood (veins from the rumen pass into the portal supply of the liver) and either peripheral venous blood or blood from arteries such as the carotid. In addition, surgically constructed pouches of rumen tissue can be used to study absorption as can the isolated rumen (perfused rumen) when maintained at the appropriate temperature and supplied with an auxilliary pump and blood supply. More recently, the isolated ventral sac has been used to collect this type of information.

Rumen Absorption of Water

Absorption of water or fluids from the rumen has been of interest for some years and methods used have varied from observation of disappearance from the rumen to sophisticated techniques involving use of isolated rumen sacs, tritium-labeled water and elaborate in vitro methods. A relatively recent review on this subject has been prepared by Engelhardt (1970) for the benefit of readers wanting more detail than is presented here.

As pointed out by Engelhardt and by

Warner and Stacy (1972), experiments dealing with the net flux of water through the rumen wall have been contradictory. A number of workers have reported data indicating a net absorption from the normal rumen. However, other investigations did not show any appreciable flux even when there was a relatively high osmotic gradient.

Studies using tritiated water have been carried out in three laboratories. In studies with goats (Engelhardt and Nickel, 1965), water exchange between rumen contents and blood was variable (4.9-49.3 ml/min), but there was little net difference in total absorption or influx into the rumen and the authors suggested that there appeared to be a wide range in osmotic pressure (265-325 m.osmol/kg) in which the net movement of water across the wall was near zero, since they found little relationship to absorption and osmotic pressure. In studies based on marker dilution, Warner and Stacy (1968) concluded, with sheep which had a rumen volume of 3.9 l., that net inflow averaged 0.29 l./hr and absorption into the blood averaged 0.05 l./hr. Wide differences were noted within and between sheep. More recently, Willes et al (1970) have studied this in sheep with isolated rumen sacs. They confirm a rapid exchange of water between rumen contents and blood. Mean water absorption ranged from 37-71 ml/min and secretion into the rumen varied from 30-65 ml/min. Net water absorption varied from 5-13.4 ml/min in several postfeeding periods. Water exchange from the rumen increased 2-3 hr postfeeding and declined after 17 hr. Net water absorption was not consistently affected by time after feeding and the rumen was consistently hypotonic to blood. Lowering the pH of rumen contents (with HCl) resulted in an increase in rate of water exchange. Dobson et al (1971) have used this technique with cattle. They observed that CO_2 and butyric acid stimulated absorption of either tritiated water or ethanol and suggest that absorption of water is highly related to blood flow in the rumen epithelial tissues.

Other studies where water flux has been related to rumen osmotic pressure include those of Parthasarathy and Phillipson (1953), Dobson and Phillipson (1958), Engelhardt (1969, 1970), Dobson et al (1970) and Warner and Stacy (1972). Except for studies from two laboratories, data show a range of absorption from 20-34 ul/min/m.osmole/kg.

Osmolality at which the water flux was near zero ranged from 295-360 (Warner and Stacy, 1972). In one marked exception, Dobson et al (1970) found water flux in the isolated ventral sac of cattle to be much greater than similar studies reported for sheep or goats. Furthermore, they noted an uptake of water against a concentration gradient, particularly when CO_2 was present.

Warner and Stacy (1972) point out that their work shows that maximal water absorption from the rumen usually coincided with minimal Na and K absorption. Based on published data, both Engelhardt (1970) and Warner and Stacy (1972) agree that the rumen wall is not very permeable to water in terms of net absorption.

Absorption of Volatile Fatty Acids

It has been known for some time (Barcroft et al, 1944) that volatile fatty acids (VFA) are absorbed through the rumen wall. Other reports from the same laboratory (Danielli et al, 1945; Kiddle et al, 1951; Masson and Phillipson, 1951; Pfander and Phillipson, 1953) confirmed these results and presented additional information demonstrating that VFA disappeared from the rumen of naturally fed sheep as well as from solutions introduced into the evacuated rumen and that the VFA are not, apparently, absorbed into the lymph system.

The effect of rumen pH on VFA absorption has been studied rather extensively, and a relatively recent review is available (Stevens, 1970). Danielli et al (ibid), Gray (1948) and Sutton et al (1963) have presented data indicating that the order of absorption was butyric > propionic > acetic acid in acidic solutions introduced into the rumen or in the naturally fed sheep or calf. For example, Sutton et al (ibid) demonstrated that absorption of VFA (pH 6.6) decreased as the chain length of the acid decreased and that a solution with a pH of 5.0-5.5 resulted in more rapid absorption than at a pH of 7.5-8.0. The depressing effect on absorption of a near neutral or alkaline solution has been shown by others (Barcroft et al, 1944; Danielli et al, 1945; Gray, 1948) as well as by in vitro studies with rumen mucosa (Bloomfield et al, 1963). Recent Canadian data (Thorlacius and Lodge, 1973) clearly substantiate suggestions that an increase in chain length results in more rapid absorption at acidic pH (Table 9-8). When expressed as ml/min, note that butyric acid is absorbed 2.5-4X faster than acetic acid. When the pH was higher (6.5), then there was much less difference in the rates of absorption. The effect of pH appears to be partly due to the presence of more free acids at a lower pH (Ash and Dobson, 1963).

Sutton et al (1963) have studied absorption from the rumen of calves fed either milk or milk, grain and hay. Averaged maximum absorption rates (mg of acid/100 ml of solution/hr) of acetic acid at 1, 4, 8 and 12 wk of age were 30, 163, 179 and 402, respectively, for MGH calves, and 21, 26, 22, and 22 for milk-fed calves. Thus, these data indicate that maturation of the rumen epithelia is necessary for appreciable absorption. Khouri (1969) has also studied absorption in calves 3-5 days or 6 wk of age. This experimenter used ^{14}C-labeled acetate and evaluated absorption on the basis of changes in venous-arterial concentrations after introducing solutions into the rinsed stomach of anesthetized animals that had been fasted. Some had been fed either milk or milk and pasture. With this technique he found ready absorption at 3-5 days and no appreciable differences between 6-wk-old calves due to diet, thus tending to contradict the data on age presented by Sutton et al (1963).

Table 9-8. Effect of pH on VFA absorption from the rumen.[a]

| pH | Absorption, ml/min | | |
	Acetic	Propionic	Butyric
5.36	52.6	116.0	202.7
5.46	68.5	100.8	160.5
mean	60.6	108.4	181.6
6.51	44.7	68.2	96.4
6.57	52.2	55.5	60.4
mean	48.5	61.9	78.4

[a]Data from Thorlacius and Lodge (1973); from cows fed hay diet.

Bull et al (1965) have presented data indicating that absorption was less from the rumen of calves which had developed rumen parakeratosis when fed pelleted rations. Hinders and Owen (1965) have reported similar results on older animals. Fasting animals also have a slower rate of absorption (Pfander and Phillipson, 1953).

The effect of diet on VFA absorption has been clearly demonstrated by Thorlacius and Lodge (1973) using cows with a temporarily isolated ventral sac (Dobson et al, 1970). Note in Table 9-9, when VFA solutions were used at the same pH, that cows fed hay had a slower rate of absorption than those fed on high concentrate rations.

Table 9-9. Effect of diet on VFA absorption.[a]

| Diet | pH | Absorption, ml/min | | |
		Acetic	Propionic	Butyric
Hay	5.32	54.0	87.7	135.3
High concentrate	5.34	77.7	106.5	157.0

[a]From Thorlacius and Lodge (1973)

Data from experiments on infusion of ^{14}C-labeled acids (Weller et al, 1967; Weston and Hogan, 1968; as well as others) indicate that the different acids disappear from the rumen at about the same rate, indicating little, if any difference in relative rates of absorption. Perry and Armstrong (1969) conclude that absorption of the VFA from the rumen is directly proportional to concentration in the rumen. Since acetic acid is usually present in much higher concentrations (molar basis) than the other acids, perhaps the relatively greater concentration of both acetic and propionic acid compensate for the normally faster absorption of butyric acid demonstrated in some of the experiments previously mentioned.

Annison et al (1957) found that considerable amounts of VFA were absorbed from the rumen and that there was a good correlation between the concentration of total VFA in rumen contents and portal blood. They also noted that less butyrate was found, relative to acetate and propionate in the portal blood and that there was a greater concentration of ketone bodies in portal than in peripheral blood. Other information along the same line has been reported by Masson and Phillipson (1951), Pfander and Phillipson (1953), and McCarthy et al (1958). This points out that data on absorption of VFA are affected by the fact that an appreciable amount of the butyric acid present is derived from acetic acid and, when coupled with the fact that the rumen epithelium actively metabolizes butyric acid, the problem of calculating absorption is complicated (see Weller et al, 1967).

Weston and Hogan (1968) estimated that ca. 76% of ruminal VFA was absorbed from the rumen, 19% from the omasum and abomasum (assuming no production in the omasum) and that 5% passed into the small intestine. Conrad et al (1958) used ^{32}P tagged red blood cells to estimate the volume of blood passing through the coeliac artery to the gastrosplenic vein. They estimated a mean rate of gastric blood flow to be 764 ml/min/100 lb of body weight in calves. With this estimate of flow rate and information on acid concentration in the vein, they calculated that ca. 63 g of acetic and 25 g of propionic acid were absorbed for each pound of dry feed (2:1 mix of alfalfa hay and grain) consumed during a 24-hr period.

Rumen perfusion has been used in a number of laboratories to study absorption. In this technique the blood supply of an isolated stomach is attached to a pump and a dialyzing apparatus to remove some of the metabolites. The whole preparation is kept at an appropriate temperature and usually in a water bath. McCarthy and others (1958) have used such a preparation in conjunction with labeled acids and could demonstrate absorption. Their data indicated that the relative quantities of acids absorbed are, in general, a reflection of acid production in the rumen. Brown et al (1960) have also used this technique. It might be noted that the technique has the same limitations as some others in that it may be able to demonstrate what can occur, but not necessarily what does occur, or, if so, in the same relative proportions.

Another method used to study absorption by the reticulo-rumen is a procedure in which isolated rumen epithelium is removed, clamped over the end of a test tube or similar apparatus. Flow through the tissue is then measured (Begovic, 1963). When using this technique, Bell and Emery (1965) demonstrated absorption by rumen epithelia. The rate of absorption increased slightly from acetate to butyrate; the authors found that absorption was a function of concentration and found some indication that propionate and butyrate may have inhibited acetate absorption. Stevens and Stettler (1966, 1967) have also reported data on permeability to acetate of the rumen epithelia.

Tsuda (1957) has used rumen pouches to study absorption in goats. As constructed, the pouch is isolated from the remainder of the rumen and exteriorized so that it can be sampled and can have material added to it. With this technique he found that the VFA were absorbed more rapidly as free acids than when in the salt form (higher pH). Using this technique, Foss (1967) found that absorption from the pouch was inhibited if blood levels of VFA were raised by intravenous administration. If blood values were higher than those in the pouch, fatty acids entered the pouch. Also, butyrate absorption was apparently inhibited by high blood levels of acetic or propionic acid. He concluded that VFA absorption is a matter of free diffusion, one that does not require a source of energy such as ATP, a conclusion also reached by Stevens (1970).

Absorption of Miscellaneous Constituents

Ammonia is one of a number of nitrogenous compounds that may be absorbed by the rumen. Lewis et al (1957) demonstrated that changes in rumen ammonia concentration were paralleled by changes in portal blood ammonia, although this was not the case when ammonium acetate was added to the rumen (an indication of effect of pH). Hogan (1961) and Bloomfield et al (1963) have also demonstrated ammonia absorption. Gartner (1963), when using rumen epithelia, placed urea on the connective tissue side of the apparatus and found that relatively small amounts of urea but large amounts of ammonia were transferred to the fluid on the epithelial side of the preparation, thus indicating that transfer of urea from the blood to rumen fluid was physiologically possible (see Ch. 13 for further details on this topic).

The effect of pH on VFA absorption was noted previously; it also influences the absorption of ammonia. Bloomfield et al (1963) reported that, when rumen pH was 7.55, 6.21, or 7.58, ammonia absorption was 26, 0, and 11 mmol/l./hr and VFA absorption was 4, 18, and 4 mmol/l./hr, respectively. Hogan (1961) found at a pH of 6.5 that the transport of ammonia across the rumen epithelium increased with the concentration gradient and that ammonia absorption was increased by absorption of VFA. Absorption of ammonia was rapid at pH 6.5, but negligible at pH 4.5.

Kameoka (1962) has demonstrated that N from ^{15}N-labeled urea was absorbed before digesta passed through an omasal cannula in goats fed a variety of diets. With animals with an isolated rumen sac, Mooney and O'Donovan (1970) found that ammonia transport was very rapid in both directions across the rumen wall. When pH was lowered on one side of the membrane, equilibrium was reached when the ammonia concentration was greater on the side of low pH, irrespective of the direction of the ammonia gradient initially. Transport of urea was very slow in both directions. In a cow with a temporarily isolated ventral sac, Thorlacius et al (1971) found that administration of CO_2 into the sac greatly increased permeability of rumen epithelium to urea. Permeability to acetamide and thiourea was also increased but there was no change for the VFA or antipyrine.

Demaux et al (1961) used isolated organs and demonstrated an increase in amino acid nitrogen in veins draining the rumen. Lewis and Emery (1962) reported that plasma lysine was increased markedly after intraruminal administration, and Leibholz (1965) found that, after feeding, free amino acids in rumen liquor increased as much as 100 fold and plasma levels 2-10 fold although intestinal absorption cannot be ruled out here. Cook et al (1965) used rumen perfusion and rumen vein catheters to demonstrate absorption of glycine, serine, threonine, methionine sulfoxide, aspartic acid, glutamine, isoleucine, and leucine from the rumen. Smith (1959) demonstrated absorption of a variety of amino acids and B-complex vitamins when introduced into the rumen of goats.

Leibholz (1971) has studied amino acid absorption from the washed rumen of sheep. The amounts of individual acids (histidine, glycine, L-amino acid mixtures) ranged from near 0 to 50%, indicating that absorption could account for ca. 6% of total N absorption from the rumen. Absorption was most rapid for branched-chain amino acids. With in vitro preparations it was shown that transfer of histidine and glycine was less than that of ammonia, but transfer (absorption) of all increased with increasing concentration. Transfer of L-histidine was unidirectional and specific and was reduced by some drugs and the presence of other amino acids in the test solution. Less than 5% of both amino acids was metabolized by the epithelium. Starvation of the sheep prior to slaughter resulted in a twofold increase in absorption of histidine and glycine, but no change in ammonia transfer. Sjaastad (1967) has shown that conjugated histamine was absorbed from in vitro rumen preparations. With respect to methionine, Lazarov and Ivanov (1970) use of ^{35}S-labeled methionine and cysteine in goats showed that the S-amino acids were absorbed to some extent, though less cysteine than methionine. Infusions of ^{35}S-methionine into the sheep rumen, in one study, resulted in recovery of 74% of the label flowing into the omasum, indicating absorption of methionine or the S in some other form (Bird and Moir, 1972).

When using rumen pouches, Tsuda (1957) found that glucose was the only organic compound studied that could be absorbed against a concentration gradient. Other compounds absorbed when at a higher concentration than in the blood included lactose, ethanol, acetone, urea and glycine (slowly). Varady et al (1969) have also used this technique to study entry of amino acids into the pouch. Entry was most rapid in the hour before feeding, declined for 2 hr after and then became stable for the remainder of the 5 hr test period.

Lactic acid, although not usually present in appreciable amounts in the rumen, apparently can be absorbed rather slowly (Hueter et al, 1956; Tsuda, 1957; Annison, 1965). Absorption of L (+) - lactate appears to be dependent upon both epithelial pH and lactate concentration, and occurs as the free acid with little conversion to any other metabolite (Jones et al, 1969).

Parthasarathy and Phillipson (1953) studied the absorption of several ions by determining the disappearance of them from solutions placed in the washed rumen and by arterial-venous differences. They found that Na and K were absorbed from the rumen when their concentrations exceeded that in the blood and that passage in the reverse direction occurred when the concentration of Na or K was lower than in the blood. Cl was absorbed from the rumen against a concentration gradient provided the concentration was 135 mg % or over, however, the change in Cl was small. At concentrations lower than this, net gains in Cl in the rumen occurred. Water absorption occurred when the solutions were of 0.165 molar (NaCl) or less. When the ionic concentration was raised to 0.33 M, water was secreted into the rumen. Dobson (1959) also demonstrated that Na could be absorbed against a higher concentration in the blood. Chloride usually moved with its electrochemical potential difference, but against it in the presence of high K and low Na concentrations (i.e., in solutions free of Cl in the rumen, Cl will flow into the rumen). In a review article, Dobson (1961) states that a number of studies have indicated that rumen epithelium is almost impermeable to P, Ca and Mg ions and that creatinine and choline can be recovered quantitatively from the rumen. Pfander et al (1956) reported that they could show no evidence of glucose, nitrate or nitrite absorption from the rumen based either on disappearance from the rumen or appearance in the blood.

More recently, Scott (1970) found that 50-60% of dietary Cl was absorbed in the rumen of sheep fed a pelleted hay diet; in most cases this occurred against the net electrochemical gradient, indicating an active transport system. Warner and Stacy (1972) noted that K absorption across the rumen wall was slow, but positively correlated to the K concentration. Na absorption appeared to depend on the Na and K concentration and on osmotic pressure in the rumen. Moderate levels of K increased Na absorption but very high levels decreased it. Ferreira et al (1970) have studied electrical flux in in vitro rumen preps. The magnitude of the flux varied according to the buffer solutions but the net flux for Na and Cl were higher from rumen to blood than from blood to rumen, whereas the reverse was true for K. Similar responses have been shown for omasal tissues in this laboratory (Harrison, 1971).

With respect to sulfide, Bray (1969) has shown that the rumen is capable of relatively rapid absorption and that small amounts may be secreted into the rumen through the rumen wall. Absorption of sulfate from the rumen was negligible.

In the guanaco, Engelhardt and Sallmann (1972) observed considerable absorption from hypotonic, isotonic and, to a lesser degree, from hypertonic solutions. Absorption of VFA was closely related to water absorption. Na, VFA and water were absorbed 2-3X faster than from the rumen of sheep.

In the omasum, Gray et al (1954) estimated that 33-64% of the water and 40-69% of the VFA were absorbed. Johnston et al (1961) demonstrated that labeled VFA injected into the exteriorized omasum of calves could be recovered in considerable quantities from veins draining the omasum. In another experiment these authors also demonstrated a decrease in VFA relative to chromic oxide; the ratios of VFA to chromic oxide indicated a decrease in VFA of 51% from the reticulum to the omasum and a further decrease of 83% from the omasum to the abomasum. Joyner et al (1963) have also demonstrated that labeled acetic and butyric acids were absorbed by omasal tissues and transferred to the blood. Oyaert and Bouckaert (1961) have published data indicating absorption of water, Na, K and ammonia by the omasum, and Engelhardt and Ehrlein (1968) have estimated that 10-15% of the fluid entering the abomasum is absorbed there. In vitro experiments with omasal epithelia show that water was transferred into pouches when they contained hypertonic NaCl solutions and was transferred out rapidly when filled with hypotonic solutions (Liker, 1971).

Absorption from the Abomasum

Very little information is available on absorptive functions of the abomasum, probably because it is generally thought that secretion is the major function of this section of the stomach (Hill, 1961b). With respect to VFA, Ash (1961) demonstrated that the abomasum can rapidly absorb the VFA, and Williams et al (1968) have shown that the rate of absorption was comparable to the reticulo-rumen. Engelhardt et al (1968) have studied absorption in goats in which the abomasum was isolated by use of inflated balloons (to restrict omasal flow) and with a snare used to close off the phlorus during experiments. Water diffusion out of the organ was determined using tritiated water. In animals with a mean abomasal volume of 606 ml, diffusion amounted to 513 ml/hr. Absorption of VFA increased with decreasing pH. At pH values of 5.2-5.6, clearance of VFA averaged 320 ml/hr; at pH 3.5-4.0, VFA clearance was 1130 ml/hr. Antipyrine diffused out of the abomasum at an average rate of 214 ml/hr. Slivicky (1970), using sheep with abomasal pouches, demonstrated rapid absorption of VFA in the order acetic < propionic < butyric. Mixtures were absorbed more rapidly and acids faster than salts.

Digestive Secretions of the Lower GIT

Information on secretion of digestive juices — abomasal or gastric juices, intestinal juice, bile and pancreatic juice — is less extensive on ruminants than on some monogastric species; nevertheless a fair amount of information is available. Hill (1961b) has presented an excellent historical review on the abomasum and other reviews that may be of interest to readers desiring more information than is presented here (Hill, 1961a, 1965).

As aptly pointed out by Hill (1961a), one of the more important features which distinguishes the ruminant animal from most monogastric animals is the continuous nature of the digestive processes. As we have seen in preceding chapters, ingestion or rumination occupy an appreciable part of the day and passage of digesta from the reticulo-rumen and the omasum on through the tract is a relatively continuous process, although apparently less so in the distal ileum and large intestine. This continuous flow of digesta into the abomasum and duodenum obviously requires a more or less continuous flow of digestive enzymes, acids and bile; whereas in a typical monogastric animal a rhythmatic cycle of periods of large output changing to low output is more typical. Studies on sheep with abomasal pouches (Hill, 1960; Ash, 1961) indicate that production of abomasal juice is a relatively continuous process, although the quantity and quality may be influenced by various factors. Hill (1965) states that the continuous production of gastric juice by the abomasum appears to be maintained by phasic activity of various cell types since the peptic cells can be seen in all stages of activity from repletion to exhaustion of their pepsinogen granules.

The mucosal folds in the abomasum serve to provide a large surface area for proliferation of glandular cells. Hill (1965) estimates that, in sheep, the fundic area without folds has a surface area of ca. 300 cm^2 and that folds have an added area of 1866 cm^2. The mucosal folds may also have a physiological function in prevention of digesta from stratifying and in ensuring rapid mixing of digesta and abomasal juices. In the monogastric stomach, incoming food tends to stratify and thus it may be some period of time before digestive juices can attack some of it. Conditions in the abomasum differ from monogastrics in that incoming digesta would tend to have a lower dry matter content (5-10% according to Oyaert and Bouckaert, 1961) and a smaller average particle size. Thus, inflowing digesta is exposed immediately to enzymatic and hydrolytic action which is presumed to require less time to complete the digestive processes for nonfibrous ingesta than in a typical monogastric stomach.

The Nature and Quantity of Abomasal Juice

Dukes (1955) and Hill (1961b) have reviewed some of the older literature which indicates that gastric juice obtained from abomasal pouches is similar to that of monogastric animals with respect to pH and freezing point (-0.555 to -0.610°C). Masson and Phillipson (1952) found that the average Cl concentration was 158 meq/l. for normally fed sheep (pouch contents), and that the total acidity averaged about 86 meq/l. The VFA concentration of abomasal effluent ranged from 3.5 to 14 meq/l. as compared to 69-103 for rumen contents. Total acidity of duodenal contents varied from 44-65 meq/l. Chloride ions made up about one half of total ash. Digesta entering the abomasum (cranial end) is said to have a pH of about 6 (Hill, 1965). Digesta leaving the abomasum usually has a pH of 2.3 (Masson and Phillipson, 1952; Ash, 1961b).

The volume of juice produced by the abomasum is not easy to estimate in view of the secretion of gastric enzymes and acid and the absorption which occurs. An appropriate method would seem to be the use of animals with omasal-abomasal and abomasal-duodenal cannulas coupled with the use of markers in the rumen. However, animals with this much artificial plumbing are difficult to maintain (Engelhardt and Ehrlein, 1968). The change in markers from the omasum to the abomasum and from the abomasum to the duodenum would seem to be one solution in the live animal. However, if the contents of these organs were the basis of evaluation, the difference in dry matter content of the omasum (18-25%) and effluent from the omasum (5-10%) would need to be accounted for. Masson and Phillipson (1952) have estimated abomasal secretion in sheep (40-45 kg) to be ca. 5-6 l./day based on dilution of Cl ions produced in abomasal pouches and Cl from omasal contents. When using marker concentration in slaughtered lambs, Vidal et al (1969) calculated that dry matter secreted by the abomasum was equivalent to 1-2X that of dietary origin. Hill (1965) suggests that an adult cow might secrete 30-35 l./day of abomasal juice, but does not elaborate on how this estimate was derived. Estimates based on abomasal pouches would, no doubt, be subject to an appreciable error because of the difficulty in determining the relative amount of active secretory tissue represented by the pouch in comparison to the intact abomasum.

Factors Influencing Flow of Abomasal Juice

When experimenting with sheep fitted with abomasal pouches and abomasal-duodenal re-entrant cannulas, Ash (1961b) found that there was a close correlation between acid secretion by the pouch and the outflow of food material from the abomasum. Increasing the food intake increased the amount of acid secreted and the volume of abomasal outflow as well as the volume of water consumed and the time spent ruminating; decreasing the food intake caused the opposite effects. The acidity of abomasal effluent varied only within narrow limits, but large changes occurred in the output of acid by the pouch. Preventing outflow did not inhibit acid production until the pH of abomasal contents declined to about 2.0. Distension of the duodenum also resulted in inhibition of acid secretion, as did the infusion of solutions containing 80-115 meq/l. of HCl. In the pouches, acid production and volume of secretion usually reached peak values about 45-90 min after feeding. In a second paper Ash (1961b) found that distension of the main body of the abomasum with a balloon stimulated acid secretion which was inhibited when acidity of the fluid reached a pH of ca. 2.0. He also reported that the introduction of buffered solutions (pH 5.7) did not stimulate acid secretion, but, when VFA were included in the buffered solutions, acid secretion by the pouch was increased, thus indicating a stimulatory effect of the VFA. Hill (1960) found that sham feeding of sheep with esophageal fistulas with normally filled stomach or feeding after the reticulo-rumen had been emptied failed to increase the secretion of acid in pouches. Insulin hypo-glycemia produced a secretory response when the stomach contained food, but after emptying the stomach the response was less, indicating that the response was due to hypermotility of the tract resulting from the hypoglycemia.

Some reports indicate increases in abomasal juice production associated with feeding; this is explained by the fact that motility of the reticulo-rumen can become conditioned to feeding accompanied by an increased passage out of the rumen at this time (Hill, 1961b). McLeay and Titchen (1970) have confirmed this reaction in sheep with abomasal pouches. Secretion (pouches in fundic region) was continuous, but it was increased by feeding and decreased by fasting. The volume, pepsin concentration and acid concentration increased within 15-30 min after the sheep was teased with food or after feeding. These responses were observed in sheep which had food available. At the same time, the authors noted an increase in reticular contractions, but they did not observe any increase in secretion when rumination occurred. However, pouches with antral mucosa included did not show these responses.

Abomasal Secretions in Preruminants

In very young animals, the acid secreting cells in the abomasal mucosa are not active and the pH of abomasal juice in newborn lambs is near neutral (Phillipson, 1955; Hill, 1956) and there is little free HCl (Sajhamanov, 1968). After birth the parietal cells develop rapidly and the growth is accompanied by a corresponding fall in pH of abomasal contents so that it is near pH 3.0 by the time the lambs are 36 hr of age (Hill et al, 1970), and there is more free HCl. Other studies (Chyla et al, 1972) indicate that pH fell with age and that protease activity increased after feeding up to 25 days of age.

Since maximal proteolysis by abomasal contents occurs at pH 2.1, Hill (1961b) suggests that the young lamb secretes pepsin and that maximum proteolysis does not occur during the early hours of life. Furthermore, this lag period, which corresponds to the period when colostral proteins are absorbed (see later section) may represent a mechanism whereby the antibodies are protected from digestion.

There is some question about enzyme secretion in early life; colostrum is clotted very efficiently in very young animals, indicating rennin secretion, although pepsin may also clot milk proteins. Early work had indicated that pepsin was not secreted until calves started to consume solid food. More recent information (Henschel et al, 1961; Hill et al, 1970; Henschel, 1973) indicates a variable secretion; some reports indicating primarily rennin secretion during the first 1-2 wk of life; others indicating primarily pepsin and some suggesting that calves may secrete both enzymes by the time they are 9-10 days of age. After weaning, however, pepsin is the primary proteolytic enzyme secreted (Hill et al, 1970).

It has been pointed out (Hill, 1961b; Hill et al, 1970) that the gastric juice of young ruminants is characterized by its milk coagulating power (extracts are used for cheese making). Rennin has maximal in vitro proteolytic activity at a pH of 4.0, and calves maintained on a milk diet tend to maintain abomasal pH at higher levels than in animals fed solid food.

Before feeding, the abomasal contents consist of fairly clear, slightly viscous fluid containing small milk clots and having a pH of ca. 2.0. During feeding, milk clots rapidly as it enters the abomasum and clotting is complete within a short time after finishing the meal. As milk is consumed, the pH of the contents rises and subsequently falls over a period of several hours (4-8) back to the initial level as a result of secretion of gastric juice (Ash, 1964; Smith, 1964; Mylrea, 1966; Hill et al, 1970). Feeding causes a considerable increase in the rate of outflow of abomasal contents which reaches a peak in the first hour after feeding. As digestion in the abomasum proceeds, the clot breaks up and the nature of the chyme passing into the duodenum changes 3-4 hr after feeding from a whey-like fluid containing predominantly carbohydrate and soluble nitrogenous compounds to a thick, white opaque material containing protein and fat (Porter, 1969). The pattern of abomasal secretion and the pH is not consistently changed from those with whole cow's milk when the concentration of fat is altered (Ash, 1964) or when milk replacers containing soy flour (Porter, 1969) or oat meal (Shaikhamanov, 1973) are fed.

In young milk-fed calves, Marchenko et al (1965) reported that the pepsin activity of the abomasal fluid was higher for calves allowed to nurse than for calves fed from a pail, suggesting that the suckling reflex is an important factor in stimulating secretion.

Grosskipf (1959) studied the proteolytic and rennin activity of calves fed with nipples or from an open bucket. Both methods of feeding caused an increase in rennin and pepsin concentration of the juice, but the effect of nipple feeding was markedly greater. During a period 7 wk, the rennin concentration and the pH of abomasal secretion of one calf fell steadily with increasing age.

Secretion in calves is said to have a diurnal pattern and secretion increases in association with feeding. Russian data (cited by Hill, 1961b) indicates a marked increase in excretion of abomasal juice by young lambs, the amount increasing 15-24 fold between the ages of 1-6 mo., reaching 4.5-6.5 l./day in lambs 6 mo. of age. In young calves, Mylrea (1968) estimates a daily chyme production of 2.8 l./12 hr/100 kg of liveweight.

Other Digestive Secretions

As noted in Ch. 5, salivary lipase from the salivary glands is apparently a factor in the hydrolysis of milk fats in young ruminants. However, activity of this enzyme is nil at pH 2.0 to 2.5, so it has relatively little time to effect hydrolysis of milk glycerides.

In nonruminant animals the pyloric antrum is the site of origin of gastrin, a hormone which stimulates the secretion of acid and water but not of pepsinogen. Anderson et al (1961) have partially characterized bovine gastrin. They found that gastrin could be obtained from both the pyloric and fundic regions of the abomasum and that their preparations had similar although longer lasting effects than porcine gastrin when administered to dogs. The fact that VFA stimulate secretion in abomasal pouches when buffered solutions without the VFA do not may be due to the mediation of gastrin (Hill, 1965).

The pH in the small intestine rises very gradually. Harrison and Hill (1962) found that the reaction of duodenal contents was 2.7 at the pylorus and rose to ca. 4 just beyond the entry of the common bile and pancreatic duct. Even 2 m further on in the upper jejunum the pH is only around 5 and neutrality is reached in the lower jejunum (Lennox and Garton, 1968; Ben-Ghedalia et al, 1974). Kay (1969) points out that the persisting acidity can be attributed to the copious secretion of acid in the abomasum and to the weakly alkaline nature of secretions entering the intestine. Bile, for example, has little bicarbonate (sheep) and diversion of it from the small intestine has only a small effect on pH (Harrison and Hill, 1962). In animals with multiple cannulas, Kay (1969) reports that intestinal contents reached a slightly alkaline pH (7.5) after passing through cannulas which were 9 m beyond the pylorus and 10 m before the cecum.

Kay goes on to point out that the slow rise in pH may have several physiological effects. Since acid provides a stimulus for pancreatic secretion, this should tend to stimulate a prolonged secretion by the pancreas. The slow rise would also prolong the conditions favorable for continued action of pepsin, but it would inhibit action by proteolytic enzymes from the pancreas.

Harrison and Hill (1962) and Harrison (1962) have studied the flow rate of duodenal juice, bile, and pancreatic juice in sheep with cannulas located at appropriate points. For periods of time varying from 4-24 hr they estimated that bile production amounted to ca. 400 ml/day; pancreatic juice to ca. 530 ml/day; and duodenal juice from 200-400 ml/day. The return of bile to the duodenum increased the volume and solid content of bile samples. Emptying the reticulo-rumen reduced the secretory rate of bile to about half that mentioned above. Caple and Heath (1971) found that pressure in the gall bladder fluctuated over a range of 18 mm Hg. During fasting, pressure waves occurred at a rate of 3-6/hr, each lasting for ca. 5 min. After feeding, the pressure waves were more frequent, sometimes lasting for 20 min. Injection of acid into the duodenum was followed by an increase in pressure in the gall bladder and the bladder contracted in response to cholecystokinin-pancreozymin. Other work from this laboratory (Heath, 1970; Caple and Heath, 1972) showed that bile secretion increased when natural secretin (a hormone which stimulates secretion of pancreatic water and electrolytes) was infused into the portal vein, the amount being similar to the amount of bile secreted when acid was infused into the duodenum. This suggests that entry of acid into the duodenum results in release of secretin, which stimulates output of water, bicarbonate and other electrolytes via the bile. In studies with mature sheep, it has been reported that inclusion of urea, ammonium carbonate or sulfate caused an increase in the volume of bile, which returned to normal when these N sources were withdrawn from the diet (Kuimov and Tituzov, 1968).

With respect to pancreatic secretions and enzymes, there have been a substantial number of papers over the past few years. McCormick and Stewart (1967) have reported data on milk-fed calves. Although considerable difficulty was encountered, observations indicated an increased production of pancreatic juice with age, some calves being 180 days old. Average flow rate was 9-10 ml/kg body weight/24 hr. In young calves the flow rate increased 2-3 ml/hr during feeding over the rate before feeding. In older calves the flow rate was more uniform after they began consuming roughage. Gorrill and Thomas (1967) and Gorrill et al (1967) indicated the volume of pancreatic juice secreted by calves was ca. 0.16 and 0.29 ml/hr/kg of body weight at 4 and 21 days of age, respectively. Although flow increased with age, the amounts of trypsin and protein were maximal at 7 days. Feeding failed to produce an increased flow rate, but output of protein, trypsin and chymotrypsin activity was correlated with protein content of pancreatic juice, rather than to volume of juice. These authors found that feeding diets containing high levels of soy protein resulted in a reduced rate of pancreatic secretion and low proteolytic activity which was attributed, in part, to the anti-trypsin inhibitor content of the soy protein. In further work (Gorrill et al, 1968) proteolytic activity was determined in digesta from the small intestine of calves and lambs fed liquid milk diets and older animals fed hay. Enzyme activity/unit of body weight increased with both age and rumen development in calves. In lambs, total enzyme activities were greater at 6 wk than at 2 wk of age, but were lower in yearling sheep. Lambs digesta had more enzyme activity/unit of body weight than digesta from calves up to 41 days of age, but less protein was digested in vitro. Except for 2-wk-old lambs, digesta in the lower small intestine had lower in vitro protein digestion than in the cranial sections. Zerebcov et al (1967) found the content of a variety of N-containing compounds to be greatest at ca. 3 mo. of age in calves. Prokudin and Tasenov (1967) estimated the volume of flow was ca. 25-30 ml/hr in lambs about 1 mo. of age. The volume increased to ca. 80 ml at 6 mo. and it was greatest before feeding. Proteolytic activity was irregular, but had declined at the time of weaning. Amylolytic and lipolytic activity tended to decline with age.

In more recent studies with milk-fed calves having appropriate cannulas, it has been shown that flow of digesta through the duodenum of milk-fed calves was 5.5, 6.3 and 7.7 l./12 hr at 7, 24 and 63 days of age, respectively (Ternouth et al, 1971; Ternouth and Buttle, 1973). At these same ages, 12-hr collections of pancreatic juice yielded 297, 441 and 602 ml. In the duodenum, they recovered 40 ml/12 hr in two calves. The rate of secretion from the pancreas varied greatly, being lowest 2-3 hr and highest 6-10 hr after feeding. In other studies, Aust and Cook (1968) reported flow rates to be 0.81 ml/min in a mo.-old-calf and 0.27 and 0.36 ml/min for a yearling sheep and goat, respectively. Other papers giving data on pancreatic secretion volume include those of Taylor (1962), Greene et al (1963) and Clary et al (1969).

Ternouth and Roy (1973) have studied the effect of severely overheated milk, no fat in the diet and partial replacement of milk protein with soy or fish protein. These dietary changes resulted in a reduced acid production in the abomasum, a reduction in protein digestion in the abomasum and reductions in the volume and enzyme activity (proleolytic) of pancreatic secretions.

In studies with young milk-fed calves, Gooden (1973) observed that pancreatic lipase had about 10 fold the activity of pregastric lipase. The lipase activity/unit of volume of pancreatic juice from 2-day-old calves was not greater than from 2-wk-old calves, but there was a substantial increase in flow in the older calves, resulting in a threefold increase in pancreatic lipase activity/kg of body weight. In ruminant calves (6-7 mo. of age) there was a further threefold increase in activity/kg of body weight. Other studies on lipase and amylase activity (Ceccarelli et al, 1973) in the gall bladder of slaughtered animals indicate a substantial variability. In sheep, pronounced amylase activity was present in 36 of 40 samples, some activity in 1 and none in 3. Lipase was present in 25 of 38 samples, slight in 6 and absent from 7. Two milk-fed lambs had little or none of either enzyme. In cattle, amylase activity was present in 15 of 25 samples, little activity in 4 and none in 6; lipase was demonstrated in only 5 of 22 samples.

The effect of absence of pancreatic juice on digestion has been studied by Jarrett and Filsell (1972). In sheep which had the pancreatic duct ligated, there was a marked reduction in wool growth and a reduction in body weight over a 6-wk period. Although there was no difference in fecal excretion of fat, the ligated sheep excreted substantially more N in the feces, indicating that pancreatic secretions have a marked effect on protein degradation in the intestine.

Huber et al (1961a) analyzed pancreatic activity from calves slaughtered from 1 to 44 days of age and fed diets with lactose or starch added. Data indicated pancreatic amylase, lipase and protease activity to be lowest at one day of age. It increased by the first week and changed little thereafter. Diet had no apparent effect on any of the pancreatic or intestinal enzymes evaluated. Morrill et al (1970) have also studied pancreatic amylase activity in calves. They found much variation in amylase concentration but with an increase with age; rate of secretion was highest 6 hr after feeding. Amylase concentrations and flow rates were higher for calves fed diets (milk, milk replacer, calf starters) in which all of the protein was from milk as compared to calves receiving some soy protein. The time for digestion of starch in vitro (g glucose formed/24 hr) was always less than 12 for calves up to 100 days of age and ranged to 220 for one calf 163 days of age. When calves were fed carbohydrate-free diets or with various sugars added (Britt and Huber, 1974), data indicated that pancreatic amylase activity was less in calves receiving a glucose-supplemented diet than for those getting the diet with no carbohydrates. With older animals, Clary (1969) found that increasing the amount of grain in rations resulted in an increased pancreatic amylase activity in both cattle and sheep. This laboratory (Call et al, 1969) also reports that raising blood glucose levels by infusions over a period of time resulted in a decrease in pancreatic amylase activity.

Huber et al (1961) did not detect any effect of diet on various enteric enzymes. Intestinal lactase activity was highest at one day of age and decreased thereafter. Intestinal maltase levels were low (as compared to lactase) and did not change with age (to 44 days of age). No intestinal sucrase was detected. Gastric protease was highest at 8 days of age and decreased with age. In a subsequent paper (Huber et al, 1964) calves were fed hay and grain after weaning from milk; whole milk; whole milk plus 5% lactose; or whole milk plus 15% lactose. When slaughtered at 11 wk of age, lactase activity in the proximal third of the small intestine was 876, 1,399, 1,881, and 2,012 units (mg glucose released/g intestinal protein) for the four diets, respectively; thus this experiment shows a pronounced effect of diet in the milk-fed animals, with declining activity when on solid rations.

In work with young calves, Toofanian et al (1973) observed that lactase activity was highest in the newborn calf, followed by cellobiase, trehalase and maltase activities. There was an initial fall in lactase and cellobiase activities during the first 4 wk of life. In ruminant calves, a further decrease in lactase, cellobiase and trehalase activities occurred at the time of weaning, but in preruminant calves the levels did not change. Maltase activity increased from birth to 8 wk and remained unchanged thereafter. The activity of lactase, cellobiase and trehalase were highest in the proximal jejunum rather than in the duodenum.

Coombe and Siddons (1973) report that isomaltase and maltase activities had a similar pattern along the small intestine, with higher activity in the jejunum than in the ileum and lowest activity in the duodenum. There was little effect of age of the animal. When calves were given none or different sugars, Britt and Huber (1974) determined that lactase activity was highest in those receiving lactose followed by galactose. Maltase activity was also higher in calves getting lactose than in those receiving no sugar in the diet.

Manunta and Nuvole (1967) reported that adult sheep (3-7 yr) had only about half as much maltase and amylase activity in intestinal mucosa as did dogs. The sheep lacked sucrase, lactase, cellobiase and inulinase, all found in the dog tissues. They do point out however, that the longer intestine of the sheep (5.5 X longer) might compensate for the lower carbohydrase activity. Henschel et al (1963) found substantial amounts of amylolytic activity (mixed duodenal and intestinal) in 4-6 mo. old steers. There was very little maltase or lactase, and no sucrase activity, but they estimated that there was sufficient carbohydrase activity (including microbial sources) to hydrolyze 120 g of starch.

Symons and Jones (1966) have partially characterized dipeptidase activity in the duodenum, jejunum, and the mid and distal ileum of sheep. They found that the activity per mg of extracted protein rose progressively from the duodenum to midileum. Activity in the distal ileum was slightly lower than that in the midileum. Data indicated a distribution similar to the rat and pig although there was some variation in individual enzymes. In sheep, Ben-Ghedalia and others (1974) found the activities of trypsin, chymotrypsin and carboxypeptidase A increased from the pylorus up to a distance of 7 m and decreased again from this point to a distance of 15 m from the pylorus.

In the large intestine, Hecker (1971a) has studied the activity of enzymes (microbial) involved in N metabolism. He demonstrated that the large intestinal contents produce ammonia, which was greater in cecal contents than in feces. Proteolytic activity of large intestinal contents was much greater than that of rumen contents and some soluble enzymes were shown to be present. Deaminase activity was present, but at a much lower order of magnitude than in rumen contents, and urease activity was much less than that of feces or rumen contents.

Absorption from the Gut

Absorption of Nitrogenous Compounds

In the case of proteins, it should be pointed out that absorption of large protein molecules can occur early in life in the young calf, a situation presumably characteristic of all young mammals. Absorption of globulins or other antibodies occurs because the young mammal's intestinal epithelial cells are able to absorb intact macromolecules (Pierce, 1962) for a limited period after birth. By this means immune globulins in colostrum are acquired and the young animal receives a degree of resistance to some common diseases, which (for the calf) cause a high incidence of mortality or morbidity, namely colisepticaemia and enteric colibacillosis (Gay, 1965).

Deutsch and Smith (1957) demonstrated globulin absorption by analyzing serum and urine of calves and goats for globulins after a meal of colostrum. Their data indicated that substantial amounts of globulins were present in these sources up to 24 hr after birth, but little was found thereafter. Smith and Erwin (1959) investigated absorption in the ligated gut of calves 6-60 hr of age. They found that calves 6 or 18 hr of age could absorb gamma globulins whereas older calves did not. Their evidence indicated that gastrointestinal enzyme development was similar in these calves; the difference apparently was due to a transitory permeability of the intestinal wall to large protein molecules. This phenomenon is very likely a protective mechanism allowing young mammals to build up their blood titer of globulins which act as antibodies. In a subsequent experiment, Smith et al (1964) found that γ-globulin was not absorbed by fetuses from the amnoitic fluid in utero or if absorbed, the titer was not retained until birth. A calf taken prematurely by Cesarean section did not absorb γ-globulin when fed 38 hr after delivery and administration of growth hormone had no effect on permeability of the gut as measured by γ-globulin absorption. Balfour and Comline (1962) have demonstrated that ^{131}I-labeled γ-globulin was absorbed via the lymph system of the small intestine and transferred to the peripheral circulation in calves 4-17 hr of age. When the labeled globulin was mixed

values were lower than when colostrum whey was used. Potassium butyrate, however, appeared to be more efficient than colostrum or whey and the other VFA were also effective, although less so than the butyrate.

More recent studies on absorption of globulins by newborn calves include those of Kruse (1970), Bush et al (1971), McEwan et al (1970a, b), Selman et al (1971) and Patt et al (1972). Kruse found that absorption during the first 24 hr was a function of the amount fed, the age at colostrum feeding and the birth weight of the calf. Age was the most important factor, his data showing that the absorption coefficient was reduced linearly to about half by delaying the feeding from 2 to 20 hr (see Table 9-10). The other papers mentioned generally agree with these data in that timing is a critical factor with respect to absorption of immunoglobulins.

Field data (Kruse, 1970; Selman, 1973) indicate that an appreciable number of calves have low blood levels of Ig; thus, there has been interest in determining what factors may be responsible for this. Kruse (1970) and Selman et al (1971) have shown that all their experimental calves were able to absorb globulins if given at an appropriate time, but

Table 9-10.   Effect of age on immunoglobulin (Ig) absorption.[a]

Item	Age (hr) when fed colostrum				
	2	6	10	14	20
Number of calves	30	24	30	23	34
Colostrum given, kg	2.2	2.7	2.6	2.9	2.9
Ig given, g	165	175	165	155	190
Serum change in Ig in 24 hr	1.49	1.40	1.15	0.89	0.86
Absorption coefficient	24	22	19	17	12

[a] Data from Kruse (1970)

with colostrum, radioactivity began to appear in the lymph after 80-120 min and reached a maximum value in about 200 min. When the globulin was administered in solution with various rations, absorption was negligible and further research indicated that a protein fraction in whey along with phosphate or glucose-6-phosphate appeared to be required for appreciable absorption. Hardy (1967) found that labeled globulin absorption could be stimulated by adding lactate or pyruvate to the medium, but the

a number of factors have been identified as being important in addition to time. The amount of colostrum (and Ig in it) is one factor. The presence of the dam and mothering by the dam appear to influence absorption. Absorption is apparently more efficient if calves nurse as opposed to bucket feeding (Selman et al, 1970). Seasonal variations have been observed (McEwan et al, 1970b) and there appears to be some differences in breeds with respect to absorption (Kruse, 1970; Selman et al, 1971;

Selman, 1973). Colostrum often contains high levels of histamine, but this is apparently not a factor in absorption (Patt et al, 1972).

Absorption of amino acids and other nitrogenous compounds (amines, purines, pyrimidines, etc.) by the ruminant is presumed to be comparable to that of monogastric species, although information on this topic is negligible. Mylrea (1966) has studied N absorption in milk-fed calves with cannulas at different levels in the small intestine. His data indicate that N (not differentiated) appeared to be absorbed over most of the length of the small intestine. This is difficult information to obtain due to the complicating factor of gastric, pancreatic and intestinal secretions and sloughing of cells in the gut. Other data obtained with markers and analyses from various parts of the gut would probably show similar trends (see first part of chapter).

Clarke et al (1966) have estimated that sheep absorbed from 3.4 to 9.8 g of α-amino nitrogen. Kay (1969), when using animals with multiple intestinal cannulas, concluded that substantial amounts of N were absorbed from each part of the small intestine, concluding that net digestion of protein continues throughout the whole length. In other data on adult sheep with multiple intestinal cannulas (Ben-Ghedalia et al, 1974), it was shown that proteolysis was very active in sections of the intestine between 1 and 3 and between 3 and 7 m from the pylorus. When using data based on use of markers, the segment of the intestine from 7 to 15 m was indicated to be the area of most intensive absorption of amino acids. In the lower intestine (15 to 25 m from pylorus) there was no apparent absorption or, if so, it was balanced by influx of N into the intestine.

Williams (1969) has investigated amino acid absorption in sheep in acute experiments wherein isolated sections of the small intestine were infused with amino acid solutions and absorption determined after 15 min. There was considerable animal variation, but isoleucine, arginine, methionine and valine were absorbed at a more rapid rate than the other acids. Glycine was absorbed at the slowest rate. There was no detectible effect of amino acid concentration. In vitro studies of amino acid uptake by the sheep intestine have been carried out by Johns and Bergen (1973). Kinetic studies

indicated the order of transport (uptake) was methionine > lysine > glycine. Data also indicated that the ileum showed maximum uptake as compared to other areas. When amino acid absorption was estimated based on portal blood flow (Hume et al, 1972), data indicated net absorption was positive at 2, 6 and 10 hr in one sheep, and 0, 2 and 10 hr after feeding in a second animal, when animals were fed 1X daily. When fed at 2 hr intervals, there was no consistent pattern in absorption. In sheep fed chopped alfalfa hay, net absorption was estimated to be 49 g/day of amino acids.

Mason and White (1971) have investigated absorption in cannulated lambs. Data on α-amino acids were obtained on sheep fed different diets with different levels of protein. Disappearance between the abomasum and end of the ileum was indicated to be from ca. 7 to 17 g/day. The previous paper and one by Mason and Milne (1971) indicate there was no net absorption of diaminopimelic acid or of muramic acid (both constituents of rumen micro-organisms), although ready absorption occurred when synthetic DAPA was introduced in the gut. They concluded that the bacterial cell wall was resistant to digestion in the small intestine. Both acids were metabolized in the large intestine.

There has been some interest in recent years in feeding of protected methionine. Neudoerffer et al (1971) found that one product (kaolin-saturated fat capsules) resulted in absorption in the distal duodenum and proximal jejunum and that 60-65% was available for absorption in the intestine.

With regard to nucleic acids, one study with tissue levels of sheep administered ^{14}C-labeled compounds indicated substantial absorption (Condon et al, 1970). Marker studies with calves (Smith and McAllan, 1971) indicated that 85 and 75%, respectively, of RNA and DNA disappeared between the duodenum and ileum. They also observed that ca. 90% of ammonia entering the duodenum was absorbed in the small intestine, and Hecker (1971b) observed that ammonia is rapidly absorbed from the cecum of sheep.

Absorption of Water from the Large Intestine

Hecker and Grovum (1971) have published an interesting paper dealing with rates of absorption of water from the large intestine of sheep. Some of their data are shown in Table 9-11. These data show that the maximum rate of absorption occurred in the centripetal and centrifugal colon. However, quantitatively, the long retention time in the cecum and proximal colon no doubt make these areas the most important. The amount

slaughtered and samples of kidney fat (perinephral) were analyzed to determine if the fatty acid composition was altered. With this technique these authors found that the unsaturated fatty acid composition of the kidney fat was increased appreciably, indicating absorption and deposition in the tissue.

Table 9-11. Water absorption from the small intestine of sheep fed 800 g of alfalfa chaff/day.[a]

Item	Intestinal section					
	Cecum and proximal colon	Centri-petal colon	Centri-fugal colon	Sub-terminal colon	Terminal colon	Total
Length, cm	80	80	86	185		430
Length, % of total	18.5	18.6	20.1	42.9		100
Wet matter, g	694	70	51	59	122	997
Dry matter, g	91	12	12	17	47	179
Total retention time, min.	531	70	68	86	295	1050
Surface area, cm^2	802	272	230	234	238	1921
Water absorbed/min, mg/100 cm^2	40	128	95	57	36	

[a]From Hecker and Grovum (1971)

of food consumed affects water absorption and consumption. When sheep were fed 400 or 1200 g of alfalfa chaff/day (Grovum and Williams, 1973), apparent water absorption (marker studies with slaughtered animals) in the small intestine of sheep was 5.8 and 13.1 l./day, respectively. Absorption in the large intestine was 2.1 and 8.5 l./day.

Absorption of VFA and Other Lipids

Williams et al (1968) have shown that the abomasum is capable of absorbing VFA at rates comparable to the reticulo-rumen. Myers et al (1967) demonstrated with an isolated cecum that VFA could be absorbed by the tissues, and Liang et al (1967) used labeled VFA administered via ileal cannulas to show that the radioactivity was almost completely absorbed in the gut posterior to the ileum.

The absorption of fats can be demonstrated in routine digestion trials with rations which contain reasonable levels of fat in the ration, although a typical ruminant ration may contain only 2-3% ether extract. Ogilvie and McClymont (1961) demonstrated absorption indirectly by administering an emulsion of linseed oil and bile to sheep with duodenal fistulas. Some time later the sheep were

Heath and Morris (1962) investigated absorption by administering ^{14}C-labeled tripalmitin and by collection of samples from sheep with chronic lymphatic fistulas. In lambs, most of the label administered into the abomasum or duodenum was recovered in the intestinal lymph, whereas in adult sheep significantly less of the label was recovered in lymph although there was appreciable variation between animals. Administration of fat via the gut temporarily reduced lymph flow; peak fat concentration was found between 3-5 hr and 5-8 hr after fat administration. When fat was given via the rumen, absorption was slow and took place over a period of several days. Most (90% +) of the label recovered was in the form of neutral glycerides. Hartmann et al (1966) have carried out experiments in which single doses of oil (480g) were given to cows orally. They found a significant increase in lymph lipids 6-7 hr after administration. The levels in the lymph began to fall by 17 hr post administration, but required 2-3 days to reach pretreatment levels. They also demonstrated that withholding feed for 24 hr resulted in a reduced lymph flow as well as a decrease in triglycerides in the lymph.

Recovery was attained within 24 hr after refeeding. Cook and McGilliard (1967) demonstrated with labeled fatty acids that very little of the label was absorbed via the stomach as compared to absorption via the intestines. Further work by Heath and Hill (1969), in which ^{14}C-labeled fatty acids were injected into the duodenum, showed that normal sheep absorbed them very well, values being: oleic acid, 92.1%; palmitic, 85.3; and stearic acid, 93.3%. Labeled tripalmitin injected into the rumen was absorbed with equal efficiency (90.1%) as intake increased from 12-44 g/day.

When working with young calves, Gooden et al (1971) observed maximum output of lipid in lymph 6 and 12 hr after feeding when given milk or colostrum, respectively. When given casein-free diets, lipid absorption was maximal at 2-3 hr.

Research in recent years has partially clarified the interaction of pancreatic juice and bile on fat absorption. Previous data (Heath and Morris, 1964) had indicated that both bile and pancreatic juice were required for fat absorption. There appears to be little doubt (Hamilton and Raven, 1973) that pregastric esterase is a factor in young preruminant animals and other research indicates that the absence of pancreatic juice (Gooden and Lascelles, 1973) or bile (Heath and Hill, 1969) may result in a reduction in fat absorption. Harrison and Leat (1970) have demonstrated that the presence of both bile and pancreatic juice allowed the recovery in lymph of 54, 69 and 83%, respectively, of the radioactivity introduced into the duodenum from stearic, palmitic and oleic acids, the rate, thus being stearic < palmitic < oleic. When the mixed secretions of bile and pancreatic juice were diverted from the intestine and bile alone infused, absorption for stearic, palmitic and oleic acids fell to 0.8, 4.2 and 24.2%, respectively. When pancreatic juice alone was infused, < 1% was recovered in the lymph duct. Leat and Harrison (1969) concluded that polyunsaturated fatty acids and lecithin, which were recovered downstream from the bile duct, might originate in the mixed secretion of bile and pancreatic juice. Diversion of bile and pancreatic juice from the intestine resulted in the disappearance of lysolecithin and a decrease in the content of unsaturated fatty acids in digesta of the jejunum. They suggested that a major function of pancreatic juice is to provide, by interaction with bilary lecithin, the lysolecithin which appears to be a major factor in micell formation (Freeman, 1969) and lipid absorption. Pancreatic juice appears to act by releasing fatty acids from food particles and allowing their solubilization in bile salts (Harrison and Leat, 1970). Scott and Lough (1971) found that unesterified fatty acids of digesta from sheep were predominately associated with particulate matter. Upon addition of bile to digesta in vitro, it was observed that unesterified fatty acids were transferred from the particulate matter to micellar solution (solubilization), thus transfer was due largely to the solubilizing effect of bile salts acting together with biliary phospholipids (lysolecithin). Thus, the interaction of these two important digestive juices, with respect to fats, appears to be rather well identified.

Carbohydrate Absorption

With respect to carbohydrate absorption, the adult ruminant animal differs from many monogastric animals in that the bulk of the readily available carbohydrates (sugars and starches) in forages are fermented in the forestomach, thus leaving very little to be absorbed in the intestine. However, in the young milk-fed ruminant and in older animals fed high-grain rations, appreciable amounts of sugars and starches, respectively, may pass into the intestine (see previous sections on partial digestion). Some of the research that has been reported on carbohydrate absorption is presented in succeeding sections:

In calves fed whole or skim milk, Rojas et al (1948) found that only a small amount of galactose was excreted in urine, the amount being equivalent to 1-3% of lactose ingested. When lactose of the milk was doubled, urinary galactose excretion increased to 8% of the lactose ingested, indicating, however, that the intestinal enzymes were still able to hydrolyze it. Flipse et al (1950) investigated the utilization of glucose, lactose or corn syrup by young calves by sampling blood after a meal. Maximum blood glucose values were attained at 4, 4, and 1 hr, respectively. Feeding starch resulted in only a moderate increase in blood sugar that was observed at 6 hr post feeding. Velu et al (1960) used a similar approach by sampling blood of calves fed sugars following a 24 hr fast. Glucose, lactose, and galactose resulted in marked elevations in blood sugars. Sucrose, however, did not result in any change, and fructose and maltose gave only slight increases in blood sugar and the feeding of these sugars resulted in diarrhea. However, sucrose inverted by invertase or citric acid was readily utilized. Huber and others (1961b) investigated carbohydrate utilization in calves when aqueous samples were introduced into the stomach in the omaso-abomasal area. Mean ages of the animals were 22, 50, 136, 227 and 600 days. Maximum increases in blood sugar (mg %) for these ages were: glucose, 134, 130, 76, 82, 50; lactose, 147, 117, 36, 37, 14; maltose, 31, 72, 30, 34, 17. Neither sucrose or starch resulted in any appreciable change in blood sugars. Ingestion of sucrose and maltose caused diarrhea, but diarrhea due to glucose or lactose was more frequent in the older animals. Absorption of ingested carbohydrates appeared to begin at about the following times (min) after ingestion: glucose, 15; maltose and lactose, 30. In a subsequent study, Huber et al (1961c) added a variety of carbohydrates to milk. Responses in blood sugar were correlated with digestibility data and they reported that the greatest increases in blood sugar resulted from lactose and maltose, the least from sucrose, with starches intermediate. Analysis of fecal samples showed that all of the soluble carbohydrate (about 25% of total carbohydrates) was glucose, indicating fermentation in the large gut. In other work from this laboratory (Natrajan et al, 1972), calves were given semi-purified diets with 62% corn starch or lactose in the form of dry milk solids. Calves gained much better on the lactose ration and blood sugar was 2.5-fold greater. Although starch digestion was relatively good (73%), data (digestibility) indicated no adaptation. A subsequent experiment indicated no response in amylase activity when given starch or cerelose.

Morrill et al (1965) have examined carbohydrate absorption in calves fitted with ileal re-entrant fistulas. They estimated that absorption anterior to the fistula for lactose was essentially complete. In the case of sucrose, estimates of flow rate and concentration indicated absorption of 41% of dietary sucrose. Preston and Ndumbe (1961) found also that milk feeding resulted in a sharp rise in blood sugar in 12-wk-old calves. Feeding dried grass resulted in no change whereas feeding concentrates resulted in an initial depression and then a gradual rise with maximum values occurring 8-12 hr after feeding.

In work with preruminant calves (10 and 50 days of age), Siddons et al (1969) noted that glucose, galactose and lactose were readily utilized; that of glucose and galactose increased with age, but lactose utilization remained constant. Maltose and fructose utilization were low in young calves and increased slightly with age. Sucrose and starch were not utilized. In older calves (53-106 days), infusion into the proximal duodenum indicated absorption of glucose, galactose, lactose and xylose, but fructose and sucrose caused little change in blood sugar. Maltose was intermediate. In cannulated calves, Coombe and Smith (1973) concluded that glucose and galactose were absorbed at about the same rate when they were present in the intestine separately; when present together, galactose absorption was greatly depressed in the proximal intestine. In the more distal intestine, where glucose concentration had fallen, galactose absorption was rapid. Since some radiolabel from galactose was recovered in glucose, they concluded that a substantial part of galactose was converted to glucose. Information on lactose indicated that hydrolysis occurred much more rapidly than absorption of its constituent monosaccharides, thus indicating that hydrolysis was not a limiting factor.

In work with isolated loops of small intestine in lambs, White et al (1971) found that glucose absorption decreased along the intestine from the duodenum to the ileum in lambs, but little change was observed in adult sheep. Absorption capacity of adult sheep appeared to be ca. 25% of that for lambs (on a basis of moles/kg of body weight).

In experiments with older animals, Porter and Singleton (1965) estimated the glucose available from rumen microorganisms from hay-fed goats. The total glucose from microbial cells and enteric liquids would amount to only about 3 g/day. Pentosans entering the duodenum were recovered quantitatively in the feces, indicating that no further hydrolysis occurred. Hogan and Weston (1967) estimated that 13-17 and 7-12 g/day of soluble carbohydrate passed from the abomasum of sheep fed alfalfa and wheaten hay, respectively, values appreciably higher than the estimates of Porter and Singleton, although representing only a small fraction of the total starch ingested in the concentrate ration. Vidall et al (1969) estimated that 10-120 g of starch/kg of diet disappeared in the lower GIT when lambs were fed rations with 100-25% hay. In the case of cattle fed high grain rations, Karr et al (1966) fed rations containing 19-63% starch and found that 16-38% passed into the abomasum, showing that appreciable amounts may enter the intestine where it would be available for hydrolysis by enteric enzymes or fermentation in the large gut by microorganisms.

Larson et al (1956) studied absorption as measured by blood sugar and digestion trials and found that glucose was readily absorbed and that maltose was hydrolyzed and absorbed in animals 8-12 mo. of age when the sugars were introduced into the omaso-abomasal area. Using the same criteria, there was little evidence of starch utilization. Experiments with isolated intestinal sections showed that glucose was absorbed readily from the jejunum and ileum and that the cecum was somewhat less efficient. Huber et al (1967) fed liquid diets to steers about 8 mo. old. They reported that maximum increases in blood sugar occurred following the administration of lactose, being three fold larger than that for starch. In addition, calves conditioned to lactose gave greater responses in blood sugar to both lactose and starch test meals than those conditioned to starch. Bensadoun et al (1962) could not detect any appreciable differences in glucose absorption in sheep 15 or 27 mo. of age fed different levels of three different rations. Although blood glucose levels were affected by diet and level of feeding in the younger animals, the differences observed were attributed to differences in metabolism and gluconeogenesis. In subsequent experiments, however, Hogue et al (1968) and Bensadoun and Ichhponani (1968) estimated that starch diets fed to sheep may result in passage of as much as 12% of the starch to the duodenum. Hogue et al calculated that as much as 120 g of glucose might thus be absorbed via the gut.

More recent data (White et al, 1971) with adult sheep (isolated intestinal loops) indicate that the absorptive capacity of the ileum was greater for sheep given wheat than that of grazing sheep. Sucrose infusion studies with sheep indicate that a large percentage of it (50-70%) passed through the ileum and

the authors suggested that any utilization in the small intestine was a result of bacterial action (Ørskov et al, 1972). Glucose absorption can be quite high. Data of Bartley and Black (1966) indicate that lactating cows could readily metabolize 1.5 kg/day when infused via the duodenum. Dirksen et al (1972) infused up to 4 kg/day into the duodenum of a cow. This caused a drop in dry matter consumption of about half. Up to 1.6 kg were said to be almost completely absorbed by the end of the ileum, and blood levels were raised from 75 to 85 mg%, but no glucose was found in the urine.

In other research with adult or non-milk-fed animals with intestinal cannulas, McAtee (1966) observed that abomasal infusion of raw starch resulted in a slight increase in blood sugar; autoclaved starch gave a greater rise in a shorter time. Henschel et al (1963) used duodenal and intestinal re-entrant cannulas to investigate carbohydrate utilization in 4-6 mo. old steers. When 10 g of carbohydrate were introduced into the duodenum, the following recoveries were found (%): raw wheat starch, 59; soluble starch, 28; maltose, 30; lactose, 14; sucrose, 62; and glucose, 0. They further found that the addition of amyloglucosidase to test suspensions reduced the recovery of raw starch appreciably. In a study with sheep (Wright et al, 1966) based on analysis of contents of the GIT after feeding high carbohydrate diets, the authors found that starch and maltose were hydrolyzed and absorbed by the small intestine. The rate of hydrolysis of maltose and absorption of glucose was appreciably faster than the rate of blood glucose clearance, whereas the rate of starch hydrolysis was only slightly faster than the rate of blood clearance (resulting in only a slight increase in blood glucose), which could be detected only when a large amount of soluble starch was administered into the abomasum of sheep.

A recap of the literature reviewed on carbohydrate absorption indicates that the young ruminant has the ability to hydrolyze and utilize lactose. Glucose is readily absorbed also. However, enteric utilization of maltose and lactose in older animals would appear to be reduced considerably. The enzyme, sucrase, is apparently lacking in ruminant species and its utilization probably depends on some hydrolysis due to acid conditions in the anterior part of the small intestine and to microbial utilization in the posterior small intestine, cecum and large intestine. Although data indicate a substantial amount of starch splitting enzymes may be present, most data indicate that enteric utilization is not high. As with sucrose, utilization in the posterior small intestine, cecum and large intestine is probably dependent upon the microbes. The fact that appreciable amounts of VFA may be produced and absorbed in these areas is probably an indication of starch utilization occurring there.

Summary and Conclusions

As the reader may have concluded, data on partial digestion are difficult to obtain except for the fibrous feed constituents which are foreign to the animal body. This is so because of the continuous absorption, secretion, and excretion occurring in various parts of the GIT. Table 9-12 is included to give the reader a summary, admittedly incomplete, of partial digestion. Data on the forestomach are more complete because of a greater research emphasis and because of relatively fewer complications from digestive secretions. Even so, there is, apparently, a wide range in digestion that occurs in the forestomach that is markedly affected by differences in ration composition, particle size and so forth.

With respect to absorption, a variety of experiments indicate that forestomach tissue is capable of absorbing a wide variety of organic compounds ranging from ammonia to lactose, although the most important components are the VFA, ammonia, and water. An approximation of the relative importance of various sites in the GIT is presented in Table 9-13. The small intestine, of course, appears to be the primary site of absorption of most organic compounds other than VFA. However, limited studies on the cecum indicate that it can absorb a variety of compounds, although its relative importance in this respect has yet to be determined. The large intestine, in addition to absorbing some mineral elements, can absorb such compounds as ammonia and the VFA, but few definitive experiments are available to allow further evaluation of its function in ruminant species.

Table 9-12. Partial digestion, adult animal.

Nutrient	Site			
	Forestomach	Small I.	Cecum	Large I.
Nitrogenous, % compounds	40-65	+ +	+	—
Lipids, %	0-40	+ + +	+ +	+
Soluble CH_2O, %	95 +	+	+	
Starches, %	50-65*	+	+ +	+ +
Celluloses, %	30-50	—	5-15	10-15
Dry matter, %	50-65	15-30	+	5-30

*Less on high starch diet

Table 9-13. Absorption from the ruminant GIT.

Nutrient	Site				
	Forestomach	Abomasum	S. Int.	Cecum	L. Int.
Nitrogenous compounds					
NH$_3$	+ +	+	+	+	+
Amino acids	+		+ + +		
Proteins			+ *		
Lipids					
VFA	+ + +	+ + +	+	+ +	+
Long-chain acids			+ + +		
Carbohydrates					
Glucose	+		+ + +		
Fructose			+ +		
Lactose	+		+ +		

*For about 1st 24 hr after birth

References Cited

Aafjes, J.H. 1967. Nutr. Abstr. Rev. 37:802.
Anderson, W.R. et al. 1961. J. Dairy Sci. 44:2218.
Annison, E.F. 1965. In: Physiology of Digestion in the Ruminant, Butterworths, London.
Annison, E.F., K.J. Hill and D. Lewis. 1957. Biochem. J. 66:592.
Armstrong, D.G. and D.E. Beever. 1969. Proc. Nutr. Soc. 28:121.
Ash, R.W. 1961a. J. Physiol. 157:185.
Ash, R.W. 1961b. J. Physiol. 156:93.
Ash, R.W. 1964. J. Physiol. 172:425.
Ash, R.W. and A. Dobson. 1963. J. Physiol. 169:39.
Aust, S.D. and R.M. Cook. 1968. J. Animal Sci. 27:1160 (abstr).
Badawy, A.M. et al. 1958a. Br. J. Nutr. 12:367.
Badawy, A.M., R.M. Campbell, D.P. Cuthbertson and W.S. Mackie. 1958b. Br. J. Nutr. 12:384; 391.
Balfour, W.E. and R.S. Comline. 1962. J. Physiol. 160:234.
Barcroft, J., R.A. McAnally and A.T. Phillipson. 1944. J. Expt. Biol. 20:120.
Bartley, J.C. and A.L. Black. 1966. J. Nutr. 89:317.
Bazanova, N.U. and V.A. Moiseev. 1967. Nutr. Abstr. Rev. 37:753.
Beever, D.E., J.F. Coelho Da Silva, J.H.D. Prescott and D.G. Armstrong. 1972. Br. J. Nutr. 28:347.
Begovic, S. 1963. Nutr. Abstr. Rev. 33:682.
Bell, J.W. and R.S. Emery. 1965. J. Animal Sci. 24:913 (abstr).
Bensadoun, A. and J.S. Ichhponani. 1968. Proc. 1968 Cornell Nutr. Conf. pp 115-118.
Bensadoun, A., O.L. Paladines and J.T. Reid. 1962. J. Dairy Sci. 45:1203.
Ben-Ghedalia, D., H. Tagari and A. Bondi. 1974. Br. J. Nutr. 31:125.
Bird, P.R. and R.J. Moir. 1972. Aust. J. Biol. Sci. 25:835.
Bloomfield, R.A., E.O. Kearley, D.O. Creach and M.E. Muhrer. 1963. J. Animal Sci. 22:833 (abstr).
Boyne, A.W., R.M. Campbell, J. Davidson and D.P. Cuthbertson. 1956. Br. J. Nutr. 10:325.
Bray, A.C. 1969. Aust. J. Agr. Res. 20:739; 749.
Britt, D.G. and J.T. Huber. 1974. J. Dairy Sci. 57:420.
Brown, R.E., C.L. Davis, J.R. Staubus and W.O. Nelson. 1960. J. Dairy Sci. 43:1788.
Bull, L.S., et al. 1965. J. Dairy Sci. 48:1459.
Bush, L.J., M.A. Aguilera, G.D. Adams and E.W. Jones. 1971. J. Dairy Sci. 54:1547.

Call, J.L., et al. 1969. J. Animal Sci. 28:135 (abstr).
Caple, I. and T. Heath. 1971. Quart. J. Expt. Physiol. 56:197.
Caple, I. and T. Heath. 1972. Aust. J. Biol. Sci. 25:155.
Ceccarelli, P., A. Debenedetti and A. Lucaroni. 1973. Nutr. Abstr. Rev. 43:958.
Chyla, M., L. Vrzgula and J. Skalka. 1972. Nutr. Abstr. Rev. 42:1634.
Clarke, E.M.W., G.M. Ellinger and A.T. Phillipson. 1966. Proc. R. Soc. B. 166:63.
Clary, J.J., G.E. Mitchell, C.O. Little and N.W. Bradley. 1969. J. Physiol. Pharmac. 47:161.
Cloete, J.G. 1966. S. African J. Agr. Sci. 9:379.
Coelho Da Silva, J.F., et al. 1972a. Br. J. Nutr. 28:43.
Coelho Da Silva, J.F., et al. 1972b. Br. J. Nutr. 28:357.
Condon, R.J., G. Hall and E.E. Hatfield. 1970. J. Animal Sci. 31:1037 (abstr).
Conrad, H.R., et al. 1958. J. Dairy Sci. 41:1.
Cook, D.A. and A.D. McGilliard. 1967. J. Dairy Sci. 50:981 (abstr).
Cook, R.M., R.E. Brown and C.L. Davis. 1965. J. Dairy Sci. 48:475.
Coombe, N.B. and R.C. Siddons. 1973. Br. J. Nutr. 30:269.
Coombe, N.B. and R.H. Smith. 1973. Br. J. Nutr. 30:131.
Danielli, J.F., M.W.S. Hitchcock, R.A. Marshall and A.T. Phillipson. 1945. J. Exptl. Biol. 22:75.
Demaux, G., et al. 1961. Bul Acad. Vet. France. 34:85.
Deutsch, H.F. and V.R. Smith. 1957. Amer. J. Physiol. 191:271.
Dirksen, G., W. Kaufmann and E. Pfeffer. 1972. Nutr. Abstr. Rev. 42:1369.
Dobson, A. 1959. J. Physiol. 146:235.
Dobson, A. 1961. In: Digestive Physiology and Nutrition of the Ruminant. Butterworths.
Dobson, A. and A.T. Phillipson. 1958. J. Physiol. 140:94.
Dobson, A., A.F. Sellers and G.T. Shaw. 1970. J. Appl. Physiol. 28:100.
Dobson, A., A.F. Sellers and S.O. Thorlacius. 1971. Amer. J. Physiol. 220:1337.
Dukes, H.H. 1955. The Physiology of Domestic Animals. 7th ed. Comstock Publ. Assoc.
Engelhardt, W.B. 1969. Zentralblatt fur Veter. A16:597.
Engelhardt, W.V. 1970. In: Physiology of Digestion and Metabolism in the Ruminant. Oriel Press, Newcastle upon Tyne, England.
Engelhardt, W.V. and H.J. Ehrlein. 1968. Pflugers Arch. Physiol. 300:R36.
Engelhardt, W.V. and W. Nickel. 1965. Pflugers Arch. Physiol. 286:57.
Engelhardt, W.V., H.J. Ehrlein and H. Hornicke. 1968. Quart. J. Expt. Physiol. 53:282.
Engelhardt, W.V. and H.P. Sallmann. 1972. Nutr. Abstr. Rev. 42:1364.
Ferreira, H.G., F.A. Harrison, R.D. Keynes and L. Zurich. 1970. J. Physiol. 222:77.
Flipse, R.J., C.F. Huffman, C.W. Duncan and H.D. Webster. 1950. J. Dairy Sci. 33:557.
Foss, D.C. 1967. Dissertation Abstr. 27:2851B.
Freeman, C.P. 1969. Br. J. Nutr. 23:249.
Gartner, K. 1963. Nutr. Abstr. Rev. 33:779.
Gay, C.C. 1965. Bacteriol. Rev. 28:75.
Goodall, E.D. and R.N.B. Kay. 1965. J. Physiol. 176:12.
Gooden, J.M. 1973. Aust. J. Biol. Sci. 26:1189.
Gooden, J.M., M.R. Brandon, P.E. Hartmann and A.K. Lascelles. 1971. Aust. J. Biol. Sci. 24:1039.
Gooden, J.M. and A.K. Lascelles. 1973. Aust. J. Biol. Sci. 26:625.
Gorrill, A.D.L., D.J. Schingoethe and J.W. Thomas. 1968. J. Nutr. 96:342.
Gorrill, A.D.L. and J.W. Thomas. 1967. J. Dairy Sci. 50:215.
Gorrill, A.D.L., J.W. Thomas, W.E. Stewart and J.L. Morrill. 1967. J. Nutr. 92:86.
Gray, F.V. 1947. J. Exptl. Biol. 24:15.
Gray, F.V. 1948. J. Exptl. Biol. 25:135.
Gray, F.V., A.F. Pilgrim and R.A. Weller. 1954. J. Exptl. Biol. 31:49.
Gray, F.V., A.F. Pilgrim and R.A. Weller. 1958. Br. J. Nutr. 12:404; 413.
Greene, L. J., C.H.W. Hirs, and G.E. Palade. 1963. J. Biol. Chem. 238:2054.
Grosskipf, J.F.W. 1959. Onderstepoort J. Vet. Res. 28:133.
Grovum, W.L. and V.J. Williams. 1973. Br. J. Nutr. 29:13.
Hale, E.B., C.W. Duncan and C.F. Huffman. 1947. J. Nutr. 34:747.
Hamilton, R.K. and A.M. Raven. 1973. J. Sci. Fd. Agr. 24:257.
Hardy, R.N. 1967. J. Physiol. 194:45 (abstr).
Harrison, F.A. 1962. J. Physiol. 162:212.
Harrison, F.A. 1971. Phil. Trans. Roy. Soc. Lond. B. 262:301.
Harrison, F.A. and K.J. Hill. 1962. J. Physiol. 162:225.
Harrison, F.A. and W.M.F. Leat. 1970. Biochem. J. 118:3.
Hartmann, P.E., J.G. Harris and A.K. Lascelles. 1966. Aust. J. Biol. Sci. 19:635.
Heath, T. 1970. Quart. J. Expt. Physiol. 55:301.
Heath, T.J. and L.N. Hill. 1969. Aust. J. Biol. Sci. 22:1015.
Heath, T.J. and B. Morris. 1962. Quart. J. Expt. Physiol. 47:157.
Heath, T.J. and B. Morris. 1964. Br. J. Nutr. 17:465.
Hecker, J.F. 1971a. Br. J. Nutr. 25:85.
Hecker, J.F. 1971b. Br. J. Nutr. 26:135.
Hecker, J.F. and W.L. Grovum. 1971. Aust. J. Biol. Sci. 24:365.
Henschel, M.J. 1973. Br. J. Nutr. 30:285.
Henschel, M.J., W.B. Hill and J.W.G. Porter. 1961. Proc. Nutr. Soc. 20:x1 (abstr).

Henschel, M.J., W.B. Hill and J.W.G. Porter. 1963. Proc. Nutr. Soc. 22:v (abstr).
Hill, K.J. 1956. Quart. J. Expt. Physiol. 41:421.
Hill, K.J. 1960. J. Physiol. 154:115.
Hill, K.J. 1961a. In: Digestive Physiology and Nutrition of the Ruminant. Butterworths.
Hill, K.J. 1961b. Vet. Rev. Annot. 7:83.
Hill, K.J. 1965. In: Physiology of Digestion in the Ruminant. Butterworths.
Hill, K.J., D.E. Noakes and R.A. Lowe. 1970. In: Physiology of Digestion and Metabolism in the Ruminant. Oriel Press, Newcastle upon Tyne, England.
Hinders, R.G. and F.G. Owen. 1965. J. Dairy Sci. 48:1069.
Hinders, R.G. and F.G. Owen. 1968. J. Dairy Sci. 51:1253.
Hogan, J.P. 1961. Aust. J. Biol. Sci. 14:448.
Hogan, J.P. 1965. Aust. J. Agr. Res. 16:179.
Hogan, J.P. and A.T. Phillipson. 1960. Br. J. Nutr. 14:147.
Hogan, J.P. and Weston. 1967. Aust. J. Agr. Res. 18:803.
Hogan, J.P. and R.H. Weston. 1969. Aust. J. Agr. Res. 20:347.
Hogan, J.P. and R.H. Weston. 1971. Aust. J. Agr. Res. 22:951.
Hogue, D.E., J.M. Elliot, E.F. Walker and H. Vidal. 1968. Proc. 1968 Cornell Nutr. Conf., pp 57-60.
Holmes, J.H.G., M.J. Drennan and W.N. Garrett. 1970. J. Animal Sci. 31:409.
Huber, J.T., N.L. Jacobson and R.S. Allen. 1961a. J. Dairy Sci. 44:1494.
Huber, J.T., N.L. Jacobson, A.D. McGilliard and R.S. Allen. 1961b. J. Dairy Sci. 44:321.
Huber, J.T., et al. 1961c. J. Dairy Sci. 44:1484.
Huber, J.T., R.J. Rifkin and J.M. Keith. 1964. J. Dairy Sci. 47:789.
Huber, J.T., S. Natrajan and C.E. Polan. 1967. J. Dairy Sci. 50:1161.
Hueter, F.G., J.C. Shaw and R.N. Doetsch. 1956. J. Dairy Sci. 39:1430.
Hume, I.D., D.R. Jacobson and G.E. Mitchell. 1972. J. Nutr. 102:495.
Jarrett, I.G. and O.H. Filsell. 1972. Aust. J. Biol. Sci. 25:405.
Johns, J.T. and W.G. Bergen. 1973. J. Nutr. 103:1581.
Johnson, R.P., E.M. Kesler and R.D. McCarthy. 1961. J. Dairy Sci. 44:331.
Jones, G.M., E.M. Kesler and R.J. Flipse. 1969. J. Animal Sci. 29:354.
Jones, O.H. and W.C. Ellis. 1971. J. Animal Sci. 32:382 (abstr).
Joyner, A.E., E.M. Kesler and J.B. Holter. 1963. J. Dairy Sci. 46:1108.
Kameoka, K. 1962. Japanese Bul. Nationl. Inst. Agr. Sci. Ser G. Animal Husbandry. 21:195. (In Japanese; English Summary).
Kameoka, K. and H. Morimoto. 1959. J. Dairy Sci. 42:1187.
Karr, M.R., C.O. Little and G.E. Mitchell. 1966. J. Animal Sci. 25:652.
Kay, R.N.B. 1969. Proc. Nutr. Soc. 28:140.
Khouri, R.H. 1969. N.Z. J. Agr. Res. 12:293; 299.
Kiddle, P., R.A. Marshall and A.T. Phillipson. 1951. J. Physiol. 113:207.
Kruse, V. 1970. Animal Prod. 12:627.
Kuimov, D.K. and I.G. Tituzov. 1968. Nutr. Abstr. Rev. 38:1200.
Larsen, H.J., G.E. Stoddard, N.L. Jacobson and R.S. Allen. 1956. J. Animal Sci. 15:473.
Lazarov, J. and N. Ivanov. 1971. Nutr. Abstr. Rev. 41:503.
Leibholz, J. 1965. Aust. J. Agr. Res. 16:973.
Leibholz, J. 1971. Aust. J. Agr. Res. 22:639; 647.
Leat, W.M.F. and F.A. Harrison. 1969. Quart. J. Expt. Physiol. 54:187.
Lennox, A.M. and G.A. Garton. 1968. Br. J. Nutr. 22:247.
Lewis, D., K.J. Hill and E.F. Annison. 1957. Biochem. J. 66:587.
Lewis, T.R. and R.S. Emery. 1962. J. Dairy Sci. 45:1487.
Liang, Y.T., J.L. Mottill and J.L. Noordsy. 1967. J. Dairy Sci. 50:1153.
Liker, B.O. 1971. Nutr. Abstr. Rev. 41:948.
MacRae, J.C. and D.G. Armstrong. 1969. Br. J. Nutr. 23:377.
Manunta, G. and P. Nuvole. 1967. Nutr. Abstr. Rev. 37:434.
Marchenko, G.M., M.V. Budnaya, E.F. Khimina and A.A. Kiyashko. 1965. Dairy Sci. Abstr. 27:125.
Mason, V.C. and G. Milne. 1971. J. Agr. Sci. 77:99.
Natrajan, S., et al. 1972. J. Dairy Sci. 55:238.
Mason, V.C. and F. White. 1971. J. Agr. Sci. 77:91.
Masson, M.J. and A.T. Phillipson. 1951. J. Physiol. 113:189.
Masson, M.J. and A.T. Phillipson. 1952. J. Physiol. 116:98.
McAtee, J.W., C.O. Little and G.E. Mitchell. 1966. J. Animal Sci. 25:262 (abstr).
McCarthy, R.D., et al. 1958. Proc. Soc. Expt. Biol. Med. 99:556.
McCormick, R.J. and W.E. Stewart. 1967. J. Dary Sci. 50:568.
McEwan, A.D., E.W. Fisher and I.E. Selman. 1970a. Res. Vet. Sci. 11:239.
McEwan, A.D., E.W. Fisher and I.E. Selman. 1970b. J. Comp. Path. 80:259.
McGilliard, A.D., C.W. Duncan and C.F. Huffman. 1957. J. Animal Sci. 16:1107 (abstr).
McLeay, L.M. and D.A. Titchen. 1970. J. Physiol. 206:605.
McNeill, J.W., G.D. Potter and J.K. Riggs. 1971. J. Animal Sci. 33:1371.
Mooney, P. and D.J. O'Donovan. 1970. Biochem. J. 119:18 (abstr).
Morrill, J.L., N.L. Jacobson, A.D. McGilliard and D.K. Hotchkiss. 1965. J. Nutr. 85:429.
Morrill, J.L., W.E. Stewart, R.J. McCormick and H.C. Fryer. 1970. J. Dairy Sci. 53:72.

Myers, L.L., H.D. Jackson and L.V. Packett. 1967. J. Animal Sci. 26:1450.
Mylrea, P.J. 1966. Res. Vet. Sci. 7:333; 394.
Mylrea, P.J. 1968. Res. Vet. Sci. 9:1.
Neudoerffer, T.S., D.B. Duncan and F.D. Horney. 1971. Br. J. Nutr. 25:333.
Nicholson, J.W.G. and J.D. Sutton. 1969. Br. J. Nutr. 23:585.
O'Dell, G.D., W.A. King, W.C. Cook and S.L. Moore. 1963. J. Dairy Sci. 46:38.
Ogilvie, B.M. and G.L. McClymont. 1961. Nature 190:725.
Ørskov, E.R., C. Fraser and R.N.B. Kay. 1969. Br. J. Nutr. 23:217.
Ørskov, E.R., C. Fraser, V.C. Mason and S.O. Mann. 1970. Br. J. Nutr. 24:671.
Ørskov, E.R., R.W. Mayes and S.O. Mann. 1972. Br. J. Nutr. 28:425.
Oyaert, W. and J.H. Bouckaert. 1961. Nutr. Abstr. Rev. 31:857.
Parthasarathy, D. and A.T. Phillipson. 1953. J. Physiol. 121:452.
Patt, J.A., A. Zarkower and R.J. Eberhart. 1972. J. Dairy Sci. 55:645.
Perry, B.N. and D.G. Armstrong. 1969. Proc. Nutr. Soc. 28:27A (abstr).
Pfander, W.H., W.C. Ellis, G.B. Garner and M.E. Muhrer. 1956. J. Animal Sci. 15:1292 (abstr).
Pfander, W.H. and A.T. Phillipson. 1953. J. Physiol. 122:102.
Phillips, G.D. and G.W. Dyck. 1964. Can. J. Animal Sci. 44:220.
Phillips, G.D., R.E. Hungate, A. MacGregor and D.P. Hungate. 1960. J. Agr. Sci. 54:417.
Phillipson, A.T. 1955 In: Advances in Veterinary Science II. Academic Press, N.Y.
Pierce, A.E. 1962. Proc. Colston Res. Soc. 13:189.
Porter, J.W.G. 1969. Proc. Nutr. Soc. 28:115.
Porter, P. and A.G. Singleton. 1965. Proc. Biochem. Soc. 96:59 (abstr).
Porter, P. and A.G. Singleton. 1971. Br. J. Nutr. 26:75.
Preston, T.R. and R.D. Ndumbe. 1961. Br. J. Nutr. 15:281.
Prokudin, A.V. and K.T. Tasenov. 1967. Nutr. Abstr. Rev. 37:757.
Putnam, P.A. and R.E. Davis. 1965. J. Animal Sci. 24:826.
Reed, W.D.C., R.C. Elliott and J.H. Topps. 1969. Rhodesian J. Agr. Res. 7:27.
Ridges, A.P. and A.G. Singleton. 1962. J. Physiol. 161:1.
Rogerson, A. 1958. Br. J. Nutr. 12:164.
Rojas, J., B.S. Schweigert and I.W. Rupel. 1948. J. Dairy Sci. 31:81.
Sajhamanov, M.H. 1968. Nutr. Abstr. Rev. 38:977.
Scott, A.M. and A.K. Lough. 1971. Br. J. Nutr. 25:307.
Scott, D. 1970. Res. Vet. Sci. 11:291.
Selman, I.E. 1973. Ann. Rech. Veter. 4:213.
Selman, I.E., A.D. McEwan and E.W. Fisher. 1970. J. Comp. Path. 80:419.
Selman, I.E., A.D. McEwan and E.W. Fisher. 1971. Res. Vet. Sci. 12:205.
Shaikhamanov, M.K. 1973. Nutr. Abstr. Rev. 43:286
Siddons, R.C., et al. 1969. Br. J. Nutr. 23:333.
Sinclair, J.H., et al. 1958. J. Animal Sci. 17:1220 (abstr).
Sjaastad, Ø, V. 1967. Acta. Vet. Scand. 8:157.
Slivickij., M.G. 1970. Nutr. Abstr. Rev. 40:121.
Smith, F.D. 1959. Thesis, Univ. of Br. Columbia.
Smith, R.H. 1964. J. Physiol. 172:305.
Smith, R.H. and A.B. McAllan. 1971. Br. J. Nutr. 25:181.
Smith, V.R. and E.S. Erwin. 1959. J. Dairy Sci. 42:364.
Smith, V.R., R.E. Reed and E.S. Erwin. 1964. J. Dairy Sci. 47:923.
Stevens, C.E. 1970. In: Physiology of Digestion and Metabolism in the Ruminant. Oriel Press, Newcastle upon Tyne, England.
Stevens, C.E. and B.K. Stettler. 1966. Amer. J. Physiol. 211:264.
Stevens, C.E. and B.K. Stettler. 1967. Amer. J. Physiol. 213:1335.
Sutton, J.D., A.D. McGilliard and N.L. Jacobson. 1963. J. Dairy Sci. 46:426.
Symons, L.E.A. and W.O. Jones. 1966. Comp. Biochem. Physiol. 18:71.
Taylor, R.B. 1962. Res. Vet. Sci. 3:63.
Ternouth, J.H. and H.L. Buttle. 1973. Br. J. Nutr. 29:387.
Ternouth, J.H. and J.H.B. Roy. 1973. Ann. Rech. Veter. 4:19.
Ternouth, J.H., R.C. Siddons and J. Toothill. 1971. Proc. Nutr. Soc. 30:89A (abstr).
Thivend, P. and M. Journet. 1968. Ann. Biol. Anim. Bioch. Biophys. 8:449.
Thivend, P. and M. Vermorel. 1971. Ann. Biol. Anim. Bioch. Biophys. 11:293.
Thomson, D.J., D.E. Beever, J.F. Coelho Da Silva and D.G. Armstrong. 1972. Br. J. Nutr. 28:31.
Thorlacius, S.O., A. Dobson and A.F. Sellers. 1971. Amer. J. Physiol. 220:162.
Thorlacius, S.O. and G.A. Lodge. 1973. Can. J. Animal Sci. 53:279.
Toofanian, F., F.W.G. Hill and D.E. Kidder. 1973. Ann. Rech. Veter. 4:57.
Topps, J.H., R.N.B. Kay and E.D. Goodall. 1968. Br. J. Nutr. 22:261; 281.
Tsuda, T. 1957. Tohoku J. Agr. Res. 7:241.
Tucker, R.E., G.E. Mitchell and C.O. Little. 1968. J. Animal Sci. 27:824.
Velu, J.G., K.A. Kendall and K.E. Gardner. 1960. J. Dairy Sci. 43:546.
Varady, J. et al. 1969. Nutr. Abstr. Rev. 39:1143.
Vidal, H.M., D.E. Hogue, J.M. Elliot and E.F. Walker. 1969. J. Animal Sci. 29:62.
Waldo, D.R. 1973. J. Animal Sci. 37:1062.
Waldo, D.R., J.E. Keys and C.H. Gordon. 1971. J. Animal Sci. 25:57 (abstr).

Warner, A.C.I. and B.D. Stacy. 1968. Br. J. Nutr. 22:389.

Warner, A.C.I. and B.D. Stacy. 1972. Quart. J. Expt. Physiol. 57:103.

Warner, R.L., G.E. Mitchell and C.O. Little. 1972. J. Animal Sci. 34:161.

Watson, M.J., G.P. Savage and D.G. Armstrong. 1972a. Proc. Nutr. Soc. 31:98A (abstr).

Watson, M.J., G.P. Savage, I. Brown and D.G. Armstrong. 1972b. Proc. Nutr. Soc. 31:99A (abstr).

Weller, R.A., F.V. Gray, A.F. Pilgrim and G.B. Jones. 1967. Aust. J. Agr. Res. 18:107.

Weller, R.A., A.F. Pilgrim and F.V. Gray. 1962. Br. J. Nutr. 16:83.

Weston, R.H. and J.P. Hogan. 1968. Aust. J. Agr. Res. 22:139.

White, R.G., V.J. Williams and R.J.H. Morris. 1971. Br. J. Nutr. 25:57.

Willes, R.F., V.E. Mendel and A.R. Robble. 1970. J. Animal Sci. 31:85.

Williams, V.J. 1969. Comp. Biochem. Physiol. 29:865.

Williams, V.J., T.R. Hutchings and K.A. Archer. 1968. Aust. J. Biol. Sci. 21:89.

Wright, P.L., R.B. Grainger and G.H. Marco. 1966. J. Nutr. 89:241.

Yadava, I.S. and E.E. Bartley. 1964. J. Dairy Sci. 47:1352.

Zerebcov, P.I., V.F. Vrakin and C.D. Tong. 1967. Nutr. Abstr. Rev. 37:78.

CHAPTER 10 — THE NATURE OF RUMEN CONTENTS

As pointed out in Ch. 11, the reticulo-rumen is host to a very diverse population of bacteria and protozoa. These organisms and their metabolites, saliva and the feedstuffs consumed appear to constitute the most important factors governing the nature of rumen contents. Absorption and passage of ingesta out of the reticulo-rumen are also important factors. There also appear to be unexplained physiological factors which may alter rumen function, but further insight into the workings of this complex system are needed for a complete understanding of it.

Some of the important physical and chemical parameters of the rumen and its contents are discussed in this chapter. In addition to these, rumen volume is an important factor. It is discussed in detail in Ch. 16. As with most other chapters, it is not intended as an exhaustive review of the available literature.

Rumen Dry Matter Content

It might be expected that rumen dry matter (%) might be one of the most variable parameters, but it usually runs between 10 and 15% of rumen contents. Warner and Stacy (1968) point out that the rumen contains approximately as much water as there is in the entire circulating blood supply and the animal, by largely unknown means, maintains this large store of water. The dry matter content will be influenced by the nature of the feed and values reported are a function of how long after drinking samples were taken. Feed ingestion is, of course, not a continuous process; salivary flow is irregular, as is rumen fermentation; passage of ingesta, both liquid and solid matter, is irregular and the volume of the reticulo-rumen is not constant. Consequently, all of these factors may influence the dry matter percentage or the amount (weight) of dry matter present in the rumen.

Burroughs et al (1946) published data illustrating the differences that might be expected when animals have been fed at different rates and watered at different times. When cattle were fed 1.47 kg of feed at 0800

and 1600 and watered at 0830, dry matter in the rumen varied from 1.25 to 3.0 kg. When the cattle were fed 2.83 kg of feed at the same times and watered at 1630, dry matter in the rumen ranged from 2.35 to 5.59 kg. More recent data (Waldo et al, 1965; Ingalls et al, 1966) are presented in Table 10-1; these data illustrate the effect of ration on the amount of dry matter that may be found in the rumen. Although the variability is, perhaps, less than one might expect when expressed as g/kg of body weight, the differences are slightly larger, percentage wise, when expressed on the basis of g/unit of metabolic size (Wt $^{0.75}$). It is also apparent that rumen dry matter varies less than does dry matter intake.

It has been mentioned previously that dry matter varies in different areas in the reticulo-rumen. This subject has been investigated by Evans and others (1973) in dairy cows fed 3, 5 or 7 kg of hay/day. Samples of digesta were taken in the reticulum, the cranial and dorsal blind sacs, and in the cranial end of the ventral sac and the ventral blind sac. Data from some of the sample sites were combined as there were no appreciable differences between them. Mean values over all levels of feeding are shown (Table 10-2). Note that the dorsal sites (cranial or dorsal blind sac) increased very little and gradually fell with time after feeding. Samples from the other sites tended to increase with time. The authors also found that there were differences in level of feeding. Mean dry matter (%) in the dorsal sites for high, medium and low feeding levels were: 14.1, 12.7 and 11.1 respectively.

Evans et al have also presented data on particle size distributions as determined by passing digesta from these different sites through screens (sieves) with different sized aperatures. The mean dimensions of digesta were described as being between 9.3 and 0.8 mm and 0.5 and 0.1 mm. Some individual particles were 30 mm long; others were microscopic in size. Data reported indicated that coarse particles were confined mainly to the dorsal sacs; the distribution of particles throughout the rumen became more uniform

Table 10-1. Effect of ration on rumen dry matter content.

| | Cattle [a] | | | | Sheep [b] | |
| | Hay | | Silage | | Alfalfa | Bromegrass |
Item	ad lib.	Maint.	ad lib.	Maint.	ad lib.	ad lib.
DM intake, g/kg of body weight	20.6	12.4	17.0	11.5	32.5	17.8
Rumen DM, g/kg BW	21.6	16.8	17.6	15.6	19.0	17.7
Rumen DM, g/kg $BW^{0.75}$	97.5	74.0	78.6	68.5		
Rumen DM, %	12.5	11.1	11.8	11.1	14.8	12.9

[a]From Waldo et al (1965). Data based on samples taken from 1 to 10 hr after feeding. The roughage was alfalfa-grass mixture.
[b]From Ingalls et al (1966). Data obtained from animals slaughtered 6 hr after feeding.

as the particles became smaller. Pronounced stratification, which persisted through the 24-hr period, was due to retention of newly ingested food in the dorsal regions.

Table 10-2. Dry matter content (%) of samples from the reticulo-rumen. [a]

| Time of sampling* | Site of sample** | | |
	A or B	C or D	E
2	13.7	3.7	3.9
4.5	13.8	3.8	4.3
7.5	13.3	3.8	4.8
11.5	12.9	4.7	4.9
19.5	11.7	5.7	6.1
23.5	10.7	5.4	5.5
Mean	12.7	4.5	4.9

*Hours, measured from time half way between beginning and end of feeding.
**A or B cranial or dorsal blind sacs;
C or D, ventral sacs; E, reticulum.

Other aspects of rumen chemistry have been investigated by Smith et al (1956). Data were obtained from the top and bottom of the rumen on the proximate chemistries, ammonia, NPN, water-soluble sugars, alcohol-soluble sugars, VFA and in vitro cellulose digestion. In all instances, except alcohol-soluble sugars, differences were observed between the top and bottom samples. All factors except ether extract and cellulose digestion were higher in top samples. In additional analyses, pH and titratable alkalinity were higher in bottom samples. Thus, the site of sampling may be critical when making comparative studies within or between animals.

Specific Gravity

The specific gravity (SG) of rumen samples has been studied by Balch and Kelly (1950). They found that the majority of digesta examined had a SG of between 1.022 and 1.055, with a mean of ca. 1.038. When cows were fed hay, there were some slight differences between the dorsal and ventral sacs; since the digesta from the ventral sac was more homogenous, it was possibly somewhat more dense. Tulloh (1966) found SG of rumen contents of grazing cows to be on the order of 0.80-0.90, values considerably lower than those given by Balch and Kelly, and Nichols (1959) reported mean SG values of 1.01. Evans et al (1973) observed that mean SG ranged from 0.860 to 1.210. In general, large particles tended to be of low density and small particles of high density. Density was least in the dorsal sites, increased in the ventral sacs and decreased in the reticulum. Mean densities tended to show two maxima and two minima during a 24 hr period.

It should be noted that data on dry matter and specific gravity may be subject to some error due to the fact that rumen contents of cattle fed forage tend to be stratified (see Fig. 7-1). The dorsal sac will have a higher content of the less dense feed particles (and be more difficult to sample), whereas the contents of the ventral and cranial sacs tend to contain the more dense material.

Rumen Temperature

Rumen temperature is generally considered to be normal at 39-41°C. Brody et al (1955) found a range of 38-40°C in normally fed cows, depending on the location in the rumen, with higher temperatures occurring as measurements were taken from ventral to dorsal locations. Feeding fasting cows resulted in an increase in rumen temperature. Active fermentation of feeds such as alfalfa hay may also result in rumen temperatures as high as 41°C (Gilchrist and Clark, 1957) with the result that rumen temperatures tend to be higher than rectal temperatures (Dale et al, 1954). Rumen temperatures also tend to be more variable than rectal temperatures. This is partly due to the ingestion of water which is at lower temperatures than the rumen. It has been observed that ingestion of water at moderate temperatures (25°C) will result in a drop in rumen temperature of 5-10°C and that as much as 2 hr may be required for rumen temperature to attain a stable level after drinking (Noffsinger et al, 1961; Cunningham et al, 1964). Other studies of this type (Dracy and Kurtenbach, 1968) with calves 6-10 wk of age show similar results, data indicating that depression of rumen temperature was a function of the temperature and quantity of fluid consumed.

Rumen pH

Rumen pH has been observed to vary in a regular manner depending on the nature of the diet and on the time that it is measured after ingestion (Phillipson, 1942). Fluctuations in rumen pH reflect the changes in the quantities of organic acids that accumulate in the ingesta (Ibid) and the amount of saliva that is produced. Rumen pH will generally reach a low from 2-6 hr after feeding (see Ch. 16 for further details), depending on the nature of the diet and the rapidity with which a meal is consumed (Briggs et al, 1957; Reid et al, 1957). With sheep, data of Briggs et al show that a diet of chopped alfalfa and cracked corn give minimum pH values of 5.2 to 5.45. The addition of feedstuffs with large amounts of starch or soluble carbohydrates will result in lower pH values than rations with a preponderence of cellulose or other carbohydrates that are metabolized slowly. The data that Briggs et al published show

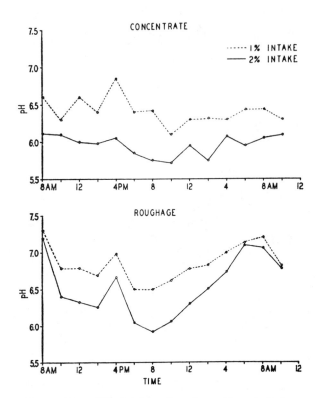

Figure 10-1. Effect of level and quality of diet on ruminal pH. Twin steers were fed either on all concentrate diet or a high-roughage pelleted diet at 0800 or 1600 hr. From Rumsey et al [1970].

minimum pH values between 4.35 and 6.5 Prefeeding values ranged from 6.25 to 7.3, depending on the diets. Beghelli et al (1959) used a recording pH meter with electrodes in the rumen and found that mean pH values in sheep on mediocre pasture to be 5.26; very good hay, mainly alfalfa, 5.20; medium hay, 5.50; poor meadow hay, 5.92; and wheat straw, 6.05. When oats were added to a poor or medium hay or to wheat straw, the pH was 5.62. Variations were shown to occur during eating and rumination. They concluded that saliva secretion rate is affected by the dryness of the feed and, in turn, it modified pH, a reasonable assumption in view of the data published on salivary production.

A variety of different reports indicates that ruminal pH increases (become less acid) as the concentration of VFA decreases; three recent examples being reports by Emmanuel et al (1969), Rumsey et al (1970), and Mullen (1973). This is not the case, however, when there is a very high level of lactic acid in the rumen (see Ch. 17). An additional example of the effect of quality of diet is shown in Fig. 10-1. In this case, steers were fed either an all concentrate diet or a high roughage pelleted diet. Rumen pH was consistently higher in animals fed the roughage diet. This figure also illustrates the effect of level of feeding on rumen pH. Data reported showed that ruminal pH went from 6.9 to 6.5 in animals fed from 0.5 to 2.0% of body weight/day of the high roughage pellet; comparable values for steers fed the concentrate diet at the same levels were 6.2 to 5.7. Other papers giving similar data include those of Balch and Rowland (1957), Woods and Luther (1962) and Bath and Rook (1963) and Mullen (1973).

Rumen pH has also been shown to vary with breed of sheep (Olson et al, 1968). Reduction in feed particle size, which would also increase the rate and probably completeness of fermentation, tends to cause a reduction in rumen pH (Cheng and Kironaha, 1973), and environmental temperatures have been reported to influence rumen pH, Mishra et al (1969) reporting values of 6.48 or 6.09 in cool and hot rooms in cows fed high roughage diets and values of 6.08 and 5.56 when fed high grain diets in cool and hot rooms, respectively. Other data relating to pH changes are discussed in Ch. 16 or 17.

A majority of reports on the subject would indicate that pH in the rumen will vary with the location of samples (Smith et al, 1956; Blake et al, 1957; Bryant, 1964; Lampila and Poutiainen, 1966; and Lane et al, 1968), although there is some disagreement by others (Balch et al, 1955; Balch and Rowland, 1957). The data, in general, indicate that pH may be expected to be somewhat higher in the dorsal and cranial sacs of the rumen and in the reticulum than in other areas. This is probably a reflection of the higher dry matter content in the dorsal sac of the rumen, washing out of the VFA and the input of saliva in the reticulum and cranial parts of the rumen. A number of these reports also show that accurate pH readings require some care and/or special apparatus. This is so because loss of CO_2 from rumen liquor will result in a reading that is higher than it should be. In addition, rumen or esophageal fistulation may result in altered rumen pH levels (Putnam et al, 1969).

Buffering Capacity

The buffering capacity of rumen contents has been well recognized. Myburgh and Quin (1943) demonstrated that rumen contents were well buffered between pH 6.8 and 7.8, but beyond this range the buffering capacity was markedly reduced when HCl or NaOH were used as titrants. Data have also been reported by Clark and Lombard (1951), Turner and Hodgetts (1955), Matscher (1959) and Bloomfield et al (1966). Turner and Hodgetts (1955) carried out rather extensive experiments on the buffering capacity of sheep rumen fluid. They found that there were considerable differences between sheep which were associated with differences in the interval after feeding, the nature of the diet and the consumption of water. The effect of diet is illustrated in Fig. 10-2. These differences were correlated with differences in total and relative concentrations of bicarbonate, phosphate and volatile fatty acids. Within the usual pH range of the rumen, the important buffering components were bicarbonate and phosphate, with the VFA having more effect at lower pH ranges. Particulate matter had little effect on buffering capacity. The effect of water consumption appeared to be due to dilution of rumen liquids. In

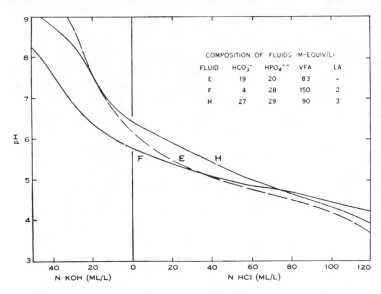

Figure 10-2. Effect of diet on rumen buffering capacity of cattle. Rations fed were: E, wheaten and oaten chaff; F, alfalfa and ryegrass pasture; H, alfalfa and oaten chaff. From Turner and Hodgetts [1955].

fasting animals, bicarbonate was more important than phosphate. During active fermentation, phosphate was relatively more important as were the VFA when the pH was < 6. They also pointed out that rumen contents were buffered to a much greater extent on the acid side than on the alkaline, results that have been confirmed by Bloomfield et al (1966).

Emmanuel et al (1969) have studied buffering capacity of rumen fluid of sheep fed a 45% roughage pellet. Buffering capacity (meq of 0.5 N acid or base/ml of rumen fluid to bring about a change of 2 pH units) in the range of pH 4-6 was low before feeding (75-80), reached a maximum 1 hr after feeding (123-134) and then gradually decreased to the original values. The response was similar, although less variable, in other pH ranges. A high correlation was found between rumen VFA and buffering capacity in the pH range of 4-6, indicating the importance of VFA as buffers in an acidic rumen environment. The authors suggested that H_2CO_3 was important within the pH range of 5-7 (as well as VFA) and that phosphate was important at pH 6-8. CO_2 levels observed range from low values of 35.3 (ml gas liberated from 1 ml rumen fluid by 1 ml H_2SO_4) at 3 hr post feeding to values of 50.7-55.6 at 6-9 hr post feeding. Kaufmann and Hagemeister (1970) concur in that they found that the rumen has a relatively stable buffer system controlled by the pH, partial CO_2 pressure and concentrations of VFA salts. However, Poutiainen (1970) states that he found a negative correlation between VFA concentration and buffering capacity. This researcher also reported that the buffering capacity of rumen fluid tended to decrease with an increase in feed consumption, with a decrease in NaCl supplement and when the proportion of long hay was reduced to 10%.

In general, it might be said that rumen buffering may be affected by factors which alter the amount or quality of salivary production, concentration of ruminal acids and CO_2, rate of absorption or passage of digesta out of the rumen.

Oxidation-Reduction Potential

Very little oxygen is found in rumen contents, although some free oxygen may be found at times (0.5-1% in rumen gas), probably coming from intake of feed or water. The rumen, consequently, is anaerobic and a reduced atmosphere is maintained. It is known from the work of Bryant and others that many strains of bacteria must have a well reduced medium in order to have appreciable growth on purified substrates. Even in the case of washed suspensions where massive inoculations are utilized in vitro, it is necessary to keep them well gassed in order to obtain rapid growth (unpublished data, author's laboratory). However, as Czerkawski and Breckenridge (1969) point out, this could be a problem of insufficient nutrient supply rather than a direct effect of oxygen.

Broberg (1957) found the oxidation-reduction potential of rumen contents to be on the order of -.35 v. and noted that oxygen was taken up rapidly by rumen contents. When measurements of redox potential and pH were combined to give the reducing power, rH, of rumen contents, he found a stable rH near 8 in rumen liquor obtained from animals on several different rations. A transient fall to 6.9 occurred soon after the feeding of concentrates. During fasting the rH rose to 11.2. When samples of rumen contents were acidified, the rH from samples from well fed animals remained constant down to about pH 5, after which it rose sharply. Samples from sheep on inadequate rations showed the rH values to rise at higher pH values. In sheep force-fed grain, a high rumen rH was found when pH dropped below 5. Eight cows with frothy bloat gave a wide range of rH from 2.8 to 17.2. Sick animals with normal appetites (?) had normal rH and rH:pH curves. Oxygen uptake was shown to be unrelated to CO_2 production, and introduction of O_2 into the rumen caused only temporary changes in rH. It has also been reported (Mishra et al, 1969) that ruminal oxidation-reduction potential may be influenced by environment (ambient temperature) and ration and that it was inversely related to rumen pH.

Broberg (1958) has shown that oxygen is actively taken up by rumen contents; data on sheep indicated that bubbling up to 40 l./day of oxygen into the rumen caused no significant changes in methane production or digestibility of dry matter (cited by Czerkawski and Breckenridge, 1969). In vitro experiments indicate that moderate amounts of oxygen do not affect VFA or ammonia production (Baldwin and Emery, 1960). More recent experiments by Czerkawski and Breckenridge (1969) indicate that addition of oxygen to mixed rumen organisms had no measurable influence on utilization of sucrose or production of CO_2 or VFA. Addition of oxygen at the beginning of incubation inhibited methane production and increased the accumulation of H_2. Similar but less pronounced changes occurred when oxygen was infused continuously. There was a net uptake of oxygen in all experiments. Thus, these various experiments show that oxygen has little apparent effect on normal rumen metabolism in contrast to studies with purified preparations used for growing isolated strains of rumen bacteria.

Baldwin and Emery (1960) reported figures for redox potentials with dead bacteria that were somewhat lower than Broberg's. They found the relationship between the redox potential and the pH of rumen fluid to be represented by the equation $Eh = 0.06$ pH (where Eh is expressed as millivolts). These authors found that only 9% of the total reductive capacity of rumen fluid was associated with the bacterial cells, whereas 47 and 38%, respectively, were associated with the large feed particles and supernatant colloidal material. They concluded that rumen bacteria utilize their substrate as an electron acceptor. Gassing in vitro fermentations with oxygen did not raise the potential or cause changes in end products produced. This result, they assumed, was due to the presence of many facultative organisms in the rumen which may survive in the presence of oxygen. They theorized that the facultative organisms utilize the highly oxidative compounds that enter the rumen as hydrogen acceptors and thereby allow the redox potential to remain at a low level so that the anaerobic organisms can continue to function.

Surface Tension and Viscosity

The surface tension of rumen fluid is on the order of 50-60 dynes/cm (Blake et al, 1957; Elam and Davis, 1962). Surface tension is reduced slightly by dilution of rumen fluid with water and by a number of surface-active agents such as detergents, silicones and fats (Blake et al, ibid; Meyer and Bartley, 1972).

Research interest in surface tension and viscosity has been primarily related to the incidence of bloat (see Ch. 17). Froth production in the rumen, a major factor in bloat, is correlated with both surface tension and viscosity, as froth formation is favored when both surface tension and viscosity are high (Blake et al, ibid; Meyer and Bartley, 1971; Cheng and Hironaka, 1973). Viscosity tends to be higher when concentrates are fed and as a result of reduction of the particle size of concentrates (Table 10-3). On fine-particle concentrates, viscosity was also affected by pH, reaching maxima between pH 5.5 and 5.8 and between 7.5 and 8.5.

Table 10-3. Effect of diet or particle size on rumen fluid (cell-free) viscosity with time after feeding. [a]

Time, hr	All-concentrate diet		Hay diet
	Coarse	Fine	
0	15.4	31.3	7.8
1	15.6	31.5	7.4
2	15.2	32.2	7.2
4	12.9	29.2	7.2
8	14.4	28.3	7.2

[a] From Cheng and Hironaka (1973); cows fed 2X daily.

Osmotic Pressure

Differences in osmotic pressure are attributed to the presence of ionized atoms or molecules present in a solute, and the pressure is believed to be equivalent to the gas pressure that would result if the ions were in gaseous form. Osmotic pressure is generally derived by determining the freezing point depression. Values for sheep have been reported to be 0.46 to 0.695°C (Parthasarathy and Phillipson, 1953; Warner and Stacy, 1965) and from 0.54 to 0.59°C for cattle (Hungate, 1942). Warner and Stacy (1965, 1968) reported that rumen liquor is generally hypotonic to blood plasma prior to feeding, information that has been confirmed by other studies (Engelhardt, 1970; Murad, 1973; Mullen, 1973). After feeding it tends to become hypertonic to blood for a period of several hours, gradually returning to the prefeeding level; typical trends are illustrated in Fig. 10-3. Osmotic pressure in the region of 350-400 m.osmol/kg may be observed in the rumen from 30 min to 2 hr after feeding (vs 300 for blood plasma) and accompanying signs of hemoconcentration indicate a transfer of body water from the blood to the gut (Warner and Stacy, 1965). There is some indication of an increased permeability of the rumen when it is quite hypertonic (Stacy and Warner, 1972). Drinking results in a marked drop in osmotic pressure, followed by a steady rise over a period of several hours. Warner and Stacy (1972) conclude that absorption of Na, the major cation in the rumen, and of the VFA are the primary means by which the animal regulates rumen osmotic pressure. Studies with sheep indicate that infusion into the rumen increased osmotic pressure, but the effect is longer lasting with NaCl than with Na acetate (Bergen, 1972).

In vitro studies indicate that osmotic pressure of 400 m.osmol/kg result in depressed cellulose digestion (Bergen, 1972). Dehority and Males (1974) have studied the effect of rumen osmotic pressure on rumen protozoa. They also showed that restricting feed intake tended to reduce osmolality and holotrich numbers but both parameters increased when sheep were returned to normal feed levels. Results with water restriction were similar to feed restriction, and these authors concluded that normal manipulation of feed and water intake did not influence numbers of holotrich protozoa.

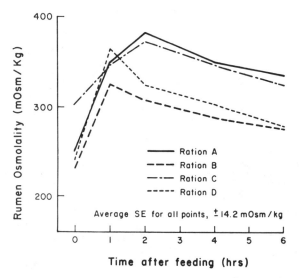

Figure 10-3. Effect of different diets on rumen osmotic pressure. Ration A, primarily corn cobs, alfalfa meal, rolled oats; B, corn cobs, ground corn [32%], ground hay; C, corn cobs, ground corn [52%], ground hay; D, alfalfa silage. From Bergen [1972].

Solutes in Rumen Liquor

It is quite obvious that many solutes, either of an organic or inorganic nature, may be found in the rumen liquor. The solutes may have originated from ingested solids or liquids, saliva, secretions into the stomach, or may be metabolites of the micro-organisms. Warner and Stacy (1965) have examined some of the solutes in the rumen of sheep that were fasted 18-24 hr (to reduce the effect of feed). In the sheep used they found the Na concentration to vary between 72 and 137 meq/l.; K from 17 to 60; NH_3 from 7 to 15, and VFA from 30 to 62. K tended to vary inversely with Na (an extract of feed contained 3.6 meq of Na and 47 of K/100 g of dry weight). The values for Na are somewhat higher (mean about 110 meq/l.) than those reported by other laboratories. For example, Emery et al (1960) reported values for about 102 meq/l. for Na and 37 for K; their samples were taken within a short time of feeding, so this may account for some of the difference. Emery and co-workers noted rather large differences between individual animals on rations which varied from 100% roughage to 80% grain.

Data are available on many organic compounds found in the rumen. Of particular importance are the nitrogenous compounds, the volatile fatty acids as well as other organic acids, and rumen gases. The reader is referred to discussions in subsequent chapters for details on these and other compounds found in the reticulo-rumen.

References Cited

Balch, C.C. and A. Kelly. 1950. Br. J. Nutr. 4:395.

Balch, C.C., et al. 1955. J. Dairy Sci. 2:27.

Balch, D.A. and S.J. Rowland. 1957. Br. J. Nutr. 11:288.

Baldwin, R.L. and R.S. Emery. 1960. J. Dairy Sci. 43:506.

Bath, I.H. and J.A.F. Rook. 1963. J. Agr. Sci. 61:341.

Beghelli, V., G. Borghi and R. Matscher. 1959. Nutr. Abstr. Rev. 29:511.

Bergen, W.G. 1972. J. Animal Sci. 34:1054.

Blake, J.T., R.S. Allen and N.L. Jacobson. 1957. J. Animal Sci. 16:190.

Bloomfield, R.A., E.G. Komer; R.P. Wilson and M.E. Muhrer. 1966. J. Animl Sci. 25:1276 (abstr).

Briggs, P.K., J.P. Hogan and R.L. Reid. 1957. Aust. J. Agr. Res. 6:674.

Broberg, G. 1957. Nord. Vet. Med. 9:918; 942.

Broberg, G. 1958. Nord. Vet. Med. 10:263.

Brody, S., R.E. Stewart and H.E. Dale. 1955. J. Animal Sci. 14:1243 (abstr).

Bryant, A.M. 1964. N.Z. J. Agr. Res. 7:694.

Burroughs, W., P. Berlaugh, E.A. Silver and A.F. Schalk. 1946. J. Animal Sci. 5:338.

Cheng, K.J. and R. Kironaha. 1973. Can. J. Animal Sci. 53:417.

Clark, R. and W.A. Lombard. 1951. Onderstepoort J. Vet. Sci. 25:79.

Cunningham, M.D., F.A. Martz and C.P. Merilan. 1964. J. Dairy Sci. 47:382.

Czerkawski, J.W. and G. Breckenridge. 1969. Br. J. Nutr. 23:67.

Dale, H.E., R.E. Stewart and S. Brody. 1954. Cornell Vet. 44:368.

Dehority, B.A. and J.R. Males. 1974. J. Animal Sci. 38:865.

Dracy, A.E. and A.J. Kurtenbach. 1968. J. Dairy Sci. 51:1787.

Elam, C.J. and R.E. Davis. 1962. J. Animal Sci. 21:327.

Emery, R.S., et al. 1960. J. Dairy Sci. 43:76.

Emmanuel, B., M.J. Lawlor and D.M. McAleese. 1969. Br. J. Nutr. 23:805.

Engelhardt, W. 1970. Nutr. Abstr. Rev. 40:852.

Evans, E.W., G.R. Pearce, J. Burnett and S.L. Pillinger. 1973. Br. J. Nutr. 29:357.

Gilchrist, F.M.C. and R. Clark. 1957. S. African Vet. Med. Assoc. 28:295.

Hungate, R.E. 1942. Biol. Bul. 83:303.

Ingalls, J.R., J.W. Thomas, M.B. Tesar and D.L. Carpenter. 1966. J. Animal Sci. 25:283.

Kaufmann, W. and H. Hagemeister. 1970. Nutr. Abstr. Rev. 40:75.

Lampila, M. and E. Poutiainen. 1966. Ann. Agr. Fenn. 5:279.

Lane, G.T., et al. 1968. J. Dairy Sci. 51:114.

Matscher, R. 1959. Nutr. Abstr. Rev. 29:511.

Meyer, R.M. and E.E. Bartley. 1971. J. Animal Sci. 33:1018.

Meyer, R.M. and E.E. Bartley. 1972. J. Animal Sci. 34:234.

Mishra, M. et al. 1969. J. Animal Sci. 29:166 (abstr).

Mullen, P.A. 1973. Br. Vet. J. 129:267.

Murad, K.M. 1973. Nutr. Abstr. Rev. 43:957.

Myburgh, S.J. and J.I. Quin. 1943. Onderstepoort, J. Vet. Sci. An. Ind. 18:119.

Nichols, R.E. 1959. Wisconsin Agr. Expt. Sta. Res. Rpt. #3.

Noffsinger, T.L., K.K. Otagaki and C.T. Furukawa. 1961. J. Animal Sci. 20:718.

Olson, J.C., D.A. Cramer and J.G. Nagy. 1968. Proc. West. Sec. Amer. Soc. Animal Sci. 19:43.

Parthasarathy, D. and A.T. Phillipson. 1953. J. Physiol. 121:452.

Phillipson, A.T. 1942. J. Expt. Biol. 19:186.

Poutiainen, E. 1970. Ann. Agr. Fenn. 9:151.

Putnam, P.A., R.R. Oltjen and E. Williams. 1969. J. Animal Sci. 28:876 (abstr).

Reid, R.L., J.P. Hogan and P.K. Briggs. 1957. Aust. J. Agr. Res. 6:691.

Rumsey, T.S., P.A. Putnam, J. Bond and R.R. Oltjen. 1970. J. Animal Sci. 31:608.

Smith, P.H. et al 1956. J. Dairy Sci. 39:598.

Stacy, B.D. and A.C.I. Warner. 1972. Comp. Biochem. & Physiol. 43A:637.

Tulloh, N.M. 1966. N.Z. J. Agr. Res. 9:252; 999.

Turner, A.W. and V.E. Hodgetts. 1955. Aust. J. Agr. Res. 6:115; 124.

Waldo, D.R., R.W. Miller, M. Okamoto and L.A. Moore. 1965. J. Dairy Sci. 48:473.

Warner, A.C.I. and B.D. Stacy. 1965. Quart. J. Expt. Physiol. 50:169.

Warner, A.C.I. and B.D. Stacy. 1968. Br. J. Nutr. 22:389.

Warner, A.C.I. and B.D. Stacy. 1972. Quart. J. Expt. Physiol. 57:103.

Woods, W. and R. Luther. 1962. J. Animal Sci. 21:809.

CHAPTER 11 — RUMEN MICROBIOLOGY

The microbiology of the rumen is an extremely complex subject due to the large numbers of organisms present, their diverse nature, and the shifting populations that result from changes in the diet of the host animal. In addition, marked changes may be noted within and between animals on the same or similar diets. As a consequence, there have not been many bacteriologists who have been interested in working in the field. In recent years, however, improved cultural technology now allows culture of many pure species and, as a result, rumen microbiology is an expanding field. Review articles by Kay and Hobson (1963) and Bryant (1959, 1963, 1970) may be of interest and the reader is referred to the detailed discussion in the book by Hungate (1966). Other reviews, such as those in the book edited by Phillipson (1970), are available on more specific subjects.

The rumen provides an environment that is very favorable for microbial growth (see Ch. 10). The pH ranges between 5.5 and 7.0 for the most part and temperature (39-41°C) is near optimum for many enzyme systems. The food supply is provided in a more or less continuous manner. Contractions of the stomach help to bring the microorganisms in contact with freshly ingested or ruminated feed and the moist conditions are favorable for many organisms. End products of fermentation, which may be inhibitory, are removed by absorption and passage out of the stomach. As a result of this favorable environment, a dense population of microorganisms thrives in the reticulo-rumen. Some estimates indicate that microbial protoplasm, at times, may be equal to 10% of rumen fluid (Warner, 1962).

Even though the rumen environment is relatively stable, a considerable diversity exists in the microbial population. Hungate (1966) suggests several possible explanations for this diversity. According to Hungate, one factor may be a selection for maximum biochemical work — the assumption of being that microorganisms accomplishing the most growth (and biochemical work) will survive in a system which is open to invasion by competing organisms. A second factor may be a result of the complexity of feedstuffs ingested by ruminants. Microorganisms may adapt themselves to utilize only a limited number of nutrients and thus become more specialized, or they may adapt to utilize a wide variety of nutrients. The former thrive under conditions best suited for them, the latter have more survival capacity under varying conditions. Examples of each type are found in the rumen.

The two major classes of rumen microorganisms are bacteria and ciliated protozoa; although other types may be found, at times, in appreciable numbers; for example, yeast-like organisms and phages. In addition, flagellated protozoa are frequently observed, particularly in young animals. Conditions in the rumen are anaerobic with the result that microbial forms found are nearly all anaerobes or facultative anaerobes. Gall and Huhtanen (1950) suggested that, to be considered a typical rumen organism, the following criteria should be satisfied: (a) the organism must be able to live anaerobically; (b) it should be able to produce the type of end product found in the rumen; (c) the rumen should contain not less than 1 mil./g of the organism (this wouldn't apply to protozoa). These criteria were suggested because it is frequently difficult to determine if an organism is a natural inhabitant of the rumen or if its presence is a result of ingestion of microorganisms by way of food, water, or other means. Hungate (1966) cites numerous examples of reports in which organisms similar to rumen microbes are found in other environments such as the cecum of the rabbit and porcupine, the feces of a wide variety of mammals and even in the human mouth. Bryant (1970) points out that many similar or identical species are present in other habitats such as the GIT of non-ruminant mammals, organic sediments of natural waters, and sewage sludge. In addition, there may be marked differences between ruminant species due to dietary habits or environmental conditions in the stomach. For example, a large oval form (Quinn's oval) is common in the rumen of sheep but is not found in cattle. In addition, the microbes of some wild species (African suni) are quite different from those of cattle.

This brings up a question. Why is greater variety not seen in the rumen? Evidence on *Escherichia coli* and *Salmonellae*, both enteric bacteria normally found only in relatively small numbers in the rumen, suggests that the VFA inhibit these organisms (Wolin, 1969). A potent pathogen, *Clostridium perfringes* type D, is not capable of maintaining itself in the rumen, but the few which reach the small intestine multiply rapidly (Bullen et al, 1953). It seems likely that rumen populations have some chemical means of restricting the growth of possible competitors. This appears to be the case with normal inhabitants, as Jarvis (1968) has shown that soluble factors may be present which stimulate lysis of cells of *Streptococcus bovis* and *Butyrivibrio* sp., both common to the rumen. The lytic activity was related to the presence of protozoal species in this study. In addition, Hoogenraad and Hird (1970) have shown substantial lytic activity by rumen fluid against *E. coli* and *Bacillus subtilis*. It seems likely that some of this activity may be due to phages as large numbers have been shown to be present in the rumen under some conditions (Ritchie et al, 1971). Rumen organisms are also known to produce toxins that affect sheep or cattle when given I.V. (Mullenax et al, 1966). Perhaps some microorganisms in the rumen produce toxins or antibiotics which affect other microbial forms, as well.

Rumen Bacteria

Identification

Publications presenting numerous pictures of rumen bacteria include those of Moir and Masson (1952) using visual light microscopy and Smiles and Dobson (1956) with ultraviolet microscopy. Hungate (1966) shows pictures of many different organisms including some taken with the electron microscope, and Hoogenraad and Hird (1970) have also presented a number of pictures using the electron microscope. Pictures representing a wide variety of organisms are shown in Plates 11-1 through 11-7.

Bryant (1963) has discussed a number of criteria that are useful in identifying rumen bacteria. A summary of some of his remarks is presented here.

The morphology (form and shape) of bacteria is useful for identifying some species but many are too similar to identify on the basis of morphology alone, partly because the most common bacteria are small cocci (Hoogenraad and Hird, 1970). Rumen cocci or short rods are often within the size range of 0.4-1.0 µ in diameter and 1-3 µ in length. Other forms such as spirochetes, rosettes, ovals and tetracocci are also found. Some species and strains can be identified by their distinctive size or shape but many others must be identified on the basis of other characteristics. As Bryant points out, the shape and size of cells within a single culture or within a group of strains may vary considerably even when observed under one set of conditions, particularly in pure culture work. In one case *Bacterioides ruminocola* cells may vary in shape from coccoid to long rods; some strains are mainly coccoid, others mainly rod-shaped and others in between. *B. succinogenes* shows similar variation and, in addition, some strains may be smaller, more slender, somewhat curved rods and show sharply pointed ends rather than the more typical rounded ends. The type of flagellation is an important means of identification in motile species, but may be difficult to detect or the point of attachment or arrangement of flagella may be difficult to determine.

Pearson (1969), while studying microbial distribution in elk, has devised a scheme for classifying rumen bacteria based on their morphology, as illustrated in Table 11-1. While this scheme might not be meaningful from the point of view of bacterial metabolism, it should provide a reasonable means of quickly classifying these organisms into recognizable groups when studying distribution as affected by season, diet and so forth.

The Gram stain reaction is useful for identification, but no ecological significance has been associated with this reaction (Hungate, 1966). Some species may include strains which give both positive and negative reaction to Gram stains. Bryant feels that more detailed cytological studies involving various staining procedures and electron microscopy should be useful means of identification. The availability of scanning electron microscopes in the past few years has facilitated identification (refer to Plates 11-3 through 11-7).

Identification can often be partially accomplished by use of various metabolism

Table 11-1.   Morphological classification of Gram-stained rumen bacteria in mule deer.[a]

Morphological groups	Bacterial type designation[b]	Bacteria described in literature
Gram-positive cocci	PC	Peptostreptococci Ruminococci Streptococci
Small (diameter up to 0.5 µm), gram-negative cocci	NSC	*Veillonella*
Large (diameter >0.5 µm), gram-negative cocci	NMC	*Neisseria*
Long (length >1.5 µm, gram-positive bacilli	PLR	Lactobacilli Cillobacteria Propionibacteria
Short (length up to 1.5 µm), gram-positive bacilli	PSR	Eubacteria
Curved, gram-positive bacilli	PCR	*Lachnospira*
Sporforming, gram-positive bacilli	PFR	Bacilli *Colostridium*
Long (length >1.5 µm), gram-negative bacilli	NLR	*Escherichia*
Short (length up to 1.5 µm) gram-negative bacilli	NSR	*Bacteroides* Fusobacteria
Cresent or moon-shaped gram-negative, gram-variable bacilli	NMR	*Selenomonas*
Oval, gram-negative bacilli	NOR	*Succinimonas*
Curved, gram-negative bacilli	NCR	*Butyrivibrio* *Succinivibrio* *Desulphovibrio*
Spiral-shaped, gram-negative bacilli	NBR	*Borrelia*

[a] From Pearson (1969)
[b] First letter: P, gram-positive; N, gram-negative. Middle letter: S, small cocci, or short bacilli; M, large cocci or moon-shaped bacilli; L, long; C, curved; F, sporeforming; O, oval, B, spiral. Last letter: C, cocci, R, bacilli.

studies and by altering cultural methods. Fermentation end products produced may be characteristic of some species, but there tends to be a great deal of overlapping, so that additional information is usually required. However, knowledge of the by-products produced is often helpful, particularly when a very specific end product such as indole, sulfide or NO_3 are produced. In addition, information on the type of substrate attacked, energy sources utilized and the nutrients required when grown in pure culture is useful, but, again, there is much duplication between different species. A study of different enzymes present may provide useful information. Serological tests involving the development of fluorescent antibodies can provide specific information, but this technique has not been used to any great extent.

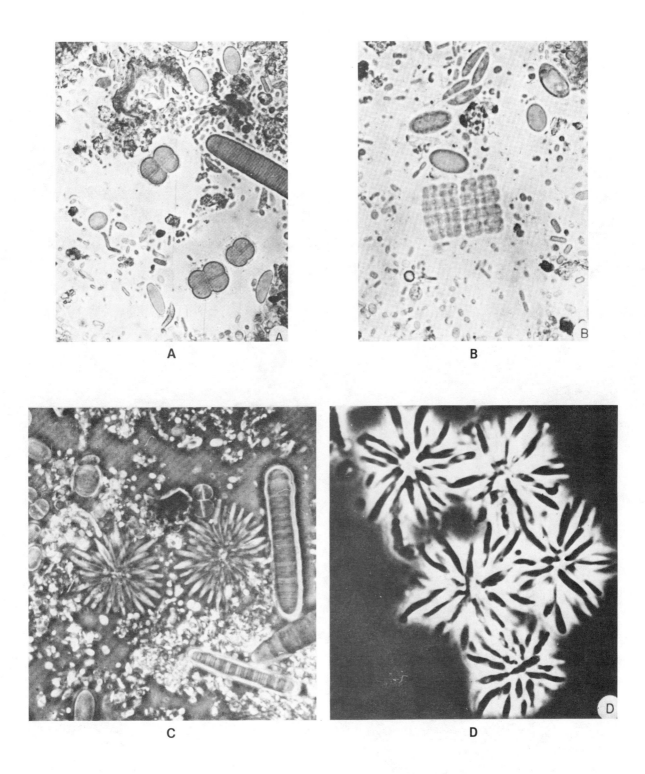

Plate 11-1. A large tetracocci resembling *Sarcina bakeri* and one end of an *Oscillospira* showing transverse septa. B. *Lampropedia* [window-pane sarcina, rectangular organism] from the sheep rumen; also long almost crescentic forms, and the oval form of Woodcock and Lapage, also called Quin's oval. C. Two rosettes from the sheep rumen, with *oscillospiras* and oval forms. D. A rosette-forming bacterium cultured concurrently with *R. albus* on rumen cellulose agar by R.A. Mah. Photography by R.A. Mah. A, B, and C after Smiles and Dobson [1956]; magnification ca. 1,830X. Ultraviolet illumination. D was made with dark-phase contrast; magnification ca. 2,200X. Courtesy of R.E. Hungate and Academic Press.

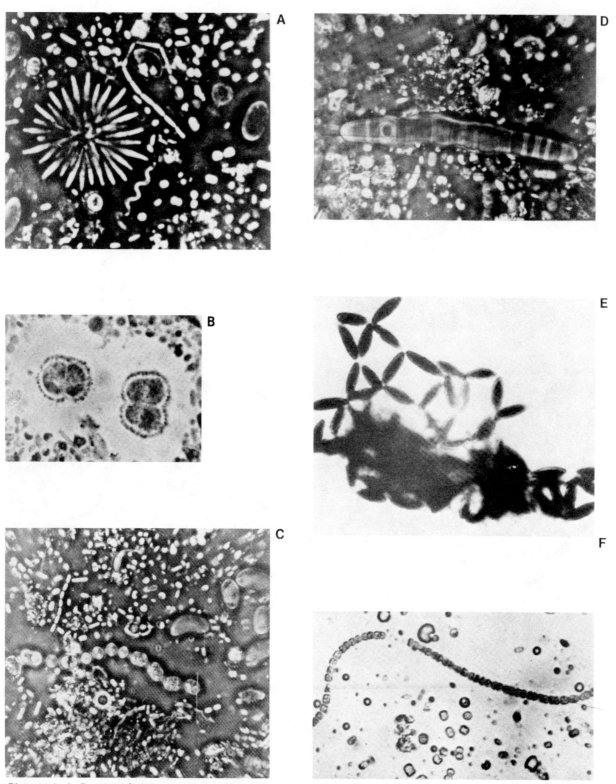

Plate 11-2. A, Rosette, Quin's organism and *Selenomonas*, and numerous small organisms. B, Sarcinae with large capsules. C, Chain of large cocci, selenomonads, and ovals. D, *Oscillospira guillermondii* [1830X]. E, clostridial forms of *Clostridium lochheadii*. F, long cocci chain. Absorbing material concentrated at edge of small bacteria. F, courtesy of R.E. Hungate; all others from Smiles and Dobson [1956].

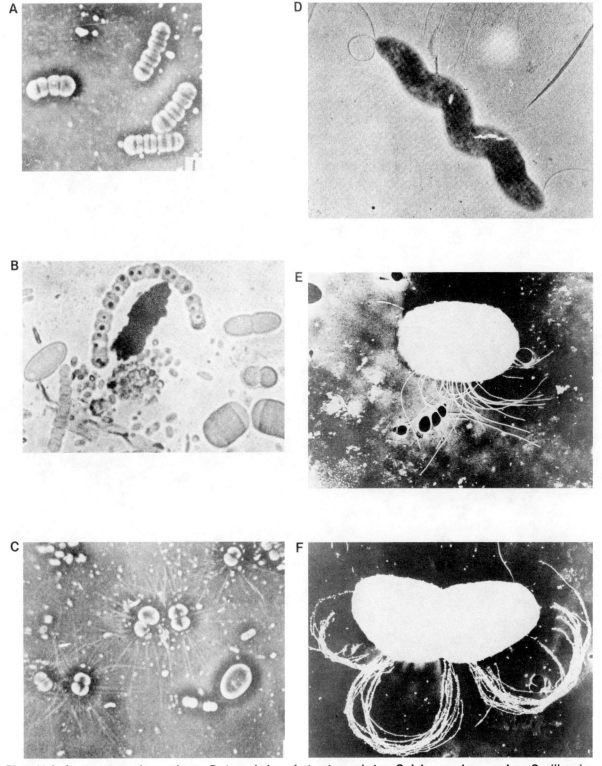

Plate 11-3. A, streptococci organisms. B, two chains of streptococci, two Quin's organisms and an Oscillospira guillermondii breaking into two parts. C, small highly refractile sarcinae with long processes. Quin's organism on bottom right. D, a cell of *Succinivibrio dextrinosolvens* strain S-4-2 [13,500X]. E, the oval form of Woodcock and Lapage [5,400X]. F, dividing oval, or possibly *Selenomonas* [5,400X]. A,B,C from Smiles and Dobson [1956]; D,E,F are electron micrographs by J. Pangborn, courtesy of R.E. Hungate and Academic Press.

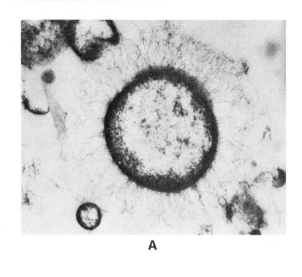

A

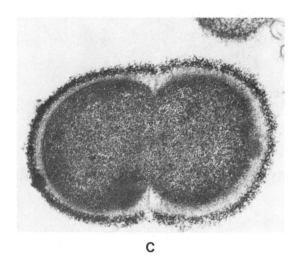

C

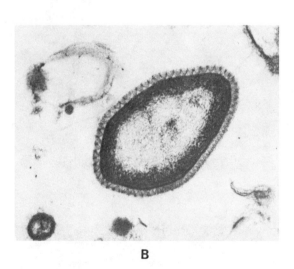

B

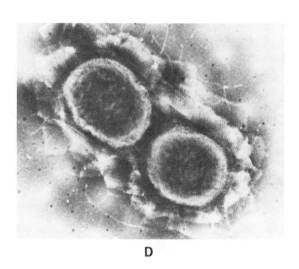

D

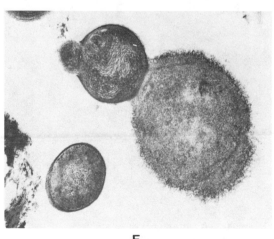

E

Plate 11-4. A, thin section of rumen bacterium illustrating its characteristic fibrillar capsule. B, thin section showing cone-shaped surface structures and typical rarefied nucleoplasm region in the cell center. C, thin section showing thickened cell wall and indentation at the plane of division. D, rumen bacterium in final stage of division illustrating its capsule of highly ordered membrane sheets. E, thin section of rumen bacterium undergoing fission into daughter cells of markedly different sizes. Electron micrographs, courtesy of Al Ritchie, ARS, USDA, National Disease Laboratory, Ames, Iowa.

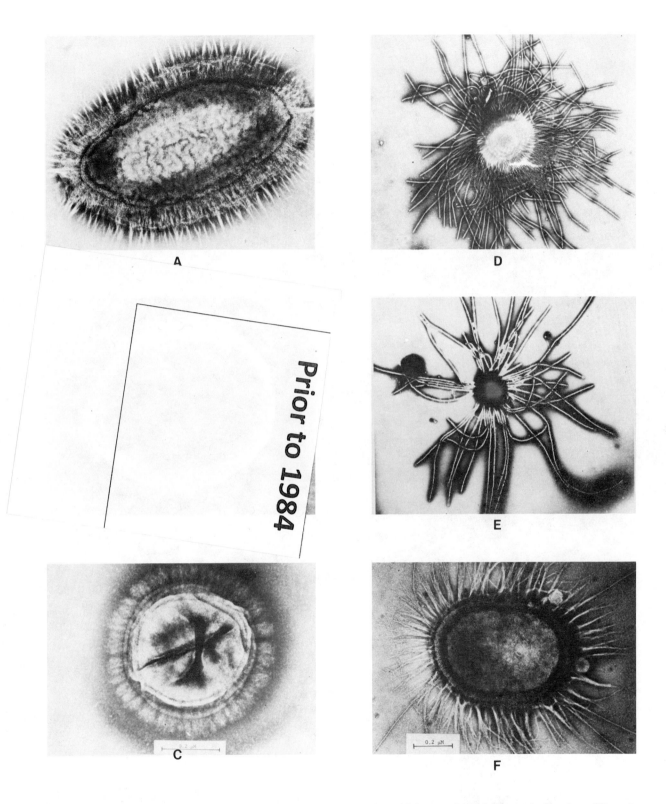

Plate 11-5. Electron micrographs of rumen bacteria illustrating A, a thick capsule and demonstrating two different lengths of capsular fibrils. B, characteristic tufts of capsular fibrils. C, surface capsular fibrils. D, hollow surface appendages. E, long hollow surface appendages. F, fibrillar capsule made up of at least two types of fibers of different length. Courtesy of Al Ritchie.

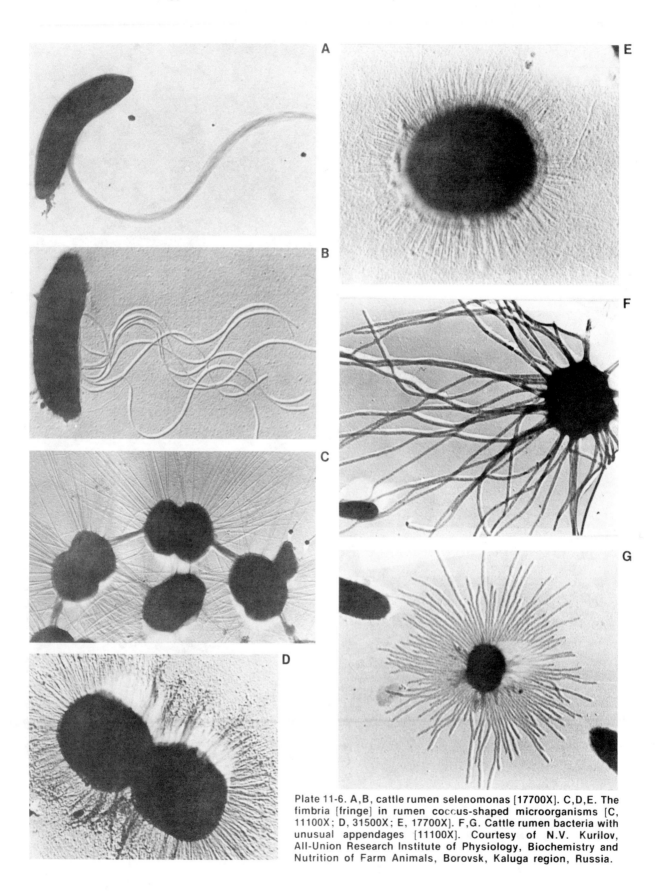

Plate 11-6. A,B, cattle rumen selenomonas [17700X]. C,D,E. The fimbria [fringe] in rumen coccus-shaped microorganisms [C, 11100X; D, 31500X; E, 17700X]. F,G. Cattle rumen bacteria with unusual appendages [11100X]. Courtesy of N.V. Kurilov, All-Union Research Institute of Physiology, Biochemistry and Nutrition of Farm Animals, Borovsk, Kaluga region, Russia.

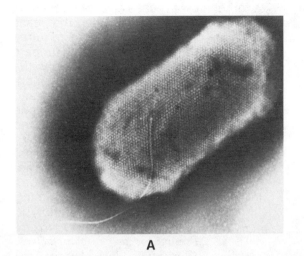

A

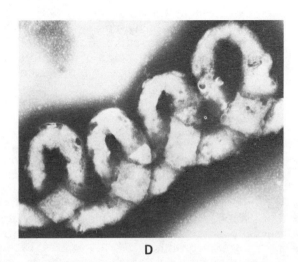

D

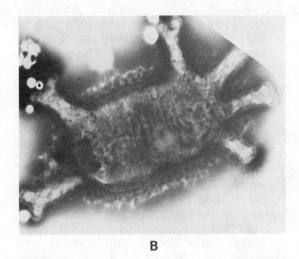

B

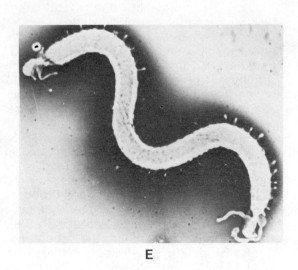

E

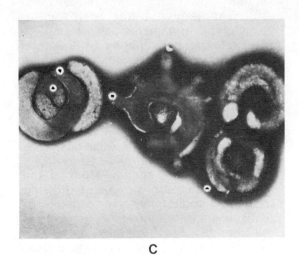

C

Plate 11-7. Electron micrographs of rumen bacteria illustrating A, single flagellum and its characteristic hollow cell wall subunits. B, unique cellular protrusions formed at the poles. C, four rumen bacteria showing common coiled morphology of the cells and pleomorphic protrusions typical of the central one. D, typical coiled morphology. E, common morphology of spirochetes and numerous small cell wall protrusions [blebs]. Courtesy of Al Ritchie.

Classification of Bacteria

There are, obviously, many ways that bacteria could be classified. Some of these could include various aspects of morphology such as cell shape and size, the presence of appendages, staining reaction, etc. They can also be classified on the basis of the substrate attacked, end products produced, cellular chemical composition, or a combination of any of these. Bacteria, although small, may be rather complex organisms and most schemes utilized for classification will either be incomplete or will result in duplications. Perhaps only a very general scheme is of value, one that will enable the reader to partially sort the complex population into recognizable groups.

For the purposes of this discussion, a method based on the type of substrate utilized as a primary source of energy is a favored method. This is a general method, but even here there may be contradictions since information from different sources is not always in agreement as to substrates utilized. This may be due to different laboratory conditions or analytical procedures or, perhaps, different strains of the same species of bacteria are involved. Hungate (1966) has classified bacteria partially on the basis of substrates utilized and partially on the basis of end products produced. The reader is referred to his book for further details.

Bacterial classification, essentially as suggested by Hungate, is discussed in subsequent paragraphs. The reader is cautioned that organisms classified on the basis of substrate utilization or end products produced are only those species that have been studied under in vitro and usually with pure culture conditions in the laboratory. Organisms identified by other techniques are not included, thus the list is far from complete.

1. Cellulolytic (cellulose digesting) bacteria. Cellulolytic organisms are widely distributed geographically and have been found in the GIT of animals other than ruminants. These bacteria have the biochemical ability to produce cellulase enzymes which can hydrolyze native cellulose. They may also have the ability to utilize cellobiose, the disaccharide containing glucose linked with beta bonds (Bryant and Burkey, 1953; Hungate, 1950). Digestion of cellulose by pure cultures appears to be a rather slow process and for some time this was believed to be the case because several species were required for digestion of cellulose. Hungate (1966) feels that this is probably the situation for plant materials (which are complex mixtures of biochemicals) and that the action by enzymes of one species on one type of chemical bond may expose other types susceptible to attack by enzymes of other species. Cellulose digesting organisms are usually found in highest concentrations in the rumen of animals consuming fibrous rations. Important cellulolytic species include: *Bacteroides succinogenes, Ruminococcus flavefaciens, R. albus, Clostridium loch headii,* and *Cillobacterium cellulosolvens.*

2. Hemicellulose digesting bacteria. Hemicellulose differs from cellulose in that it contains pentose as well as hexose sugars and usually contains uronic acids. Hemicellulose is an important plant constituent and organisms which are capable of hydrolyzing cellulose are usually capable of utilizing hemicellulose. However, a number which can utilize hemicellulose cannot utilize cellulose (Dehority and Scott, 1967). Some of the species which digest hemicellulose include: *Butyrivibrio fibrisolvens, Lachnospira multiparus* and *Bacteroides ruminicola.*

3. Amylolytic (starch digesting) bacteria. Quite a number of cellulolytic organisms are also capable of digesting starch; however, some of the amylolytic organisms cannot reciprocate. Amylolytic organisms are found in much larger percentages of the total microbial population when rations high in starch are fed. Important species which digest starch include: *Bacteroides amylophilus, Succinimonas amylolytica, Butyrivibrio fibrisolvens, B. alactacidigens, Bacteroides ruminicola, Selenomonas ruminantium, S. lactilytica,* and *Streptococcus bovis.*

4. Bacteria utilizing sugars. Most of the bacteria which are capable of utilizing polysaccharides are also capable of utilizing disaccharides or monosaccharides. Plant material, particularly from young plants, contains a relatively large amount of water soluble carbohydrates and these would be

available to bacteria. Presumably, sugars from dead and lysing bacteria cells or from capsular material (mostly carbohydrates) of bacterial cells would be available. If not, the rapid fermentation of soluble carbohydrates would make survival difficult for organisms that depend on sugars for their energy source. Cellobiose may be a source of energy for some of these organisms since it has been demonstrated that many noncellulolytic organisms have the β-glucosidase enzyme required to hydrolyze cellobiose (Conchie, 1954). High concentrations of organisms utilizing lactose are found in the rumen of young ruminants.

5. Bacteria utilizing acids. Quite a number of organisms are known to utilize lactic acid although it is not normally present in appreciable amounts in the rumen except in abnormal situations. Others utilize succinic acid or similar acids such as malic or fumaric. Formic acid is utilized by some organisms and acetic by others, although probably not as a primary energy source. Oxalic acid is another example of an acid that is decomposed by rumen organisms. Some species which utilize lactate include: *Veillonella gazogenes, V. alacalescens, Peptostreptococcus elsdenii, Propioni bacterium* sp., *Desulphovibrio* and *Selenomonas lactilytica.*

6. Proteolytic bacteria. A number of rumen bacteria are known to utilize amino acids as primary energy sources; one proteolytic organism studied by Hungate did not utilize sugars. *Bacteroides amylophilus, Clostridium sporogenes* and *Bacillus licheniformis* are three species known to have proteolytic capability.

7. Ammonia-producing organisms. This class may be a duplication to some extent of No. 6. However, a number of organisms are known to produce ammonia from various sources, and ammonia is almost invariably found in rumen fluid, indicating that its production is an important reaction in the rumen. Species known to produce ammonia include: *Bacteroides ruminicola, Selenomonas ruminantium, Peptostreptococcus elsdenii* and some strains of *Butyrivibrio.*

8. Bacteria producing methane. Methanogenic bacteria have been difficult to culture in vitro; consequently, very little is known about such organisms with respect to their specific requirements, even though the rumen must harbor a large number as about 25% of the gas produced in the rumen is methane. Methanogenic bacteria that have been identified include: *Methanobacterium ruminantium,* and *M. formicicum;* species believed to be of lesser importance include: *M. sohngenii, M. suboxydans* and *Methanosarcina* sp.

9. Lipolytic bacteria. Mixed suspensions of bacteria are capable of utilizing glycerol and of hydrolyzing glycerol from a fat molecule. An organism studied by Hobson and Mann (1961) could utilize only a few sugars in addition to glycerol. Other organisms hydrogenate unsaturated fatty acids and some apparently metabolize long-chain fatty acids to ketones.

10. Vitamin-synthesizing organisms. The synthesis of vitamins by individual species of rumen bacteria has not been studied extensively; however, a number are known to synthesize various members of the vitamin B complex.

A number of ruman bacteria are listed in Table 11-2, and some of their important characteristics have been tabulated (after Hungate, 1966, and Bryant, 1963). Rumen bacteria have often been grouped according to their function in attacking particular substances or with respect to the end products produced (as was done in the table). However, most species of rumen bacteria ferment more than one kind of substrate. As shown in the table, many bacteria are variable in specificity of substrate attacked. Some are specific. *Bacteroides amylophilus* is specific for maltose and starch and *Anaerovibrio lipolytica* for fructose and glycerol. Those species that attack cellulose also utilize various other carbohydrates. Species such as *Butyrivibrio fibrisolvens Selenomonas lactilytica* are very versatile with respect to the substrate that is attacked. Others are intermediate in ability to attack substrates. As a further example, Bryant and Burkey (1953) isolated 896 strains of different organisms from cattle on different diets. Of these, 98% were

Table 11-2. Characteristics from some rumen bacteria that have been cultured *in vitro* (after Hungate, 1966, and Bryant, 1963).

Organism	Shape of cells	Gram stain	Size, μ	Motility	Important function	Glucose	Cellulose	Xylan	Starch	Lactate	Glycerol	Some energy sources used
1. *Bacteroides succinogenes*	rods to coccoid	−	0.3-0.4 by 1-2	−	Attacks resistant cellulose	+	+	−	+−	−	−	
2. *Ruminococcus flavefaciens*	cocci, usually in chains	+−	0.8-1.0	−	Fiber digestion	+−	+−	+−	−	−	−	
3. *Ruminococcus albus*	cocci	+−	0.8-2.0	−	Fiber digestion	+−	+−	+−	−	−	−	
4. *Bacteroides amylophilus*	rods to coccoid	−	0.9-1.6 by 1.6-4.0	−	Starch digestion	+	−	+−	+−	−	−	
5. *Succinimonas amylolytica*	coccoid to rod	−	1.0-1.5 by 2.2-3.0	+	Starch digestion	+	−	−	+	−	−	
6. *Veillonella alcalescens*	cocci	−	0.3-0.6	−	Lactate fermenter	−	−	−	−	+	−	
7. *Methanobacterium ruminantium*	curved rod	+	0.7-0.8 to 1.8	−	Methane production	−	−	−	−	−	−	($H_2 + CO_2$)
8. *Anaerovibrio lipolytica*	rods	−	0.4 by 1.2-3.6	+	Lipolytic	−	−	−	−	−	+	(Fructose)
9. *Peptostreptococcus elsdenii*	cocci to chains	−	1.2-2.4	−	Lactate fermenter	+	−	−	+	+	+−	(Sucrose)
10. *Clostridium lochheadii*	rods	−	0.7-1.7 by 2.0-6.0	−	Cellulose digester poor forage	+	+	+	−	−	−	(Fructose)
11. *Clostridium longisporum*	rods	−	1.0 by 7-12 or 2.3 by 7.0	+	?	+	+	+	−	−		
12. *Borrelia* sp.	spirochete	−	0.3-0.5 by 4.0-7.0	+	?	+	−	−	−	+	+−	(Sugars)
13. *Lachnospira multiparus*	curved rod	+−	0.4-0.6 by 2.0-4.0	+	Pectin digester	+	−	−	+−	−	+	(Pectins)
14. *Cillobacterium cellulosolvens*	coccoid to rod	−	0.5-0.7 by 1.0-2.0	+	Cellulose digestion	+	+	+	−	−	−	
15. *Butyrivibrio fibrisolvens*	curved rod	−	0.4-0.6 by 2.0-5.0	+	Starch digestion to widely adapted	+	+−	+−	+−	−	−	(Saccharides)

	Glucose cellulose	Xylan	Starch	Lactate	Glycerol (Disaccharides) (Sugars)		Shape	Size (μm)		
16. *Butyrivibrio alactacidigens*	+ −	+	+	−		+	curved rod	0.5–1.0 by 1.5–8.0	+	Starch digestion to widely adapted
17. *Bacteroides ruminicola*	+ −	+	−	+	−	−	coccoid to rod to irregular	0.8–1.0; 0.8–30.0	−	Widely adapted
18. *Selenomonas ruminantium*	+ −	−	+	−	+	+	crescentic	0.8–2.5 by 2.0–7.0	+	Widely adapted
19. *Selenomonas lactilytica*	+ −	−	+	−	+	+	crescentic	0.4–0.6 by 1.8–3.0	+	Lactate fermenter to widely adapted
20. *Succinivibrio dextrinosolvens*	+ −	−	−	−	−	−	spiral	0.3–0.5 by 1.0–1.5	+	Dextran fermenter
21. *Streptococcus bovi*	+ −	−	+	+	−	−	cocci	0.7–0.9	−	Starch digestion to various
22. *Eubacterium ruminantium*	+ −	+	+	−	−	−	coccoid to rod	0.4–0.7 by 0.7–1.5	−	Sugars, xylan
23. *Sarcina bakeri*							cocci	1.0–4.0	−	?
24. *Lactobacilli* sp.	+ −	−	+	+	−	−	rods	0.7–1.0 by 1–6	+	Widely adapted under acidic conditions

+ = fermented by most strains;
± = fermented by few strains.

anaerobic, 6% produced H_2S; 21% liquified gelatin; 39% utilized starch; 14% utilized cellulose (5.2% from cows on concentrate diets and 27.9% from cattle consuming wheat straw); 72% used glucose; 54% used xylose; and 71% used cellobiose. As you will note in Table 11-1, seven of the 24 species are cellulolytic whereas at least 19 can utilize glucose, 15 use cellobiose, 13 use starch, and 10 use dextran. Many species can utilize carbohydrates that are not included in this table (see Hungate, 1966, pp 86-87 for further detail).

Moir and Masson (1952) catalogued 33 different types of rumen bacteria on the basis of microscopic observations without any attempt to classify the bacteria on the basis of physiological differences. Bryant (1959) noted that, of bacteria that have been cultured in vitro, 29 genera and 63 species had been described, of which 16 genera and 28 species were almost certainly of functional significance. In addition, within most species there are numerous strains that have been cultured which differ in some respect from other closely related organisms. Pictures of some rumen bacteria representing different morphological forms are shown in Plates 11-1 through 11-6.

Other Nutrients Utilized or Required

As might be expected, the requirements for nutrients other than energy sources are quite variable among bacterial species. Bryant and co-workers have probably published more on this subject that any other group. In one example Bryant and Robinson (1962) used a basal medium containing glucose, cellobiose, or maltose as energy sources, minerals, cysteine and sulfide salts as reducing agents and bicarbonate as a buffer. They worked with 89 freshly isolated strains of predominant culturable bacteria. Of these strains, 13% grew poorly or not at all in the medium plus casein hydrolysate; 6% (one morphological group) required casein hydrolysate; 56% grew with either ammonia or casein hydrolysate as the main source of nitrogen; and ammonia, but not casein hydrolysate, was essential for 25% of the strains. The volatile acid mixture supplied (acetic, n-valeric, isovaleric, 2-methylbutyric, and isobutyric), excluding acetate, was essential for 19% of the strains; this mixture and acetate were necessary for good growth of 23% of the strains when casein hydrolysate was excluded from the medium; 30% of the

strains required hemin. Most cellylolytic organisms seemed to require ammonia.

In addition to these nutrients, many bacteria require CO_2, some require peptides or amino acids, and some of the B-complex vitamins are required by several species. For example, *Bacteroides succinogenes* required biotin and PABA; *Ruminococcus flavefaciens* required biotin, folic acid or PABA, and some strains may require pyridoxamine, thiamin or riboflavin. Many species, however, do not require vitamins. Mineral requirements have not been well defined for organisms cultured as pure strains. However, Bryant gets good growth for many organisms on media containing Ca, Mg, Na, K, Mn, P, Co, S and Fe (in hemin). Some organisms seem to require rumen fluid in the media. Whether rumen fluid supplies unknown factors or an optimum combination of growth factors is an unresolved question. Specific examples of nutrient requirements are cited in subsequent chapters.

Fermentation Products

The fermentation products resulting from bacterial action are quite varied and depend somewhat on the nature of the substrate and on the species of bacteria. Hungate (1966) has tabulated data on 22 of the species listed in Table 11-2 and the results are shown:

Product	Produced by [No. species]
Formate	16
Acetate	21 (2 species may use acetate)
Propionate	6
Butyrate	7
Higher acids	1
Lactate	13
Succinate	12
Ethanol	8
Carbon dioxide	9 (8 used CO_2)
Hydrogen	10 (1 used hydrogen)
Methane	1
H_2S	9

The fermentation products of mixed cultures or products from the rumen may be quite different from that resulting from pure cultures grown on synthetic media. For example, 13 of the 22 species produced lactate and 12 produced succinate; however, neither of these acids are usually found in any significant quantities in the rumen. Rather, they are utilized as energy sources by other organisms since they are compounds that are readily fermented by many bacteria. In the rumen, the bulk of the acids are represented by acetic, propionic and butyric with lesser amounts of other volatile acids. The concentration of acids varies with several factors, but may be expected to be on the order of 80-180 µmol/ml (see Ch. 16). More specific data on fermentation products will be mentioned in other chapters.

Cultural Methods

An appreciable amount of information has been published on rumen microbiology which was derived from sampling rumen contents, analysis of rumen fluid, etc. However, the interest of many bacteriologists in recent years has turned to the development of techniques which allow bacterial species to be isolated and cultured in pure cultures under controlled laboratory conditions. As example of a nonselective medium used by Caldwell and Bryant (1966) is shown in Table 11-3. This medium can be simplified considerably for some organisms; it can also be made more selective in terms of the energy or nitrogen source.

For those interested in the techniques used for preparation of culture media, inoculation and transfer of rumen organisms, Hungate (1966) goes into considerable detail on these subjects. Avoiding contamination is always quite a problem. With rumen bacteria one of the biggest problems is to maintain sufficiently anaerobic conditions to support and sustain growth, even though studies with crude mixed cultures do not indicate that strict anaerobic conditions are nearly this important.

Total Numbers of Rumen Bacteria

The number of bacteria found in the rumen may be estimated by several methods. The methods commonly used by bacteriologists are:

Direct Count. According to Hungate this is the most reliable method for determining the total numbers of bacteria, although it measures the dead as well as the living organisms. In addition, unknown organisms which cannot be grown in the laboratory can be counted readily. Since a large percentage of bacteria are normally attached to solids in the rumen, rather than being found free in rumen liquids, direct counts may not be an accurate reflection of total numbers. In direct counting it is necessary to dilute rumen contents because of the large number of cells. The cells are frequently killed with formalin and stained to make them more visible. The diluted fluid may then be counted in a counting chamber designed for bacteria (similar to blood counting chambers) or spread on a slide and the fluid is then dried, fixed, and stained (less accurate method).

Table 11-3. Non-selective medium for rumen bacteria.

Component	% composition
Glucose	0.05
Cellobiose	0.05
Soluble starch	0.05
Minerals	3.75
$Na_2S \cdot 9H_2O$	0.025
Cysteine $\cdot$ HCl $\cdot$ H_2O	0.025
Resazurin	0.0001
Na_2CO_3	0.04
Trypticase	0.2
Yeast extract	0.05
Volatile fatty acids	0.31
Hemin	0.0001
Agar	2.0
CO_2 gas phase	100

Optical Density. A colorimeter or spectrophotometer can be used to obtain approximate counts of organisms in suspension. When using a wavelength of 600 µ, a rule of thumb is that an optical density of 0.3 is equal to about 1 billion cells per ml. O.D. is not a very precise measure of numbers, but it is a quick and easy way to obtain information.

Culture Counts. Culture counts are obtained by making appropriate dilutions of rumen contents and inoculation of known quantities into culture media, usually on roll tubes. After a period of time colony counts are made on organisms in the medium. Culture counts usually yield numbers that are much lower than direct counts, although the relative values are believed to be reasonably accurate. Bryant (1970) states that such techniques may account for 10-30% of those organisms seen in a direct microscopic count. This discrepancy is due partially to the difficulty in growing rumen microorganisms in these conditions; those more difficult to grow do not show up in colonies, so the count is less than it would otherwise have been. Another reason is that not all of the organisms seen in the microscope are alive; there may be substantial numbers that are not capable of producing colonies.

Hungate (1966, pp 34-35) has tabulated published data from a number of laboratories on rumen bacterial counts. These data were obtained on rumen organisms of sheep and cattle fed under a wide variety of conditions and were reported by many different authors. Direct counts (mean values of all examples) ranged from a low value of 16.2 bil./ml to a high value of 40.8 bil./ml. The extreme range varied from a low of 4 bil./ml for animals fed on wheat straw plus various nitrogen sources to a high of 88 bil./ml for sheep on pasture. Some counts as high as 100 bil./ml have been reported, but most bacteriologists tend to discount such high values. Bryant (1970) suggests that the usual range is 15-80 bil./ml, with variability in numbers being due to nature of the diet, feeding regimen, time of sampling after feeding, individual animal differences and the presence or absence of ciliate protozoa. Other factors that have been observed include seasonal differences, availability of green feed and animal species. Bryant also points out that the number of bacteria/unit weight may give very little information as to their total metabolic activity, due to such factors as variation in rumen volume and because metabolic activity/unit of cells can vary greatly depending on factors such as the growth rate and stage of growth.

Culture counts tabulated by Hungate were much lower than direct counts, ranging from a low of 8 mil./ml to a high of 23 bil./ml. Mean low values averaged 1.2 bil./ to mean high values of 7.9 bil./ml.

Rumen Protozoa

Rumen protozoa have been known to exist since the mid 19th century, since they are much larger than bacteria and can easily be seen with the aid of a microscope. Information on classification, morphology and occurrence of rumen ciliates has been available for many years, with the years in the late 1920's and early 30's being particularly productive. Data on nutrition, metabolism and related subjects are of more recent origin. Review papers on rumen ciliates include: Oxford (1955), Hungate et al, (1964), Hungate (1955, 1966) and Eadie and Howard (1963). Articles discussing classification include Kofoid and Maclennon (1930, 1932, 1933), Oxford (1955), Corliss (1961), Clarke (1964), and Hungate (1955, 1966).

Classification

Protozoa in the rumen are primarily ciliated species although a few organisms with flagella rather than cilia are found, particularly in young ruminants before ciliates become established or in animals which have lost their ciliate population for one reason or another (Eadie, 1962a).

Classification of the protozoa is based on cell morphology since the organisms are large enough to readily visualize many distinguishing cellular structures even with simple microscopes. There is some disagreement on classification and not all authorities agree on how many genera there should be nor on the number of species. In the past, they were commonly divided into two orders, the holotrichs and the oligotrichs. As classified by Corliss (1961), a comparable grouping would be the subclass holotricha and spirotricha. Four genera are commonly included in the holotricha (6 species), and about nine genera which are found in domestic ruminants under the order entodiniomorphida (about 30 species). Tabulated in Table 11-4 are most of the common protozoa classified essentially as suggested by Hungate (1966). Some of the different species are shown in Plates 11-10 through 11-15.

The holotrich species are large (see next section) and are somewhat similar to paramecium, being more or less egg-shaped. The cell surface is covered with cilia in contrast to the oligotrichs which have tufts of cilia on the anterior parts. The oligotrichs are represented by a great variety of species with a variety of sizes, shapes and organelles which distinguish them. They tend to be oval to elongate in shape.

Size and Numbers

Protozoa are relatively large, varying in size from 38 μ in length and 15 in width for *Charon equi* to 195 μ in length and 109 In width for *Metadinium medium* (Clarke, 1964). This size makes them somewhat difficult to count accurately in a typical counting chamber, with the partial result that much of the data in the literature has a rather low repeatability on numbers counted. Counts vary from none to as high as 5 mil./ml; however, total counts would usually be within the range of 200,000-2 mil./ml (see Hungate, 1966, p 126 for tabulated results).

Table 11-4.   Ciliates found in ruminants.[a]

Class: Ciliata*
   Sub-class: Holotrichia (move about more rapidly; usually are larger; have rows of cilia over
       entire body).
      Genera and specie: *Isotricha intestinalis*
                       Isotricha prostoma
                       Dasytricha ruminantium
                       Blepharocorys bovis (rare)
                       Charon equi (rare; also found in the horse)
                       Charon ventriculi (rare)
                       Buetschilla (rare)

   Sub-class: Spirotrichia; Order, Entodinimorpha (commonly called oligotricha; have tufts of
       cilia on anterior parts)
      Genera and specie: *Caloscolex* (camel)
                       *Diplodinium***

                Sub-species: *Diplodinium dentatum* (consumes cellulose)
                               Diplodinium posterovesiculatum [*Eodinium*]
                               Diplodinium crista-galli
                               Diplodinium psittaceum
                               Diplodinium elongatum
                               Diplodinium polygonale
                               Eudiplodinium neglectum (syn. *Eremoplastron*];
                        several forms such as *bovis* and *giganteum*
                               Eudiplodinium magii (syn. *Metadinium medium*)
                               Eudiplodinium medium (syn. *Metadinium tauricum*]
                               Eudiplodinium bursa (syn. *Diplodinium neglectum*]
                               Eudiplodinium affine
                               Eudiplodinium rostratum
                               Polyplastron multivesiculatum
                               Elystroplastron bubali
                               Ostracodinium obtusun
                               Ostracodinium gracile
                               Ostracodinium uncinucliatum
                               Ostracodinium dentatum
                               Enoploplastron triloricatum

          Entodinium bursa (ingests plant material and small protozoa)
          Entodinium caudatum (very common)
           Numerous other species have been suggested such as *E. minimum,
          rostratum, longinucleatum, elongatum, simplex,* etc. See Dogiel (1927)
          for details.
          Epidinium ecaudatum   (many different forms observed)
          Ophryoscolex purkynei   (numerous different forms)
          Opisthotrichum   (found in African antelopes)

[a]Classification essentially as suggested by Hungate (1966).
*Flagellates sometimes found in the rumen include *Monocercomonas ruminantium,
Callimastix frontalis, Chilomastix,* two species of *Tetratichomonas, Pentatrichomonas
hominis* and *Monocercomonas bovis.*
**Note: Considerable confusion or difference of opinion exists as to classification of species
   in this genera. Some authorities consider some of these sub-genera as separate genera or
   classify them in a different manner.

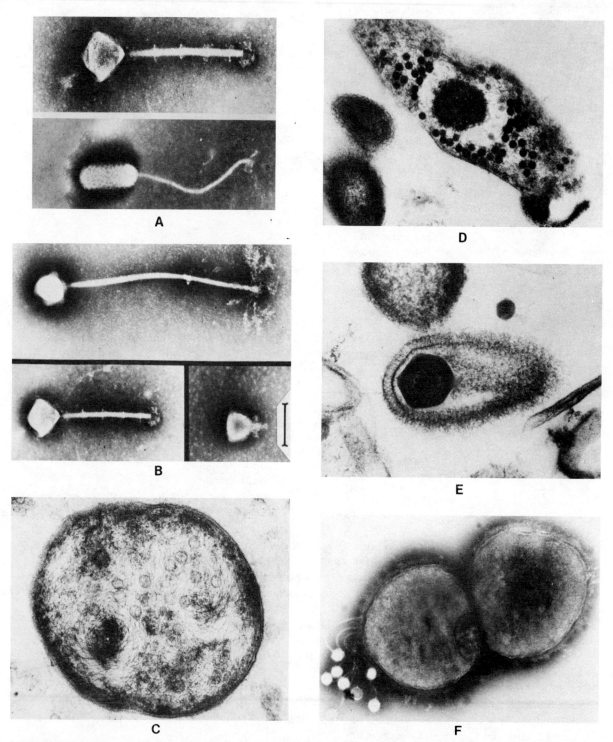

Plate 11-8. Electron micrographs illustrating A, two bacteriophages from the bovine rumen which show different structures of the head and tail. B, three bacteriophages [bovine] showing the typical range of morphological varieties present. C, thin section of rumen bacterium illustrating the fibrillar character of its nucleoplasm. The small hollow structures are phage head membranes. D, thin section of rumen bacterium infected with bacteriophage [small dense bodies are phage heads]. The large central mass represents an organized body of gene products associated with the phage tails. E, thin section of rumen bacterium showing a large complex phage head inside. F, rumen bacterium with attached bacteriophages. Phages appear to attach at selective areas rather than at random. Courtesy of Al Ritchie.

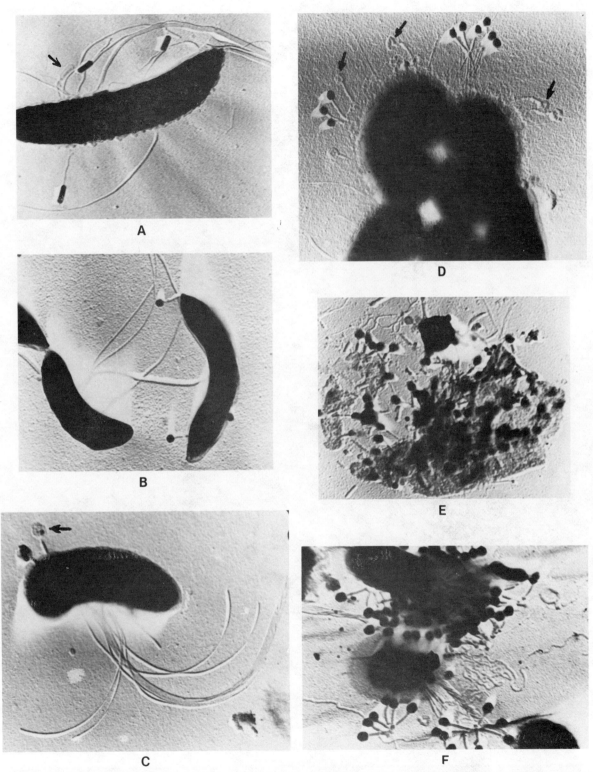

Plate 11-9. Rumen bacteriophages. A-D, bacteriophage adsorption on the selenomonas and kidney-shaped cocci. A tungsten oxide shading effect [24000X except C which is 17700X]. Arrow marks show phages with an empty capsid. E,F, Lysis of rumen microorganisms showing the large number of phages involved. [E, 24000X; F, 17700X]. Courtesy of N.V. Kurilov, All-Union Research Institute of Physiology, Biochemistry and Nutrition of Farm Animals, Borovsk, Kaluga region, Russia.

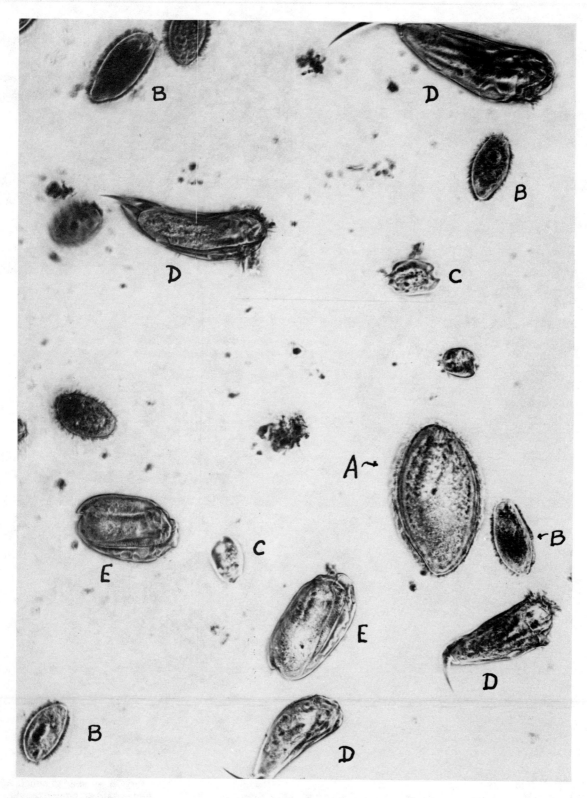

Plate 11-10. Mixture of rumen protozoa. Shown are [A] *Isotricha intestinalis,* **[B]** *Dasytricha ruminantium,* **[C]** *Entodinium* **sp., [D]** *Epidinium ecaudatum* **, and [E]** *Ostracodinium* **sp. Magnification ca. 280X. Courtesy of R.T. Clarke, New Zealand.**

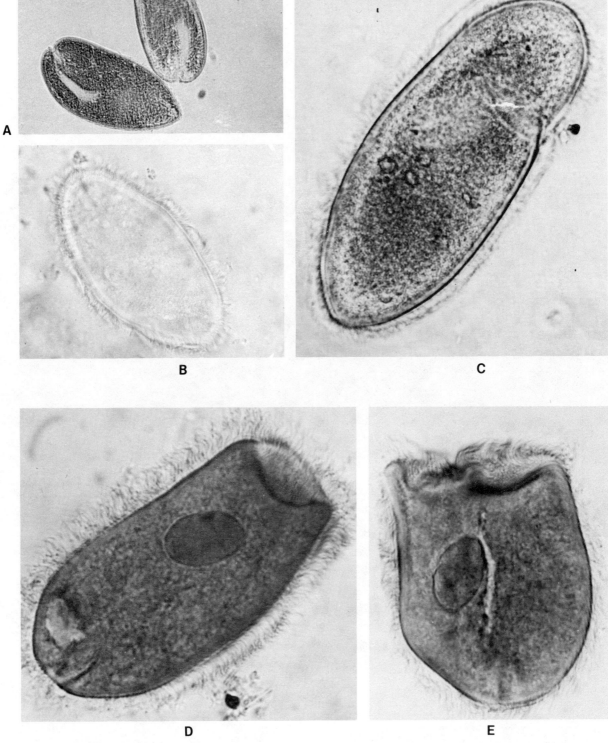

Plate 11-11. Some of the holotrich species. A, *Isotricha prostoma;* **the picture shows the gullet quite well [375X]. B, same species, but focused to show the ciliary activity [400X]. C,** *I. intestinalis* **[690X]. D,E, two excellent photographs of** *Buetschlia parva* **[1,350X]. A, courtesy of R.E. Hungate; B, A.J. Kutches; C, R.T. Clarke; D, E, B.A. Dehority.**

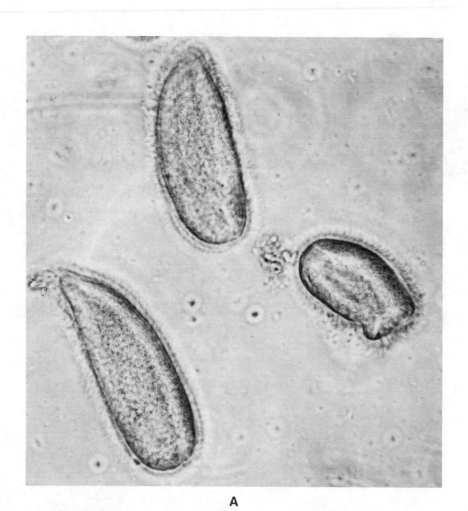

A

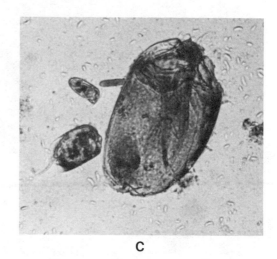

B   C

Plate 11-12. A, single *Buetschilia parva* shown with two *Dasytricha ruminantium* [690X]. Buetschilia has only rarely been photographed. B, *D. ruminantium* [1100X]. C, *Polyplastron multivesiculatum* and *Entodinium* sp. Dilute iodine has been used to show up large skeletal plates of *Polyplastron.* A, courtesy of R.T. Clarke; B, courtesy of G.S. Coleman; C, courtesy of J.M. Eadie.

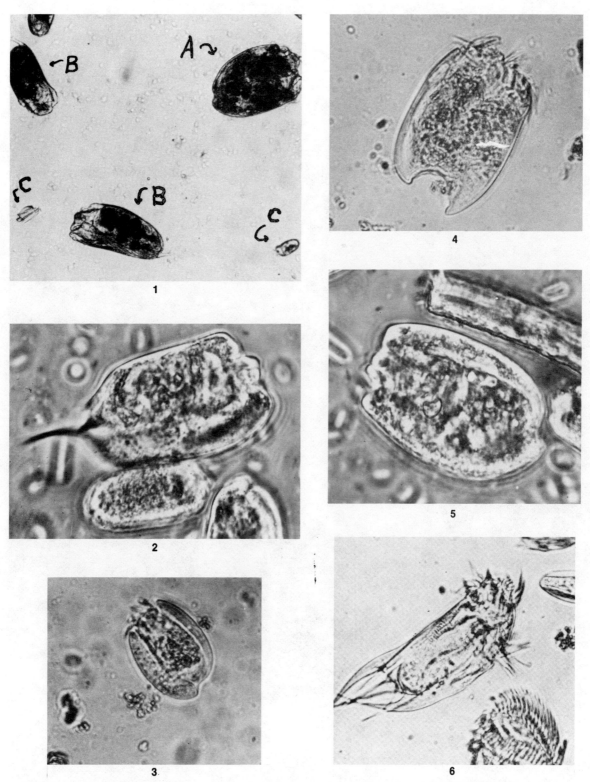

Plate 11-13. 1, A, *Eudiplodinium magii;* **B,** *Epidinium ecaudatum.*m; **C** *Entodinia;* **these organisms have had access to starch and are well filled. 2,** *Entodinium caudatum* **[with spine] [1000X]. 3,** *Entodinium* **sp. 4,** *Ostracodinium gracile.* **5,** *Entodinium longinucleatum* **[1000X]. 6,** *Epidinium ecadatum.* **form** *Cattanei.* **[594X]. 1 courtesy of J.M. Eadie; 2, 5 courtesy of G.S. Coleman; 3, 4 and 6 courtesy of R.E. Hungate.**

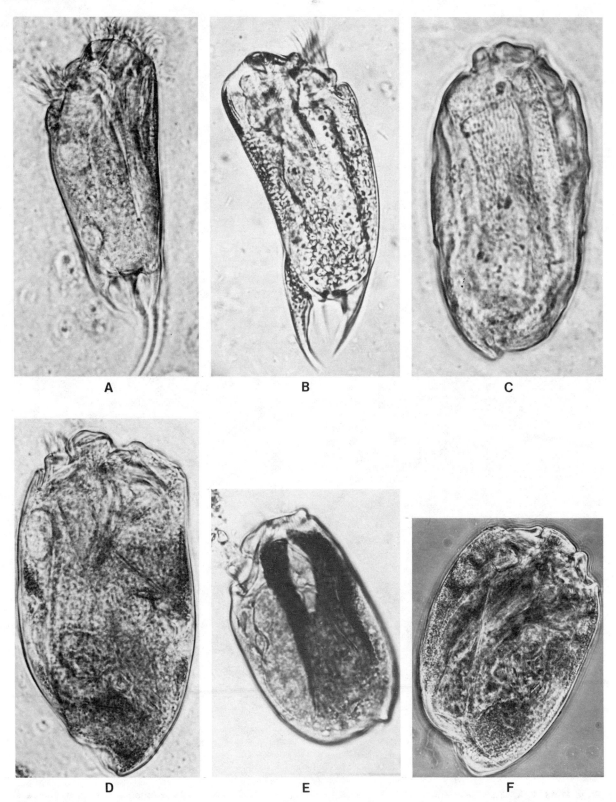

Plate 11-14. A, *Epidinium ecaudatum trichaudatum.* **B,** *Epidinium caudatum;* **C,** *Ostracodinium rugoloricatum.* **D,** *Eudipoldinium magii.* **E,** *Ostracodinium,* **probably** *O. triloricatum.* **F,** *Polypastron multivesiculatum.* **A, E and F, courtesy of G.S. Coleman. B, C and D, courtesy of R.T. Clarke.**

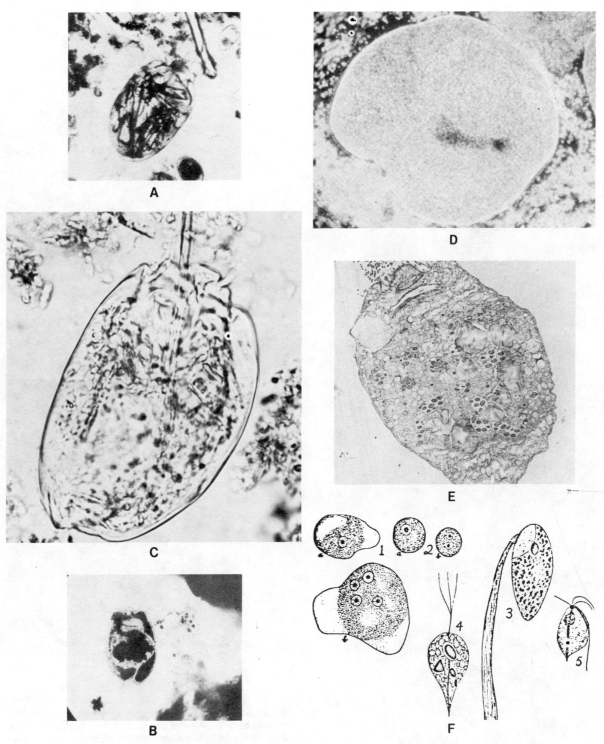

Plate 11-15. A, ingestion of cellulose fibers by *Metadinium medium.* **B,** *Entodinium longinucleatum* **digesting rice starch; stained with iodine to show ingested starch concentrated in the 'gastric sac' and storage starch around the periphery [from Sugden, 1953]. C,** *Diplodinium* **sp engulfing a fiber of plant material. D, Bursting** *Isotricha intestinalis* **due to excessive storage starch formation in a carbohydrate-rich medium. E,** *Entodinium caudatum* **that has been engulfing** *E. coli* **bacteria for 5 min. F, Noncilliated species of rumen protozoa; 1,** *Vahkampfia lobospinosa;* **[a] uninucleated form and [b] large individual with 4 nuclei. ca. 1,240X. 2,** *Vahlkampfia lobospinosa* **cysts. 3,** *Callimastix frontalis.* **4,** *Eutrichomastix ruminantium.* **5,** *Trichomonas ruminantium.* **Drawings from Becker and Talbott [1927]. B, E courtesy of G.S. Coleman.**

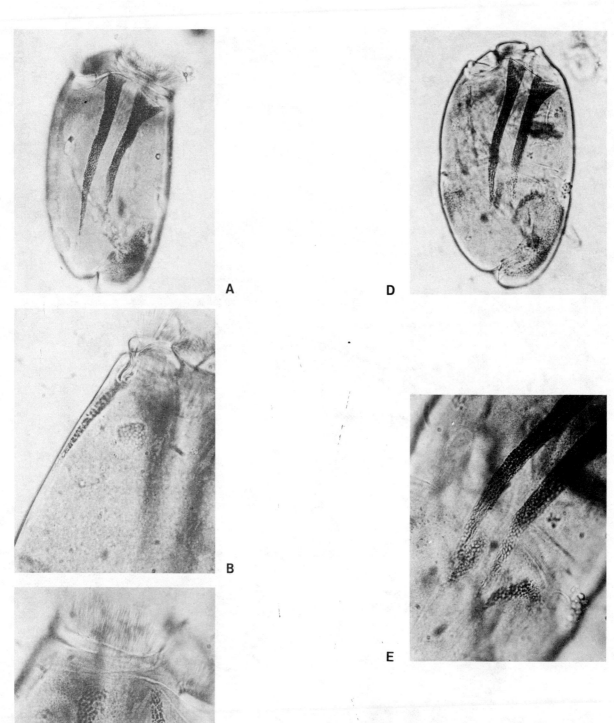

Plate 11-16. Photographs of *Polyplastron multivisiculatum.*
**A, the two main skeletal plates. The first plate is on the left
and the second plate is on the right. B, enlarged view from
the left side showing the third skeletal plate. C, the same
cell as in B showing the 4th and 5th plates on the left side.
Plates 1 and 2 are visible on the opposite side of the cell. D,
a cell just starting to divide. Small skeletal plates are visible
on daughter cell. E, enlarged view of cell in D. Magnification ca. 435X in A & D; 970X in B, C and E. Courtesy of B.A.
Dehority.**

Protozoal Culture

A knowledge of protozoal function and physiology has been rather slow in developing. This is so because of the difficulty in culturing these organisms. Hungate (1955) achieved partial success in the early 1940's. Other investigators have worked on the problem with only limited success (for example, see papers by Mah, 1964; Clark and Hungate, 1966; Tompkin et al, 1966; Jarvis and Hungate, 1968). Coleman (1960, 1962) has been able to maintain some species for a prolonged period of time. He has successfully cultured *Entodinium caudatum* on a medium containing a salt solution, dried grass, rice starch, rumen fluid and chloramphenicol or various other antibiotics to control bacterial growth. In such a procedure it was necessary to centrifuge, remove the supernatant liquid and add fresh medium every two days in order to keep the protozoa alive and active. More recently (Coleman, 1969; Coleman et al, 1972) this laboratory has grown *Epidinium ecaudatum* or *Entodinium simplex* in the presence of bacteria on a medium containing salts, autoclaved rumen fluid, wholemeal flour and dried grass. Another species, *Polyplastron multivesticulatum,* could be maintained if other species were available, the minimum daily requirement for growth of *P. multivesticulatum* being one epidinium per polyplastron.

Clarke and Hungate (1966) have reported that *Dasytricha ruminantium* could be cultured in a medium of salts and clarified rumen fluid, with periodic addition of sucrose. When the organisms were transferred to a medium free of those nutrients, rumen fluid was essential. Omission of protozoal extracts resulted in gradual death, although bovine serum could be satisfactorily substituted for the protozoal extract but various rumen bacteria, extracts of rumen bacteria and extracts of plant material could not substitute satisfactorily.

More recently Hino et al (1973) have grown *Entodinia* sp on a medium containing whole egg protein, proteose-petone, rice starch, yeast extract, cellulose powder and white clover juice. Of these, the proteose-peptone, yeast extract and cellulose powder could be omitted, but omission of the clover juice resulted in death of the protozoa. Studies on the clover demonstrated that the water-soluble fraction was stimulatory but could be replaced by soluble starch, glucose, ribo-nucleic acid, vitamins and minerals. The lipid fraction was essential and the essential factors were identified as sterols. Of these, β-sitosterol, when given along with other nutrients previously identified, would maintain *Entodinia* for more than 100 days.

Anyone familiar with culture of bacteria will recognize that the media described for culture of protozoa can hardly be classified as purified. A major problem has been to grow protozoa in the absence of bacteria. Some data indicate that holotrichs may not require the presence of bacteria, but the current evidence is that oligotrichs probably do — at least they are impossible to culture in the absence of bacteria. Removal of bacteria is difficult due to the presence of bacteria inside the bodies of the protozoa as well as those that adhere to the external surface. If bacteria are required, it may be that the bacteria are contributing some enzymes or other organic molecules vital to protozoal survival.

Nutrition and Metabolism

Due to the difficulty in culturing protozoa, much of the information on nutrition and metabolism of nutrients has been obtained by carrying out short term (a few hr) experiments or by preparing enzyme extracts of isolated protozoa. Most of the information available has to do with carbohydrate utilization, although some information is available on other nutrients. All species produce large amounts of a starch-like reserve polysaccharide, an energy reserve that may be drawn on during periods of nutrient shortage.

Holotrichs — *Isotricha prostoma* and *I. intestinalis.* Both species are found when the diet contains relatively large amounts of soluble sugars. They metabolize glucose, fructose, sucrose, inulin, levans (polyfructosan), granular starch (if grains are not too large) and pectins, but cannot use mannose, maltose or glucosamine. Carbohydrates are stored as amylopectin. They will ingest sugars until the cells burst (no control mechanism). They form acetic, butyric and lactic acids with traces of propionic. Hydrogen and CO_2 are also produced.

Dasytricha ruminantium. This organism is biochemically more versatile than the *Isotricha* species with respect to carbohydrate metabolism. Except for granular starch, it can ferment the same carbohydrates, plus maltose, galactose, cellobiose and other β-glucosides such as salacin. It also appears to produce liberal quantities of methane.

The *Oligotricha* (entodinimorphs). These organisms utilize very little, if any, soluble carbohydrate; however, nearly all ingest granular starch. *Entodinia* are usually the predominant genera found in animals fed high-starch rations. Some species ingest holotrich starch. Many species actively ingest plant fiber, and, although hemicellulases have been found, evidence is lacking to prove whether cellulose digestion is accomplished by the protozoa or by bacteria species. Fermentation products of some species studied are similar to those of the holotrichs.

References applicable to information cited on carbohydrate metabolism include: Oxford (1955), Guiterrez (1955) Abou Akkada and Howard (1960, 1961), Bailey et al (1962), Bailey and Clarke (1963), Bailey and Howard (1963a, b), Mah (1964), Clarke and Hungate (1966), Hungate (1966), and Naga and el-Shazly (1968).

Studies with mixed cultures of oligotrichs plus *Dasytricha* indicate that they utilized glucose, fructose, mannose, sucrose, cellobiose, maltose and raffinose, but did not utilize arabinose, ribose, xylose, melibiose and lactose (Kubo and Kandatsu, 1969). Data also indicate that the type of carbohydrate deposited in storage polysaccharide was dependent upon the type of dietary carbohydrate. Storage polysaccharide (glucose polymers) increased rapidly after the beginning of the meal (except for cellulose), sometimes reaching 40% of protozoan dry matter by ca. 2 hr. Smaller quantities of mannose, arabinose and galactose polymers were found (Jouany and Thivend, 1972).

There is ample evidence to show that many of the holotrichs and oligotrichs actively ingest bacteria of one type or another and most of the studies on the culture of protozoa clearly indicate problems when the bacterial population is kept low by washing and treatment with antibiotics to inhibit growth. References showing active ingestion or presence of identifiable bacteria include: Sugden (1953), Guiterrez (1958), Guiterrez and Davis (1959), Kandatsu and Takahashi (1963), Mah (1964), Coleman (1964, 1967), White (1969) and Coleman and White (1970). In studies with *Entodinium caudatum*, Coleman and White (1970) isolated bacteria

from the bodies of protozoa after washing and disintegrating the cells. The average number of bacteria found was 22 which consisted of three main types, small Gram-negative cocci resembling *Veillonella* sp., small curved or curled Gram-negative bacteria resembling *Butyrivibrio* and Gram-positive cocci resembling *Streptococcus bovis*.. Thus, there seems to be little doubt that protozoa actively prey on bacteria as well as other protozoan species (see later section).

With respect to N metabolism, studies with *Entodinium* indicate that they rapidly hydrolyze a variety of different proteins, producing ammonia from amide groups along with liberation of amino acids and peptides. There appears to be very little, if any, metabolism of amino acids (Abou Akkada and Howard, 1962; Kandatsu and Takahashi, 1963; Coleman, 1964, 1967). With *Isotricha* species, Harmeyer (1972) found that amino acids were excreted into the medium and that concentration in the medium had little effect. The protozoa survived longer in a medium lacking amino acids than in one containing 19 different amino acids.

Distribution

Protozoal species found in the rumen of domestic ruminants are known to vary according to diet, season of the year (partially diet) and geographical location. An example of this is shown in Table 11-5, taken from Clarke's data (1964) obtained from samples collected from twin cows in New Zealand on various diets. The data shown in Table 11-5 illustrate a very common phenomenon of rumen microbial populations; that is, the change in composition resulting from a change in diet.

In addition to the data shown above, Clarke gives protozoal composition by species of entodinimorphs (oligotrichs) from samples taken from animals on the diets listed in the table. On 9/8/62, samples from cows on grass hay showed that only a few species accounted for most of the ciliates. For example: *Entodinium ovinum*, 6.8%; *E. Biconcavum*, 18.8%; *E. Bicarinatum*, 6.4%; *E. lobatum*, 6.8%; *Eremoplastron bovis*, 20.8%; *E. Brevispinum*. 8.4%; and *Diplodinium monacanthum*, 4.4%. All other species (23 others) were 3.0% or less each. A goodly number of papers are available in the literature which provide information on the

Table 11-5. Ciliate composition from twin cows.[a]

| | Composition, % of total | | |
| | Grass hay | | Fresh clover |
Genus	9/8/62	1/6/63	2/26/63
Entodinium	32.6	8.0	35.4
Eodinium [*Diplodinium*]	9.4	14.4	1.6
Eremoplastron [*Eudiplodinium*]	27.2	23.2	22.4
Epidinium	0.9	6.4	22.0
Eudiplodinium	1.9	3.0	2.2
Metadinium [*Eudiplodinium*]	0.2	0.8	—
Ostracodinium	3.4	4.2	1.2
Diplodinium	12.5	—	—
Isotricha	6.0	1.6	4.2
Dasytricha	5.5	23.2	10.8
Buetschlia	0.2	2.4	0.2
Charon	0.2	12.8	—

[a] Two genera, *Polyplastron* and *Ophryoscolex*, common in other countries, were not found.

different species which may be found, particularly in domestic ruminants. In most cases, the research has dealt with one ruminant host. In one example of a relatively recent paper where studies were made on both sheep and cattle, 20 species were observed in sheep and 31 in cattle, 15 being common to both (Constantinescu and Palfy, 1967).

Limited data on feral ruminant species indicate that most species of protozoa are common to more than one ruminant species, although at times only a limited number of protozoan species may be found. *Ophryoscolex* have been found in primates and *Charon* is more commonly found in horses. Different species of cattle appear to have different populations, but comparisons between ruminant species are frequently confounded because of diet and geographical differences. Although information is limited, studies with feral ruminants indicate that protozoans found in white-tailed deer (Pearson, 1965), mule deer (Pearson, 1969), fallow deer (Crha, 1972), bison (Pearson, 1967) and elk (McBee et al, 1969) are, in general, similar to those found in domestic ruminants. Holotrichs in the giraffe are the same as those in domestic ruminants (Noirot-Timothee, 1963). Nonruminant species with stomach fermentation, such as the hippopotamus, have a very diverse population of both holotrichs and oligotrichs, but the species seen are different than those in ruminants, resem-

bling those seen in the horse or related animals (Thurston and Grain, 1971; Thurston and Noirot-Timothee, 1973). A diverse population of ciliates have been noted in other nonruminant species (Thurston and Noirot-Timothee, 1973). Information on flagellated protozoan species appears to be restricted to a limited number of observations on their occurrence. Although they are present in larger numbers in young animals which are ciliate-free, there is no information on their physiological function or any idea of their relative importance in the total picture of rumen ecology and metabolism.

Other Rumen Microorganisms

Bacteriophages, sometimes referred to as bacterial viruses, have been known to exist for some time, but information on ruminal phages is of much more recent origin. Information at this point is based primarily on a limited number of studies using electron microscopy (Adams et al, 1966; Hoogenraad et al, 1967; Brailsford and Hartman, 1968; Paynter et al, 1969; Ritchie et al, 1971; and Tarakanov, 1971 — reference only in Russian). Ritchie et al have identified more than 125 morphologically distinct types and more than 65 distinct rumen bacteria were found to contain intracellular phage. Counts indicated that phages exceeded bacteria in the ratio of 2:1 to 10:1. Photographs of phages are shown in Plates 11-8, 9.

It was noted previously that other microorganisms may, at times, be found in the rumen — species of bacteria that are not considered to be normal inhabitants. Likewise, yeast-like organisms are sometimes found in the rumen in appreciable numbers (Clarke and DiMenna, 1961), particularly when animals have been subjected to sudden ration changes involving the ingestion of large amounts of cereal grains (see Ch. 17). In addition, Brewer and Taylor (1969) have isolated fungi from rumen contents and found that they were facultative anaerobes.

Development of Rumen Microorganisms in Young Ruminants

Bacteria

Warner (1965) points out that nearly all of the typical rumen microorganisms appear to be specific to the rumen, although there are many exceptions to this general statement. Bacteria in other habitats may resort to the production of spores which may be resistant to various environmental hazards and which aid in spreading and propagating the species. However, this does not appear to be the case for the majority of rumen bacteria (Bryant, 1959). Some organisms produce an abundance of spores, but they do not appear to be persistent (Hungate, 1957). Consequently, it is assumed that the young ruminant normally acquires its microbial population by oral contact with older animals, or possibly by inhalation of organisms temporarily suspended in the air. Some species can survive for a limited period of time when suspended in air (Mann, 1963).

Bryant and Small (1960) have studied microbial development by isolating calves from other ruminants immediately after birth. These calves were maintained in isolated quarters for 17 wk at which time they were inoculated with rumen fluid. They found that the bacterial flora of the isolated calves was modified considerably, although some typical species were found. When colony counts were made on rumen contents, the isolated calves generally had higher levels of anaerobes, lower levels of cellulolytic organisms, but markedly higher levels of lactate fermenters than normal. They found various strains of typical rumen bacteria such as *Bacteroides ruminicola*, *Butyrivibrio*, *Selenomonas* and *Borrelia*; however, unknown organisms accounted for a large proportion of the total isolated. Of the known organisms, their fermentation characteristics did not appear to be typical of those from inoculated calves or mature animals. No explanation could be offered for the presence of the known organisms in these isolated animals. Growth of the calves did not appear to be affected. Pounden and Hibbs (1950) have reported somewhat similar experiences on isolated calves, although the data presented were less complete with respect to bacterial identification.

Information from a number of sources indicates that bacteria become established in the rumen of young animals at an early age whether they are isolated, kept with other young animals, or left with their dam. Data on calves (Bryant et al, 1958; Eadie, 1962; Lengemann and Allen, 1959; Perry and Briggs, 1957; and Zoilecki and Briggs, 1962) indicate that a large population of *lactobacil-* develops within a week of age. The numbers tend to decline after 3 wk of age, reaching adult levels by 3-4 mo. of age. Anaerobes tend to be at higher levels than in adult animals and cellulolytic organisms may be found at high levels even at 1 wk of age. In the case of lambs, an essentially adult type of flora may be established by the time lambs are 2 wk of age provided rumen conditions are not too acid (Eadie, 1962a). In young lambs, based on VFA analyses, Oh et al (1972) have demonstrated that fermentation in the hind gut preceded the development of functional rumen fermentation, and VFA levels in the cecum were higher than those in the rumen in lambs 2-3 wk of age. Mann et al (1954) observed that feeding chlortetracycline tended to promote intensive rumen bacterial action at an earlier age, whereas Lengemann and Allen (1959) reported that feeding this antibiotic or a liberal milk ration tended to slow development of adult-type organisms and cellulose digestion.

Williams and Dinusson (1972) have reported results of experiments in which calves were isolated from their dams within 24-48 hr after birth and thereafter housed in facilities allowing rather complete isolation. In calves kept free of ciliate protozoa, aerobic and facultative anaerobic organisms reached high counts by 7-9 days of age and then gradually declined. Cellulolytic bacteria were found in concentrations of $10^4/g$ of sample by 5-7 days and ruminal fluid degraded cellulose in vitro. The authors concluded that these organisms were obtained from the dam (or from feed and water supplies) as the

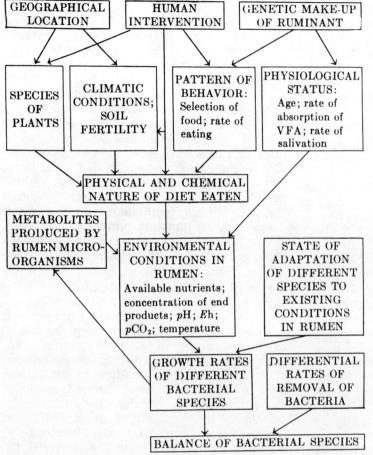

increased in the ileum to $10^7/g$ by ca. 8 days. The streptococci, usually rare in the abomasum, increased progressively toward the posterior parts of the gut. The dominant microflora isolated and identified included *Lactobacillus* , *Bifidobacterium*, *Bacteroides* , *Eubacterium* and *Clostridium* . Total strict anaerobes reached counts of 10^8 to 10^{10} in the cecum from 3 days of age. Similar data of this type are presented by Hartman et al (1966), and Mann and Ørskov (1973) found that bottle feeding (older sheep) solutions of glucose, sucrose or maltose resulted in a marked increase in the number of cecal bacteria. Bottle feeding also caused a redistribution of bacterial types and VFA distribution.

Protozoa

In contrast to the situation with rumen bacteria, establishment of rumen ciliate populations in the young ruminant requires contact with older animals with a protozoal population (Pounden and Hibbs, 1950; Bryant et al, 1958; Eadie, 1962a; Ziolecki and Briggs, 1962; and Borhami et al, 1967). Isolation of newborn animals from older animals will prevent the ciliates from developing, although some of the flagellated species apparently do not require such contact (Eadie, 1962a) if rumen pH is relatively high (above 6.5). If young animals are kept with older animals or if artificial transplantation is carried out by man, protozoal populations may develop within 1 to 2 wk in sheep, cattle, or buffalo provided rumen pH is about 6.0 or higher. Lengemann and Allen (1959) observed that ciliates became established within the first 3 wk of life in calves and reached adult levels by 6 wk. High intakes of milk or grain tend to inhibit development of a ciliate population, presumably because of a low rumen pH. Bryant et al (1958) found that *Entodinia* were first to become established, followed by *Diplodinia* and holotrichs and Eadie (1967) noted that it took *Ophryoscolex tricoronatus* and *Epidinium* longer to

Figure 11-1. Factors which may influence the balance of bacterial [or protozoal] species in the rumen. From Kistner [1965]. Courtesy of Butterworths.

facilities would likely preclude airborne transfer. The general conclusion was that ruminal bacterial populations shifted to levels comparable to mature animals as the calves matured.

Development of organisms in the hind gut of young ruminants has received considerably less attention than the rumen. The paper of Oh et al has been referred to. Smith (1965) noted that viable bacterial counts in the rumen of lambs were on the order of 10^4 to 10^5 as compared to 10^6 to $10^9/g$ of gut contents at 8 hr after birth. In studies by Contrepois and Gouet (1973), it was observed that *E. coli* was very rare in the abomasum, the duodenum and the jejunum, but was found from the 3rd day beginning in the ileum. In animals with diarrhea, *E. coli* proliferated abnormally in the jejunum and/or duodenum. Lactobacilla were found in the abomasum in relatively large numbers ($10^3/g$ at 3 days; $10^7/g$ at 7 days) and become established than certain other organisms. With buffalo calves, Borhami et al (1967) found that inoculation at 2-3 wk of age allowed establishment of a thriving population. *Entodinium* was first established, followed by *Eudiplodinium*, *Diplodinium* and *Isotricha*.

Factors Affecting the Population of Rumen Microorganisms

There are many factors that have been shown to affect the rumen microbial population, both quantitatively and qualitatively. Some of these are discussed in succeeding paragraphs. For further information, the reader is referred to reviews by Warner (1965), Kistner (1965) and Hungate (1966).

Kistner (1965) has presented a diagram (Fig. 11-1) which illustrates some of the factors likely to interact to bring about a given balance of rumen microorganisms. As he points out, growth rates at a particular time will depend on the adaptation of an organism to its environment and to the nature and concentration of available nutrients. Furthermore, the nutrients required by some organisms may not be present in the diet, but are end products of fermentation by other organisms, examples being water-soluble vitamins, branched-chain VFA, and probably other growth factors.

Other variables that he mentions which could certainly be a factor would include such things as the rapidity of eating, selectivity when grazing, soil fertility, the geographical location, and the climate — all factors which may influence the quality and quantity of nutrients presented to the rumen microorganisms. A more detailed discussion of certain factors is presented in succeeding sections.

Incompatibility of Various Protozoa

Eadie (1962a, 1967, 1968) has studied the occurrence of various types of protozoa in cattle and sheep. She found the ciliate populations to consist of a mixture of *Entodinium* sp., holotrich sp. and either (type A) large *Ophryoscolecids, Polyplastron multivesiculatum* with other species such as *Diploplastron affine* and *Ophryoscolex tricoronatus* or (type B) large *Ophryosco-*

lecids, Eudiplodinium maggi and *Epidinium* sp. together or alone. Types A and B appeared unable to form a stable population after artificial inoculation although they were not host-specific. In sheep, type A was always dominant, but not always in cattle. The apparent cause for this antagonism is the predation by *Polyplastron multivesiculatum* on *Epidinium Eudiplodinium*, *Eremoplastron* and *Ostracodeinium*, resulting in loss of these ciliates from the population. Other factors such as food competition, gross bacterial change or specific rations were more or less ruled out. Neither *Entodina* or holotrich ciliates were involved. Data showing similar information in lactating cows fed a variety of different diets have been published by Abou Akkada et al (1969).

Effect of the Absence of Ciliates on the Rumen and the Animal

There has been a considerable interest in the past few years in determining the effect of protozoa on rumen fermentation. To accomplish this objective, young ruminants have been raised in isolation or they have been defaunated by various procedures such as administering copper sulfate, acids, gelatinized corn (Clemens et al, 1974) or chemicals such as dioctylsodium-sulfosuccinate (Abou Akkada et al, 1968) or dimetridazole (Clarke and Reid, 1969). Following defaunation, the animals can then be kept free of ciliates or inoculated with one or more specific species of organisms. The latter method (defaunation) would be expected to result in a normal rumen bacterial population as compared to complete isolation from an early age.

Eadie and Hobson (1962) have observed that no large change occurred in the numbers of rumen bacteria when protozoa were introduced into the rumen of isolated calves. The number of small bacteria decreased as did the number of flagellated protozoa. In a comparable situation, Bryant and Small (1960) observed reduced numbers of bacteria. When lambs, presumably with normal rumen populations, have been defaunated (Barringer et al, 1966; Klopfenstein et al, 1966), marked increases in number of bacteria were seen. This would, perhaps, be a better estimate of the effect of protozoa since isolated young ruminants may be expected to have atypical populations of rumen bacteria. More recent information on this subject has been provided by Kuirhara et al (1968), Eadie and Gill (1971) and Williams and Dinusson (1972). These reports essentially confirm the earlier results, although Kuirhara et al point out that the differences in bacterial numbers were not always clear cut since the protozoa changed the patterns of diurnal variation in bacterial numbers. Eadie and Gill (1971) point out that, in isolated lambs, large numbers of flagellate protozoa populations developed in ciliate-free animals after flagellates had been introduced into the building in which the lambs were housed.

Observations on isolated ciliate-free calves (Pounden and Hibbs, 1950; Bryant and Small, 1960; Eadie, 1962; Borhami et al, 1967; el-Sayed Osman et al, 1970; and Williams and Dinusson, 1973) indicate that they grow normally, although they tend to have a rougher hair coat and be "pot-bellied." Long term studies (up to 400 days of age) by Williams and Dinusson (1973) did not show any effect on growth in the absence of ciliates, although short-term studies with buffalo calves indicated a growth response in inoculated calves (Borhami et al, 1967) as did the data of el-Sayed Osman et al (1970) with Zebu calves. In the case of lambs, Abou Akkada and el-Shazly (1964) hand raised lambs to 5 wk of age in isolation at which time half were inoculated with rumen contents from mature sheep. The noninoculated lambs were ciliate-free. Inoculated lambs gained more weight from 50 to 168 days of age. Eadie and Gill (1971) found that faunated lambs gained more only between the 14th and 21st wk when lambs were carried through a 61-wk study.

In experiments beginning with isolated young ruminants, part of which may be inoculated with rumen contents of older animals to establish rumen protozoa, it seems likely that inoculation would also result in the establishment of normal rumen bacteria. Since some reports indicate atypical rumen flora in isolated animals, it is logical to believe that differences observed in such cases may be a result of both the absence of protozoa and an atypical bacterial population. Abou Akkada and el-Shazly (1964) stated, however, that ". . . the groups of bacteria in the ciliate-free lambs made up an 'adult-type' population which is remarkably similar to those found in the inoculated controls." No data were presented, however. This would appear to be in contradiction to some of the previous literature cited.

A variety of different changes have been noted in rumen or blood chemistry or body metabolism when ciliate-free animals have been studied. For example, Abou Akkada and el-Shazly (1964) found that inoculated lambs showed greater increases after feeding in reducing sugars, ammonia and VFA in rumen fluid. Blood sugar levels were higher, also, and they tended to have lower hemoglobin values. In addition, blood protein levels were higher, but NPN was lower. Average daily N retention was higher (ca. 51%) as compared to ciliate-free lambs (40%), mainly because of greater N loss in urine in ciliate-free lambs. In the young lambs studied by Eadie and Gill (1971), only minor differences were observed in calorimetric trials, digestibility and N balances. There were no differences between groups in total protein N and soluble sugar in the rumen, but the ammonia and VFA concentration was higher in the faunated group. In the blood, there were no differences in blood sugar or hemoglobin.

In older lambs, Christiansen et al (1965) inoculated previously defaunated lambs with *Entodinium*, *Diplodinium*, *Isotricha*, and *Ophryoscolex* and a combination of these species. Faunated lambs gained more rapidly and efficiently than protozoa-free lambs. Rumen pH was also lower, and VFA and ammonia levels were higher in the inoculated lambs. A narrower acetate-propionate ratio was observed in rumen ingesta of faunated lambs. Inoculation with single genera of protozoa resulted in rumen changes approaching those observed with the inoculum including all four genera. When lambs were fed 80% roughage, inoculated lambs showed higher levels of ruminal VFA and ammonia, but when fed 80% concentrates, the presence of protozoa resulted in more ruminal propionic acid although no greater concentration of total VFA (Luther et al, 1966). In calves inoculated with *Entodinium* or *Isotricha* sp. or mixtures of both, it was noted that either genera resulted in rumen samples with higher propionic acid than calves with mixtures of these two genera or from ciliate-free calves. Calves with the mixture had higher levels of n-butyric acid, results similar to those reported by Klopfenstein and others (1966). In vitro preps with bacteria and protozoa (Youssef and Allen, 1968) have shown higher levels of total VFA with generally more acetate and butyrate, but less propionate than with bacteria only. The pH was also lower in the presence of the protozoa.

As noted, numerous reports indicate an increase in ruminal ammonia in the presence of ciliates. The plasma urea does not necessarily show a corresponding increase, however. Klopfenstein et al (1966) suggested that lysine may have been a limiting factor when lambs were defaunated as plasma amino acids were lower in faunated lambs. Purser et al (1966) also noted that faunated lambs had lower plasma amino acids.

Other data showing similar responses in rumen VFA and ammonia have been reported by Luther et al (1966), Kuirhara et al (1968) and Males and Purser (1970). In the later study, defaunation resulted in higher rumen dry matter and lower rumen pH and ammonia but the molar % of propionate was higher in the rumen.

With regards to digestibility, Luther et al (1966) found that protozoa had little effect, however, Klopfenstein et al (1966) noted greater dry matter digestion with two of three rations and Perkins and Luther (1967) found that digestibility of dry matter, protein, fiber and organic matter were higher for faunated lambs, and Males and Purser (1970) observed higher N digestibility and retention in faunated sheep. Lindsay and Hogan (1972) could not detect any differences in apparent digestion in the stomach and intestines between normal controls and defaunated sheep.

It is known that rumen protozoa are capable of hydrogenating unsaturated fatty acids (see Ch. 14). Thus, Klopfenstein et al (1966) found more oleic acid and less linoleic acid in the plasma of faunated lambs and Clemens et al (1974) noted less linoleic acid in body fats of cattle which had a normal rumen population as compared to defaunated cattle.

The literature that has been reviewed indicates that protozoa do result in some differences in rumen metabolism and animal performance. Live weight gain would appear to be improved, possibly as a result of greater digestibility accompanied by higher levels of ruminal VFA — indicating more complete ruminal digestion. The higher levels of ruminal ammonia observed in some cases might be indicative of greater protein digestion, but it might also be indicative of greater wastage. Reduced propionate levels associated with ciliates might be expected to be a negative effect also; animals fed high grain rations tend to have high propionate levels and either none or very few ciliates — perhaps the lack of protozoa is a partial explanation for the difference. The literature indicates some contradictory situations in faunated vs. defaunated animals; obviously, more research is required to define clearly the contribution of the ruminal protozoa to total ruminal and host metabolism, but results obtained to date clearly do not indicate that protozoa are vital to the host.

Cyclical Variations

Protozoal populations tend to have rather definite cycles. Moir and Somers (1957) found that feeding once daily resulted in the greatest fall in rumen pH and in bacterial counts as compared to other methods where the ration was fed at more frequent intervals. Clarke (1965) has also studied the diurnal (daily) variation in protozoal concentrations in cows. When the animals were fasted for 18-24 hr and then fed once or twice daily, protozoal concentrations were usually highest at 2 hr after feeding (sampled at 0, 2, 5, 8, and 14 hr). Corrections were made for the weight of rumen contents which were removed and weighed at each sampling time. Some of his data are shown in Fig. 11-2 and it is apparent that, under these conditions, the oligotrichs did not contribute greatly to variation in numbers, but the holotrich numbers fluctuated greatly. Another example of diurnal variation is shown in Fig. 11-3 from Warner (1965). Clarke observed that protozoal counts may not always be a good measure of protozoal activity since the holotrichs ingest soluble sugars until the cells burst when an excess of sugar is available, often (presumably) resulting in a rapid decline in numbers following feeding. This reaction may be related to the osmotic pressure of rumen contents. Warner (1965) points out that, during periods of maximum holotrich multiplication, rumen contents tend to be hypotonic to plasma.

Data on diurnal variation of rumen bacteria are less prevalent than for protozoa; however, papers by Moir and Somers (1956, 1957), Purser and Moir (1959), Warner (1965) and Nottle (1956) indicate a substantial variation, although perhaps less than observed for protozoa. Figure 11-3 shows variations observed by Warner. Moir and Somers (1956) have studied the diurnal trend in rumen bacteria as affected by frequency of feeding. Although the data are not con-

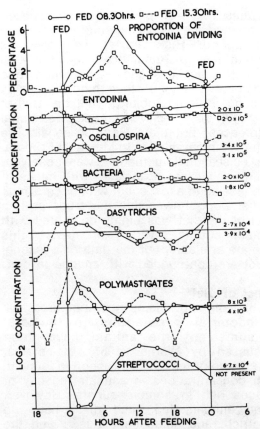

Figure 11-3. Graphical data illustrating diurnal variation in rumen microbial populations in a sheep fed alfalfa and wheaten hay once [solid line] or twice [dotted line] daily. The actual number of organisms are shown on the right side, the counts at 0830 being above the line and the counts at 1530 being below the line. From Warner [1965]. Courtesy of Butterworths.

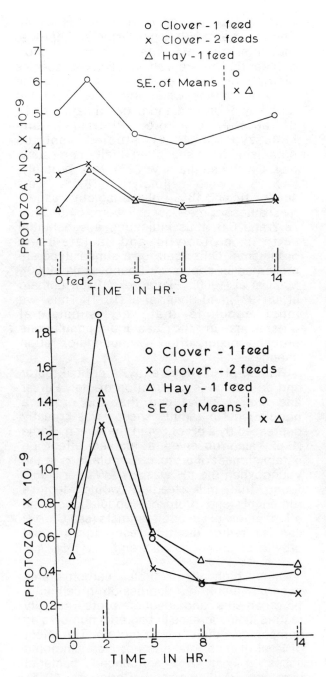

Figure 11-2. Top. Mean numbers of total ciliate protozoa in the rumen liquor of two cows fed fresh red clover. Bottom. Mean numbers of holotrich protozoa in the same cows. Note the marked peak in numbers compared to the total population shown in the top graph. From Clarke [1965].

clusive, they indicate that there was less variation in numbers when animals were fed frequently. Peak numbers occurred 4-8 hr after feeding, depending upon the nature of the diet.

Bryant and Robinson (1968) have made culture counts at intervals after feeding in cattle that were fed different rations at 12-hr intervals. Counts were made from samples obtained at 1, 2.5, 5.5 and 10 hr after feeding. Under these conditions, counts were highest for the hay and pelleted hay ration at 5.5 hr, for a hay-grain ration at 5.5 or 10 hr and for a silage ration at 5.5 or 10 hr. These workers also made counts in the dorsal and ventral rumen and near the reticulo-omasal orifice. For all of the rations, counts were appreciably higher in the dorsal rumen, indicating a more favorable environment for the rumen bacteria. In the reticulum, counts were appreciably higher than in the ventral rumen when the cattle were fed pellets.

In addition to daily cycles, Moir (1951) and Nottle (1956) among others have observed substantial seasonal variation, much of which would probably be attributed to changes in feed. Nottle (1956), however, maintained sheep on a constant ration over a 2-yr period. His data showed seasonal fluctuations in rumen pH and bacterial numbers, and he suggested that light and temperature, among other things, probably influenced the microbial population. Gall et al (1949) observed very marked seasonal differences, but diets were seasonal. The same comment applies to Moir's (1951) data. Marked seasonal fluctuations were observed. A high count was associated with intake of green feed and a low count with dry grazing; further work showed that the crude protein level of the diet was highly correlated with bacterial counts. A variety of papers of this type are available, but the data on seasonal effect are confounded with change in diet.

Effect of Diet

Some of the problems in relating protozoal or bacterial populations to the diet consumed by the animal have been discussed by Warner (1965). He states, ". . . the holotrich protozoa are often found in high concentrations in animals fed hay or forages rich in soluble sugars. However, some animals fed such diets have no holotrich, and some only a few; and the different holotrich species may be affected differently. On the other hand, sheep fed a diet rich in grain have been observed with a high holotrich count. Again, animals fed diets rich in starch often have high concentrations of *Entodinia* in their rumens. These are sometimes the only opryoscolecids or even the only ciliates present, but again, animals with few or no *Entodinia* can be found. The position is even more confused with the bacteria, where there have been few detailed counts of species or even of functional groups. . . . no clear principles have emerged except that alterations in the diet are accompanied by alterations in the microbial population, and diets richer in readily fermented nutrients support greater total numbers." These observations are borne out by bacterial data published by Hungate (1957) on animals fed constant amounts of a variety of rations. He reported that there was no correlation between the different rations and differences in the observed bacterial colony counts. Giesecke et al (1966) also concluded that differences in bacterial populations from sheep fed semi-purified or roughage-concentrate rations were primarily of a quantitative nature rather than of a qualitative nature. However, Thorley et al (1968), when using an improved media for culture counts, were able to show substantial differences in bacterial species distribution between individual cows and between rations when the cows were fed long hay or ground and pelleted hay. By way of another example, Pietraszek and Maluszynska (1970) studied isolated organisms from sheep fed alfalfa or meadow hay. On the alfalfa hay, 72% were proteolytic, 25.3 were cellulolytic, 78.0% were amylolytic and 16% utilized lactate; respective values for meadow hay were: 54.0, 21.3, 76.2 and 6.6, thus indicating a substantial shift in proteolytic and lactate-using organisms. Other data of a similar type are presented in papers by Sosnovskaja (1960), Maki et al (1969), Pietraszek (1970), Latham et al (1971) and Slyter et al (1971). Thus, we must conclude that very substantial differences in the bacterial populations probably occur, often without major ration changes.

Rumen pH is, apparently, a critical factor and one which is a reflection of diet. Purser and Moir (1959) found that the protozoa population in adult sheep was greatly depressed by a pH of 5.4 in the rumen. Eadie (1962) also observed a marked effect on establishment of protozoa populations in the young when the pH was low. Warner (1962) found that milk feeding would depress rumen pH and protozoal populations. The effect of low pH in adult animals (see Ch. 17) can be rather drastic, resulting in rapid growth of *Streptococcus* and *Lactobacillus* sp.

Diets high in soluble carbohydrates generally result in a depression in cellulolytic organisms, and adequate protein usually results in an increase in bacterial numbers as compared to diets low in protein. The effect of level of feed intake is not clear. In some cases it has not influenced bacterial numbers (Williams and Christian, 1956; Gilchrist and Kistner, 1962), while in others (Christiansen et al, 1964) the full feeding of a pelleted low-fiber ration resulted in a marked reduction in rumen protozoa, whereas two thirds of a full feed had less effect. In steers fed all-concentrate diets, restricted feeding increased both the number of protozoa and cellulolytic bacteria as compared to animals full fed (Slyter et al, 1970). In sheep fed pelleted moderate roughage (65%) rations, Dearth et al (1974) found that increasing the level of feeding from maintenance to 1.8 maintenance resulted in a decrease in total numbers of rumen ciliates [*Dasytricha, Entodinium, Ophryoscolex*], but caused an increase in total anaerobic bacteria. Grinding the roughage in a ration also is said to result in fewer protozoa (Christiansen et al, 1964), as does pelleting (Chalupa et al, 1965).

The use of diethylstilbestrol has been a standard practice for feedlot cattle. Some reports indicate a marked response on protozoal numbers in lambs and dairy cattle, respectively (Christiansen et al, 1964; Ibrahim et al, 1970), but other papers on steers or lambs (Slyter et al, 1970; Dearth et al, 1970b) have not shown any effect.

The holotrich protozoa generally appear in largest numbers in grazing ruminants and in animals on a diet containing a considerable amount of hay (Hungate, 1966), presumably due to the presence of dissolved sugars from ingested plant material. A number of authors have noted differences in the ability of different forages to support a population of a given organism. Starch diets, in general, promote the development of species such as *Entodinia*, sometimes to the exclusion of other genera, and it has frequently been noted that "better" rations result in greater concentrations of protozoa. As suggested, older studies generally show that starch in the diet promotes larger numbers of *Entodinium* sp., data confirmed by more recent studies as well (Nakamura and Kanegasaki, 1969; Abe et al, 1973; Eadie, 1973). However, all-concentrate diets may result in such an acid rumen that the protozoa do not survive. Eadie (1973) points out that the level of feeding of grains is a factor and her results show that survival of *Entodinium* and *Isotricha* sp. is much greater in sheep fed whole barley as compared to pelleted barley.

Purser and Moir (1966) have studied the effect of a number of feedstuffs on rumen protozoa. Unextracted linseed added to a basal ration caused a decrease in protozoal concentration, and daily infusion of 60 g of linseed oil had the same effect on sheep. A urea supplement supplying 8 g of N was fed resulting in a greater protozoal concentration than when one half or three quarters of the supplement was infused into the rumen 10 hr after feeding, or when the urea supplement was infused continuously. When urea and gluten were added (isonitrogenous) to the basal ration, protozoal concentration with the urea was greater than with gluten supplementation which, in turn, was greater than with the basal ration. In each case, greater protozoal concentrations were associated with high levels of rumen ammonia. Other data of this type (Devuyst et al, 1973) show that inclusion of sucrose or lactose with alfalfa stimulated *Entodinium* numbers as did additions of barley to grass silage.

The rumen microorganisms disappear at different rates when animals are starved. Warner (1965) has presented graphical data showing that some organisms, such as Oscillospirae and the polymastigates (flagellates) disappear very rapidly and the ciliates decline, although bacteria numbers did not appear to be markedly affected. Rumen fermentation, as measured by cellulose digestion or VFA production declines rapidly (Meiske et al, 1958; Fowle and Church, 1973). Protozoa numbers drop off, of course, during starvation, although Potter and Dehority (1973) found that their generation rate decreased as rumen turnover rate decreased. Restriction of water intake also results in a gradual decrease in holotrich species.

Gnotobiotic Animals

Studies with gnotobiotic (germ-free) animals have been carried out with a number of different animals species, but relatively little information is available on young ruminants, primarily because they are difficult to keep alive without becoming contaminated with bacterial sources (Coates, 1973). Soares et al (1970) point out that some of the first work with gnotobiotics was done with goats in 1912 and give two other references indicating that gnotobiotic lambs had lower levels of hemoglobin, blood glucose, serum protein and rate of growth. In the experiments of Soares et al, experimental lambs showed a marked lack of stomach development, the weights being 139-160 g as compared to 432-726 g in conventionally-fed lambs. The ruminal lining was thinner, only rudimentary papillae were present and the color was pink. Digestibility of purified diets (24% cellulose) was appreciably lower and there was no apparent digestion of acid detergent fiber. After 2 wk of age, blood glucose tended to be higher, and body fats had very high levels of unsaturated fatty acids present (diet had 5% corn oil), indicating none of the typical hydrogenation seen in normal ruminants. Most of the lambs in this study were contaminated by 4 wk of age. Data on germ-free rabbits indicate that they, too, digest carbohydrates very poorly (Yoshida et al, 1968).

Conclusions

A variety of factors has been mentioned that affect the numbers and kinds of rumen microorganisms found at a given time. These include the relative amount and nature of the diet of the host animals, seasonal and diurnal cycles as affected by periodic food intake, rumination, feed processing, incompatability of certain protozoa types, competition between protozoa and bacteria, geographical distribution of protozoa and bacteria, the species of host, and unexplained factors accounting for differences in similar animals treated alike.

Warner (1965) points out that just because a microorganism is introduced into the rumen does not mean that it will become established. A number of organisms found in soil, water, or on feedstuffs seem to have the capability to exist in the rumen, but they do not become established. One paper indicates that natural antibiotics may be produced by rumen microorganisms that may prevent invasion by other forms. Some organisms have been observed to disappear from the rumen for no apparent reason and they have been shown to return after an interval of months or years. However, loss of one or more species tends to result in an increase in concentration of other species (at least when protozoa are lost this is the case). In addition, there must be minor differences in the physiology of the host which influence the rumen population since the microbial population may be quite different in animals kept under the same conditions and fed the same diet.

References Cited

Abe, M., H. Shibui, T. Iriki and F. Kumeno. 1973. Br. J. Nutr. 29:197.
Abou Akkada, A.R., E.E. Bartley and L.R. Fina. 1969. J. Dairy Sci. 52:1088.
Abou Akkada, A.R. and K. el-Shazly. 1964. Appl. Microbiol. 12:384.
Abou Akkada, A.R. and K. el-Shazly. 1965. J. Agr. Sci. 64:251.
Abou Akkada, A.R. and B.H. Howard. 1960. Biochem. J. 76:445.
Abou Akkada, A.R. and B.H. Howard. 1961. Biochem. J. 78:512.
Abou Akkada, A.R. and B.H. Howard. 1962. Biochem. J. 82:313.
Abou Akkada, A.R. et al. 1968. Appl. Microbiol. 16:1475.
Adams, J.C., et al. 1966. Experientia 22:717.
Bailey, R.W. and R.T.J. Clarke. 1963. Nature. 198:787.
Bailey, R.W., R.T.J. Clarke and D.E. Wright. 1962. Biochem. J. 83:517.
Bailey, R.W. and B.H. Howard. 1963a. Biochem. J. 87:146.
Bailey, R.W. and B.H. Howard. 1963b. Biochem. J. 86:446.
Barringer, R., A. Trenkle and W. Burroughs. 1966. J. Animal Sci. 25:1257 (abstr).
Becker, E.R., J.A. Schulz and M.A. Emmerson. 1929. Iowa State College J. Sci. 4:215.
Becker, E.R. and M. Talbott. 1927. Iowa State College J. Sci. 1:345.
Borhami, B.E.A., K. el-Shazly, A.R. Abou Akkada and I.A. Ahmed. 1967. J. Dairy Sci. 50:1654.
Brailsford, M.D. and P.A. Hartman. 1968. Can. J. Microbiol. 14:397.
Brewer, D. and A. Taylor. 1969. J. Gen. Microbiol. 59:137.
Bryant, M.P. 1959. Bact. Rev. 23:125.
Bryant, M.P. 1963. J. Animal Sci. 22:801.
Bryant, M.P. 1970. In: Dukes' Physiology of Domestic Animals. 8th ed. Comstock Publ. Assoc., Ithaca, N.Y.
Bryant, M.P. and L.A. Burkey. 1953. J. Dairy Sci. 36:218.
Bryant, M.P. and I. Robinson. 1962. J. Bact. 84:605.
Bryant, M.P. and I. Robinson. 1968. J. Dairy Sci. 51:1950.
Bryant, M.P. and N. Small. 1960. J. Dairy Sci. 43:654.
Bryant, M.P., N. Small, C. Bouma and I. Robinson. 1958. J. Dairy Sci. 41:1747.
Bullen, J.J., R. Scarisbrick and A. Maddock. 1953. J. Path. Bact. 65:209.
Caldwell, D.R. and M.P. Bryant. 1966. Appl. Microbiol. 14:794.
Chalupa, W., A.J. Kutches, R. Lavker and G.D. O'Dell. 1965. J. Animal Sci. 24:876 (abstr).
Christiansen, W.C. and W. Burroughs. 1962. J. Animal Sci. 21:990 (abstr).
Christiansen, W.C., R. Kawashima and W. Burroughs. 1965. J. Animal Sci. 24:731.
Christiansen, W.C., W. Woods and W. Burroughs. 1964. J. Animal Sci. 23:984.

Clarke, R.T.J. 1964. N.Z. J. Agr. Res. 7:248.
Clarke, R.T.J. 1965. N.Z. J. Agr. Res. 8:1.
Clarke, R.T.J. and M.E. DiMenna. 1961. J. Gen. Microbiol. 25:113.
Clarke, R.T.J. and R.E. Hungate. 1966. Appl. Microbiol. 14:340.
Clarke, R.T.J. and C.S.W. Reid. 1969. N.Z. J. Agr. Res. 12:437.
Clemens, E.T., W. Woods and V.H. Arthaud. 1974. J. Animal Sci. 38:640.
Coates, M.E. 1973. Proc. Nutr. Soc. 32:53.
Coleman, G.S. 1960. J. Gen. Microbiol. 22:555.
Coleman, G.S. 1962. J. Gen. Microbiol. 28:271.
Coleman, G.S. 1964. J. Gen. Microbiol. 37:209.
Coleman, G.S. 1967. J. Gen. Microbiol. 47:433; 449.
Coleman, G.S. 1969. J. Gen. Microbiol. 57:81.
Coleman, G.S., J.I. Davies and M.A. Cash. 1972. J. Gen. Microbiol. 73:509.
Coleman, G.S. and R.W. White. 1970. J. Gen. Microbiol. 62:265.
Conchie, J. 1954. Biochem. J. 58:552.
Constantinescu, E. and F. Palfy. 1967. Nutr. Abstr. Rev. 40:1338.
Contrepois, M. and P. Goet. 1973. Ann. Rech. Veter. 4:161.
Corliss, J.P. 1961. The Ciliated Protozoa: Characterization, Classification and Guide to the Literature. Pergamon Press.
Crha, J. 1972. Acta Vet. Brno. 41:355.
Dearth, R.N., B.A. Dehority and E.L. Potter. 1974. J. Animal Sci. 38:991.
Dehority, B.A. and D.B. Purser. 1970. J. Animal Sci. 30:445.
Dehority, B.A. and H.W. Scott. 1967. J. Dairy Sci. 50:1136.
Devuyst, A. et al. 1973. Nutr. Abstr. Rev. 43:997.
Dogiel, V.A. 1927. Arch. Protistenk. 5:1.
Eadie, J.M. 1962a. J. Gen. Microbiol. 29:563.
Eadie, J.M. 1962b. J. Gen. Microbiol. 29:579.
Eadie, J.M. 1967. J. Gen. Microbiol. 49:175.
Eadie, J.M. 1968. J. Physiol. 194:8 (abstr).
Eadie, J.M. 1973. Proc. Nutr. Soc. 32:64A (abstr).
Eadie, J.M. and J.C. Gill. 1971. Br. J. Nutr. 26:155.
Eadie, J.M. and P.M. Hobson. 1962. Nature 193:503.
Eadie, J.M. and B.H. Howard. 1963. In: Progress in Nutrition and Allied Sciences. pp 57-68. Oliver and Boyd Pub. Co.
el-Sayed Osman, H., A.R. Abou Akkada and K.A. Agabawi. 1970. Animal Prod. 12:367.
Fowle, K.E. and D.C. Church. 1973. Amer. J. Vet. Res. 34:849.
Gall, L.S., W. Burroughs, P. Gerlaugh and B.H. Edginton. 1949. J. Animal Sci. 8:441.
Gall, L.S. and C.N. Huhtanen. 1950. J. Animal Sci. 9:656 (abstr).
Giesecke, D., M.J. Lawlor and K. Walser-Karst. 1966. Br. J. Nutr. 20:383.
Gilchrist, F.M.C. and A. Kistner. 1962. J. Agr. Sci. 59:77.
Gutierrez, J. 1955. Biochem. J. 60:516.
Gutierrez, J. 1958. J. Protozool. 5:122.
Gutierrez, J. and R.E. Davis. 1959. J. Protozool. 6:222.
Harmeyer, J. 1972. Nutr. Abstr. Rev. 42:609.
Hartman, P.A., J.L. Morrill and N.L. Jacobson. 1966. Appl. Microbiol. 14:70.
Hino, T., M. Kametaka and M. Kandatsu. 1973. J. Gen. Microbiol. 19:325; 397.
Hobson, P.N. and S.O. Mann. 1961. J. Gen. Microbiol. 25:227.
Hoogenraad, N.J., F.J.R. Hird, I. Holmes and N.F. Millis. 1967. J. Gen. Virol. 1:575.
Hungate, R.E. 1950. Bact. Rev. 14:1.
Hungate, R.E. 1955. In: Biochem. & Physiol. of Protozoa. 2:159. Academic Press.
Hungate, R.E. 1957. Can. J. Microbiol. 3:289.
Hungate, R.E. 1966. The Rumen and Its Microbes. Academic Press.
Hungate, R.E. 1972. Amer. J. Clin. Nutr. 25:1480.
Hungate, R.E., M.P. Bryant and R.A. Mah. 1964. The Rumen Bacteria and Protozoa. Ann. Rev. Microbiol. 18:131-166.
Ibrahim, E.A., J.R. Ingalls and N.E. Stanger. 1970. Can. J. Animal Sci. 50:101.
Jarvis, B.D.W. 1968. Appl. Microbiol. 16:714.
Jarvis, B.D.W. and R.E. Hungate. 1968. Appl. Microbiol. 16:1044.
Jouany, J.P. and P. Thivend. 1972. Ann. Biol. Anim. Bioch. Biophys. 12:673.
Kandatsu, M. and N. Takahashi. 1963. Japanese J. Zootech. Sci. 34:143; 148.
Kay, R.N.B. and P.N. Hobson. 1963. J. Dairy Res. 30:261.
Kistner, A. 1965. In: Physiology of Digestion in the Ruminant. Butterworths.
Klopfenstein, T.J., D.B. Purser and W.J. Tyznik. 1966. J. Animal Sci. 25:765.
Kofoid, C.A. and R.F. MacLennan. 1930. Univ. Calif. Pub. Zool. 33:471.
Kofoid, C.A. and R.F. MacLennan. 1932. Univ. Calif. Pub. Zool. 37:53.
Kofoid, C.A. and R.F. MacLennan. 1933. Univ. Calif. Pub. Zool. 39:1.
Kubo, T. and M. Kandatsu. 1969. Nutr. Abstr. Rev. 39:1241.
Kuirhara, Y., J.M. Eadie, P.N. Hobson and S.O. Mann. 1968. J. Gen. Microbiol. 51:267.
Latham, M.J., M.E. Sharpe and J.D. Sutton. 1971. J. Appl. Bact. 34:425.
Lengemann, F.W. and N.N. Allen. 1959. J. Dairy Sci. 42:1171.

Lindsay, J.R. and J.P. Hogan. 1972. Aust. J. Agr. Res. 23:321.
Luther, R., A. Trenkle and W. Burroughs. 1966. J. Animal Sci. 25:1116.
Mah, R.A. 1964. J. Protozool. 11:546.
Maki, L.R., L.K. Devlin, K. Sheehan and G.E. Smith. 1969. Proc. West. Sec. Amer. Soc. Animal Sci. 20:205.
Males, J.R. and D.B. Purser. 1970. Appl. Microbiol. 19:485.
Mann, S.O. 1963. J. Gen. Microbiol. 33:IX.
Mann, S.O., F.M. Masson and A.E. Oxford. 1954. Br. J. Nutr. 8:246.
Mann, S.O. and E.R. Ørskov. 1973. J. Appl. Bact. 36:475.
McBee, R.H., J.L. Johnson and M.P. Bryant. 1969. J. Wildl. Mgt. 33:181.
McNaught, M.L., E.C. Owens, K.M. Henry and S.K. Kon. 1954. Biochem. J. 46:32.
Meiske, J.C., R.L. Salsbury, J.A. Hoefer and R.W. Luecke. 1958. J. Animal Sci. 17:774.
Moir, R.J. 1951. Aust. J. Agr. Res. 2:322.
Moir, R.J. and M.J. Masson. 1952. J. Pathol. Bact. 64:343.
Moir, R.J. and M. Somers. 1956. Nature 178:1472.
Moir, R.J. and M. Somers. 1957. Aust. J. Agr. Res. 8:253.
Moir, R.J. and V.J. Williams. 1950. Aust. J. Sci. Res. 3:381.
Mullenax, C.H., R.F. Keeler and M.J. Allison. 1966. Amer. J. Vet. Res. 27:857.
Naga, M.A. and K. el-Shazly. 1968. J. Gen. Microbiol. 53:305.
Nakamura, K. and S. Kanegasaki. 1969. J. Dairy Sci. 52:250.
Noirot-Timothee, C. 1963. L.C.R. Acad. Sci. 256:5400.
Nottle, M.C. 1956. Aust. J. Biol. Sci. 9:593.
Oh, J.H., I.D. Hume and D.T. Torell. 1972. J. Animal Sci. 35:450.
Oxford, A.E. 1955. Exper. Parasitol. 4:569.
Paynter, M.J.B., D.L. Ewert and W. Chalupa. 1969. Appl. Microbiol. 18:942.
Paynter, M.J.B. and R.E. Hungate. 1968. J. Bact. 95:1943.
Pearson, H.A. 1965. J. Wildl. Mgt. 29:493.
Pearson, H.A. 1967. Appl. Microbiol. 15:1450.
Pearson, H.A. 1969. Appl. Microbiol. 17:819.
Perkins, J.L. and R.M. Luther. 1967. J. Animal Sci. 26:928 (abstr).
Perry, K.D. and C.A.E. Briggs. 1957. Appl. Bact. 20:119.
Phillipson, A.T. (ed.) 1970. Physiology of Digestion and Metabolism in the Ruminant. Oriel Press, Newcastle upon Tyne, England.
Pietraszek, A. 1970. Acta. Microbiol. Polonica 2:193; 205.
Pietraszek, A. and G.M. Maluszynska. 1970. Biol. Inst. Genet. Hodowli Zwierzat PAN 19:51.
Potter, E.L. and B.A. Dehority. 1973. Appl. Microbiol. 26:692.
Pounden, W.D. and J.W. Hibbs. 1950. J. Dairy Sci. 3:639.
Purser, D.B., T.J. Klopfenstein and J.H. Cline. 1966. J. Nutr. 89:226.
Purser, D.B. and R.J. Moir. 1959. Aust. J. Agr. Res. 10:555.
Purser, D.B. and R.J. Moir. 1966. J. Animal Sci. 25:668.
Ritchie, A.E., I.M. Robinson and M.J. Allison. 1971. J. Animal Sci. 33:298 (abstr).
Sijpesteijn, A.K. 1949. J. Microbiol. Serol. 15:49.
Slyter, L.L., R.R. Oltjen, D.L. Kern and F.C. Blank. 1970. J. Animal Sci. 31:996.
Slyter, L.L., et al. 1971. J. Nutr. 101:847.
Smiles, J. and M.J. Dobson. 1956. J. Royal Microscop. Soc. 75:244.
Smith, H.W. 1965. J. Path. Bact. 90:495.
Soares, J.H., E.C. Leffel and R.K. Larsen. 1970. J. Animal Sci. 31:733.
Sosnovskaja, E.A. 1960. Nutr. Abstr. Rev. 30:172.
Sugden, B. 1953. J. Gen. Microbiol. 9:44.
Sugden, B. and A.E. Oxford. 1952. J. Gen. Microbiol. 7:145.
Thorley, C.M., E. Sharpe and M.P. Bryant. 1968. J. Dairy Sci. 51:1181.
Thurston, J.P. and J. Grain. 1971. J. Protozool. 18:133. .
Thurston, J.P. and C. Noirot-Timothee. 1973. J. Protozool. 20:562.
Tompkin, R.B., D.B. Purser and H.H. Weiser. 1966. J. Protozool. 13:55.
Warner, A.C.I. 1962. J. Gen. Microbiol. 28:129.
Warner, A.C.I. 1965. In: Physiology of Digestion in the Ruminant. Butterworths.
White, R.W. 1969. J. Gen. Microbiol. 56:403.
Williams, P.P. and W.E. Dinusson. 1972. J. Animal Sci. 34:469.
Williams, P.P. and W.E. Dinusson. 1973. J. Animal Sci. 36:588.
Williams, V.J. and K.R. Christian. 1956. N.Z. J. Sci. Tech. A38:194.
Wolin, M.J. 1969. Appl. Microbiol. 17:83.
Yoshida, T., J.R. Pleasants, B.S. Reddy and B.S. Wostmann. 1968. Br. J. Nutr. 22:723.
Youssef, F.G. and D.M. Allen. 1968. Nature. 217:777.
Ziolecki, A. and C.A.E. Briggs. 1962. J. Appl. Bact. 24:148.

CHAPTER 12 — RUMEN METABOLISM OF CARBOHYDRATES

Quantitatively, carbohydrates are very important to the ruminant animal. Plant tissues contain about 75% carbohydrates of one kind or another, the amount and distribution depending on the age, agronomic and environmental factors, and species of plant in question. Consequently, carbohydrates provide the primary source of energy for both the rumen organisms and the host animal.

The carbohydrates found in plant tissues are primarily polysaccharides — cellulose, hemicelluloses, pectins, fructans and starches with minor amounts of a wide variety of other compounds containing carbohydrate molecules. Of these, cellulose is by far the most abundant. Only in a few plants is there any appreciable concentration of disaccharides such as sucrose. In addition, most plants have only very small amounts of glucose in their tissues, particularly in mature or dried plant tissue is this so.

Knowledge of utilization of a variety of carbohydrates by the animal has been available for many years based on results of digestion and balance trials, including calorimetry studies. However, only in relatively recent years has it been possible to determine the scope of activity occurring in the reticulo-rumen in relation to carbohydrate utilization. The majority, although not all, of the research on carbohydrate utilization by rumen microorganisms has been carried out under in vitro conditions. There is a wealth of literature on this subject, particularly so with regard to the fibrous carbohydrates — cellulose and hemicellulose — as might be expected in view of the high degree of utilization of cellulose by the ruminant animal as compared to most monogastric species. Consequently, the data presented and the papers discussed represent only a sampling of the available literature. Reviews that may be of interest to the reader would include those of Hungate (1966, pp 36-90, 128-140, 245-280), Barnett and Reid (1961, pp 89-106) and more recent and briefer reviews by Bryant (1970), Dehority (1973) and Van Soest (1973).

Fermentation of Carbohydrates

Fermentation data with crude suspensions, washed suspensions and pure cultures of bacteria or protozoa are available in relatively large number. Some of the bacterial data are shown in Table 11-2. These data clearly show a marked difference in the ability of pure cultures to ferment various carbohydrates, although these data are not necessarily indicative of fermentation by the complex population found in the rumen. Information is also presented in Ch. 11 relative to utilization of some carbohydrate sources by protozoa. Consequently, this chapter will be less detailed than it otherwise might be. Some relatively recent papers dealing with the metabolism of specific carbohydrates by pure cultures of bacteria would include those of Thomas (1960), Hobson and Purdom (1961), Kistner et al (1962), Walker and Hope (1964), Dehority (1966), Clarke et al (1969), Coen and Dehority (1970), Slyter and Weaver (1971), Gradel and Dehority (1972), and Smith et al (1973). For the protozoa, the reader is referred to papers by Abou Akkada and Howard (1960, 1961), Naga and el-Shazly (1968), Coleman (1969), and Kubo and Kandatsu (1969).

Carbohydrates Metabolized and End Products

One of the earlier papers demonstrating the disappearance of carbohydrates from the reticulo-rumen was that of Phillipson and McAnally (1942). Sheep with rumen and abomasal fistulas were utilized and were administered doses of a variety of mono- and disaccharides. The data, partially substantiated with in vitro experiments, indicated that glucose, fructose and sucrose underwent rapid fermentation giving rise to lactic acid and volatile fatty acids. Glucose disappearance could not be related to the amount found in the abomasum. Maltose, lactose and galactose disappeared less rapidly with no accumulation of lactic acid. Starch and cellulose were fermented slowly and the production of the volatile fatty acids was prolonged.

Table 12-1.   Distribution of carbon of three sugars fermented by rumen organisms.[a]

Final products formed	Percentage distribution of carbohydrate carbon		
	Maltose	Arabinose	Xylose
Volatile fatty acids	34.7	41.3	48.4
Lactic acid	8.0	0.7	0
Carbon dioxide	8.0	4.0	4.8
Methane	3.1	1.3	2.1
Bacterial protein	11.8	16.7	16.1
Bacterial polysaccharide	28.1	18.7	16.5
Undetermined carbon	6.3	17.3	12.1

[a] McNaught (1951)

Table 12-2.   Effect of carbohydrate or acid substrate on the amount and distribution of VFA produced.[a]

Substrate (155 M)	M volatile fatty acids				Iodine test
	Total	Acetic	Propionic	Higher	
Cellobiose	180	110	40	30	+
Maltose	240	87	99	57	+
Glucose	148	86	39	23	+
Xylose	114	45	34	35	+
Pyruvate	116	78	23	15	0
Lactate	—*	—	—	—	0
Oxaloacetate	24	—	—	—	0
Succinate	176	21	141	15	0
Fumarate	24	24	0	0	0
Malate	125	68	48	9	0
Formate	15	15	0	0	0
Acetate	100	100	0	0	0
Propionate	137	14	123	0	0
Butyrate	285	262	0	23	0
β-hydroxy butyrate	39	25	8	6	0

[a] Doetsch et al (1953)
*Yield too small for further fractionation.

The utilization of the carbon in three different carbohydrates by in vitro rumen suspensions was investigated by McNaught (1951). Some of the published data are shown in Table 12-1. These data show that the carbohydrates supplied as substrates influenced the amount and distribution of the end products as well as the synthesis of bacterial protein and bacterial polysaccharide. McNaught presented other data indicating that a variety of polysaccharides and sugars were readily utilized. However, oxidized compounds such as gluconic and glucuronic acids or manitol resulted in no noticeable activity. D and L isomers of various sugars varied in fermentation activity produced. McNaught also reported that succinic acid was not fermented, but later reports indicate that this is not the case. Further evidence of the effect of the carbohydrate (or acid) source on amount and relative proportion of VFA produced is shown in Table 12-2. These data were collected using washed suspensions of rumen bacteria. They clearly show that the carbohydrate or organic acid supplied resulted in marked differences in the fermentation products recovered. The data also illustrate the fact that what is a waste product for one species may be a usable energy source for another species. Lactic and succinic acids are very good examples of this situation. A number of organisms are known to produce one or the other of these acids but since others can readily utilize them as substrates, only very small amounts of these acids are normally found in mixed cultures of rumen organisms. There are exceptions to this statement, but the exceptions usually occur during a period of adaptation to changing rations (see Ch. 16 and 17 for details).

On the basis of published data, it seems likely that almost any naturally occurring carbohydrate (or carbohydrate derivative) is apt to be fermented in the rumen. A sampling of the literature indicates that the following compounds are fermented: propylene glycol, various lactic acid salts (Waldo and Schultz, 1960); glycerol (Johns, 1953; Wright, 1969); lactic acid (Knox, 1966; Czerkawski and Breckenridge, 1969); D-xylose (Pazur et al, 1958; Czerkawski and Breckenridge, 1969); other sugars such as cellulobiose, arabinose, galactose, mannose; and inulin (Czerkawski and Breckenridge, 1969); xylan (Heald, 1953; Dehority, 1966); glucuronic acid (Heald, 1952); pectin (Wright, 1961; Gradel and Dehority, 1972); salicin (Prins, 1971); oligoglacturonides (Wojciechowicz, 1972); rutin (Cheng et al, 1969); pentosans from wheat and xylans from red seaweed (Howard, 1957); pyruvate (Peel, 1960); succinic acid (Blackburn and Hungate, 1963); citric acid (Packett and Fordham, 1965; Wright, 1971); soluble cellulose (Underkofler et al, 1953); and a wide variety of starches, hemicelluloses and celluloses. Other compounds such as methanol and ethanol are produced in the rumen at times by some bacterial species. Methanol may appear as a result of pectin fermentation (Vantcheva et al, 1970); in vivo data indicate adaptation to ethanol infusions with a resultant reduction in propionate and an increase in valerate (Pradhan and Hemken, 1970).

As pointed out in preceding paragraphs (and in Ch. 16), the specific carbohydrate fermented has a marked effect on the end products produced. This is undoubtedly a reflection of (a) a different route of metabolism undergone by different compounds or (b) a selective increase in mixed cultures of organisms capable of fermenting the particular substrate. In addition to carbon dioxide and the VFA and lactic or succinic acids, other end products may include ethanol, methane, hydrogen, and hydrogen sulfide which may originate wholly or partially from microbial fermentation of carbohydrates.

With respect to the fibrous carbohydrates, data published by Gray and Pilgrim (1952), Barnett and Reid (1957), Bath and Head (1961) and Satter et al (1964) indicate that molar proportions of VFA produced from cellulose or hemicellulose were similar. Both Bath and Head (1961) and Satter et al (1964) used ^{14}C-labeled material. Satter et al used inoculum from cows fed either alfalfa hay or a grain-alfalfa hay mixture. Some of their data are shown in Table 12-3. These data indicate no marked difference in VFA produced from cellulose or hemicellulose, although there is some indication of a change in relative amounts of butyric and propionic acids, and the acetic:propionic ratios are somewhat different, reflecting the different metabolism of microbial populations adapted to a high cellulose vs. a moderate level of starch.

Table 12-3. Recovery of ^{14}C in VFA produced from cellulose or hemicellulose.[a]

| Labeled acid | Alpha-cellulose | | Hemicellulose | |
	Hay inoculum	G-H inoculum	Hay inoculum	G-H inoculum
	molar %		molar %	
Valeric	1.1	0.6	0.5	0.8
Butyric	13.1	5.7	6.9	7.4
Propionic	18.6	30.1	23.3	27.5
Acetic	67.1	62.9	69.3	64.5
Acetic/propionic ratio	3.6	2.1	3.0	2.4

[a]Satter et al (1964)

Carbohydrases Present in Rumen Organisms

The ability of an individual organism or of the rumen population to ferment any specific carbohydrate is dependent upon the presence of the appropriate enzyme required to utilize any specific carbohydrate (or other energy source). In view of the fact that there has been a considerable amount of literature on this subject, it seems pertinent to this discussion to include a review of the literature.

Sometime ago Nasr (1950) demonstrated that rumen liquor contained appreciable quantities of an α-amylase which was presumed to be of ruminal origin since no such enzyme had been detected in ruminant saliva. Hobson and MacPherson (1952) isolated extracellular amylases from two rumen bacteria and Bailey and Roberton (1962) isolated isomaltodextrinase from *Lactobacillus bifidus.* This enzyme was capable of degrading dextrins having 2 to 9 molecules of glucose to glucose and could attack a variety of β-linked sugars. Bailey (1963) also isolated an intracellular α-galactosidase, amylase, sucrose phosphorylase and, occasionally, isomaltase from *Streptococcus bovis.* Sugars of the raffinose series were hydrolyzed to galactose and sucrose. The α-galactosidase readily hydrolyzed melibiose and other oligosaccharides containing α-1,6 linked galactose as well as other carbohydrates of a similar linkage.

Howard et al (1960) isolated two enzymes having activity on carbohydrates containing xylan. One acted on inner linkages producing xylobiose as the main product and the other acted by removing single molecules. A similar enzyme was indicated which removed side chains containing arabinose. Walker and Hopgood (1961) have isolated enzymes which hydrolyze hemicellulose preps to xylose, xylobiose, xylotriose and higher oligosaccharides together with glucose and arabinose. Gillard et al (1965) isolated hemicellulases from bacteria which had varying degrees of activity in releasing pentoses as compared to galactose and uronic acids. An enzyme from *Butrivibrio fibrisolvens* had more rapid activity on linear chains of hemicellulose than on branched chains. With regard to cellulases, Stanley and Kesler (1959) isolated enzymes from rumen fluid which could hydrolyze cellulose, as did Festenstein (1959). King (1959) presented data which indicated that cellulases may be bound to the surface of bacteria. Leatherwood (1965) found that cellulase from *Ruminococcus albus* produced cellobiose as the main product of swollen cellulose, but glucose was the product of cellulase from mixed organisms. Miscellaneous carbohydrases such as fumaric reductase, succinic dehydrogenase, lactyl-coenzyme A dehydrase and lactic dehydrogenase have been isolated by Baldwin and Palmquist (1965).

With respect to protozoa, Mould and Thomas (1958) demonstrated that *Isotricha* and *Dasytricha* produced α-amylase. Howard (1958) found that extracts of mixed *I. intesinalis* and *I. prostona* contained very little maltase, a trace of cellobiase and small amounts of β-glucosidase and moderate amounts of maltase. Neither genus yielded extracts able to hydrolyze lactose, melibiose, trehalose or xylobiose. Sucrose, raffinose, inulin and a bacterial levan were all hydrolyzed. Abou Akkada and Howard (1961) found that *Entodinium caudatum* extracts contained no pectin esterase or polygalcturonase activity. Extracts of mixed *Isotricha* species or *Dasytricha ruminatium* decomposed pectin or polygalcturonic acid, principally to oligouronides. Bailey (1958) found that extracts of *Epidinium ecaudatum* contained amylase, maltase and, possibly, cellobiase. When exposed to starch, the reaction product was mainly maltose with some glucose and maltotriose. Intact starch granules from red clover were hydrolyzed but not those from potato starch. Further studies on this organism by Bailey et al (1962), Bailey and Howard (1963a, 1963b) and Bailey and Gaillard (1965) demonstrated that it could hydrolyze plant hemicellulose, α-galactosides, isomaltose and β-linked glucose polymers.

Coleman (1964) demonstrated with ^{14}C-labeled carbohydrates that very little carbon from starch, maltose or glucose was incorporated into cellular material by *Entodinium caudatum,* although soluble starch and glucose were incorporated into storage starch. Further research on this species (Coleman, 1969) showed that it hydrolyzed starch to maltose and glucose; that the amount of sugars in the medium had a controlling effect on the hydrolysis of starch, being inhibitory at higher levels. Studies with *Eudipolodinium medium* show that it did not metabolize sugars, but utilized starch and had high activity on hemicellulose; xylanase was purified from cell-free extracts (Naga and el-Shazly, 1968).

It might be noted that some caution is required in interpreting data from these experiments where enzymes have been extracted. If an extract does hydrolyze a specific substrate, it is reasonably safe to conclude that the cell has the same function; however, if no activity is detected, it may not, necessarily, be correct to conclude that the reaction does not occur inside the cell since disruption of the cell and other manipulations may have resulted in inactivation of the enzyme.

Optimum pH Values

The pH of a medium is known to have a marked effect on enzyme activity. In the case of rumen organisms, it might be of interest to list some of the observed results on pH optima of various carbohydrases from different sources. These are shown in Table 12-4.

The optimal pH of most of these enzymes would appear to be within the normal range of rumen pH with the exception of the two enzymes studied by Abou Akkada and Howard (1961); in this case, the methods used may have been responsible for the apparent high estimates of pH optima. Thus, low rumen pH, except in situations such as acute indigestion, would not appear to be a limiting factor as far as the carbohydrases are concerned.

Factors Influencing Carbohydrate Fermentation

Quite a number of factors have been demonstrated to influence the extent of carbohydrate fermentation and the end products produced. The example shown previously from Satter et al (1964) indicating an effect due to feedstuffs fed the host (with a resultant modification of the flora and fauna) is one factor that has been shown by a number of laboratories including reports by Eusebio et al (1959), Church and Petersen (1960), and Donefer et al (1961) as well as many others. These papers indicate, essentially, that adaptation of rumen micro-organisms to a ration has a marked effect on the metabolism of nutrients in that ration.

With respect to readily available carbohydrates — sugars, starches, nonfibrous polysaccharides, there is no reason to believe that these compounds are not readily utilized, providing some vital nutrient is not absent and that the rumen microbial population is adapted to the particular compound in question.

Only limited amounts of glucose or other free sugars are present in rumen fluid (Takashashi and Nakamura, 1968; Walker and Monk, 1971). In vitro data (Sutton, 1968, 1969), where different sugars were added at rates equivalent to 200 g/hr for 8 hr for rumen infusions in cows, indicate that 97-100% of sucrose, glucose and fructose were

Table 12-4.   The pH optima for various rumen carbohydrases.

Source of enzyme	Enzyme	Optimum pH	Literature source
Mixed bacteria	cellulase	5.5	Kitts and Underkofler (1954)
Cell-free rumen fluid	cellulase	5.5-6.0	Stanley and Kesler (1959)
Rumen microorganisms	hemicellulase	6.0	Walker and Hopgood (1961)
Ruminococcus albus	produced epimer of cellobiose	6.5-7.0	Tyler and Leatherwood (1966)
Streptococcus bovis	α-galactosidase	5.6-6.3	Bailey (1963)
Lactobacillus bifidus	isomaltodextrinase	5.5-6.5	Bailey and Roberton (1962)
Dasytricha ruminantium	maltase	5.5	Bailey and Howard (1963b)
Entodinium caudatum	maltase	5.7-6.1	Bailey and Howard (1963b)
Isotricha sp	polygalacturonase	8.7-9.9	Abou Akkada and Howard (1961)
	pectinesterase	8.6-8.8	
Epidinium ecaudatum	α-amylase	5.3-6.5	Bailey (1958)
	α-galactosidase	5.0-5.5	Bailey and Howard (1963a)
	maltase	6.7	Bailey and Howard (1963b)
	isomaltase	6.0	Bailey and Howard (1963a)
	hemicellulase	5.8-6.2	Bailey et al (1962)
	xylobiase	5.8-6.2	
Eudiplodinium medium	xylanase	7.5	Naga and el-Shazly (1968)

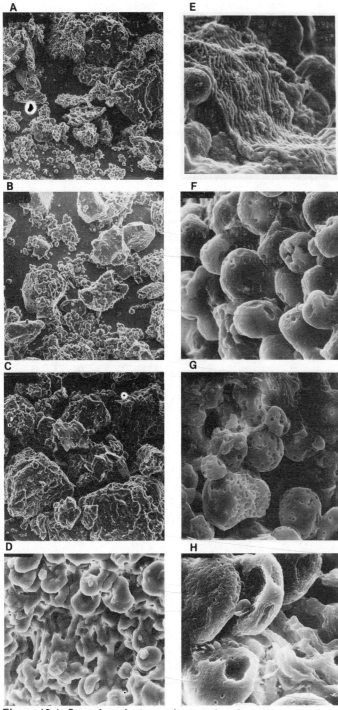

Figure 12-1. Scanning electron micrographs of cereal starch. Left. A,B,C, ground corn, milo and wheat, respectively [75X]. In C note lack of individual starch granules seen in A and B. D, gelatinized starch granules of steam-flaked milo [390X]. Right. E, split corn kernal exposed to rumen bacteria of steer on high-roughage ration [1080X]. F, soft endosperm starch of split corn exposed to rumen bacteria of steer on high-concentrate ration [2040X]. G, soft endosperm of split milo kernel exposed to rumen contents of steer on high-concentrate ration [870X]. H, wheat starch in split kernal exposed to rumen contents of steer on high-concentrate ration [1000X]. E, courtesy of A.B. Davis and L.H. Harbers. All others, L.H. Harbers, Kansas State University.

fermented within 2 hr, but only 42-56% of other sugars (galactose, xylose, arabinose). VFA produced varied with the sugar source (as indicated previously), clearly indicating that results obtained with soluable carbohydrates should not be extrapolated to studies with polysaccharides without evidence of comparable fermentation patterns. Other recent papers giving data on rumen fermentation of soluable or readily available carbohydrates include those of Marty and Sutherland (1970), Danilenko and Mirosnki (1971), Bolduan et al (1972) and Vuyst et al (1972, 1973).

With readily available carbohydrates there is ample evidence that feed preparatory methods, involving moist heat accompanied by flaking, result in more rapid and complete fermentation of cereal grains and resultant changes in VFA ratios. These effects are apparently caused by some fragmentation of the starch granules and by partial hydrolysis of the starch molecules (Frederick et al, 1968, 1973, Osman et al, 1966; Holmes et al, 1970).

It is well known that starch from different sources has different physical characteristics. Recent studies on rumen digestion of starches from the sorghum grain (waxy, yellow endosperm, bird resistant varieties), indicate different modes of attack on the starch (Fig. 12-1) depending on the type (Davis and Harbers, 1974). Surface attack on the waxy starch was mainly point hydrolysis with alternate layers digested inside the starch granule. Yellow endosperm starch was digested without structural resistance, and the bird resistant starch showed a mixture of both types of hydrolysis on the surface with preferential layer digestion internally.

In the case of fibrous carbohydrates, a number of factors other than nutrient deficiencies, etc., are known to influence the rate and/or completeness of rumen utilization (see Kistner, 1965, for details). For example, Balch and Johnson (1950) found that the rate of digestion of cotton thread in the rumen was more rapid in the ventral than in the dorsal rumen sac. Furthermore, the rate of breakdown was found to be indirectly related to the dry matter content of the surrounding digesta, and the authors suggested that this may be a factor explaining the reduced digestion of ground hay, which tends to result in higher rumen dry matter content (it would also result in more rapid rumen turnover time).

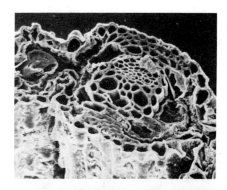

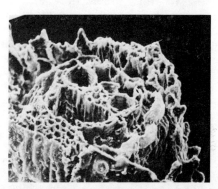

Figure 12-3. Scanning electron micrographs showing cross sections of Coastal Bermudagrass leaves. Top, leaf section incubated without rumen microorganisms. Bottom, leaf section fermented with rumen microorganisms for 12 hr. Note the degradation that has occurred as a result of rumen fermentation. Upper photo, ca. 425X; lower, ca. 400X. Courtesy of D.E. Akin, USDA, ARS, Athens, Ga.

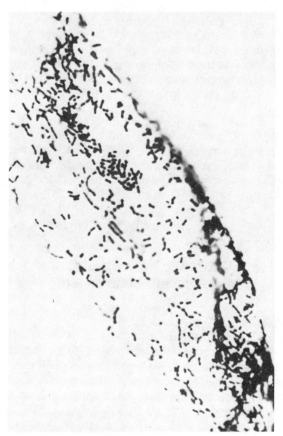

Figure 12-2. Cells of a pure culture of *Ruminococcus flavefaciens* illustrating close attachment to cotton fiber. After Sijpesteijn [1949], Courtesy of R.E. Hungate.

The physical nature of fibrous feedstuffs has been shown to have an appreciable effect on rumen fermentation. Baker et al (1959) found that the susceptibility of purified celluloses to hydrolysis could be related to differences in X-ray diffractometer patterns; differences that were not due to particle size or degree of polymerization of the cellulose.

Church and Petersen (1960) and Dehority and Johnson (1961) have observed that the particle size of forage influences cellulose digestion in vitro, perhaps partly due to an initial higher rate of attack on the smaller particles (Dehority, 1961).

Although it is assumed that cellulase and hemicellulase enzymes are primarily extra-cellular (Hungate, 1966), it is also evident that most cellulolytic organisms are found in close proximity to fibrous material in the rumen (Fig. 12-2), resulting in gradual hydrolysis and disolution of digestible plant fiber as illustrated in Fig. 12-3.

There are many reports in the literature indicating that maturity of forage results in reduced utilization of fibrous carbohydrates, but the subject is far from completely understood. It is also well known that the lignin content of forage generally increases with maturity. Van Soest (1973) points out that availability of native celluloses varies from 0-100%, depending on factors such as the crystallinity of cellulose, its association with lignin, cutin, and silica. In addition, the characteristics of cellulose vary widely among plant species and ratios of hemicellulose and proportions of lignin and cellulose differ. Van Soest also goes on to point out, since some cellulose is relatively available and some is not in the same plant tissue, that cellulose cannot be regarded as a single substance.

Wilkins (1972) has shown that potential cellulose digestibility in grasses, as determined by long-term fermentation, decreases in the order of: leaf blade, inflorescence, leaf sheath, and stem. Lignified tissue, which increased with age, did so mainly through an increase in the number of sclerenchyma cells, but was also affected by the formation of cavities between the vascular bundles in leaf blades of one species and in leaf sheaths of all species studied. Other work indicates that incomplete digestion of hemicelluloses in the rumen is due to physical protection (by lignin) rather than to structural differences between different components of the hemicelluloses (Beveridge and Richards, 1973). There was no difference between rates of digestion of branched and linear hemicelluloses. Smith et al (1972) point out that cell wall digestion rates were more highly correlated with soluble dry matter percentage than with lignin percentage. Legumes were higher in percentage of soluble dry matter and lignin and lower in hemicellulose than grasses. Legume cell walls were also more lignified and less digestible, but were digested at faster rates than grass cell walls. Waldo et al (1972) also suggest that lignin influences the amount of digestion, but increasing lignin content did not slow rate of digestion.

In studies with red clover, ca. 40% of the clover hemicellulose was undigested in the rumen of sheep (Bailey and Macrae, 1970) and little of this was digested post-ruminally, although cecal microflora yielded enzyme extracts capable of hydrolyzing isolated hemicellulose, but not hemicellulose from undelignified digesta.

Not to be overlooked is the possibility that some plants may contain inhibitors of one kind or another. Sidhu and Pfander (1968) have implicated orchard grass (*Dactylis glomerata*) as containing cellulose inhibitors and Autry et al (1973) have also found that *Serala sericea* may also contain cellulose inhibitors.

There appear to be complementary effects between different rumen microorganisms. In work in Dehority's laboratory (Dehority and Scott, 1967; Coen and Dehority, 1970), it has been observed that there were marked differences in the ability of different purified strains of *Ruminococcus, Bacteroides* and *Butyrivibrio* organisms to digest forage cellulose or hemicellulose and marked differences on the digestion of cellulose or hemicellulose from different plant sources. They observed that strains of *B. ruminicola*, which digested hemicellulose but not cellulose, resulted in a marked increase in cellulose digestion when combined with any of four cellulolytic organisms. Perhaps this is an indication that attack by a variety of organisms is required for rapid or complete digestion; those digesting cellulose could be removing tissue that is inhibitory to the hemicellulose digesters and vice versa. Dehority (1973) also points out that some organisms may degrade hemicellulose, but may not have the capability of utilizing isolated hemicellulose. Definite synergism was observed with intact forages when an organism which degraded hemicellulose but did not utilize it was combined with an organism which utilized isolated hemicellulose but had limited capability of degrading it.

Metabolic Pathways of Carbohydrate Metabolism

Although a detailed discussion of the metabolic pathways of carbohydrate metabolism is beyond the scope of this text, a simplified presentation might be in order. Shown in Fig. 12-4 are the commonly accepted routes believed to be prevalent in the rumen. For further details on this topic see the review article by Baldwin (1965).

The relative importance of these various pathways is unknown except under rather specific in vitro conditions. The pathway may be influenced by the relative amounts of various carbohydrates present (Satter et al, 1967), the utilization of end products of one organism as a substrate by another, and the relative importance of microbial polysaccharides (Baldwin, 1965). The complexity of the problem might be compared to a study of the utilization of glucose when administered orally or intravenously. Otagaki et al (1963) have done this with labeled glucose and found a much different labeling pattern

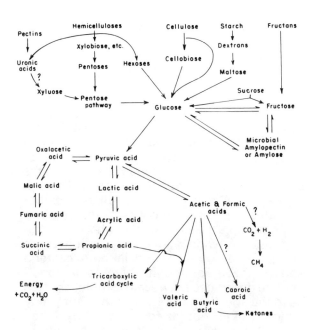

Figure 12-4. Commonly accepted metabolic pathways of carbohydrate metabolism in the rumen.

in milk constituents when the two methods were compared, presumably due to a much greater production of VFA by rumen fermentation than by tissue metabolism and due to a different pattern of VFA production.

It might be appropriate to use some specific examples to illustrate the effect of certain factors on various metabolic pathways. When Satter et al (1964) investigated the fermentation of cellulose and hemicellulose (see Table 12-3), they degraded labeled propionic acid produced, and from the data obtained, calculated that 92 and 82%, respectively, was formed from dicarboxylic acids (succinate pathway) when hay inoculum was used to ferment cellulose and hemicellulose. Comparable values for grain-hay inoculum were 83 and 77%, respectively. Blackburn and Hungate (1963) also found that succinic acid was the major precursor of propionic acid in the rumen, and Baldwin et al (1963) reported that the amount of propionate formed via acrylic acid increased when carbohydrate intake in the diet was increased. A more recent paper by Satter et al (1967) indicated that 82% of the propionate was formed via the succinate pathway from hay ingesta as compared to 63% from grain ingesta. The addition of sodium lactate to the media with either grain or hay inocula resulted in a marked increase in molar percentage of butyrate — a change that was considered to be direct evidence of

the effect which ration constituents could have on metabolic routes. In the case of lactic acid, Bruno and Moore (1962) estimated that 35% of the ^{14}C from lactic acid was converted to acetic acid, 33% was recovered in ether-extracted aqueous residues and 9% in propionate. The remainder was distributed in other fatty acids and fermentation gases. The production of lactic acid was stimulated by adding alfalfa meal to the ration or by glucose or heated starch. When using ^{14}C-labeled glucose, Feaster (1968) found that 86% of the label recovered in ether extract of rumen fluid was in acetic acid, 13-25% was in a solid precipitate, and 11-17% in CO_2. More recent experiments (Walker and Monk, 1971) showed that most of the label from glucose was recovered in acetate when small amounts were added to in vitro fermentations. If, however, a relatively large amount was introduced, then there was a marked increase in propionate production. Removal of protozoa resulted, in one experiment, in a reduction of label in butyrate.

Baldwin et al (1962) found that the major amount of lactic acid was synthesized via acrylate, but this could be increased by using rumen inoculum from cattle given more carbohydrate or lactic acid in the diet. A later paper from the same laboratory (Palmquist and Baldwin, 1966) indicated that the proportion of concentrates in the diet affected the relative activities of a number of enzymes required for normal metabolic activities as well as resulting in greater butyrate production.

Microbial Polysaccharides

Information on the quantitative deposition of microbial polysaccharides or other carbohydrates by rumen microorganisms seems to be in rather short supply although some information is available. Smith and Baker (1944) reported that rumen bacteria contained about 47% polysaccharide (dry basis) and McNaught et al (1950) found about 40% in their preps. Masson and Oxford (1951) observed that they could recover about 1 g of polysaccharide per kg of rumen contents from holotrich protozoa obtained from sheep fed primarily on hay. The polysaccharide was characterized as an amylopectin by these authors. A number of the holotrich protozoa deposit storage polysaccharide following ingestion of soluble carbohydrates; *Isotricha* and various oligotrichs can be observed rapidly depositing storage polysaccharides after ingesting starches (Oxford, 1955). Steyert and Emery (1965) observed that mixed protozoa stored about 20 times as much labeled glucose as did bacteria, thus indicating that the protozoa are much more important for the host as a potential source of microbial polysaccharide.

Gibbons et al (1955) found that rumen bacteria could utilize either D-xylose or D-glucose to synthesize a storage polysaccharide containing only D-glucose. The compound was believed to be of the starch-glycogen class but no definite proof was obtained on this. It is known (Hungate et al, 1955; Bailey and Oxford, 1958) that a number of bacteria produce dextrans which form slime under some conditions. Heald (1951) found that microbial carbohydrates also included quantities of arabinose, xylose, ribose and rahmnose in addition to glucose, and Thomas (1960) has indicated that bacteria or holotrich protozoa converted about 30-32% of sucrose or fructan from grass to storage polysaccharides.

In studies with mixed rumen organisms, Walker (1968) observed that ca. 80% of the energy from glucose, maltose, cellobiose and xylose was used for polysaccharide synthesis, depending upon the assumptions made in the calculations. It might be pointed out that the sugars added were said to supply < 10% of total energy available to the organisms. In studies with sheep fed hay or restricted hay and glucose, Hobson and Thompson (1970) recovered only small amounts of polysaccharides (56 mg/100 ml). These contained rahmnose, starch-like polysaccharides and xylose polymers. When resting or growing cell suspensions were incubated with sugars, Thompson and Hobson (1971) noted rapid synthesis of intracellular polysaccharide. Relative to glucose, other compounds were used to synthesize polysaccharides in the order of: sucrose, 80%; fructose, 75%; soluble starch 19%; maltose, 7%; cellobiose, 4%; and xylose, 2%. No microbial starch was formed from galacturonic, acetic, propionic, butyric, lactic or succinic acids. The utilization of microbial starch and lactic acid, formation of which often accompanied starch synthesis, gave rise to VFA in a ratio similar to that from fermentation of glucose. The maximum amount of starch, in cultures with an excess of glucose, amounted to 25 g/day in the sheep's rumen.

Summary

Carbohydrates represent the most important organic nutrient presented to rumen microorganisms on a quantitative basis, accounting for about 75% of plant tissues. Data published from a variety of sources indicate that all plant carbohydrates are metabolized by rumen microbes although the soluble and readily available carbohydrates are, for the most part, metabolized at more rapid rates than the fibrous carbohydrates. A wide variety of carbohydrase enzymes have been found in both bacteria and protozoa, although there is a considerable difference between microbial species as to the specific carbohydrate that they may attack. The pH optima for the carbohydrases studied would not appear to be a limiting factor with regard to carbohydrate utilization with the possible exception of the very acid conditions that may develop during acute indigestion. Solubility and physical nature of carbohydrates would appear to be the principal factors affecting rate or completeness of utilization, although adaptation to a given carbohydrate is certainly important at times. Carbohydrates may be metabolized to a variety of end products. Several reports indicate that a substantial amount of labeled carbon may be utilized to synthesize cellular protein; labels may also be recovered in the form of storage polysaccharide, the VFA, carbon dioxide and methane, or any of a variety of other compounds. Data on microbial polysaccharides indicate that only moderate amounts may be passed into the lower GIT.

References Cited

Abou Akkada, A.R. and B.H. Howard. 1960. Biochem. J. 76:445.
Abou Akkada, A.R. and B.H. Howard. 1961. Biochem. J. 78:512.
Autrey, K.M., T.A. McCaskey and J.A. Little. 1973. J. Dairy Sci. 56:643 (abstr).
Bailey, R.W. 1958. N.Z. J. Agr. Res. 1:809.
Bailey, R.W. 1963. Biochem. J. 86:509.
Bailey, R.W., R.T.J. Clarke and D.E. Wright. 1962. Biochem. J. 83:517.
Bailey, R.W. and B.H. Howard. 1963a. Biochem. J. 87:146.
Bailey, R.W. and B.H. Howard. 1963b. Biochem. J. 86:446.
Bailey, R.W. and B.D.E. Gaillard. 1965. Biochem. J. 95:758.
Bailey, R.W. and J.C. Macrae. 1970. J. Agr. Sci. 75:321.
Bailey, R.W. and A.E. Oxford. 1958. J. Gen. Microbiol. 19:130.
Bailey, R.W. and A.M. Roberton. 1962. Biochem. J. 82:272.
Baker, T.I., et al. 1959. J. Animal Sci. 18:655.
Balch, C.C. and V.W. Johnson. 1950. Br. J. Nutr. 4:389.
Baldwin, R.L. 1965. In: Physiology of Digestion in the Ruminant. Butterworths, London.
Baldwin, R.L. and D.L. Palmquist. 1965. Appl. Microbiol. 13:194.
Baldwin, R.L., W.A. Wood and R.S. Emery. 1962. J. Bact. 83:907.
Baldwin, R.L., W.A. Wood and R.S. Emery. 1963. J. Bact. 85:1346.
Barnett, A.J.G. and R.L. Reid. 1957. J. Agr. Sci. 49:180.
Barnett, A.J.G. and R.L. Reid. 1961. Reactions in the Rumen. Edward Arnold LTD.
Bath, I.H. and M.H. Head. 1961. J. Agr. Sci. 56:131.
Beveridge, R.J. and G.N. Richards. 1973. Carbohydrate Res. 29:79.
Blackburn, T.H. and R.E. Hungate. 1963. Appl. Microbiol. 11:132.
Boulduan, G., J. Voigt, B. Piatkowski and H. Steger. 1972. Nutr. Abstr. Rev. 42:311.
Bruno, C.F. and W.E.C. Moore. 1962. J. Dairy Sci. 45:109.
Bryant, M.J. 1970. In: Dukes' Physiology of Domestic Animals. 8th ed. Comstock Publ. Assoc., Ithaca, N.Y.
Cheng, K.J., G.A. Jones, F.J. Simpson and M.P. Bryant. 1969. Can. J. Microbiol. 15:1365.
Church, D.C. and R.G. Petersen. 1960. J. Dairy Sci. 43:81.
Clarke, R.T.J., R.W. Bailey and B.D.E. Gaillard. 1969. J. Gen. Microbiol. 56:79.
Coen, J.A. and B.A. Dehority. 1970. Appl. Microbiol. 20:362.
Coleman, G.S. 1964. J. Gen. Microbiol. 35:91.
Coleman, G.S. 1969. J. Gen. Microbiol. 57:303.
Czerkawski, J.W. and G. Breckenridge. 1969. Br. J. Nutr. 23:925.
Danilenko, I.A. and I.A. Mirosnki. 1971. Nutr. Abstr. Rev. 41:1093.
Davis, A.B. and L.H. Harbers. 1974. J. Animal Sci. 38:900.
Dehority, B.A. 1961. J. Dairy Sci. 44:687.
Dehority, B.A. 1966. J. Bacteriol. 91:1724.
Dehority, B.A. 1973. Fed. Proc. 32:1819.
Dehority, B.A. and R.R. Johnson. 1961. J. Dairy Sci. 44:2242.
Dehority, B.A. and H.W. Scott. 1967. J. Dairy Sci. 50:1136.
Doetsch, R.N., R.O. Robinson, R.E. Brown and J.C. Shaw. 1953. J. Dairy Sci. 36:825.
Donefer, E., L.E. Lloyd and E.W. Crampton. 1961. J. Animal Sci. 20:959 (abstr).
Eusebio, A.N. et al. 1959. J. Dairy Sci. 42:692.
Feaster, W.H. 1968. Dissert. Abstr. 29:1102B.
Festenstein, G.N. 1959. Biochem. J. 72:75.
Frederick, H.M., B. Theurer and W.H. Hale. 1968. Proc. West. Sec. Amer. Soc. Animal Sci. 19:91.
Frederick, H.M., B. Theurer and W.H. Hale. 1973. J. Dairy Sci. 56:595.
Gibbons, R.J., R.N. Doetsch and H.C. Shaw. 1955. J. Dairy Sci. 38:1147.
Gillard, B.D.E., R.W. Bailey and R.T.J. Clarke. 1965. J. Agr. Sci. 64:449.
Gradel, C.M. and B.A. Dehority. 1972. Appl. Microbiol. 23:332.
Gray, F.V. and A.F. Pilgrim. 1952. Nature. 170:375.
Heald, P.J. 1951. Br. J. Nutr. 5:75; 84; 92.
Heald, P.J. 1952. Biochem. J. 50:503.
Heald, P.J. 1953. Br. J. Nutr. 7:124.
Hobson, P.N. and M. MacPherson. 1952. Biochem. J. 52:671.
Hobson, P.N. and M.R. Purdom. 1961. J. Appl. Bact. 24:188.
Hobson, P.N. and J.K. Thompson. 1970. J. Agr. Sci. 75:471.
Holmes, J.H.G., M.J. Drennan and W.N. Garrett. 1970. J. Animal Sci. 31:409.
Howard, B.H. 1957. Biochem. J. 67:643.
Howard, B.H. 1958. Biochem. J. 71:675.
Howard, B.H., G. Jones and M.R. Purdom. 1960. Biochem. J. 74:173.
Hungate, R.E. 1966. The Rumen and Its Microbes. Academic Press.
Hungate, R.E., D.W. Fletcher, R.W. Dougherty and B.F. Barrentine. 1955. Appl. Microbiol. 3:161.
Johns, A.T. 1953. N.Z. J. Sci. Tech. 35:262.
King, K.W. 1959. J. Dairy Sci. 42:1848.
Kistner, A. 1965. In: Physiology of Digestion in the Ruminant, Butterworths.

Kistner, A., L. Gouws and F.M.C. Gilchrist. 1962. J. Agr. Sci. 59:85.
Knox, K. 1966. J. Dairy Sci. 49:715 (abstr).
Kubo, T. and M. Kandatsu. 1969. Nutr. Abstr. Rev. 39:1241.
Leatherwood, J.M. 1965. Appl. Microbiol. 13:771.
Marty, R.J., and T.M. Sutherland. 1970. Revista Cubana Cien. Agr. 4:45.
Masson, F.M. and A.E. Oxford. 1951. J. Gen. Microbiol. 5:664.
McNaught, M.L. 1951. Biochem. J. 49:325.
McNaught, M.L., J.A.B. Smith, K.M. Henry and S.K. Kon. 1950. Biochem. J. 46:32.
Mould, D.L. and O.J. Thomas. 1958. Biochem. J. 69:327.
Naga, M.A. and K. el-Shazly. 1968. J. Gen. Microbiol. 53:305.
Nasr, H. 1950. J. Agr. Sci. 40:308.
Osman, H.F., B. Theurer, W.H. Hale and S.M. Mehen. 1966. Proc. West. Sec. Amer. Soc. Animal Sci. 17:271.
Otagaki, K.K., et al. 1963. J. Dairy Sci. 46:690.
Oxford, A.E. 1955. Expt. Parasitol. 4:569.
Packett, L.W. and J.R. Fordham. 1965. J. Animal Sci. 24:488.
Palmquist, D.L. and R.L. Baldwin. 1966. Appl. Microbiol. 14:60.
Pazur, J.H., E.W. Shuey and C.E. Georgi. 1958. Arch. Biochem. Biophys, 77:387.
Peel, J.L. 1960. Biochem. J. 64:525.
Phillipson, A.T. and R.A. McAnally. 1942. J. Expt. Biol. 19:199.
Pradhan, K. and R.W. Kemken. 1970. J. Dairy Sci. 53:1739.
Prins, R.A. 1971. J. Bacteriol. 105:820.
Satter, L.D., J.W. Suttie and B.R. Baumgardt. 1964. J. Dairy Sci. 47:1365.
Satter, L.D., J.W. Suttie and B.R. Baumgardt. 1967. J. Dairy Sci. 50:1626.
Sidhu, K.S. and W.H. Pfander. 1968. J. Dairy Sci. 51:1042.
Slyter, L.L. and J.M. Weaver. 1971. Appl. Microbiol. 22:930.
Smith, J.A.B. and F. Baker. 1944. Biochem. J. 38:496.
Smith, L.W., H.K. Goering and C.H. Gordon. 1972. J. Dairy Sci. 55:1140.
Smith, W.R., I. Yu and R.E. Hungate. 1973. J. Bacteriol. 114:729.
Stanley, R.W. and E.M. Kessler. 1959. J. Dairy Sci. 42:127.
Steyert, D.H. and R.S. Emery. 1965. J. Animal Sci. 24:904 (abstr).
Sutton, J.D. 1968. Br. J. Nutr. 22:689.
Sutton, J.D. 1969. Br. J. Nutr. 23:567.
Takahashi, R. and K. Nakamura. 1968. Agr. Biol. Chem. 33:619.
Thomas, G.J. 1960. J. Agr. Sci. 54:360.
Thompson, J.K. and P.N. Hobson. 1971. J. Agr. Sci. 76:423.
Underkofler, L.A., W.D. Kitts and R.L. Smith. 1953. Arch. Biochem. Biophys. 44:492.
Van Soest, P.J. 1973. Fed. Proc. 32:1804.
Vantcheva, Z.M., K. Pradhan and R.W. Hemken. 1970. J. Dairy Sci. 53:1511.
Vuyst, A.D., et al. 1972. Nutr. Abstr. Rev. 42:339.
Vuyst, A.D., D. Jaramillo, M. Vanbelle and R. Arnould. 1973. Nutr. Abstr. Rev. 43:957.
Waldo, D.R. and L.H. Schultz. 1960. J. Dairy Sci. 43:496.
Waldo, D.R., L.W. Smith and E.L. Cox. 1972. J. Dairy Sci. 55:125.
Walker, D.J. 1968. Appl. Microbiol. 16:1672.
Walker, D.J. and M.F. Hopgood. 1961. Aust. J. Agr. Res. 12:651.
Walker, D.J. and P.R. Monk. 1971. Appl. Microbiol. 22:741.
Walker, G.J. and P.M. Hope. 1964. Biochem. J. 90:398.
Wilkins, R.J. 1972. J. Agr. Sci. 78:457.
Wojciechowicz, M. 1972. Acta. Microbiologica Polonica 4:189.
Wright, D.E. 1961. N.Z. J. Agr. Res. 4:203.
Wright, D.E. 1969. N.Z. J. Agr. Res. 12:281.
Wright, D.E. 1971. Appl. Microbiol. 21:165.

CHAPTER 13 — RUMEN METABOLISM OF NITROGENOUS COMPOUNDS

Metabolism of nitrogenous compounds by rumen microorganisms has received an appreciable amount of attention by numerous scientists interested in either the microorganism or the ruminant animal. Review articles on this topic that would be recommended include Phillipson (1964), Hungate (1966, pp 281-330), some of the papers in the book edited by Briggs (1967), Waldo (1968), Allison (1969), Smith (1969) and some of the papers in Federation Proceedings (1970, pp 33-54). Due to the large volume of literature on this subject, the papers reviewed in this chapter will be very selective.

Nitrogenous Compounds in the Rumen

The variety of nitrogenous compounds presented to rumen microorganisms is quite large. Such compounds will include proteins of a varied nature which differ markedly in solubility and amino acid content, nuclear proteins containing a variety of pyrimidine and purine bases, many different nonprotein-nitrogen compounds such as amino acids, peptides, amides, amines, volatile amines, ammonium salts, nitrates and nitrites, as well as compounds such as urea and biuret which may be included intentionally in ruminant rations. Natural feedstuffs vary widely in the amount of total N found as NPN compounds. The range is said to vary from 4-5% in some seeds to as high as 60-75% in some unwilted silages (Waldo, 1968). Fertilization will affect the amount of soluble N in grasses and the seasonal changes in plant compounds, no doubt, result in marked changes in the nature and solubility of the nitrogenous components. The consequence of this diversity is that N metabolism in the reticulo-rumen may vary considerably due to environmental influences.

Concentrations of various nitrogenous compounds in the rumen are, obviously, quite variable. Ranges found include: 0.1-1.5 mg% as free amino acids; 0.2-1.0 mg% as diffusible peptides; 0-130 mg% ammonia N; 100-400 mg% protein N, and 1.5-40 mg% as nucleotide N (Johns, 1955; Lewis, 1955, 1957; Annison, 1956; Williams and Christian, 1956; Ellis and Pfander, 1965; Smith and McAllan, 1970).

It has been estimated by Weller et al (1958) that the microbes in the rumen contain between 63 and 81% of the N. Blackburn and Hobson (1960b) found 47-77% in protozoa and bacteria, and Weller et al suggest that 54-74% of the total N is found in rumen liquid. The amount found in the microbes will vary, obviously, with the amount of N in the diet, solubility of the protein, and time after feeding (Blackburn and Hobson, 1960b).

Ammonia is also quite variable, typical values for ammonia N being on the order of 10-50 mg% (Lewis, 1955, 1957; Ciszuk, 1973; numerous other papers). The amount of ammonia found is largely a reflection of N content of the feed, solubility and the rapidity with which N-containing compounds are attacked. An example of diurnal variation in rumen ammonia of sheep fed different diets is shown in Fig. 13-1; the values represent means for two sheep on each diet.

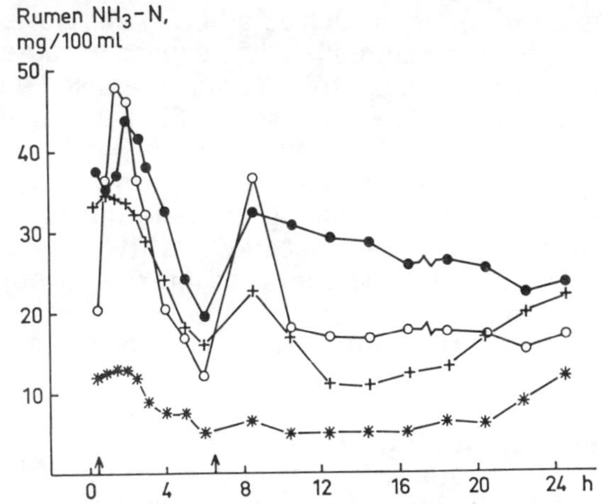

Figure 13-1. Diurnal variations in the NH_3-N content of rumen fluid on 4 different rations. * grass hay, low crude protein; + high temperature dried grass, high crude protein; • hay, grain and soy meal; o hay, grain and urea. Feeding times are marked with an arrow. ⁄⁄ interval of 1 day. From Ciszuk [1973].

Free amino acids are found in the rumen only in very limited quantities, although the concentration tends to vary with diet (Gutowski et al, 1960; Hoshima and Hirose, 1964; Prokudin, 1967). Leibholz (1969) found the maximum amino acid N in the rumen was reached 60 min after feeding as compared to 90-130 min for ammonia. The amount present in the rumen was related to dietary protein intake, although the proportions of the individual free amino acids were relatively constant. In centrifuged rumen fluid, Harmeyer (1972) found total N to be between 8.3 and 20.2 mg%. The different fractions varied but were on average: ammonia, 15%; peptide N, 14%; amino acids, 8%; and residual N, 63%. Amino acid N content rose with time after feeding and the peptide fraction fell slightly. Harmeyer also identified 18 amino acids in free form, concentrations ranging from 0.1 to 1.0 mg%. Those present in highest concentrations were aspartic and glutamic acids, alanine, ornithine and lysine. No tryptophan was found. He also noted 40 unidentified ninhydrin-positive peaks when using column chromatography to separate the amino acids.

Catabolism of Ingested Proteins

In order to utilize large molecules such as intact plant proteins, it is necessary to degrade them before they can be utilized by microorganisms or by the host's tissues (with exceptions such as globulin absorption in the young animal). With respect to rumen microorganisms, this basic premise has been recognized for some 30 years (see Blackburn, 1965), although experimental proof has been somewhat slow in developing. Factors influencing passage out of the rumen — such as specific gravity, particle size, solubility, and level of intake — would be expected to have an important effect on the amount of protein metabolism that may occur in the rumen.

Proteolytic Activity

The proteolytic bacteria have probably been studied more by Blackburn and colleagues than by anyone else. Blackburn and Hobson (1960a) studied changes of certain nitrogenous compounds in the rumens of sheep fed casein preparations differing in solubility. They found that total N decreased faster than did added PEG (indicated loss via ammonia) and that the decrease was most rapid after meals with the more soluble forms of casein. Protozoal and bacterial N remained relatively constant throughout. Proteolytic activity of rumen

microorganisms varied with the diet, but did not change appreciably after the sheep were fed. In other papers (Blackburn and Hobson, 1960b) they reported that proteolytic activity of rumen fluid from sheep did not depend on the diet but the pH seemed to be a major factor. The optimum pH value for maximum proteolytic activity was between 6 and 7, with an irregular maximum at ca. pH 6.5. The number of culturable proteolytic bacteria was relatively low at all times, although greater after feeding. Abou Akkada and Blackburn (1963) studied bacterial isolates from sheep on a variety of diets and observed that not more than 10% of the culturable species were proteolytic, although Fulghum and Moore (1963) reported that about 38% of culturable bovine rumen organisms had proteolytic activity. More recently, Isaacs and Owens (1971) published data which indicate that extra-cellular enzymes, other than amino peptidase, could hydrolyze protein rapidly, although proteolysis was extremely low in the cell-free fluid.

When using a relatively refined medium, the data obtained are a reflection of the medium utilized and the methods employed to culture the microorganisms. Perhaps a relatively high percentage of rumen organisms may be proteolytic, but they may not be culturable by the methods used.

Research data leaves little doubt that the proteolytic activity of the rumen may be substantial, resulting in hydrolysis of protein to peptides and amino acids and subsequent deamination of a high percentage of the amino acids to ammonia and organic acids. For example, Hogan and Weston (1967) found in sheep that up to 25% of the N was lost between the diet and duodenal digesta. In sheep which were fed alfalfa hay or pellets, Pilgrim et al (1969) estimated that 23-27% of dietary N in alfalfa hay was converted to ammonia as compared to 17% from the pellets; 59-66% of the ammonia N was absorbed from the rumen and the remainder passed into the omasum. In another study based on relatively long-term infusion of ^{15}N-labeled ammonia, Mathison and Milligan (1971) concluded that 50-65% of bacterial N and 31-55% of protozoal N were derived from rumen ammonia; that 60-92% of the dietary N, which was chopped hay or barley and chopped hay, was transformed into ammonia in the rumen; also, that 17-54% of the ammonia was absorbed from the rumen. Nolan and Leng (1972) have used a similar technique with sheep fed chopped alfalfa hay. They calculated that 80% of microbial N was derived from ammonia and 20% more directly from amino acids. Of the dietary N entering the rumen, estimates were that 59% was digested there; 29% of digested N was utilized as amino acids and 71% was degraded to ammonia.

When studying pure cultures, Abou Akkada and Blackburn (1963) examined a number of types of proteolytic bacteria — *Bacteroides amylophilus, B. ruminocola, Butyrivibrio* sp., *Selenomonas ruminatium,* and gram-positive rods and cocci — for enzymes concerned with different proteolytic reactions. Proteolytic activity varied with the strains in each group of bacteria and all possessed exo- and endo-peptidase activity, i.e., enzymes which act to some degree on peptide bonds adjacent to a terminal NH_2 or carboxyl group. Significant deaminase activity was confined to *B. ruminicola* and *S. ruminantium*, but many strains possessed amidase activity. No strain showed significant urease activity. Bladen et al (1961) reported that *Bacteroides ruminicola* was usually the most important ammonia-producing bacterium in cattle, based on the number of strains and the amount of ammonia produced from casein hydrolysates. Other species of probable significance

included *Selenomonas ruminantium, Peptostreptococcus elsdenii* and some strains of *Butyrivibrio.* There appeared to be little difference between rumen contents of different animals examined. In young calves many predominant bacteria produced ammonia. While working with *B. amylophilus*, Blackburn (1968) has determined that protease obtained from it had a broad area of activity between pH 5.5 and 9.5.

With respect to protozoa, Abou Akkada and Howard (1962) reported that suspensions of *Entodinium caudatum* readily hydrolyzed casein yielding peptides and amino acids as the principal products. Ammonia was formed as a result of hydrolysis of amide groups in the casein, but not from deamination of amino acids. However, Warner (1956) thought that ammonia was the end product of N metabolism of mixed suspensions of protozoa and papers by Purser and Moir (1966) and Abou Akkada and el-Shazly (1964), to mention only two, clearly indicate higher concentrations of ammonia in the rumen of animals containing protozoa as compared to defaunated animals. An example of the difference in rumen ammonia between faunated and defaunated animals is shown in Fig. 13-2. Kandatsu and Takahashi (1956) also reported that cultures of *Entodinium* always produced ammonia, so it seems likely that both bacteria and protozoa contribute to the degradation of proteins and the production of end products such as ammonia. Blackburn (1965) states that various proteolytic enzymes have been extracted from protozoa, however, it should be noted that it is almost impossible to grow such organisms free of bacteria, thus there is usually some uncertainty regarding the true source of the enzyme.

There is information on protozoa (see Ch. 11) which indicates that they take up very little N from amino acids. When rumen protozoa had access to either ^{14}C-labeled amino acids or rumen bacteria, Onodera and Kandatsu

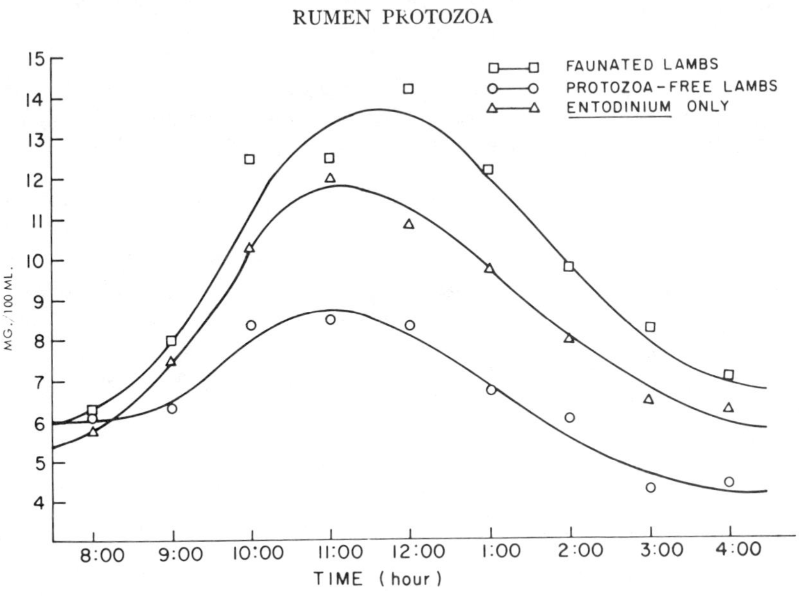

Figure 13-2. Diurnal variation of ammonia in the rumen of faunated and cilate-free lambs. From Christiansen et al [1965]

(1970) found that several amino acids — aspartic acid, valine, alanine, arginine and phenylalanine — were well utilized when incorporated into bacteria, but not when given as the free acid. They concluded that amino acids may not be the main N nutrient for rumen ciliates, but more likely ciliates obtain most of their N directly from rumen bacteria.

Degradation of Amino Acids

el-Shazly (1952) was one of the first to report that degradation of protein by rumen microorganisms resulted in the production of more branched-chain VFA and higher fatty acids as indicated by a correlation between ammonia concentration and concentrations of isobutyric and of the C6 acids. Sirotnak et al (1953) investigated the metabolism of amino acids by mixed suspensions of rumen microorganisms. Of 22 amino acids tested, aspartic, glutamic, serine, arginine, cysteine and cystine were found to be attacked. The principal products detected were CO_2, NH_4 and acetic, propionic and butyric acids. Optimum pH for this activity was about 6.9. Lewis (1955) investigated amino acid metabolism by placing solutions in the rumen of sheep. Data indicated that ammonia production was greatest when DL-glutamic acid was added, followed by glycine, DL-alanine and DL-methionine when the sheep were fed hay. When the sheep were fed hay and casein hydrolysate, the order of ammonia production was DL-alanine, DL-methionine, DL-glutamic acid and glycine. A hay and grass-fed sheep gave different results, also, the order being DL-glutamic acid, DL-methionine, glycine and DL-alanine. Studies with in vitro suspensions indicated that aspartic acid resulted in greatest ammonia production. Amino acids gave rise to VFA, CO_2 and H_2. Mixtures of amino acids were rapidly deaminated with the optimum pH being about 6.5 for ammonia formation.

Lewis and Emery (1962) have also carried out extensive experiments in which solutions of amino acids have been added to the rumen. Rumen ammonia concentrations were the highest 6 hr following arginine administration although tryptophan and lysine yielded smaller, but detectable amounts of ammonia. Arginine yielded ornithine. Lysine administration was accompanied by an increase in Δ-amino valeric acid. Plasma lysine increased markedly after its administration. In another experiment, Lewis and Emery (1962) studied relative deamination rates of amino acids fermented with crude or washed suspensions of rumen organisms. They found that individual amino acids could be divided into three groups with regard to relative rate of deamination. Serine, cysteine, aspartic acid, threonine and arginine were attacked most completely, followed by glutamic acid, phenylalanine, lysine and cystine and those attached least were tryptophan, Δ-amino valeric acid, methionine, alanine, valine, isoleucine, ornithine, histidine, glycine, proline and hydroxyproline. Deamination rates were more rapid and complete in the crude rumen liquor. Mixtures of three or four amino acids were not attacked to any greater degree than the summation of activity for each individual acid. The D and L forms of serine and tryptophan were catabolized at the same relative rates, whereas the D isomers of aspartic acid, lysine, threonine, and phenylalanine were not attacked. Other research (Portugal and Sutherland, 1966) indicates that ^{14}C-labeled glutamic and aspartic acids were rapidly metabolized by sheep rumen fluid. Only a small percentage of the label was recovered in the same amino acid from bacterial protein; the amounts being recovered were about 10 and 4%, respectively, thus indicating that most of these amino acids were degraded by the rumen organisms. Amos et al (1971b) found that proline additions to a medium for washed suspension stimulated digestion of cellulose. It resulted in a marked increase in valeric acid levels with about 47% of the carbon label being recovered in VFA after 24 hr. Other radioactivity was found in the protein and lipid fractions of the bacterial cells.

One recent study shows that aspartic acid, glutamate and arginine were extensively decomposed (90%). Phenolic amino acids were reduced by ca. 50%, but valine, leucine, isoleucine, methionine, alanine and glycine appeared to be relatively stable toward microbial action (Isaacs and Owens, 1971).

In studies where single amino acids were infused into the rumen, Chalmers and Hughs (1969) observed that glycine produced no increase in ruminal ammonia over a 24-hr period and it passed out of the rumen at the same rate as a marker (PEG). Both alanine and lysine resulted in an increase in ruminal ammonia and lysine infusion caused a sharp increase in blood lysine levels. Other reports on lysine (Lord et al, 1972) indicate that ca. 50% was degraded by whole rumen fluid during a 6-hr in vitro incubation and Onodera and Kandatsu (1972) have shown that some L-lysine was converted to pipecolate by rumen ciliates.

Metabolism of tryptophan in the rumen is of interest because some data indicate that large doses of tryptophan or oral doses of 3-methylindole cause pulmonary emphysema in cattle and goats, a disease which appears to be increasing in incidence (Carlson et al, 1972). Candlish et al (1970) have shown rapid absorption of tryptophan from the rumen and Yokoyama and Carlson (1974) found that incubation of L-tryptophan, which was carbon labeled in the ring, resulted in 39% of the label being recovered in skatole, 7% in indole and 4% in indole-acetate. D-tryptophan was not degraded to any of these metabolites. Addition of glucose reduced the formation of both skatole and indole from L-tryptophan as did the addition of antibiotics.

With respect to methionine, Zikakis and Salsbury (1969) published data indicating that methionine is metabolized to S-methyl-L-cysteine and methanethiol. Methionine hydroxy analog has been of interest in recent years as one possible means of improving protein utilization in ruminants. Although some data indicated that the analog was more resistant to rumen degradation than methionine (Belasco, 1972), other data indicate that it is degraded or disappears at about the same rate (Emery, 1971; Gil et al, 1973). Langar et al (1973) show that N-steroyl-DL-methionine is resistant to rumen degradation and suggest its use in ruminant feeds. Older papers dealing with amino acid metabolism by rumen microorganisms include those of Van Den Hende et al (1963, 1964) and Warner (1964).

As mentioned previously, el-Shazly (1952) found that fermentation of amino acids resulted in the formation of some branched-chain fatty acids. Two other papers of interest on this topic might be mentioned. Dehority et al (1958) demonstrated with washed cell suspensions that valine was deaminated and decarboxylated by rumen microorganisms to give rise to isobutyric acid and that proline could give rise to valeric acid. As much as 43% of the ^{14}C label in DL-valine-1-^{14}C was recovered as $^{14}CO_2$. Menahan and Schultz (1964) studied the metabolism of L-leucine and DL-valine and found that these acids resulted in large quantities of isovaleric and isobutyric acids, respectively. References on other examples of degradation are referred to in the section on protein synthesis.

With regard to the nucleotide bases, Jurtshuk et al (1958) demonstrated that rumen organisms could metabolize xanthine, uric acid, guanine and, to a lesser extent, hypoxanthine. VFA and CO_2 were the primary products produced. More recent data show that pure nucleic acids, when added to the rumen, were rapidly degraded (Smith and McAllan, 1970). Other data from this laboratory indicate rapid degradation of RNA, DNA and nucleic acids in hay (McAllan and Smith, 1973). With one species of rumen protozoa, Coleman (1968) demonstrated that they would take up labeled adenine, guanine and uracil into the cell and that there was some interconversion of the nucleic acid bases.

The Value of Protein Degradation in the Rumen

There can be no doubt that soluble proteins can be degraded by rumen micro-organisms with the resultant production of ammonia, VFA, carbon dioxide and other metabolites. However, there is some question as to how much degradation of natural feedstuffs may occur and the value of it. The degradation of proteins is complicated by secretion of urea into the rumen via saliva and of ammonia through the rumen epithelia, absorption of ammonia and other nitrogenous compounds by rumen epithelia, and recycling of bacterial and protozoal proteins in the rumen.

Proteins such as zein from corn are relatively insoluble in rumen liquor as compared to casein (McDonald, 1952; Annison, 1956; Lewis, 1962; Ely et al, 1967). For example, where casein was 92-93% soluble in rumen fluid diluted with buffer, the solubility of isolated proteins from alfalfa, oats, and field beans was 43, 38 and 20%, respectively (Proksova, 1968).

McDonald (1952) and McDonald and Hall (1957) calculated that about 40% zein was converted to microbial protein as compared to 90% of the casein. However, these calculations assumed that all dietary protein left the rumen either as microbial protein or undigested food, that the protein other than zein consisted of microbial protein only, and that the rate of flow of digesta from the abomasum was constant (an unlikely situation). McDonald's data on zein diges-tion did not indicate any increase in rumen ammonia following ingestion. Ely et al (1967) estimated that 24-30% of zein was converted to microbial protein, depending on the ration fed and the method used to estimate the amount of microbial protein and Hume (1970) found that only 13% of zein was degraded. Annison (1956) found with in vitro fermen-tations that casein, arachin and soy protein were readily degraded, but bovine albumin, zein and wheat gluten were less extensively attacked. Data published by Lewis (1962) were similar in this respect. More recently, Mangan (1972) showed that casein was rapidly degraded with a half life of 5.6-21.5 min and up to 43% of the casein N was found as ammonia in rumen fluid. Ammonia formation was also quite rapid when acid-hydrolyzed casein was given via a rumen fistula. However, ovalbumin was degraded slowly with a half life of 175 min, although this was reduced to 132 min after feeding the cattle with ovalbumin for 5 days, thus showing the effect of adaptation.

Some of the differences in solubility and rumen utilization of native plant proteins may be due to the presence of inhibitors in the plant tissue. A paper by Leroy et al (1965) is of interest in that their data indicate that tannin prevented some deamination in in vitro fermentations without interfering with cellulose digestion. Proksova (1969) found, also, that solubility of isolated proteins from alfalfa or field beans was reduced as pH was decreased from 6.7 to 3.75 with acetic acid.

Weller and others (1958) have calculated the conversion of ingested protein to micro-bial protein, basing estimates on the fact that diaminopimelic acid is found in the proteins of bacteria and not in plant or protozoal protein (see later section). When rumen contents of sheep fed wheaten hay were sampled from 2-24 hr after feeding, these authors estimated that 63-82% of the total N was present as microbial N, 11-27% as plant N, and 5-10% as soluble N. In studies with sheep fed forage oats varying in maturity, Hogan and Weston (1969) concluded that appreciable quantities of plant protein must have passed through the stomach, indicating relatively less protein degradation than did Weller et al (1958). In a recent paper reporting results with sub-terranean clover, Hogan (1973) calculated that 60% of the N passing from the stomach was in the form of bacterial cells and

Leibholz (1972) calculated that microbial protein in the rumen and duodenal contents ranged from 43-97% in diets containing alfalfa, casein or wheat gluten. Amos et al (1971a) have also shown that the source of protein in the diet affects the N components in the duodenum. For example, when corn gluten meal provided the supplemental N, total N, protein, essential and nonessential amino acids were higher than when distillers' dried solubles or soybean meal were the supplemental N sources. Thus, these various examples clearly show that the amount of protein degradation in the rumen is affected by diet, solubility of the protein and, no doubt, by other factors such as level of intake and adequacy of the total diet to support a thriving rumen population.

Chalmers (1961) points out that there is not a good correlation between degradation of protein in the rumen and N utilization by the ruminant animal. Casein, which is made less soluble in the rumen by heating or chemical treatments, usually results in greater N retention than more soluble forms of casein. Comparison of other feedstuffs, such as herring meal and peanut meal, shows that peanut meal is hydrolyzed more extensively in the rumen, but results in lower N retention. Comparisons of cottonseed meal of different solubilities indicate little difference in N retention (Woods et al, 1957). Little et al (1963) also compared proteins of different solubilities with in vitro and in vivo methods. Lambs receiving corn gluten meal as a supplement gained less and digested less cellulose than those receiving soybean meal, although N retention was not different. Heat-treated soybean meal resulted in gains as rapid as untreated meal, indicating that difference in solubility of the same protein source was not a major factor, although the heat-treated soybean meal was less soluble in rumen fluid and produced less free ammonia on fermentation. The addition of urea to corn gluten meal improved in vitro cellulose digestion and lamb gain, however. Some of the data reported by Little et al are shown in Table 13-1.

Data in a paper by Davis and Stallcup (1967) show some marked differences in rumen ammonia and protein as a result of feeding isonitrogenous rations with a variety of different N sources. In the first experi-ment, steers were fed N from soybean meal, raw soybeans or corn gluten feed. In the second experiment, they were fed soybean

Table 13-1. Effect of protein source on nitrogen utilization.

Item	In vivo digestion				In vitro digestion	
	CP	Cellulose, %	Organic matter, %	N balance, % of intake	Cellulose, %	Free ammonia, mg % ammonia N
Corn gluten meal	67.5	50.5*	71.1	32.8	15.1	1.6
Soybean oil meal	65.5	61.2**	75.0	31.7	28.5	10.2
Heated SOM					14.4	3.0
Urea					23.0	
Casein					25.5	12.5

*Statistically different than **

meal, urea or urea and soybean meal. Some of the data (shown in Fig. 13-3) from the first experiment (graphs A and B) indicate that supplements resulting in high levels of rumen ammonia (soybean meal) do not necessarily result in the highest level of rumen protein, although there was no attempt to distinguish between microbial and ingested protein. In the second experiment, supplementation with urea resulted in the highest level of rumen ammonia, but the lowest level of rumen protein. Unfortunately, no data were available on digestibility or N retention. Total VFA levels found in the rumen in experiment 1 were (μmol/ml): soybean meal, 110; raw soybeans, 92; and corn gluten feed, 109. In experiment 2 the VFA levels were: soybean meal, 110; urea, 73; urea and soybean meal, 87. These VFA levels might be a reasonable estimate of the degree of utilization of these various N sources by the rumen microbes. However, a comparison of the results of these two experiments would lead to the conclusion that one cannot safely extrapolate results from one N source to another, if the intent is to infer rumen protein levels from rumen ammonia levels.

In the rumen it seems likely that there may be a great deal of recycling of N. As cells divide, grow, die and lyse, they release cell contents into the rumen fluid, thus providing a source of nutrients for the living organisms. In addition, predation of protozoa on bacteria and other protozoa results in a considerable amount of recycling. Unfortunately, quantitative estimates of the amount of protein degradation and resynthesis are limited. Borchers (1965) has provided some information on the subject. In this case strained rumen fluid was incubated with casein and several other normal feedstuffs. Thymol was added to prevent deamination of hydrolyzed protein. The amounts of amino acids liberated (μmol/min/l.) were: casein, 165; alfalfa, 44; corn, 25; soybean meal, 52; no substrate, 37. When thymol was not added, an appreciable amount of ammonia and free amino acids were produced from casein but not from corn. Subsequent experiments with microbial protein indicated that it was readily hydrolyzed and deaminated, thus indicating that microbial recycling or synthesis from urea and/or ammonia and free amino acids may be relatively more important than the degradation of ingested proteins. Nolan and Leng (1972) estimate that ca. 4.3 g of N/day might be recycled within the rumen of sheep. They suggested that 30% of ammonia continually being incorporated into ruminal protein may have recycled through the amino acid and ammonia pools.

Chalmers (1961) states that the ideal ration for maximum use of N should contain protein of good digestibility with a low solubility in the rumen. This assumption is based on the premise that high rumen ammonia values are indicative of poor N utilization by the host. However, the data of Little et al (1963) would tend to refute this belief, at least in regard to digestion and retention of N. Obviously, there must be an adequate amount of N in required forms for the growth and activity of rumen microorganisms — i.e., a net balance between salivary urea, ammonia passage through the rumen wall and passage of N down the GIT — which will allow for microbial growth and reproduction. Any excessive degradation over this requirement would tend to be wasteful since a highly digestible protein probably can be more efficiently utilized by the host if digestion takes place in the low GIT. It is certain that degradation of proteins, peptides, amino acids, etc., is an expensive

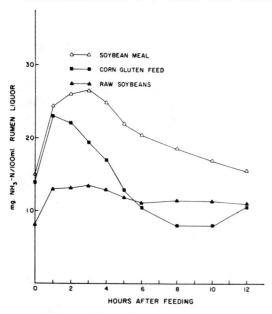

A. Concentration of ammonia-N from soybean meal, raw soybeans, and corn gluten feed in the rumen of fistulated steers.

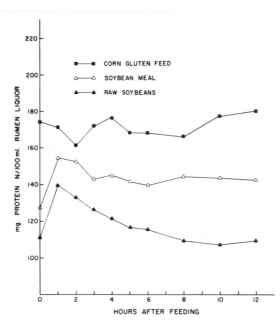

B. Level of protein N in the rumen liquor of fistulated steers fed various N sources.

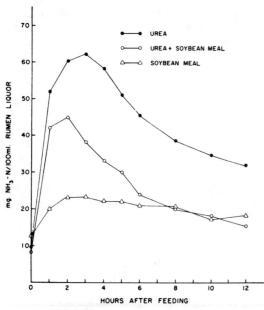

C. Concentration of ammonia-N from soybean meal, urea, and urea + soybean meal in the rumen of fistulated steers.

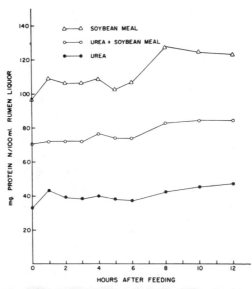

D. Level of protein N in the rumen liquor of fistulated steers fed various N sources.

Figure 13-3. Effect of various N sources on rumen ammonia-N and on protein found in rumen liquor. From Davis and Stallcup [1967].

process from an energetic point of view unless some added benefit is derived. Of course, the quality of protein produced by rumen microorganisms is one added benefit that may accrue from rumen fermentation — one which may be of very substantial value to animals consuming low quality protein.

Proteins Protected Against Rumen Fermentation

Protein supplements are generally the most expensive ingredients in ruminant rations, thus there is interest in maximizing their utilization. A considerable body of evidence has been accumulated in recent years to clearly show that infusions via the abomasum of high quality protein, such as casein, will result in improved N retention, more rapid wool growth, greater milk production, and so forth (Reis and Schinckel, 1964; Egan, 1965; 1970; Schelling and Hatfield, 1968; Colebrook and Reis, 1969; Ørskov and Fraser, 1969; Reis and Colebrook, 1972; Black and Tribe, 1973; Derrig et al, 1974). These data indicate that rumen degradation and resynthesis into bacterial and protozoal proteins (or loss of ammonia) has been detrimental to maximum utilization. This statement is partially substantiated by the fact that some of the less soluble or poor quality proteins produce less of a response than soluble or high quality proteins (Reis and Schinckel, 1964; Colebrook and Reis, 1969; Reis and Colebrook, 1972).

Severely heat damaged proteins are generally not attacked by rumen microorganisms because they form insoluble complexes which are not digested in the lower GIT; thus, this is not a feasible method of reducing rumen degradation. Moderate heating, however, may improve utilization of proteins for many monogastric species. For ruminants a moderate amount of heating may reduce solubility of soybean protein, but it does not appear to alter animal performance (Ely et al, 1963; Hudson et al, 1969). Excessive heating may reduce availability of some essential amino acids as well as total digestibility (Goering et al, 1972).

Encapsulation of specific nutrients which are deficient may be one method of bypassing rumen action. This method is widely utilized in human medicine. With ruminants, Neudoerffer et al (1971) have shown that it could be used to increase availability of methionine to the lower gut.

Treatment of proteins or plant protein concentrates with tannic acid has been used to protect protein from rumen degradation (Leroy et al, 1964; Delort-Laval and Zelter, 1968; Leroy and Zelter, 1970; Zelter et al, 1970). Data from these experiments indicate that plant protein concentrates can be protected from drastic degradation (90% protection) without a marked effect on rumen function although protein digestibility by the animal was reduced.

Aldehydes have also been used to protect protein from rumen fermentation. Formaldehyde has been favored because of cost (Ferguson et al, 1967; Reis and Tunks, 1969; Zelter et al, 1970; Faichney, 1972; Faichney and Davies, 1973; Schmidt et al, 1973; 1974; Dinius et al, 1974; many other papers). The results with formaldehyde treatment of casein indicate a response equivalent to giving casein via the abomasum. Formaldehyde treatment may reduce casein solubility from 85-90% to 4-8%. Treatment of plant protein concentrates such as soybean, sunflower, safflower and peanut meal also results in reduced rumen attack, but performance of animals has not been markedly improved. Data in Table 13-2 show calf performance on rations containing peanut meal. Although gain tended to be increased on diet LTP as compared to LPU (both ca. 12% crude protein), there was little effect on the diets MPU and MPT with higher protein. Also, treatment appeared to reduce N digestibility. In vitro data comparing tannin to aldehydes (Zelter et al, 1970) showed that the minimum dose of aldehyde which would protect the protein resulted in a 13-20% depression of cellolytic activity whereas tannin did not have this negative effect. At this point it appears that this method needs more research before it is feasible for commercial use.

Table 13-2. Effect of treating proteins with formaldehyde.[a]

Item	Diet*			
	LPU	LPT	MPU	MPT
Digestibility, %				
Dry matter	76	73	74	73
Organic matter	77	74	75	74
Nitrogen	72	66	75	67
Liveweight gain, kg/day	0.74	0.81	0.92	0.94
Feed conversion, kg DM/ kg of gain	3.48	3.41	2.94	2.94

[a]Data from Faichney and Davies (1973)
*Diets LPT and MPT were treated by spraying during mixing with 10% w/v formaldehyde (2 g formaldehyde/100 g crude protein); the composition of LPU and LPT was similar as was that of MPU and MPT; protein content increased from the L to the M rations.

Secretion of Nitrogen
into the Reticulo-Rumen

It has been known for some years that urea passed into the rumen via saliva (see Ch. 5) and in recent years there has been a considerable interest manifested in studying the passage of N from the blood into the rumen through the rumen wall. A variety of experiments has been carried out in order to obtain results that might provide data on the nature of the transfer and to provide quantitative data on the amount of N secreted into the rumen. Older papers relating to this topic include those of Schmidt-Nielsen et al (1957), Houpt (1959), Decker et al (1960), Kameoka (1962), Engelhardt (1963), Gartner (1963), Engelhardt and Nickel (1965), Packett and Groves (1965), Cocimano and Leng (1967), Varady et al (1967) and Houpt and Houpt (1968). Many more have been published since this book was first published in 1969. Some of these will be referred to in subsequent paragraphs.

Experiments which have been carried out include those in which the tissues have been flooded with urea using intravenous infusions, use of labeled compounds introduced in the lower GIT, sampling of rumen contents after intravenous infusions, use of rumen pouches or isolated perfused rumens, sampling of rumen or pouch contents after replacement of digesta with saline solutions and studies with rumen epithelia.

Data published on ruminal arterio-venous differences in blood urea and ammonia indicate that urea concentration is usually less and ammonia is usually found in greater concentration in the veins (Packett and Groves, 1965), thus indicating secretion into the rumen or tissue metabolism. Hecker and Nolan (1971) found the same relationship but, when blood concentrations were corrected for water absorption, differences were insignificant.

In studies with rumen epithelia, Gartner (1963) was able to show that N could be transferred from the connective tissue side to the epithelial side of the rumen wall. His data indicated that N passed through the rumen wall until the concentration on the connective tissue side reached levels of 10-20 mg%, but not at higher levels, thus indicating a tissue block of some type. When doing infusion studies in sheep, Weston and Hogan (1967) found that rumen N was not

increased when blood urea was > 16-18 mg% N. Similar results have been observed in sheep by Thornton (1970) and McIntyre (1971) and in cattle by Vercoe (1969).

All of the published reports indicate that N may be transferred into the rumen in greater or lesser degree. In many cases, the amount contributed by saliva has been included with that which crosses the rumen wall. In fact, some Russian data indicate that plasma proteins may be detected in the rumen (Kurilov et al, 1972). As a general rule, data indicate that rather rapid passage of N occurs when animals are fed low-N diets or when they are starved. In the early stages of starvation, blood urea increases sharply and rumen ammonia tends to decrease, followed by an increase in rumen ammonia in subsequent days (Varady et al, 1970; Harmeyer et al, 1973; Szanyiova et al, 1974). Harmeyer et al suggest that the reduction of ruminal ammonia in starving animals is a result of a reduced permeability of the GIT during this stage, and data published by Harrop and Phillipson (1971) indicate that pentagastrin increased urea transfer in sheep fed low-protein diets.

Passage of urea N into the rumen appears to be a result of diffusion since little or no passage occurs when there is no gradient between blood urea and ruminal ammonia (Varady et al, 1967; Houpt and Houpt, 1968). Houpt and Houpt suggest that some of the conflicting results which show an increased transfer into the rumen may be due to removal of urease from the tissues — a situation which could take place with tissue studies or when the rumen or a rumen pouch have been washed out and filled with saline solutions.

The fact that the gradient between blood urea and ruminal ammonia may be of great importance was illustrated in data presented by Varady et al (1967). They found in starving sheep that secretion of N into the rumen increased during the first few days of starvation even though ruminal ammonia and blood urea levels were lower than in fed animals. These authors rationalize the conflicting data in the literature by concluding that ruminal N levels are probably highly dependent upon blood and tissue urea levels when ruminal ammonia levels are low.

If ruminal levels of N are dependent upon blood levels, this would be a useful mechanism to increase the utilization of N and would act as a backup source to assure rumen microorganisms a limited supply of N during time of need. Such a mechanism would probably be relatively more important during ingestion of proteins of low solubility but good digestibility, during periods of starvation or interrupted feed intake or low N intake.

The earlier reports suggest that blood urea N is transferred to the rumen as ammonia. However, when efforts have been made to inhibit urease activity in ruminal contents or rumen epithelia (Houpt and Houpt, 1968), it appears that urea can be transferred. Under normal situations, however, the high urease activity of ruminal contents would result in rapid hydrolysis of the urea.

Estimates of the amount of N recycled into the rumen have been made by a number of investigators. One of the interesting papers in this respect is that of Kameoka (1962). In this case ^{15}N-labeled ammonium sulfate was administered via an abomasal cannula and digesta samples coming from the omasum were subsequently taken. He found that ca. 14% of the labeled N was recycled into the rumen. Unfortunately, no attempt was made to determine how much of this occurred via the saliva.

In other reports where ^{15}N and/or ^{14}C have been used, Aliev et al (1971) used sheep fed a grass ration. Of the ^{15}N introduced directly into the rumen, 4% entered the abomasum in 24 hr compared to 2.8% of that given by vein. On a hay ration, 7.1% of the ^{15}N given by vein reached the abomasum, perhaps due to greater secretion of saliva. Data from the same laboratory (Aliev and Radchenkova, 1972) showed that ^{15}N entered a rumen pouch most rapidly 4-6 hr after urea was given by vein, corresponding to the time of greatest labeling in rumen contents. When renal excretion was prevented, there was a marked increase of entry of protein and NPN into the pouch and ammonia entry into the rumen increased 20 fold. In work with sheep fed alfalfa (Nolan and Leng, 1972), 1.2 g of rumen ammonia were derived from plasma urea.

In other experiments, Houpt (1959) estimated that 8-13 µmol of urea N/hr were transferred to the rumen when estimates were based on urea body pool size and 3-5 µmol/hr when based on accumulation of ammonia in the rumen. Packett and Groves (1965) found that 17-50 mg of ammonia N/hr accumulated in rumen solutions and Juhasz (1965) calculated that 5-10 times as much ammonia entered the rumen by diffusion as

in saliva. Houpt and Houpt (1968) calculated that about 80 mg of urea N/hr were transferred into the rumen; the values in this case involved estimating the relative area of the rumen pouches used.

Thornton et al (1970) suggest that appreciable amounts of urea N (as ammonia) may be transferred to the hind gut, and it is known that high urease levels may be found in the ileum. Hecker and Nolan (1971) and Nolan et al (1973) tend to discount data showing large transfers of urea N to the rumen, pointing out that many of the experiments have been carried out under unphysiological conditions, concluding that most of the urea N is probably derived from saliva. Thus, at this time, it seems likely that passage of urea N into the rumen is of most physiological significance in animals on a low protein diet.

Utilization of Nitrogenous Compounds by Rumen Microorganisms

Ureolytic and Biuretolytic Activity of the Rumen

It is known that urea is usually hydrolyzed rather rapidly to ammonia in the rumen (Pearson and Smith, 1943; Huntanen and Gall, 1955). The rumen epithelia apparently hydrolyze urea to ammonia as it passes through the tissues (Gartner, 1963; Houpt and Houpt, 1968), although this activity may be derived from urease secreted by rumen microbes (Abdel Rahman and Decker, 1966).

Jones et al (1964) isolated bacteria from the rumen of sheep fed hay, barley and urea and reported that about 35% of the bacteria produced urease; this estimate is somewhat higher than values usually quoted (Hungate, 1966). Abou Akkada and Blackburn (1963) found that no urease was produced by strains of culturable proteolytic bacteria, and Abou Akkada and Howard (1962) and Jones et al (1964) observed that protozoal suspensions had very little, if any, urease activity. Clifford et al (1968) and Wortham et al (1968) have demonstrated that urease activity may vary with the diet fed. Ruminal pH appears to be an important factor in urease activity as optimal values in one report were said to be 8.35 for an animal fed concentrate and 8.17 when fed roughage (Prokop et al, 1971). Changing rations from roughage to concentrate resulted in a marked drop in urease activity. Total ureolytic activity was observed to be between 6 and 10 g of urea/min for mature sheep and 75-125 g for steers.

Muller and Kirchner (1971, 1972) report that urease was active over a pH range of 5.4 to 7.3. Activity appeared to be associated with particulate matter and was lowest in the first 3 hr following feeding. Their data indicate that urea dissolves rapidly in rumen fluid although liberation from large, hard pellets took 1 hr or longer. Binding urea to beet pulp or gelatinized starch granules also delayed release of urea.

In recent years there has been interest in biuretolytic activity as biuret has a number of features that warrant its use in ruminant rations. Gilchrist (1968) noted there was a marked dietary effect on activity and that activity of the enzyme was negligible except when biuret was included in the ration. Clemens and Johnson (1973) and Johnson and Clemens (1973) have noted similar findings in that it takes some time, perhaps as long as 30 days or more, for full biuretolytic activity to develop; in addition, it is lost very quickly when biuret is removed from the diet.

Biuret is much less soluble in the rumen than urea. One study indicated that 65% was degraded in the rumen and 35% passed out of the rumen; it was also shown that protozoa probably do not degrade biuret (Tiwari et al, 1973). Biuretase appears to be associated with microorganisms closely associated with plant debris. Evidence indicates that the enzyme is distinct from urease, with an intermediate step in degradation involving a complex with some soluble component(s). Urease appears to be required for complete hydrolysis to ammonia and water (Craig et al, 1969; Bauriedel, 1971; Tiwari et al, 1973). Additional evidence indicates that most of the biuret passing out of the rumen or intestine is likely to be excreted unchanged in urine; some could be degraded in the gut, but the rumen was the main site of degradation (Schroder, 1970). Older papers dealing with ureolytic activity are discussed by Jones (1967).

Nitrogenous Compounds Used for Microbial Growth

From papers reviewed in preceding sections we have seen that rumen microorganisms are capable of degrading ingested proteins to varying degrees, that most of the amino acids can be metabolized to some extent, that nitrogenous bases such as the pyrimidines and purines can be metabolized,

and that urea and biuret are hydrolyzed to ammonia. It is obvious that the presence in rumen fluid of a variety of nitrogenous sources makes evaluation of the nitrogen requirements somewhat difficult.

It has been known for many years that rumen microorganisms are capable of utilizing some NPN compounds for at least part of their metabolic requirements (Wegner et al, 1940; Pearson and Smith, 1943). More recent data show that ruminants can subsist and maintain moderate levels of production on diets containing only NPN sources (Virtanen, 1966; Oltjen et al, 1969). Rumen microorganisms may even be able to fix small amounts of N_2 (Postgate, 1970; Mathison and Milligan, 1971; Hobson et al, 1973). For a compilation of references on NPN utilization the reader is referred to the publication by Stangel et al (1963) or the book edited by Briggs (1967).

The bulk of the information on N requirements or utilization of different N-containing compounds has been obtained using in vitro techniques. An appreciable number of studies have been done using pure cultures or washed suspensions and other information has been obtained using crude suspensions. These are discussed in subsequent paragraphs.

Pure Cultures or Washed Suspensions. One of the earlier papers on utilization of N compounds by pure cultures was a paper by Bryant et al (1959). In these experiments strains of *Bacteroides succinogenes* were utilized. The authors found that ammonia was essential for growth even in the presence of 19 amino acids, a mixture of purines and pyrimidines and all B-complex vitamins. None of the amino acids were essential for growth. Cysteine or sulfide could serve as the only source of sulfur.

Bryant and Robinson (1961) have studied N requirements of several cellulolytic bacteria — strains of *Ruminococcus flavefaciens* and *R. albus.* These organisms grew with ammonia as the sole source of N other than that in vitamins added to the medium. Ammonia was essential for growth in the presence of 17 amino acids, 3 purines and 2 pyrimidines. *Bacteroides succinogenes* strain S85 grew with asparagine and glutamine but at slower rates than with ammonia. Dehority (1963) has also reported data on cellulolytic bacteria. Four of 5 strains studied required ammonia. As for the other strain, he concluded that it required one or more amino acids because no growth occurred when casein hydrolysate was left out of the medium.

In another example Bryant and Robinson (1962) studied the nutritional characteristics of predominant bacteria that could be cultured. At least 9 different genera were included in 89 freshly isolated strains. Of these organisms, 13% grew poorly or not at all on defined medium plus casein hydrolysate; 6% required casein hydrolysate; 56% grew with either ammonia or casein hydrolysate as the main source of N; and ammonia, but not casein hydrolysate, was essential for 25% of the strains. Hemin was required by some species. The apparent need for peptides has been partially clarified by a report of Pittman and others (1966). In this experiment it was shown, using ^{14}C-labeled peptides, that *Bacteroides ruminicola* organisms would take up labeled peptides with molecular weights up to about 2,000, whereas they did not take up labeled proline or glutamic acid. Their data indicated that the peptides were hydrolyzed during or after uptake and that the oligopeptides function only to supply amino acids in a form available to the organism.

Hoover and Lipari (1971) observed that *Ruminococcus flavefaciens* would grow only on a cellobiose-casein medium if methionine was added. *Bacteroides ruminicola* would grow on this media without methionine; when these two organisms were grown together, it was shown that *R. flavefaciens* accounted for 20-40% of the bacterial count after 96 hr, indicating that *B. ruminicola* liberated sufficient methionine to support growth of the other organism.

Papers from other laboratories such as the report by Leru and Raynaud (1964) and Beauville et al (1962) indicate that washed suspensions utilized N from amino acids in proportion to the amount of ammonia liberated. Acids such as aspartic acid and histidine were rapidly deaminated and the ammonia utilized. Urea was superior to all amino acids tried except aspartic acid and glutamine (Beauville et al, 1962).

It is interesting to note that Abou Akkada and Blackburn (1963) observed that many strains of proteolytic bacteria used ammonia N in preference to amino acid N. Organisms that digest starch apparently are less dependent upon ammonia as the sole source of N than are most cellulolytic organisms (Provost and Doetsch, 1960). With respect to N requirements of rumen microbes, Hungate

(1966) points out that ammonia is probably relatively more important for the nutrition of the fiber and starch-digesting bacteria than for those utilizing soluble sugars. Since it appears to take fiber-digesting organisms longer to become established on particles of newly ingested feed and since cellulose degradation is slow compared to metabolism of soluble carbohydrates, Hungate feels that the fiber digesters must, more or less, utilize forms of N that are not immediately utilized by bacteria which attack the soluble nutrients. In some respects, the cellulolytic organisms would be considered scavengers insofar as utilization of N sources is concerned.

Crude Suspensions. One of the earlier papers comparing in vitro utilization of different N sources is that of Burroughs et al (1951). These authors reported that urea stimulated cellulose digestion by crude suspensions about as effectively as a variety of protein sources. Belasco (1954) reported similar results when urea and a variety of protein sources were compared. Belasco (1954) also compared a variety of inorganic N sources (ammonium succinate and lactate, salts of guanidine, amides of mono- and dicarboxylic acids) and found that most were available to rumen organisms to varying degrees, as measured by cellulose digestion, except amides of dicarboxylic acids. Henderickx (1961) has also studied a series of ammonium salts of inorganic acids (sulfate, succinate). Several amides, biuret and thiourea all gave results similar to those obtained with urea, from which an average of 46% of the N was converted to bacterial protein. Henderickx and Martin (1963) have reported similar results. With respect to starch digestion, a paper by Acord et al (1966) reported that ammonium salts of sulfate, chloride, acetate and phosphate were equivalent to urea. Aspartic acid was inferior to urea, but was more effective than other amino acids tested. Arginine, serine, methionine, valine, and glutamic acid additions resulted in moderate to slight increases in starch digestion. Lysine was not effectively utilized. Acetamide, propionamide, butyramide, succinamide, malonamide, guanidine acetate or aminoguanidine bicarbonate did not consistently stimulate starch digestion.

Brent et al (1966) have studied NPN utilization in a continuous flow in vitro system, a laboratory situation which should be more typical of the animal's physiology than most in vitro systems. Under the conditions used, only urea was hydrolyzed completely. NPN compounds such as biurea, guanidine hydrochloride, guanylurea sulfate and thiocarbanalide depressed VFA levels. Another report using continuous in vitro cultures (Vatthauer et al, 1968) indicated that urea fed cultures had higher bacterial populations and produced higher levels of VFA as compared to biuret fed cultures although the latter supported higher protozoal populations.

Papers indicating a growth promoting effect of amino acids, peptides and other nitrogenous compounds include those of Bentley et al (1954), Hall et al (1954), Dehority et al (1957), Salsbury and Haenlein (1964), and Lampila (1967).

David et al (1955) and Hershberger and others (1959) have shown that bound ammonia in ammoniated feedstuffs such as molasses, corn cobs, etc., could not be utilized by rumen organisms to any appreciable degree.

Continued research on a variety of NPN compounds still proceeds as proteins are expensive feedstuffs. For example, Lilligan et al (1972) have demonstrated that glucosyl-urea is substantially degraded. Lengerken et al (1970) have shown that acetyl urea, formyl urea and acetamide have good potential, particularly acetamide. Barbituric acid and methylene urea had a negative effect on in vitro digestibility. Munchow et al (1973) point out that acetyl urea can be utilized, but not as the sole source of N. Abe et al (1973) found that compounds such as succinic diamide, transcyclopropane dicarboxylic diamide, α-amino nitriles, ethyl and n-propyl hydantoins and 1,1-diureidoisobutane could be utilized by rumen microorganisms.

The need for specific N sources in the diet of the host animal has been shown to be very modest, at least for maintenance or low levels of production. It would seem that this is probably so because of recycling of N compounds within the rumen. As bacteria or protozoa die and the cells lyse, this would make the cell contents available to other organisms — thus they would have a source of preformed compounds available. However, the importance of rumen recycling has not been clearly established.

Effect of Carbohydrates on Nitrogen Utilization

A major factor influencing the utilization of ruminal ammonia is the availability of carbohydrates to rumen organisms. As early as 1943, Pearson and Smith (1943) indicated that in vitro fermentations utilized urea to a greater extent when carbohydrates were available. Mills et al (1944) demonstrated greater N retention in animals receiving urea plus soluble carbohydrates. Arias et al (1951) reported that a variety of soluble carbohydrates improved N utilization by in vitro fermentations and suggested that a small amount was necessary since the rumen bacteria probably needed a readily available energy source until cellulose could be partially digested. Warner (1956) noted that starch or other polysaccharides reduced the production of ammonia by in vitro fermentations and reported that this was not due to any effect on proteolysis or reduced amount of deamination, but was believed to be due to an increased utilization of the ammonia for microbial growth. Belasco (1956) compared starch to other polysaccharides (xylan, pectin) when the primary substrate was cellulose, and found that starch resulted in somewhat better N utilization. Lewis and McDonald (1958) found that the greatest utilization of protein in the rumen occurred when a carbohydrate was present that could be fermented at a comparable rate to the protein. When using casein, they determined that levan and starch were more effective than glucose or xylan and that the effect of cellulose was negligible. Kameoka (1962) noted that N utilization in the rumen was markedly reduced as the amount of soluble carbohydrate decreased in feedstuffs labeled with ^{15}N (however, the soluble protein was also reduced). Schwartz et al (1964) reported that soluble starch remained in the rumen two to three times as long as did glucose, and Robertson and Hawke (1965) observed that infusion of starch into the rumen of cows on high-N pasture resulted in consistently lower rumen ammonia levels than in negative control cows. In vitro data indicated that ammonia production was reduced by addition of galactose, sucrose, lactose or glucose.

More recently, Meyer et al (1967) have demonstrated some effect of feed processing methods on N utilization. Finely ground hay and expanded grain were compared to unprocessed feed. The expansion process results in almost complete gelatinization of starch. The results showed that the processed feed lowered rumen ammonia concentration ca. 50%, yet resulted in an increased bacterial N level of

50% — thus indirectly indicating more efficient utilization of N due to greater carbohydrate utilization. Similar results from the same laboratory were published by Helmer and others (1970). Arthur et al (1967) observed that N utilization in in vitro fermentations tended to increase with time in fermentations carried for 9 hr. N was utilized at a rate of about 0.35 mg N/hr during the first 3 hr; 0.44 mg N/hr in the next 3 hr; and about 0.99 mg N/hr during the final 3 hr (these data may merely be a reflection of a lag phase in growth). These authors determined that ca. 50 to 80 mg of glucose were utilized for each mg of N taken up.

Continued effort in recent years has been placed on utilization of N in the presence of low quality roughages. When using straw, Ichhponani et al (1969) observed that addition of molasses, starch or both decreased in vitro cellulose digestion. The decreases were almost entirely overcome by the addition of urea. In addition, adding molasses or starch or both increased the production of microbial protein. When using urea or biuret supplemented to a diet with 87% wood pulp or wood pulp with 13% starch, Slyter et al (1971) observed that addition of starch decreased fiber digestion and increased N retention. Other work with biuret (Bauriedel et al, 1971) indicated that biuret hydrolysis was not affected by energy sources, but incorporation of ^{15}N-labeled ammonia into microbial protein was promoted by addition of carbohydrate substrate.

Potter et al (1971) noted that N entering the abomasum was only 79.4% as great when urea was fed as compared to soybean meal; when 2.5% molasses and urea were fed, N entering the abomasum increased to 93% of the soy diet. Increasing molasses to 10% of the diet did not further increase abomasal N. In an experiment where 2% urea was fed, Tandon et al (1972) determined that 15% molasses in a concentrate mixture resulted in the best N utilization based on rumen VFA, ammonia N, and microbial N formed. In work where lambs were fed hay and concentrates supplemented with either casein or urea (Barej et al, 1970), results indicated that ruminal protein N and ammonia N accounted for 38 and 31% in sheep given casein and 52 and 20%, respectively, when given casein with starch. When given urea, values were 22 and 70% without starch and 30 and 63% with starch; thus, even with casein, the results show the valuable effect of starch in promoting more efficient N utilization.

Other studies of this type showing differences in the carbohydrates of different feedstuffs on N utilization in the rumen include those of Ørskov et al (1971), Winter and Pigden (1971), Griffiths and Bath (1973) and Oldham et al (1973).

Synthesis of Amino Acids and Proteins in the Rumen

As we have seen in discussions in previous sections, the requirement of mixed cultures of rumen organisms can be met with ammonia. Since rumen microbes synthesize a large variety of proteins for cellular growth, enzymes, etc., it is obvious that an appreciable amount of synthesis must occur, although there is some indication that a small amount of synthesis may take place in the rumen wall (Kurilov and Kosarov, 1970). One of the earliest reports on this topic was that of Loosli et al (1949). In this research sheep and goats were fed a purified diet containing urea as the only supplemental N source. Analyses were carried out after several days on the diet for the 10 amino acids considered to be essential for the rat. Rumen material contained 9-20 times more of the amino acids than was found in the diet — indicating that all of these acids could be synthesized in appreciable quantities. Duncan et al (1953) also demonstrated appreciable quantities of the same amino acids in the rumen of calves fed rations containing urea.

An estimate of ruminal synthesis was made by Barej (1965) by sampling duodenal contents. He reported that the duodenal concentration of aspartic acid, serine, alanine, threonine, glutamic acid, valine and methionine was higher than in the rumen contents, thus giving an indirect estimate of synthesis if the amino acid content of duodenal and abomasal juice was ignored. Temler-Kucharski et al (1966) have made somewhat similar estimates in young calves which were fed low lysine rations. They found that total and protein N contents of the duodenal ingesta increased with increasing protein content of the diet up to 20% of the diet and NPN increased from ca. 36 to 50% of total N during the first 3 wk after weaning. The lysine content of duodenal digesta was higher than that of the feeds and ranged from about 4.6 to 6.4 mg/16 mg of N. DNA levels in the digesta were much higher than in the diet. Ely et al (1967) estimated that 26 and

30% of the N in abomasal contents was microbial protein in lambs fed zein and high cellulose and high starch diets, respectively, based on physical fractionation. When estimates were based on changes of lysine ratios between the diet and abomasal fluid, 24 to 28% was estimated to be microbial protein.

With respect to pure culture studies, Allison and Bryant (1963) demonstrated that valine was synthesized by *Ruminococcus flavefaciens* and Allison (1965) demonstrated synthesis of phenylalanine by *Bacteroides succinogenes*. Subsequent research from this laboratory (Allison et al, 1966) indicated that *B. ruminicola, Peptostreptococcus elsdenii* and *Ruminococcus flavefaciens* organisms utilized isovalerate to synthesize leucine, a pathway that is different than that used by many other nonruminal microorganisms. Robinson and Allison (1969) have also shown that isoleucine may be synthesized from 2-methyl-butyric acid by rumen anaerobes. Other data of this type have been discussed in detail by Allison (1969).

Conrad et al (1965) found that an appreciable amount of methionine synthesis (6-15 g) occurred in the rumen of dairy cows, based on the incorporation of ^{35}S into the amino acid molecule. A subsequent paper from the same laboratory (Conrad et al, 1967a) indicated that methionine synthesis increased as the level of dry matter and protein intake increased, and synthesis was also increased as protein degradation in the rumen was decreased. Estimates of methionine synthesis (Conrad et al, 1967a, 1967b) indicated synthesis at a rate of from 30-60 mg/kg of body weight. Data on cysteine and methionine, when added as the free acids to rumen fluid, indicate that at most 1% of cysteine and 11% of methionine was incorporated unchanged into microbial protein (Nader and Walker, 1970).

Ulbrich and Scholz (1967) found that ^{15}N-labeled ammonia was rapidly incorporated into bacterial and protozoal protein. The half life of labeled N in bacterial N was estimated to be 19-20 hr as compared to 37-42 hr in protozoal N. These values compare to a half life in bacterial protein of 38 and 42 hr in sheep given barley and hay diets by Mathison and Milligan (1971).

Hoover et al (1963) have studied the utilization of some of the VFA and glucose with respect to in vitro protein synthesis by bacterial cultures. Evaluation of VFA utilization is complicated, of course, by production of VFA and estimates were made on the basis of decline in radioactivity and on the radioactivity found in cellular protein and DNA. They found that small amounts of label from the VFA could be recovered in protein, but about 85% of this was calculated to have been derived from acetate. Glucose resulted in higher levels of labeled protein. With respect to DNA, only acetate and glucose resulted in other than a trace of label and the values for glucose were on the order of 20 fold of those for acetate. Otagaki et al (1955) studied the utilization of ^{14}C-labeled casein, glutamic acid, leucine or carbonate by rumen bacteria. Their data indicated that most of the label from casein was in the VFA fraction with little in bacterial protein. Glutamate label was recovered in carbon dioxide and VFA — indicating degradation of the acid. In the case of leucine, most of the label was recovered in VFA. An appreciable amount of labeled carbonate was utilized in amino acid synthesis. Portugal and Sutherland (1966) observed that labeled glutamic and aspartic acids were rapidly metabolized to CO_2 and VFA. About 17% of the carbon label of glutamic acid was recovered from bacterial protein, about half as glutamic acid. Values for aspartic acid were much lower. Borchers (1967) has studied the utilization of carbon-labeled glucose as compared to carbon-labeled amino acids for the synthesis of protein by in vitro preparations. His data indicated that very little label from the amino acids appeared in TCA precipitates whereas a substantial amount of the label from glucose was found to be incorporated into TCA precipitates. Studies by Harmeyer and Jezkova (1972) indicate that 90% of the activity of ^{14}C-labeled glucose which was recovered in microbial cell components was in the protein and 10% in the amino acid fraction. Label was found in all of the amino acids of the microbial protein; specific activity of individual amino acids was 50-100% greater in proteins from a goat fed on urea than in those from a goat fed soy protein. The data from the experiments cited indicate that a very substantial amount of some of the amino acids are degraded rather than being incorporated directly into bacterial protein.

Experiments covering a wide range of carbon sources and organisms indicate that the carbon in amino acids may be derived from many different compounds. Recent data, however, suggest that <1% of carbon from urea or $NaHCO_3$ was recovered in

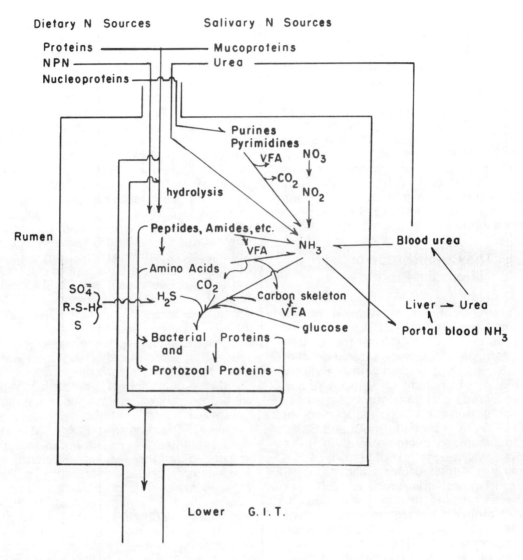

Figure 13-4. A tenative scheme of N metabolism in the rumen.

amino acids (Isaacs and Owens, 1971). Further details on this subject have been discussed by Allison (1969).

Information on the synthesis of purine and pyrimidine bases into polynucleotides by rumen microorganisms is relatively scarce. Ellis and Pfander (1965), for example, found that microbial polynucleotide N represented from 5.0 to 13% of ingesta N in sheep, depending upon the ration fed (all were low in nucleotides); they also observed that nucleotide N was highly correlated with the amount of microbial N. Arthur et al (1966) observed that the adenine-guanine ratios were 0.51 in sheep fed in dry lot and 0.81 in sheep fed on pasture — a difference probably reflecting the diversity in microbial

species found on the two diets. However, Wortham et al (1968) did not find any difference in DNA levels in sheep fed different dry rations. It would seem that substantial amounts of the nucleotides must be synthesized in view of the fact that Temler-Kucharski et al (1966) observed that the DNA content of duodenal contents was much higher than that of diets fed to calves. Topps and Elliott (1965) have observed that urinary excretion of allantoin and uric acid ranged from 76-187 µg/ml. In calves or cows on natural diets, Smith and McAllan (1970, 1971) calculated that 8-12% of N entering the small intestine was bound in nucleic acids and that it accounted for 8-15% of the nonammonia N in rumen fluid. Furthermore, nucleic acid content in the rumen of calves was as much as 5 fold greater than could be explained by the dietary concentration, thus synthesis of these bases would not appear to be a limiting factor for rumen microbial growth.

An overall scheme of nitrogen metabolism in the rumen is shown in diagrammatic form in Fig. 13-4 for the benefit of those who like this type of presentation. It is, admittedly, incomplete. For further reading on this subject, Nolan and Leng (1972) have presented a model of N metabolism in sheep illustrating different routes of N metabolism and have presented some quantitative estimates.

The Composition of Microbial Protein

Crude Protein

The protein content of ruminal micro-organisms has been reported in a number of papers. Johnson et al (1944) found that rumen protozoa had a crude protein content of ca. 55%. Bacteria isolated with a relatively high amount of contamination from rumen fluid had a crude protein content of ca. 44% and those cultured on a synthetic medium had ca. 59% crude protein. Smith and Baker (1944) found mixed microbial protein to be ca. 36%. McNaught et al (1950, 1954) reported that rumen bacteria had ca. 42% crude protein as compared to 26% for protozoa and stated that this was due, in part, to a higher polysaccharide content of the rumen protozoa. Weller (1957) analyzed the crude protein content of bacteria and protozoa from animals fed a variety of diets and reported that the crude protein content of bacteria ranged from 58-77% and that of protozoa from 24-49%, with the highest values being for microorganisms from animals on grass. Abdo and others (1964) found the crude protein content of mixed organisms to be from 38-49% when they were freeze-dried and acetone-dried, respectively. Thus, these various reports indicate appreciable differences which are probably due to contamination of the microbial preparations with ingesta and other organisms, differences in chemical technique, and differences due to rations and the resultant differences in organisms in the reticulo-rumen. Other values are given in later sections.

Amino Acid Composition

The amino acid composition of rumen microbes has been determined by a number of laboratories. Examples of data from three sources are shown in Table 13-3, with comparisons given on casein and two leaf protein sources.

The data shown in the table from Weller (1957) were obtained by sampling bacteria and protozoa from sheep fed on four rather different diets: (1) wheat hay chaff, (2) alfalfa hay chaff, (3) wheat straw, crushed oats and urea, and (4) mixed green pasture. He found the N content to vary but the range in amino acid composition was rather small as shown in Table 13-3, thus indicating no appreciable effect of diet on amino acid composition. The data of Purser and Buechler (1966) were obtained on 22 strains representing 9 species of rumen bacteria grown in pure cultures and a nonselective medium. These authors observed very little difference for different organisms even though the age of the cultures varied somewhat (which would influence the number of dying cells). They found that amino acid N averaged 86% of total N, although the range varied from 56-100% amino acid N. The protozoal preps were from sheep maintained on a natural ration of corn, alfalfa, corncobs and molasses. The data from Bergen et al (1968) were obtained on microorganisms from sheep fed rations varying in alfalfa, corn, soybean meal and other ingredients. Recent data on sheep microbes from animals fed semipurified or conventional diets (Ibrahim and Ingalls, 1972) also show no effect of diet or diethylstilbestrol on the amino acid composition. It is apparent that the analyses shown in Table 13-3 are not identical; however, the analyses are reasonably similar, particularly since different analytical methods were utilized for the amino acids and since the sources of the bacteria were quite different. Protozoa would appear to be substantially higher in lysine content and somewhat higher in various amino acids such as glutamic acid. Bacteria, on the other hand, tend to be higher than protozoa in histidine, threonine, serine, cystine and methionine (Ibrahim and Ingalls, 1972). Regardless of these minor differences, the information at hand clearly indicates that the amino acids presented to the lower GIT are remarkably constant. Hutton and Annison (1972) suggest that the N content of ruminal microbes is ca. 10%, on average, of which 85% is true protein. Other relatively recent reports providing data on amino acid

Table 13-3. Amino acid content (%) of casein, two leaf proteins and of rumen bacteria and protozoa.[a]

Amino acid	Casein	Leaf proteins Barley	Alfalfa	Weller Bacteria	Protozoa	Purser and Buechler Bacteria	Protozoa	Bergen et al Bacteria	Protozoa
Aspartic acid	6.64	9.57	9.70	6.7-6.8	7.4- 8.4	11.1	12.4	11.1-12.1	11.9-13.5
Threonine	4.20	5.07	4.99	3.5-3.8	3.1- 3.7	5.5	5.1	6.0- 7.8	4.8- 6.5
Serine	5.75	4.40	4.22	2.5-3.0	2.6- 3.2	3.8	3.6	4.2- 5.1	4.4- 5.1
Glutamic acid	21.46	11.28	11.55	6.6-7.5	7.9- 8.7	11.9	12.5	13.5-14.4	15.0-16.3
Proline	10.29	4.98	4.55	2.1-2.8	1.9- 2.9	4.1	3.7	2.4- 2.9	2.9- 6.0
Glycine	1.66	6.53	5.40	5.9-6.3	4.7- 5.7	6.1	5.0	6.0- 7.6	4.1- 5.5
Alanine	2.54	6.45	6.27	6.4-6.5	4.1- 4.6	6.5	5.2	7.2- 7.6	4.4- 6.1
Cystine	0.33		1.54	0.7-0.8	1.1- 1.3	1.0	1.0		
Valine	7.52	5.64	6.45	4.4-4.5	3.6- 4.1	6.6	5.2	4.7- 5.2	4.0- 4.2
Methionine	2.99	2.11	2.05	1.5	1.1- 1.4	2.6	2.2	2.0- 2.2	1.3- 1.9
Isoleucine	6.31	5.03	5.21	3.6-3.8	4.3- 4.9	6.4	6.9	5.2- 6.3	5.8- 6.3
Leucine	9.51	10.40	9.43	4.5-4.7	5.0- 5.7	7.3	8.1	7.7- 8.7	7.4- 8.2
Tyrosine	5.20	4.19	4.73	2.0-2.2	2.0- 2.4	4.2	5.4	4.1- 4.5	4.2- 5.2
Phenylalanine	5.09	6.85	6.11	2.3-2.5	2.8- 3.3	5.1	6.2	4.4- 5.1	5.0- 6.0
Histidine	2.77	2.00	2.45	2.6-3.0	2.6- 3.4	2.3	2.1	1.8- 2.0	1.6- 2.2
Lysine	7.74	5.23	6.83	7.5-8.2	10.6-12.6	9.3	10.1	7.6- 9.0	9.4-13.0
Arginine	3.76	6.33	6.77	8.6-9.3	8.0-10.2	5.4	4.9	5.0- 5.3	3.7- 4.8
Diaminopimelic acid						0.8			
Ammonia			1.75						

[a]Casein data from NRC; leaf protein analyses from Byers (1971); Source of data on rumen microbes is indicated.

composition of rumen microorganisms include those of Abdo et al (1964), Hoeller and Harmeyer (1964) and Meyer et al (1967).

It has been shown (Weller et al, 1958) that rumen bacteria contain relatively high levels of 2,6-diaminopimelic acid in their tissues. The acid has the structural formula as shown:

$$HOOC-\underset{\underset{NH_2}{|}}{CH}-CH_2-CH_2-CH_2-\underset{\underset{NH_2}{|}}{CH}-COOH$$

Since this acid is not found in plant, animal or protozoal tissues, it has been used as a marker and as a means of estimating the conversion of plant proteins to bacterial proteins (Weller et al, 1958).

Protozoa also have an amino acid not characteristic of bacteria. It is ciliatine (aminoethylphosphonic acid), shown below:

$$NH_2-CH_2-CH_2-P(OH)_3 = 0$$

Abou Akkada et al (1968) have reported the occurrence of ciliatine in holotrich species of rumen protozoa and in *Entodinium* . The levels found were (mg/g of dry matter): *Isotricha* , 1.12; *Entodinia* , 0.30; mixed protozoa, 1.02. This amino acid also offers the opportunity to use it as a marker if the distribution in protozoa is satisfactory for such a purpose.

Onodera and Kandatsu (1972) have shown that rumen ciliates produce appreciable amounts of pipecolic acid (2-piperidine-carboxylic acid) and that most of this originated from ^{14}C-labeled lysine. Production of other naturally occurring less common amino acids by microorganisms has been discussed by Murti and Seshadri (1967).

Digestibility and Biological Value of Microbial Protein

There has been interest in determining the feeding value of rumen microbes for some years. Johnson et al (1944) were among the first to study this problem. Digestibility has, for the most part, been determined with rats or mice and the biological value has usually been calculated from such data. Some authors have calculated biological value using the index of Oser (1951) which is based on amino acid composition. In either case one must assume that the tissues of the ruminant animal are utilizing amino acids in a manner comparable to that of the rat or mouse, an assumption that is not necessarily valid since the ruminant's tissues can apparently synthesize adequate amounts of arginine, an essential amino acid for the young rat (Black et al, 1957; Downes, 1961).

In early work, Uselli and Fiorini (1938) found that protozoa gave better growth in chicks than did rumen bacteria. In the report of Johnson et al (1944) it was determined that dried protozoa had a true digestibility of 86.2

and a biological value of 68, whereas the digestibility of dried bacteria grown on synthetic mediums was 82.4 and with a biological value of 66%. McNaught et al (1950) grew up batches of rumen organisms on maltose and urea and determined that the sludge obtained had a true digestibility of 73.2 and a biological value of 88.2%. In another experiment McNaught et al (1954) determined that the true digestibilities of rumen bacterial and protozoal protein and yeast protein were 74, 91 and 84% and the biological values were 81, 80 and 72, respectively. If N utilization is expressed as net utilization (biological value x true digestibility), the estimated values were 60, 73 and 60%, respectively. Reed et al (1949) collected bacteria from sheep fed on dry feeds or on pasture and compared these preparations to casein. The average true digestibility of protein of bacteria from animals fed on pasture was 62.1 as compared to 64.8% from those fed dry feeds. These values compared to a value of 101.2% for casein. Average biological values for the three protein sources were 79.9, 77.9 and 79.6%, respectively, when they provided the sole source of supplemental N. Purser and Buechler (1966) used the index method of Oser to calculate biological value of the pure strains they worked with. When using the average composition of all strains, the calculated biological value was 69%. The same value was obtained for protozoal samples.

Bergen et al (1967) calculated a protein quality index based on distribution of amino acids in various fractions of egg protein compared with amino acid distribution in the equivalent fraction following digestion with enzymes. When this index was applied to strains of rumen bacteria, this index was 60 or less in 9 of 10 strains. Enzymatic digestibility of cellulolytic and noncellulolytic strains averaged 69 and 77%, respectively. The protein utilization index for pooled strains of cellulolytic and noncellulolytic strains was 72 for each and 74 when all were combined; this compared to a value of 74 for casein. These data indicate a complementary effect of the amino acid distribution in different organisms. On this basis of their calculations, methionine was indicated as the limiting amino acid in pooled cellulolytic strains and leucine as the limiting amino acid for pooled noncellulolytic strains and for a combination of both.

More recently, Mason and Palmer (1971)

isolated rumen bacteria from cattle fed a barley-soybean diet. These were freeze-dried and fed to rats. True digestibility was calculated to be ca. 80% and net protein utilization was 57%. They concluded that ca. 20% of the bacterial N, which was mainly incorporated in the cell wall, was not absorbed by the rat.

The digestibility of ^{14}C-labeled *E. coli* cells has been evaluated by Hoogenraad and Hird (1970). They concluded that ca. 20% of the label was released as a result of autolytic enzymes in the bacterial cells, and that additional lysis occurred when incubated in whole rumen fluid. When incubated with trypsin, chymotrypsin and pepsin, additional label was released but that in the cell walls was resistant to digestion.

In studies where ^{35}S-labeled rumen microorganisms were infused into the abomasum of sheep (Bird, 1972), data indicated a true digestibility of 71.3% or 73.6% if corrected for the difference in inorganic S present. Net protein utilization was calculated to be 52% in this experiment.

The data from studies of biological value and digestibility of microorganisms with rats or the report of Bergen et al (enzymatic digestibility) show that the quality of protein produced by rumen bacteria and protozoa is quite good, as a general rule. Most bacterial-protozoal comparisons indicate that digestibility of the protozoa is higher, but that the biological value of the two is similar and that the net protein utilization of protozoa is somewhat greater than for bacteria. Certainly, the organisms are capable of upgrading low quality N sources such as urea. It is also likely that some very high quality proteins are downgraded as a result of the proteolysis, deamination and resynthesis of protein that occurs in the rumen. Studies on protein quality of common supplementary sources of protein and of leaf proteins would, in some cases, indicate a reduction of quality as a result of rumen metabolism.

Estimates on the Amount of Protein Synthesis in the Rumen

The amount of microbial protein that might pass into the lower GIT is of interest with respect to evaluation of the animal's requirements as well as its utilization of proteins in the digesta. Estimates of the amount of microbial protein have been made on the basis of how much of the ration proteins have been converted to microbial proteins, with the use of in vitro studies, and with experiments which provide data on rumen turnover time. Hungate (1966, pp 312-328) has discussed the subject in detail.

In vitro data (see Hungate, 1966, pp 315, 316) suggest that about 10-15% of carbohydrate fermented may be recovered as bacterial cells which may have a content of about 10-11% N; thus, estimates could be made on the amount of protein that might be made available to the host. On this basis, if a sheep consumed 1,000 g of a ration containing 70% carbohydrate of which 50% was available carbohydrate (350 g), we would estimate a cell yield of 35 to 52 g with a N yield of about 3.5 to 5.2 g or a crude protein yield of 21.9-32.5 g/day.

Data published by Gray et al (1958) indicate that rumen microorganisms will utilize N in the diet in an amount not exceeding about 1.1% of the ration. Digestion of carbohydrates in the rumen was calculated to be 50% with a yield of microbial protein of 11 g/100 g of fermentable carbohydrate. When compared to the previous example, if the available carbohydrate is 350 g, the yield of microbial protein would be about 38 g.

Other examples (McDonald and Hall, 1957; Weller et al, 1958) indicate that 40-80% of ingested protein may be converted to microbial protein by sheep rumen microorganisms. Thus, if we assume an intake of 150 g of crude protein per day, these estimates would suggest that from 70 to 120 g of microbial protein might be available to the lower GIT, of which about 80% might be digestible. This estimate would, then, indicate that 56 to 96 g of digestible protein would be available to the host.

These estimates may or may not be very accurate. It is apparent that estimates made in several different ways lead to somewhat similar approximations of the amount of protein that may be available from microbial sources. Further work utilizing markers such as diaminopimelic acid and ciliatine coupled with analyses in rumen fluid, and analyses from other sites in the lower GIT might be expected to result in more reliable calculations when combined with estimates of flow through the GIT.

There have been a number of recent papers dealing with total protein synthesis in the rumen. A series of papers by Hume (1970) and Hume et al (1970) are of interest. In one experiment when sheep were fed on a protein-free purified diet, increasing the daily N from 2 to 9 g/day increased production of protein in the rumen from 32 to 50 g/day; there was no further increase in protein when N intake was raised to 16 g/day. The author calculated that 9.1 g of protein were produced/100 g of digested organic matter when N was most limiting; this increased to 13.3 g/100 g when N was in excess. In a second experiment on the same type of diet, sheep were given 1.8% dietary N (14.9 g/day). Ruminal synthesis of protein was calculated to be 71 g of microbial protein/day; addition of a mixture of branched-chain VFA increased this to 81 g daily. The yield of protein was calculated to be ca. 13 g/100 g of digested organic matter. In a third experiment, N was provided from urea, gelatin, casein or zein. With urea protein synthesis was 90 g/day. When gelatin was substituted for the VFA and half of the urea N, little increase in protein synthesis occurred. With casein and zein, protein synthesis increased to 101 and 104 g/day, respectively. The authors suggested that the maximum possible yield of protein may exceed 20 g/100 g of digested organic matter/day.

In other research, Roberts and Miller (1969) suggest that bacterial protein ranged from 53 to 73% of dietary protein intake in sheep fed a high-energy diet. Mathison and Milligan (1971) have calculated that rumen protein amounted to 10.6-16.2 g/day in sheep, and Al-Rabbat et al (1971) suggest that ca. 15 g of ruminal protein is synthesized/100 g of digestible organic matter. Ibrahim and Ingalls (1972) found that ruminal microorganisms contributed 54-92% of total amino acids in rumen digesta with 24-31% as bacterial amino acids. Protozoal amino acids were markedly increased when stilbestrol was included in the diet of dairy cows. Total amino acids passing into the gut were estimated to be 937 and 882 g/day on purified diets with and without stilbestrol as compared to 1,271 and 1,108 g/day when conventional diets were fed. Nikolic and Jovanovic (1973) suggest that bacterial N may account for 61-94% of total rumen N 3 hr after feeding and point out that the proportional contribution of bacteria increased as the digestible energy was decreased. However, since the ruminal total protein N concentration fell as the digestible energy of the diet was reduced, the actual concentration of bacterial N decreased with decrease in dietary digestible energy.

Bucholtz and Bergen (1973) note that P

uptake and incorporation into microbial phospholipids is highly related to ruminal protein synthesis. Their calculations, based on in vitro data, indicate that 16 g of protein were synthesized/100 g of organic matter digested.

Summary

The literature reviewed clearly indicates that rumen organisms actively degrade a large percentage of ingested proteins, the amount being dependent upon the solubility of the protein, the amount of protein in the ration and probably other factors such as level of dry matter intake and other unknown variables. Furthermore, amino acids and other N sources are apparently further deaminated to a large extent with the result that an extensive amount of resynthesis must take place to provide the amino acids and nucleotide bases required for microbial proteins. It seems likely that the ruminant animal might utilize proteins more efficiently, especially those of high quality, if a substantial amount passed intact into the lower GIT. Of course, a sufficient amount for microbial activity must be made available.

With respect to N requirements, adequate data are available to show that individual organisms may have relatively complex requirements with some species requiring peptides and hemin, although many species can make do with ammonia. Mixed cultures, on the other hand, can utilize very simple sources of N such as ammonia, probably because of recycling of microbial protein within the rumen.

A substantial amount of ammonia absorption is known to occur from the rumen when ammonia levels are high. Recent data indicate, however, that the net flow of N into the rumen may be at relatively high levels only when ruminal ammonia level is low. This would serve as a means of conserving N and act as a secondary source of N for the rumen organisms.

As mentioned, a substantial amount of resynthesis of amino acids has been shown to occur. Apparently, the organisms do not have the appropriate enzyme systems to utilize most of the amino acids intact. Results indicate that they seem to prefer glucose carbon to amino acid carbon for synthesis of amino acids. The amino acid composition of rumen bacteria and protozoa does not differ greatly and appears to be affected relatively little by the diet of the host, thus indicating a rather constant quality. Estimates of the digestibility of rumen microorganisms by ruminants and data obtained on rats indicate relatively high digestibility, with protozoa being somewhat more completely digested than bacteria. Estimates of the amount of microbial protein synthesized in the rumen have been derived in various ways with data indicating that 40-80% of ingested protein may be converted to microbial protein and potential microbial production is on the order of 15-20 g/100 g of digested organic matter.

References Cited

Abe, A., S. Horri and M. Yoshida. 1973. Nutr. Abstr. Rev. 43:305.
Abdel Rahman, S. and P. Decker. 1966. Nature 109:618.
Abdo, K.M., K.W. King and R.W. Engel. 1964. J. Animal Sci. 23:734.
Abe, A., S. Horri and M. Yoshida. 1973. Nutr. Abstr. Rev. 43:305.
Abou Akkada, A.R. and T.H. Blackburn. 1963. J. Gen. Microbiol. 31:461.
Abou Akkada, A.R., D.A. Messmer, L.R. Fina and E.E. Bartley. 1968. J. Dairy Sci. 51:78.
Acord, C.R., G.E. Mitchell, C.O. Little and M.R. Karr. 1966. J. Dairy Sci. 49:1519.
Aliev, A.A., I.G. Belogrudov and A.N. Kosarov. 1971. Nutr. Abstr. Rev. 41:70.
Aliev, A.A. and T.A. Radchenkova. 1972. Nutr. Abstr. Rev. 42:999.
Allison, M.J. 1965. Biochem. Biophys. Res. Comm. 18:30.
Allison, M.J. 1969. J. Animal Sci. 29:797.
Allison, M.J. and M.P. Bryant. 1963. Arch. Biochem. Biophys. 101:269.
Allison, M.J., J.A. Bucklin and I.M. Robinson. 1966. Appl. Microbiol. 14:807.
Al-Rabbat, M.F., R.L. Baldwin and W.C. Weir. 1971. J. Dairy Sci. 54:1150.
Amos, H.E., D. Burdick and T.L. Huber. 1974. J. Animal Sci. 38:702.
Amos, H.E., C.O. Little, D.G. Ely and G.E. Mitchell. 1971a. Can. J. Animal Sci. 51:51.
Amos, H.E., C.O. Little and G.E. Mitchell. 1971b. Agr. Fd. Chem. 19:112.
Annison, E.F. 1956. Biochem. J. 64:705.
Arthur, R.D., R.A. Bloomfield and M.E. Muhrer. 1966. J. Animal Sci. 25:1275 (abstr).

Arthur, R.D., M.E. Muhrer and R.A. Bloomfield. 1967. J. Animal Sci. 26:1488 (abstr).
Arias, C., W. Burroughs, P. Gerlaugh and R.M. Bethke. 1951. J. Animal Sci. 10:683.
Bailey, R.W. and A.E. Oxford. 1958. J. Gen. Microbiol. 19:130.
Barej, W. 1965. Nutr. Abstr. Rev. 35:984.
Barej, W., S. Garwacki and G. Kulasek. 1970. Nutr. Abstr. Rev. 40:74.
Bauriedel, W.R. 1971. J. Animal Sci. 32:704.
Bauriedel, W.R., L.F. Craig, J.C. Ramsey and E.O. Camehl. 1971. J. Animal Sci. 32:711.
Beauville, M., A.M. Lacoste and P. Raynaud. 1962. Nutr. Abstr. Rev. 32:849.
Belasco, I.J. 1954. J. Animal Sci. 13:601; 739.
Belasco, I.J. 1956. J. Animal Sci. 15:496.
Belasco, I.J. 1972. J. Dairy Sci. 55:353.
Bentley, O.G., A. Lehmkuhl, R.R. Johnson and A.L. Moxon. 1954. J. Animal Sci. 13:1015 (abstr).
Bergen, W.G., D.B. Purser and J.H. Cline. 1967. J. Nutr. 92:357.
Bergen, W.G., D.B. Purser and J.H. Cline. 1968. J. Animal Sci. 27:1497.
Bird, P.R. 1972. Aust. J. Biol. Sci. 25:195.
Bladen, H.A., M.P. Bryant and R.N. Doetsch. 1961. Appl. Microbiol. 9:175.
Black, A.L., M. Kleiber, A.H. Smith and D.N. Stewart. 1957. Biochem. Biophys. Acta 23:54.
Black, J.L. and D.E. Tribe. 1973. Aust. J. Agr. Res. 24:763.
Blackburn, T.H. 1965. In: Physiology of Digestion in the Ruminant. Butterworths.
Blackburn, T.H. 1968. J. Gen. Microbiol. 53:37.
Blackburn, T.H. and P.N. Hobson. 1960a. Br. J. Nutr. 14:445.
Blackburn, T.H. and P.N. Hobson. 1960b. J. Gen. Microbiol. 22:272; 290.
Borchers, R. 1965. J. Animal Sci. 24:1033.
Borchers, R. 1967. J. Dairy Sci. 50:242.
Brent, B.E., H.W. Newland, D.E. Ullrey and B.L. Bradley. 1966. J. Animal Sci. 25:1247 (abstr).
Briggs, M.H. (ed.). 1967. Urea as a Protein Supplement. Pergamon Press.
Bryant, M.P. and I.M. Robinson. 1961. Appl. Microbiol. 9:96.
Bryant, M.P. and I.M. Robinson. 1962. J. Bact. 84:605.
Bryant, M.P., I.M. Robinson and H. Chu. 1959. J. Dairy Sci. 42:1831.
Bucholtz, H.F. and W.G. Bergen. 1973. Appl. Microbiol. 25:504.
Burroughs, W., et al. 1951. J. Animal Sci. 10:672.
Byers, M. 1971. Leaf Protein: Its Agronomy, Preparation, Quality and Use. IBP Handbook No. 20. Blackwell Scientific Publ., Oxford, England.
Candlish, E., N.E. Stanger, T.J. Devlin and L.J. LaCroix. 1970. Can. J. Animal Sci. 50:337.
Carlson, J.R., M.T. Yokoyama and E.O. Dickinson. 1972. Science 176:298.
Chalmers, M.I. 1961. In: Digestive Physiology and Nutrition of the Ruminant. Butterworths.
Chalmers, M.I. and A.D. Hughes. 1969. Proc. Nutr. Soc. 28:34A (abstr).
Christiansen, W.C., R. Kawashima and W. Burroughs. 1965. J. Animal Sci. 24:731.
Ciszuk, P. 1973. Swedish J. Agr. Res. 3:167.
Clemens, E.R. and R.R. Johnson. 1973. J. Animal Sci. 37:1027.
Clifford, A.J., J.R. Bourdette and A.D. Tillman. 1968. J. Animal Sci. 27:814; 1073.
Cocimano, M.R. and R.A. Leng. 1967. Br. J. Nutr. 21:353.
Coleman, G.S. 1968. J. Gen. Microbiol. 54:83.
Colebrook, W.F. and P.J. Reis. 1969. Aust. J. Biol. Sci. 22:1507.
Conrad, H.R., J.W. Hibbs and A.D. Pratt. 1965. J. Dairy Sci. 48:793 (abstr).
Conrad, H.R., J.W. Hibbs and A.D. Pratt. 1967a. J. Nutr. 91:343.
Conrad, H.R., R.C. Miles and J. Burdorf. 1967b. J. Nutr. 91:337.
Craig, L., J.C. Ramsey and E.O. Camehl. 1969. J. Animal Sci. 29:151 (abstr).
Davis, G.V. and O.T. Stallcup. 1967. J. Dairy Sci. 50:1638.
Davis, R.F., R.H. Wasserman, J.K. Loosli and C.H. Grippin. 1955. J. Dairy Sci. 38:677.
Decker, P., H. Hill, K. Gartner and H. Hornicke. 1960. Deut. Tieraerztl. Wochschr. 67:539.
Dehority, B.A. 1963. J. Dairy Sci. 46:217.
Dehority, B.A., O.G. Bentley, R.R. Johnson and A.L. Moxon. 1957. J. Animal Sci. 16:502.
Dehority, B.A., R.R. Johnson, O.G. Bentley and A.L. Moxon. 1958. Arch. Biochem. Biophys. 78:15.
Delort-Laval, J. and S.Z. Zelter. 1968. Proc. 2nd World Conf. Animal Prod. p 457.
Derrig, R.G., J.H. Clark and C.L. Davis. 1974. J. Nutr. 104:151.
Dinius, D.A., C.K. Lyon and H.G. Walker. 1974. J. Animal Sci. 38:467.
Downes, A.M. 1961. Aust. J. Biol. Sci. 14:254.
Duncan, C.W., I.P. Agrawala, C.F. Huffman and R.W. Leucke. 1953. J. Nutr. 49:41.
Edwards, D.C. and R.A. Darroch. 1956. Br. J. Nutr. 10:286.
Egan, A.R. 1965. Aust. J. Agr. Res. 16:169.
Egan, A.R. 1970. Aust. J. Agr. Res. 21:85.
Ellis, W.C. and W.H. Pfander. 1965. Nature 205:974.
el-Shazly, K. 1952. Biochem. J. 51:640.
Ely, D.G., C.O. Little, P.G. Woolfolk and G.E. Mitchell. 1967. J. Nutr. 91:314.
Emery, R.S. 1971. J. Dairy Sci. 54:1090.
Engelhardt, W.V. 1963. Naturwissenschaften. 50:357.
Engelhardt, W.V. and W. Nickel. 1965. Arch. Ges. Physiol. 286:57.
Faichney, G.J. 1972. Aust. J. Agr. Res. 23:859.
Faichney, G.J. and H.L. Davies. 1973. Aust. J. Agr. Res. 24:613.

Federation Proceedings. 1970. Amino Acids in Ruminant Nutrition. 29:33-54.
Ferguson, K.A., J.A. Hemsley and P.J. Reis. 1967. Aust. J. Sci. 30:215.
Fulghum, R.S. and W.E.C. Moore. 1963. J. Bact. 85:808.
Gartner, K. 1963. Nutr. Abstr. Rev. 33:779.
Gil, L.A., R.L. Shirley and J.E. Moore. 1973. J. Dairy Sci. 56:757.
Gilchrist, F.M.C. 1968. J. Agr. Sci. 70:157.
Gibbons, R.J., R.N. Doetsch and J.C. Shaw. 1955. J. Dairy Sci. 38:1147.
Goering, H.K., et al. 1972. J. Dairy Sci. 55:1275.
Gray, F.V., A.F. Pilgrim and R.A. Weller. 1958. Br. J. Nutr. 12:413.
Griffiths, T.W. and I.H. Bath. 1973. J. Agr. Sci. 80:89.
Gutowski, B., W. Barej, A. Temler and I. Nowosieska. 1960. Nutr. Abstr. Rev. 30:1290.
Hall, G., E.A. Cheng, W.H. Hale and W. Burroughs. 1954. J. Animal Sci. 13:985 (abstr).
Harmeyer, J. 1972. Nutr. Abstr. Rev. 42:513.
Harmeyer, J. and D. Jezkova. 1972. Nutr. Abstr. Rev. 42:218.
Harmeyer, J., J. Varady and R. Birck. 1973. Arch. fur Tierernahrung. 23:461.
Harrop, C.J.F. and A.T. Phillipson. 1971. Proc. Nutr. Soc. 30:3A (abstr).
Heald, P.J. 1951. Br. J. Nutr. 5:75; 84.
Hecker, J.F. and J.V. Nolan. 1971. Aust. J. Biol. Sci. 24:403.
Helmer, L.G., et al. 1970. J. Dairy Sci. 53:330.
Henderickx, H. 1961. Nutr. Abstr. Rev. 35:566.
Henderickx, H. and J. Martin. 1963. C.R. Rech. Inst. Encour. Rech. Scient. Ind. Agr. 31:9.
Hershberger, T.V., O.G. Bentley and A.L. Moxon. 1959. J. Animal Sci. 18:663.
Hobson, P.N., R. Summers, J.R. Postgate and D.A. Ware. 1973. J. Gen. Microbiol. 77:225.
Hoeller, H. and J. Harmeyer. 1964. Zentr. Vet. Med. Reihe. A., Band II. 3:244.
Hogan, J.P. 1973. J. Agr. Res. 24:587.
Hogan, J.P. and R.H. Weston. 1967. Aust. J. Agr. Res. 18:973.
Hogan, J.P. and R.H. Weston. 1969. Aust. J. Agr. Res. 20:347.
Hoogenraad, N.J. and F.J.R. Hird. 1970. J. Gen. Microbiol. 62:261.
Hoover, W.H., E.M. Kesler and R.J. Flipse. 1963. J. Dairy Sci. 46:733.
Hoover, W.H. and J.J. Lipari. 1971. J. Dairy Sci. 54:1662.
Hoshina, S. and Y. Hirose. 1964. Jap. J. Zootech. Sci. 35:271.
Hoshina, S., K. Sarumaru and K. Morimoto. 1966. J. Dairy Sci. 49:1523.
Houpt, T.R. 1959. Amer. J. Physiol. 197:115.
Houpt, T.R. and K.A. Houpt. 1968. Amer. J. Physiol. 214:1296.
Hudson, L.W., H.A. Glimp, C.O. Little and P.G. Woolfolk. 1970. J. Animal Sci. 30:609.
Huhtanen, C.N. and L.S. Gall. 1955. J. Bact. 69:102.
Hume, I.D. 1970. Aust. J. Agr. Res. 21:297; 305.
Hume, I.D., R.J. Moir and M. Somers. 1970. Aust. J. Agr. Res. 21:283.
Hungate, R.E. 1966. The Rumen and Its Microbes. Academic Press.
Hungate, R.E., D.W. Fletcher, R.W. Dougherty and B.F. Barrentine. 1955. Appl. Microbiol. 3:161.
Hutton, K. and E.F. Annison. 1972. Proc. Nutr. Soc. 31:151.
Ibrahim, E.A. and J.R. Ingalls. 1972. J. Dairy Sci. 55:971.
Ichhponani, J.S., G.S. Makkar and G.S. Sidhu. 1969. Indian J. Animal Sci. 39:27.
Isaacs, J. and F.N. Owens. 1971. J. Animal Sci. 33:287; 1168 (abstr).
Johns, A.T. 1955. N.Z. J. Sci. Tech. 37A:323.
Johnson, B.C., T.S. Hamilton, W.B. Robinson and J.C. Garey. 1944. J. Animal Sci. 3:287.
Johnson, R.R. and E.T. Clemens. 1973. J. Nutr. 103:494.
Jones, G.A. 1967. In: Urea as a Protein Supplement. Pergamon Press.
Jones, G.A., R.A. MacLeod and A.C. Blackwood. 1964. Can. J. Microbiol. 10:371.
Juhasz, B. 1965. Nutr. Abstr. Rev. 35:709.
Jurtshuk, P., R.N. Doetsch and J.C. Shaw. 1958. J. Dairy Sci. 41:190.
Kameoka, K. 1962. Jap. Bul. Natl. Inst. Agr. Sci. Ser. G. Animal Husbandry. 21:195.
Kandatsu, M. and N. Takahashi. 1965. Jap. J. Zootech. Sci. 34:143.
Kurilov, N.V. and A.N. Kosarov. 1970. Nutr. Abstr. Rev. 40:517.
Kurilov, N.V., et al. 1972. Nutr. Abstr. Rev. 42:1365.
Lampila, M. 1967. Ann. Agr. Fenn. 6:14.
Langar, P.N., P.J. Buttery and D. Lewis. 1973. Proc. Nutr. Soc. 32:86A (abstr).
Lengerken, J.V., H. Wetterau, V. Muller and A. Schellenberger. 1970. Arch. fur. Tierernahrung. 20:641.
Leibholz, J. 1969. J. Animal Sci. 29:628.
Leibholz, J. 1972. Aust. J. Agr. Res. 23:1073.
Leroy, F. and S.Z. Zelter. 1970. Ann. Biol. Anim. Biochem. Biophys. 10:401.
Leroy, F., S.Z. Zelter and A.C. Francois. 1964. C.R. Acad. Sci. 259:1592.
Leroy, F., S.Z. Zelter and A.C. Francois. 1965. Nutr. Abstr. Rev. 35:444.
Leru, Y. and P. Raynaud. 1964. Nutr. Abstr. Rev. 34:156.
Lewis, D. 1955. Br. J. Nutr. 9:215.
Lewis, D. 1957. J. Agr. Sci. 48:438.
Lewis, D. 1962. J. Agr. Sci. 58:73.
Lewis, D. and W.I. McDonald. 1958. J. Agr. Sci. 51:108.
Lewis, T.R. and R.S. Emery. 1962. J. Dairy Sci. 45:765; 1487.
Lilligan, L.P., et al. 1972. Proc. West. Sec. Amer. Soc. Animal Sci. 23:372.

Little, C.O., W. Burroughs and W. Woods. 1963. J. Animal Sci. 22:358.
Loosli, J.K., et al. 1949. Science. 110:144.
Lord, P.J.E., G.T. Schelling and G.E. Mitchell. 1972. J. Animal Sci. 34:361 (abstr).
Mangan, J.L. 1972. Br. J. Nutr. 27:261.
Mason, V.G. and R. Palmer. 1971. J. Agr. Sci. 76:567.
Masson, F.M. and A.E. Oxford. 1951. J. Gen. Microbiol. 5:664.
Mathison, G.W. and L.P. Milligan. 1971. Br. J. Nutr. 25:351.
McAllan, A.B. and R.H. Smith. 1973. Br. J. Nutr. 29:331; 467.
McDonald, I.W. 1952. Biochem. J. 51:86.
McDonald, I.W. and R.J. Hall. 1957. Biochem. J. 67:400.
McIntyre, K.H. 1971. Aust. J. Agr. Res. 22:429.
McNaught, M.L., E.C. Owen, K.M. Henry and S.K. Kon. 1954. Biochem. J. 56:151.
McNaught, M.L., J.A.B. Smith, K.M. Henry and S.K. Kon. 1950. Biochem. J. 46:32.
Menahan, L.A. and L.H. Schultz. 1964. J. Dairy Sci. 47:1080.
Meyer, R.M., E.E. Bartley, C.W. Deyoe and V.F. Colenbrander. 1967. J. Dairy Sci. 50:1327.
Mills, R.C., C.C. Lardinois, I.W. Rupel and E.B. Hart. 1944. J. Dairy Sci. 27:571.
Muller, R. and I. Kirchner. 1971. Nutr. Abstr. Rev. 41:961.
Muller, R. and I. Kirchner. 1972. Nutr. Abstr. Rev. 42:514.
Munchow, H., H. Bergner and J.N. Gupta. 1973. Arch. Tierernahrung 23:133.
Murti, V.V.S. and T.R. Seshadri. 1967. Nutr. Abstr. Rev. 37:667.
Nader, C.J. and D.J. Walker. 1970. Appl. Microbiol. 20:677.
Neudoerffer, T.S., D.B. Duncan and F.D. Horney. 1971. Br. J. Nutr. 25:333.
Nikolic, J.A. and M. Jovanovic. 1973. J. Agr. Sci. 81:1.
Nolan, J.V. and R.A. Leng. 1972. Br. J. Nutr. 27:177.
Nolan, J.V., B.W. Norton and R.A. Leng. 1973. Proc. Nutr. Soc. 32:93.
Oldham, J.D., H. Swan and D. Lewis. 1973. Proc. Nutr. Soc. 32:98A (abstr).
Oltjen, R.R., J. Bond and G.V. Richardson. 1969. J. Animal Sci. 28:717; 29:81.
Onodera, R. and M. Kandatsu. 1970. Nutr. Abstr. Rev. 40:572.
Onodera, R. and M. Kandatsu. 1972. Agr. Biol. Chem. 36:1989.
Ørskov, E.R. and C. Fraser. 1969. J. Agr. Sci. 73:469.
Ørskov, E.R., C. Fraser and I. McDonald. 1971. Br. J. Nutr. 26:477.
Oser, B.L. 1951. J. Amer. Dietetic Assoc. 27:396.
Otagaki, K.K., A.L. Black, H. Goss and M. Kleiber. 1955. J. Agr. Fd. Chem. 3:943.
Oxford, A.E. 1955. Expt. Parasitol. 4:569.
Packett, L.V. and T.D. Groves. 1965. J. Animal Sci. 24:341.
Pearson, R.M. and J.A.B. Smith. 1943. Biochem. J. 37:148; 153.
Phillipson, A.T. 1964. In: Mammalian Protein Metabolism. Academic Press.
Phillipson, A.T., M.J. Dobson, T.H. Blackburn and M. Brown. 1962. Br. J. Nutr. 16:151.
Pilgrim, A.F., F.V. Gray and G.B. Belling. 1969. Br. J. Nutr. 23:647.
Pittman, K.A., S. Lakshmanan and M.P. Bryant. 1966. J. Bact. 93:1499.
Porter, P. and A.G. Singleton. 1965. Proc. Biochem. Soc. 96:59P (abstr).
Portugal, A.V. and T.M. Sutherland. 1966. Nature 209:510.
Postgate, J.R. 1970. J. Gen. Microbiol. 63:137.
Potter, G.D., C.O. Little, N.W. Bradley and G.E. Mitchell. 1971. J. Animal Sci. 32:531.
Prokop, M.J., W. Woods and T.J. Klopfenstein. 1971. J. Animal Sci. 33:1169 (abstr).
Prokosva, M. 1968. Nutr. Abstr. Rev. 38:471.
Prokosva, M. 1969. Nutr. Abstr. Rev. 39:442.
Prokudin, A.V. 1967. Nutr. Abstr. Rev. 37:755.
Provost, P.J. and R.N. Doetsch. 1960. Biochem. J. 22:259.
Purser, D.B. and S.M. Buechler. 1966. J. Dairy Sci. 49:81.
Purser, D.B. and R.J. Moir. 1966. J. Animal Sci. 25:668.
Reed, R.M., R.H. Moir and E.J. Underwood. 1949. Aust. J. Sci. Res. B 2:304.
Reis, P.J. and W.F. Colebrook. 1972. Aust. J. Biol. Sci. 25:1057.
Reis, P.J. and P.G. Schinckel. 1964. Aust. J. Biol. Sci. 17:532.
Reis, P.J. and D.A. Tunks. 1969. Aust. J. Agr. Res. 20:775.
Ridges, A.P. and A.G. Singleton. 1962. J. Physiol. 161:1.
Roberts, S.A. and E.L. Miller. 1969. Proc. Nutr. Soc. 28:21A (abstr).
Robertson, J.A. and J.C. Hawke. 1965. J. Sci. Fd. Agr. 16:268.
Robinson, I.M. and M.J. Allison. 1969. J. Bact. 97:1220.
Salsbury, R.L. and G.F.W. Haenlein. 1964. J. Animal Sci. 23:891 (abstr).
Schelling, G.T. and E.E. Hatfield. 1968. J. Nutr. 96:319.
Schmidt, S.P., N.J. Benevenga and N.A. Jorgensen. 1973. J. Animal Sci. 37:1258.
Schmidt, S.P., N.J. Benevenga and N.A. Jorgensen. 1974. J. Animal Sci. 38:646.
Schmidt-Nielsen, B., et al. 1957. Amer. J. Physiol. 188:477.
Schroder, H.H.E. 1970. J. Agr. Sci. 75:231.
Schwarz, H.M., C.A. Schoeman and M.S. Faber. 1964. J. Agr. Sci. 63:289.
Sirotnak, F.M., R.N. Doetsch, R.E. Brown and J.C. Shaw. 1953. J. Dairy Sci. 36:1117.
Slyter, L.L., R.R. Oltjen, E.E. Williams and R.L. Wilson. 1971. J. Nutr. 101:839.
Smith, J.A.B. and F. Baker. 1944. Biochem. J. 38:496.
Smith, R.H. 1969. J. Dairy Res. 36:313.

Smith, R.H. and A.B. McAllan. 1970. Br. J. Nutr. 24:545.

Smith, R.H. and A.B. McAllan. 1971. Br. J. Nutr. 25:181.

Stangel, H.J., R.R. Johnson and A. Spellman. 1963. Urea and Non-protein Nitrogen in Ruminant Nutrition. Nitrogen Division, Allied Chem. Corp.

Szanyiova, M., M. Bajo, J. Varady and J. Fejes. 1974. Nutr. Abstr. Rev. 44:182.

Tandon, R.N., D.D. Sharma and V.D. Mudgal. 1972. Indian J. Animal Sci. 42:174.

Temler-Kucharski, A., et al. 1966. Nutr. Abstr. Rev. 36:95.

Thornton, R.F. 1970. Aust. J. Agr. Res. 21:323; 337.

Thornton, R.F., P.R. Bird, M. Somers and R.J. Moir. 1970. Aust. J. Agr. Res. 21:345.

Tiwari, A.D., F.N. Owens and U.S. Garrigus. 1973. J. Animal Sci. 37:1390; 1396.

Topps, J.H. and R.C. Elliott. 1965. Nature 205:498.

Ulbirch, M. and H. Scholz. 1967. Nutr. Abstr. Rev. 37:795.

Uselli, F. and P. Fiorini. 1938. Bool. Sac. Ital. Biol. Spec. 13:11.

Van Den Hende, C., W. Oyaert and J.H. Bouchaert. 1963. Res. Vet. Sci. 4:89.

Van Den Hende, C., W. Oyaert and J.H. Bouchaert. 1964. Res. Vet. Sci. 5:491.

Varady, J., K. Boda, J. Fejes and M. Bajo. 1970. Phys. Bohem. 19:519.

Varady, J., K. Boda, I. Havassy, M. Bajo and J. Tomas. 1967. Physiol. Bohemoslovaca. 16:571.

Vatthauer, R.J., F.C. Hinds, and U.S. Garrigus. 1968. J. Animal Sci. 27:1178 (abstr).

Vercoe, J.E. 1969. Aust. J. Agr. Res. 20:191.

Virtanen, A.I. 1966. Science. 153:1603.

Waldo, D.R. 1968. J. Dairy Sci. 51:265.

Warner, A.C.I. 1956. J. Gen. Microbiol. 14:749.

Warner, A.C.I. 1964. Aust. J. Biol. Sci. 17:170.

Wegner, M.I., A.N. Booth, G. Bohstedt and E.B. Hart. 1940. J. Nutr. 23:1123.

Weller, R.A. 1957. Aust. J. Biol. Sci. 10:384.

Weller, R.A., F.V. Gray and A.F. Pilgrim. 1958. Br. J. Nutr. 12:421.

Weston, R.H. and J.P. Hogan. 1967. Aust. J. Biol. Sci. 20:967.

Williams, V.J. and K.R. Christian. 1956. N.Z. J. Sci. Tech. 38A:194.

Winter, K.A. and W.J. Pigden. 1956. N.Z. J. Sci. 51:777.

Woods, W.R., W.D. Gallup and A.D. Tillman. 1957. J. Animal Sci. 16:675.

Wortham, J.S., et al. 1968. J. Animal Sci. 27:1180 (abstr).

Yokoyama, M.T. and J.R. Carlson. 1974. Appl. Microbiol. 27:540.

Zelter, S.Z., F. Leroy and J.P. Tissier. 1970. An. Biol. Anim. Biochem. Biophys. 10:111.

Zikakis, J.P. and R.L. Salsbury. 1969. J. Dairy Sci. 52:2014.

CHAPTER 14 — RUMEN METABOLISM OF LIPIDS

Plant Lipids

Forage plants (and many seeds) do not contain a large quantity of lipid material. The usual amount will be about 4-6% which is made up of 1.5-4% glycerides, 0.5-1% waxes, 0.5-1% sterols and 0.5-1% phospholipids with salts of phosphatidic acid (Hilditch, 1956). The assumption used to be that most of the glyceride fraction was triglyceride in nature, but Weenink (1959) found that ca. 60% of the lipid fraction was made up of galactosyl glyceryl esters of fatty acids, primarily linolenic acid. Garton (1960a) also found this to be the case and that triglyceride fatty acids represented only 3.3% of total fatty acids. Bailey (1964) reported that the leaves of red clover [*Trifolium pratense L.*] contained much larger amounts of lipid-bound sugars than did other parts of the plant and that seasonal trends in concentration occurred that were unrelated to stage of maturity of the plant. The relative dietary importance of lipids is illustrated by calculations of Garton (1960b), who estimated that a cow consuming 100 lb (46.5 kg) of pasture forage would consume as much as 500 g of plant lipids. Examples of the fatty acid composition of several forages are shown in Table 14-1.

Metabolism of Dietary Lipids by Rumen Microorganisms

It has been known for many years that the depot fat of ruminant species is subject to little modification by dietary changes or the feeding of relatively large amounts of unsaturated fats or oils. In monogastric species, in contrast, the feeding of large amounts of unsaturated fats can markedly affect depot fat. The depot fat of ruminants contains rather large amounts of stearic acid (C18:0), substantial amounts of *trans* isomers, as well as quantities of branched-chain acids. Milk fat, particularly, contains appreciable quantities of odd-length acids as well. The *trans* , odd-length and branched-chain acids are not characteristic of plant lipids, thus it was evident that synthesis of these acids must take place in the rumen, the lower GIT or the body tissues. Recent research has indicated that most of this activity takes place in the rumen, resulting in characteristic modifications of dietary fat as well as synthesis of the odd-length and branched-chain acids.

Hydrolysis of Fatty Acid Esters

Garton et al (1959) were the first to demonstrate that rumen microbial suspen-

Table 14-1. Fatty acids found in pasture forage or hay.[a]

Fatty acid	Clover-rich pasture	Mixed pasture grasses	Timothy, sun-cured	Timothy, dehydrated	Red clover, sun-cured
Saturated acids					
C14 (myristic)	—	1.1	1-2	1.9	0.5
C16 (palmitic)	8.9	15.9	22-26*	26.0*	22.7*
C18 (stearic)	2.8	2.0	1-2	1.9	1.1
Higher than C18	3.9	0.5			
Unsaturated acids					
C16:1 (palmitoleic)	7.9	2.5	*	*	*
C18:1 (oleic)	9.5	3.4	5-6	12.0	5.3
C18:2 (linoleic)	8.1	13.2	21-24	36.5	23.4
C18:3 (linolenic)	58.9	61.3	44-50	21.8	46.9

[a]Data from Shorland et al (1955), Garton (1960a) and Oksanen and Thafvelin (1965)
*C16 and C16:1 not differentiated

sions could hydrolyze triglycerides. In one experiment they found that ca. 95% of fatty acids from linseed oil were hydrolyzed and ca. 70% of those in olive oil. A subsequent paper from the same laboratory (Garton et al, 1961) revealed that linseed oil, olive oil and coca butter were hydrolyzed to the extent of 95, 68 and 40%, respectively. Wright (1961), Hawke and Robertson (1964) and Miller and Cramer (1969) have also demonstrated that a variety of glycerides could be hydrolyzed. Miller and Cramer observed that the extent of hydrolysis of a variety of different oils or fats (both plant and animal) ranged from a maximum of ca. 93% (linseed oil) to a low of ca. 35% (fish oil). Plant oils were, in general, hydrolyzed more completely than animal fats or fish oils.

Hawke and Silcock (1970) observed, following incubation of labeled triglyceride in vitro, that ca. 80% of the linolenate from the glyceride was present as free acid after 100 min. There was no detectable linolenic acid in triglycerides which remained unhydrolyzed nor in mixtures of mono- and diglycerides. Japanese research with forage-fed goats has demonstrated, also, that hydrolysis of triglycerides in the rumen is a rapid process. When 50 g of safflower oil was fed daily, the mono- and diglycerides accounted for 8-11% of total rumen lipid (Watanabe et al, 1969; Tanaka and Hayashi, 1972). Clarke and Hawke (1970) have determined that organisms responsible for hydrolysis of triglycerides were closely associated with the particular matter and that homogenization released much of the lipolytic activity.

In the milk-fed calf, information on stomach hydrolysis of lipids is vague. Felinski and Toullec (1972) found a high proportion of free fatty acids in chyme from the abomasum. Gastric juice did not hydrolyze milk triglycerides; thus, it may be that salivary lipase may be responsible (see Ch. 5).

Phospholipids may account for 8-11% of rumen lipids in some circumstances (Watanabe et al, 1969). Dawson (1959) has shown that a number of phospholipids were hydrolyzed. Bailey (1964) observed that galactolipids in the rumen were rapidly released and degraded, thus demonstrating that the galactosyl glyceryl esters found in plants can be readily metabolized. As a result of these experiments, it can be concluded that plant lipids of various forms can be readily hydrolyzed from the glycerol molecule. Other sources of triglycerides may be less completely hydrolyzed.

Data published by Johns (1953), Garton et al (1961) and Wright (1969) indicate that glycerol can be metabolized by such organisms as *Selenomonas ruminantium* with propionic acid as the main production of fermentation.

Hydrogenation of Dietary Lipids

As pointed out before, it has been known for some time that the depot fats of ruminants contain mostly saturated fatty acids. The fat of other herbivorous animals will have appreciable amounts of unsaturated fatty acids and omnivores may have very high levels of unsaturated fats in their tissues, so that the body fats tend to resemble dietary fats.

Reiser (1951) first showed that incubation of linseed oil in vitro with rumen liquor resulted in a marked reduction in linolenic acid (C18:3) content. This finding was confirmed in other research by Reiser and Reddy (1956), Shorland et al (1955), Garton et al (1958, 1959) and others. When fatty acids present in the diet were compared to those present after fermentation, these research reports showed a marked change, indicating either selective metabolism of some of the acids or hydrogenation of some of the unsaturated acids. Wood et al (1963) investigated this by infusing labeled linoleic acid into the rumen of sheep. They recovered 85-96% of the dose (the reticulo-omasal orifice was ligated) of which 3-6% was linoleic acid; about 45% was hydrogenated to saturated acids, and 33-50% was hydrogenated to oleic or elaidic acids. A more recent example of the type of change to be expected is shown in Table 14-2, using data from the paper of Macleod et al (1972). Note in this example that there is generally an increase in rumen fluid and milk in the content of C14 and C16 acids. With respect to C18:0, there is a substantial increase in rumen fluid content with a corresponding decrease in C18:2 and C18:3. This change is not necessarily reflected in milk fat however, as milk fat is complicated by synthesis of the mammary gland. The data illustrate, however, that very little C18:2 acid is found in rumen fluid and almost no C18:3.

Other investigators including Ward et al (1964), Polan et al (1964) and Wilde and Dawson (1966) have demonstrated hydro-

Table 14-2. Fatty acids found in the diet, rumen fluid and milk fat.[a]

Fatty acid	Dietary Composition*			Rumen fluid			Milk fat		
	A	C	D	A	C	D	A	C	D
					%				
C14:0	0.2	2.3	0.3	5.9	5.4	9.0	15.6	18.6	14.0
C16:0	15.8	22.8	14.0	21.9	30.7	25.1	35.4	48.2	31.7
C18:0	1.0	35.2	5.9	29.9	49.3	19.2	12.4	8.5	14.1
C18:1	21.3	10.8	22.5	29.1	10.9	34.7	34.8	23.2	37.6
C18:2	56.2	26.3	50.3	12.6	3.1	11.1	1.8	1.5	2.6
C18:3	5.5	2.6	7.0	0.6	0.6	0.9	0	0	0
% dietary fat	2.8	4.2	4.2						

*Diet A was hay; C contained hydrogenated tallow and D contained soybean oil.
[a]From Macleod et al (1972)

genation with ^{14}C-labeled fatty acids using in vitro techniques. Polan et al and Wilde and Dawson both reported that *Butyrivibrio fibrisolvens* in pure culture would actively hydrogenate C18:2 acid to one of several octadecenoic isomers, whereas mixed suspensions of rumen organisms will hydrogenate a large quantity of C18:3 or C18:0. *B. fibrisolvens* apparently lacks the cellular enzymes required to hydrogenate C18:1 acids. Therefore, since mixed cultures rapidly hydrogenate C18:3 or C18:2 acids to C18:0, it is apparent that other organisms must be able to hydrogenate monoene acids. Whether any given specie can hydrogenate a C18:3 or C18:2 to C18:0 remains to be seen since data are lacking on this point. More recent evidence bears out the suggestion that individual species may not hydrogenate C18:3 to C18:0. For example, Mills et al (1970) found that a micrococcus hydrogenated 50-75% of added C18:3 to mono- and dienoic acids during a 24-hr incubation, but neither C18:3 nor C18:2 were completely hydrogenated to C18:0. Yokoyama and Davis (1971) have published similar results using a strain of *Borrelia*.

When cows have been fed fish oils, which contain substantial amounts of fatty acids with C20 and C22 carbon chains, data indicate that many of these long-chain polyunsaturated acids are recovered in the blood plasma lipids, suggesting that these acids are not easily hydrogenated in the rumen (Brumby et al, 1969; Nicholson and Sutton, 1971).

Data published by Hawke and Silcock (1970) and Hawke (1971) clearly show that hydrogenation of glycerides does not take place and that free fatty acids must be present. When using ^{14}C-labeled triglycerides, they could not detect any label in mono-, di- or triglycerides isolated after incubation. Data of Hawke and Silcock and Harfoot et al (1973) indicate that removal of particulate matter reduced the extent of hydrogenation. It may be that organisms capable of hydrogenating fatty acids adhere to these particles; on the other hand, the food particles might be involved in the reaction. Smith and Lough (1973) note that free long-chain fatty acids in the digesta are associated with particulate matter. Based on studies of solubility, they concluded that these acids are absorbed on the surfaces of the particles; thus this may be the explanation relating particulate matter to hydrogenation. It might also be noted that hydrogenation is prevented by protecting dietary fats with formaldehyde-treated casein or similar preparations (Scott et al, 1970, 1971). Other papers providing data on hydrogenation of dietary fatty acids include those of Miller and Cramer (1969), Sutton et al (1970), Tanaka and Hayashi (1972) and Tanaka et al (1974).

With respect to protozoa, Wright (1959) was probably the first to demonstrate that ciliates could hydrogenate plant lipids; in this case lipids from chloroplasts. Williams et al (1963) observed that *Isotricha intestinalis* could hydrogenate fatty acids as could rumen bacterial suspensions. Further research by Chalupa and Kutches (1968) pointed out that hydrogenation actively occurred in suspensions of oligotricha species; however, their research with suspensions of about ⅔ holotrich and ⅓ oligotrich species indicated very little, if any, hydrogenation. They felt that hydrogenation occurring in oligotrich suspensions was probably similar to that suggested for bacteria. Dawson and Kemp (1969) found that hydrogenation was less complete in defaunated sheep than in those with protozoa, and Sklan et al (1971) found that protozoa-rich fractions had a much more intense hydrogenation activity than protozoa-free fractions of rumen liquor from calves, cows or sheep.

The results of these experiments, although not in complete agreement, indicate that rumen ciliates, as a group, have the capability of hydrogenating unsaturated fatty acids. Indirect evidence has also been presented in several situations. For example, Klopfenstein et al (1966) observed that defaunated lambs had higher levels of linoleic acid and less oleic acid in blood plasma than faunated lambs. Likewise, Chalupa et al (1967) reported that almost no protozoa were present in the rumen of cows during a time when they were producing milk with high levels of unsaturated fatty acids.

In the lower GIT, Ward et al (1964) found that unsaturated C18 acids present in ileal digesta were hydrogenated in the cecum and colon with the result that nearly all of the acids in the excreta were saturated. Similar data have been reported by Zerebocov and Listunov (1972).

Fatty Acid Isomers Produced in the Rumen

Unsaturated fatty acids found in plants are almost all of a *cis* configuration whereas *trans* isomers are a result of microbial metabolism or are artifacts of catalytic hydrogenation. Hartman et al (1954) demonstrated that *trans* fatty acids were characteristically much higher in ruminant fats than in other animals and Shorland et al (1955, 1957) showed that rumen fermentation was the probable source of these isomers. When they incubated oleic, linoleic and linolenic acids with rumen contents in vitro, they found that about 23, 16 and 17%, respectively, of these acids were converted to stearic acid and 59, 45 and 72%, respectively, to a monoenoic acid. *Trans* monoenoic isomers represented 17, 48 and 67% of the total acids recovered. In the case of linolenic acid, *trans* isomers represented 91% of the unsaturated acids. Shorland et al (1957) point out that this compares to about 66% *trans* acids produced when catalytic

hydrogenation is carried out. It might be noted that commercially hydrogenated fat products are said to have large amounts of *trans* isomers in them.

In addition to the geometric isomers [*cis-trans*] , Shorland et al found that several positional isomers (those having one or more double bonds in a different location than the original acid) were produced during rumen fermentation. This migration of double bonds in long-chain fatty acids is, apparently, a situation which also occurs during catalytic hydrogenation (Allen and Kiess, 1955). Shorland et al went on to point out that some of the isomers found after rumen fermentation were conjugated acids which appeared to resist further hydrogenation. They further showed that carotene did not disappear during fermentation and speculated that the conjugated structure of carotene may be the reason that it is resistant to hydrogenation — obviously a useful protective mechanism insofar as the host is concerned.

Wood et al (1963) also concluded that appreciable amounts of *trans* acids and unidentified acids were formed during rumen fermentation. Ward and others (1964) found that linolenic acid uniformly labeled with radioactive carbon was rapidly hydrogenated to two types of dienoic acids, subsequently to a C18:1 acid, and finally to C18:0 (stearic acid). The isomers in the dienoic acid fraction had *cis-cis* nonconjugated configurations with double bonds largely at carbon atoms 11:12 or 12:13 and 15:16 or 16:17 (linoleic acid has bonds at 9:10 and 12:13). The monoenoic acids were largely *trans* with the double bond predominantly at 12:14 or 14:15 (oleic acid has a double bond at 9:10). Rapid hydrogenation of linoleic and oleic acids occurred. The former gave rise to a *trans* C18:1 as an intermediary, also observed by Harfoot et al (1973). The *trans* acids passing from the rumen were absorbed almost quantitatively in the ileum. Wilde and Dawson (1966) reported that linolenic acid appeared to be isomerized in the rumen to a diconjugated *cis-cis-cis* C18:3 (octadecatrienoic) acid, then to a non-conjugated *trans-cis* or *cis-trans* C18:2 acid, and then to a *trans* C18:1, although other pathways were indicated. When Kepler et al (1966) used *Butyrivibrio fibrisolvens* to study hydrogenation, they identified intermediates of linoleic acid *cis-cis* 9:10, 12:13 C18:2 as *cis-trans* and *trans-cis* C18:2 and a mixture of *trans* -9:10 C18:1 and *trans* -11:12 C18:1.

When different positional isomers of cis-trans conjugated C18:2 were incubated, various trans C18:1 acids were produced which reflected the double bond positions of the conjugated substrates. In studies with a micrococcus organism (Mills et al, 1970), it was shown that linolenic acid was first isomerized mainly to cis-9, trans-11, cis-15 C18:3. This was probably hydrogenated to trans-11, cis-15 C18:2. The principal monoene isolated was trans-11 C18:1, suggesting hydrogenation of the double bond with the cis configuration. Linoleic acid was metabolized almost exclusively to trans-11 C18:1 with small amounts of a conjugated diene identified as cis-9, trans-11. Oleic acid was not hydrogenated.

Katz and Keeney (1966) analyzed rumen digesta at different times after a cow was fed alfalfa hay and found no significant changes in total lipid, fatty acid concentrations, types of fatty acids or the concentration of trans-octadecenoic acids. The C18:1 acids from the rumen (about 7% of the total) consisted of 75% trans acids, trans-11:12 being the major component. Rumen bacterial C18:1 acids consisted of a mixture of 23 geometrical and positional isomers, the major acids being trans-11, cis-9, and cis-11. Data indicated that rumen bacteria preferentially esterify the cis isomers into polar lipids (phospholipids).

Czerkawski and Blaxter (1965) have studied isomerization of fatty acids in the rumens of sheep continuously infused with emulsions of fatty acids. Results of experiments when only grass lipids were present indicated that the predominant monoenoic acid (C18:1) was in the trans form. The infusion of a small amount of oleic acid — which introduced several times as much fatty acid as was derived from the grass — led to an accumulation of the cis form, together with somewhat smaller amounts of the trans form as well as accumulation of C18:0. When larger amounts of oleic acid (60 g/day) were infused, no accumulation of oleic acid was observed, but a further increase in elaidic acid (trans form of oleic) occurred. The infusion of linoleic and linolenic acids gave rise to an increase in all C18 acids; in the case of linolenic acid, trans acids were present in much greater concentration than were cis forms. There was little evidence of double bond migration under normal conditions or when oleic acid was infused. Conjugated acids accounted for 5-10% of the polyenoic acids during infusion of small amounts of nonconjugated linoleic or linolenic acids and rose to 12-25% during infusion of the large amounts. Ulyatt et al (1966) reported, in studies with sheep, that 85% of the double bonds of unsaturated acids from grass or added linseed oil were hydrogenated before reaching the pylorus; however, Czerkawski et al (1966) indicated that the rumen, if overloaded with fat, will hydrogenate less than maximal amounts. On purified rations Tove and Matrone (1962) found that sheep produced body fats that were highly unsaturated, indicating incomplete hydrogenation in the rumen.

An indirect method of showing the effect of rumen fermentation on unsaturated lipids is to infuse fats intravenously or administer them via the duodenum (Ogilvie and McClymont, 1961; Tove and Mochrie, 1963; Moore et al, 1969). Data of this type generally show that unsaturated acids in the blood may give rise to much higher levels of unsaturated acids in body depot fat or milk fat thus indicating that most, if not all, of the hydrogenation occurs in the reticulo-rumen.

Several scientists have theorized why rumen microorganisms hydrogenate unsaturated fatty acids. One theory which seems reasonable is that hydrogenation may be a convenient means of disposing of excess hydrogen that might accumulate during anaerobic fermentation. Czerkawski et al (1966) have studied methane production in sheep to which they administered various fatty acids intraruminally. They found that methane production was reduced somewhat by infusion of all the acids tested, although there was somewhat less production of methane as a result of infusing the more unsaturated acids. Further data reported by this laboratory (Czerkawski and Breckenridge, 1969; Czerkawski, 1973) confirms the inhibition of methane production by fatty acids of linseed oil. This is illustrated in Fig. 14-1. Czerkawski (1973) has discussed this subject in detail with accompanying calculations. He suggests, when methane production is inhibited, that part of the hydrogen, which might otherwise accumulate in rumen gas, is utilized in the hydrogenation process for saturating the double bonds in unsaturated acids. It also seems likely that some hydrogen is utilized for synthesis of palmitic acid (see section on synthesis), but he goes on to suggest that other lipid synthesis may take up some of the hydrogen. The complete answer to this must await further research.

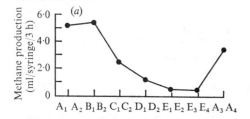

Figure 14-1. Effect of linseed oil fatty acids on in vitro methane production. Diets were: A, basal primarily grass cubes; B,C,D,E, 20, 40, 60 and 80 g of fatty acids/day. From Czerkawski [1973].

Fatty Acid Content of Rumen Microorganisms

Data on the fatty acid content of rumen microorganisms are relatively limited in the literature, although several papers are available. Williams et al (1963) found the lipid content of *Isotricha intestinalis* to be about 9.1% and that of *Entodinium simplex* about 6.3%. The lipid content of bacteria associated with these protozoa was about 6.8%, but quantitative data on fatty acids were not given. Keeney et al (1962) have determined the fatty acid distribution in neutral lipids, free fatty acids and polar lipids (phospholipids) of mixed rumen bacteria and of protozoa and Ifkovits and Ragheb (1968) have examined the fatty acid content of a variety of rumen bacteria. Some of the data from the latter two papers are shown in Table 14-3.

With respect to the data presented by Keeney et al, the authors stated that the protozoal fraction was contaminated with bacteria and feed particles, so these data are, no doubt, less accurate than those for the bacteria. The data show that rumen bacteria have larger concentrations of some of the odd-length or branched-chain fatty acids than do protozoa, particularly C15:0 and C15:0 iso acids. These marked differences may be indicative that protozoa do not synthesize the C15 acids. These data would also seem to be good proof of the suggestion of Keeney et al that the rumen microorganisms are the source of the odd-length and branched-chain fatty acids found in the milk and body fat of ruminants.

The detailed analyses of fatty acid composition of different species of rumen bacteria by Ifkovits and Ragheb (1968) clearly show a vast difference between species in the composition of fatty acids. These authors also reported that the fatty acid composition may be expected to vary within a given species during different phases of a growth cycle and when grown on different media. Other papers giving data on fatty acid composition of rumen microbes include those of Katz and Keeney (1966) and Viviani et al (1965). In the latter paper it was pointed out that protozoal lipids differed from bacterial lipids in having appreciable amounts of linolenic acid and more linoleic acid than bacteria. Furthermore, protozoa have only *cis* unsaturated acids whereas bacteria contain mainly *trans* acids (Katz and Keeney, 1966).

Kunsman (1967) has characterized some of the lipids of several pure cultures of rumen bacteria. Polar lipids constituted the major fraction of *Bacteroides amylophilus, B. succinogenes, Butyrivibrio fibrisolvens, Selenomonas faciens* and *Ruminococcus albus*. Lipids from *Peptostreptococcus elsdenii* were found to be high in hydrocarbons. When a pure culture of *B. ruminicola* was grown on media with either branched-chain VFA or acetate, lipids from the medium containing acetate had a higher proportion of polar lipids through the same phospholipids. The major phospholipid was phosphatidyl ethanolamine. In the nonpolar fractions, diglyceride was the main component; other constituents were free fatty acids, triglyceride, monoglyceride and hydrocarbons.

In sheep that were defaunated, Dawson and Kemp (1969) noted the almost complete absence of the choline-containing phospholipids, phosphatidylcholine and sphingomyelin. Also absent was phosphatidylhydroxyethylalanine, confirming that this phospholipid is a characteristic lipid in protozoa.

Synthesis of Fatty Acids by Rumen Microbes

Research from a variety of laboratories on the synthesis of fatty acids has resulted in a number of interesting papers, particularly those dealing with the odd-length or branched-chain acids (see Table 14-4). Allison et al (1962) grew *Ruminococcus flavefaciens* on isovalerate-1-[14]C. Most of the ^{14}C was recovered in a branched-chain C15 acid and some in a C17 acid. In addition, about 7% of the label was recovered in a branched-chain C15 aldehyde from the phospholipid fraction. In another case when a strain of *R. albus* was grown in a medium containing isobutyrate-1-^{14}C, 86% of the

Table 14-3. Percent fatty acid composition of rumen organisms as compared to ruminant subcutaneous and milk fat.

Fatty acid[a]	Sub-Q fat[b]	Milk fat[c]	Protozoa[d] neutral lipids	Protozoa[d] phospho-lipids	Mixed bacteria[d] neutral lipids	Mixed bacteria[d] phospho-lipids	Bacterial species 1[d]	Bacterial species 2[e]	Bacterial species 3[e]	Bacterial species 4[e]
10:0 or less		19.7								
11:1									2.6	
12:0	tr	3.6			0.6	1.5	0.7	2.5	3.2	7.0
13:0 iso					tr	1.2	1.5		2.8	
13:0		tr		0.7	tr	0.7	tr	2.2		1.2
14:0 iso		tr			0.7	1.3	2.0	1.9	4.7	
14:0	3.0	10.5	1.0	1.6	2.0	3.8	2.5	2.5	22.4	18.2
14:1	1.6	2.1							4.2	2.4
15:0 iso			0.5	3.7	6.7	20.3	43.7	2.6	21.8	
15:0		0.9	1.1	2.0	4.5	8.2	4.3	3.6	10.8	1.4
unidentified										2.8
16:0 iso	tr	tr	2.2	1.1	2.9	1.6	9.3		10.8	
16:0	25.9	25.6	26.5	37.5	26.1	30.6	19.0	34.0	7.2	31.7
16:1	4.6	2.7	0.7	1.2	1.5	1.3		8.0		5.6
17:0 iso			1.2	2.8	1.5	1.2	3.4	6.0	8.8	
17:0	2.1	0.7	tr	0.8	0.4	0.8	1.8	4.9		
18:0 iso	1.4	0.1						8.5	2.3	
18:0	15.5	8.7	12.3	10.3	10.7	6.5	4.1	3.8		
18:1	44.1	20.7	17.1	20.3	16.2	10.2	6.9	11.8		22.5
18:2	1.7	2.9	27.5	14.6	18.1	10.7	0.8			
18:3	tr	1.8								
18:4 or 20:1			9.7	3.2	7.9	—				
19:0 iso								7.7		
19:0										4.8
19:cy										1.6

[a] Iso acids are branched chain acids, and, perhaps keto acids; cy is a cyclopropane acid;
[b] Author's laboratory, beef steers, (figures for C14:1 include C15:0)
[c] Smith, 1961; [d] Keeney et al (1962); [e] Ifkovits and Ragheb (1968); 1, *Ruminococcus flavefaciens*; 2, *Butyrivibrio fibrisolvens*; 3, *Succinivibrio dextrinsolvens*; 4, *Bacteroides amylophilus*.

cellular ^{14}C was recovered in the lipid fraction, most of which was in branched-chain C14 and C15 acids with another 11% in other C14 and C16 compounds thought to be aldehydes.

Wegner (1962) and Wegner and Foster (1963) have investigated the synthesis of long-chain fatty acids from certain VFA by *Borrelia* and *Bacteroides succinogenes* organisms, respectively. When labeled isobutyric acid was added to the medium, both organisms synthesized the label into C14 iso and C16 iso acids with some aldehyde production. When n-valerate was added, *B. succinogenes* produced primarily C13 and C15 acids plus aldehydes and *Borrelia* produced primarily C15 and C17 acids. *B. succinogenes* produced primarily C14 and C16 acids from n-caproic acid. Kanegasaki and Takahashi (1968) have

examined lipids of *Selenomonas ruminantium* grown with labeled VFA. In the phospholipid fraction, labeled carbon from n-valerate was incorporated into C13, C15 and C17 acids and that from caproate was recovered in C12, C14 and C16 acids. Although C13 and C15 acids were present in cells grown on caproate, they had little radioactivity. The fatty acids in the bound lipid fraction (chloroform-methanol extract) were odd numbered when cells were grown with n-valerate, but were even numbered when grown with n-caproate. In the case of mixed suspensions of rumen microorganisms, Tweedie et al (1966) found that isobutyrate was incorporated into branched long-chain fatty acids with both odd and even numbers, primarily into C13:0, C13:0 br, C14:0 br and C15:0 br. Data also indicated that label from DL-valine was incorporated into both long-

Table 14-4. Synthesis of long chain acids from VFA.

Acid substrate	Organisms[a]	Products
Propionic	*Bacillus subtillis*	C15:0
Butyric	*B. subtillis*	C14:0 iso, C16:0 iso
Isobutyric	*Ruminococcus albus*	C14 br, C15 br, aldehydes
	Borellia	C14 iso, C15 iso, aldehydes
	Bacteroides succinogenes	C14 iso, C15 iso, aldehydes
	Mixed rumen bacteria	C13:0, C13:0 br, C14:0 br, C15:0 br
	B. subtillis	C14 iso, C16 iso
2-Methylbutyric	*B. subtillis*	12-methyl C14:0, 14-methyl C16:0
n-Valeric	*B. succinogenes*	C13, C15, aldehydes
	Borellia	C15, C17
	Selenomonas ruminantium	C13, C15, C17
	Mixed organisms	C18:1
Isovaleric	*R. flavefaciens*	C15 br, C17, aldehydes
	B. subtillis	C15:0 iso, C17:0 iso
n-Caproic	*B. succinogenes*	C14, C16
	S. ruminantium	C12, C14, C16

[a] *Bacillus subtillis* is included along with the various rumen species for comparative purposes.

chain branched acids and in straight-chain odd numbered acids (C13:0, C13:0 br, C14:0 br and C17:0 br). Labeled isobutyrate and propionate were synthesized from valine and probably represented intermediates in the synthesis of the branched- and straight-chain fatty acids, respectively. When using mixed organisms fermented with labeled valeric acid, Hidiroglou and Lepage (1967) recovered most of the label in C18:1, especially in the phosphatidyl ethanolamine fraction.

With respect to synthesis of branched-chain fatty acids, it might be of interest to mention a paper on *Bacillus subtillis,* a nonrumen organism. Kaneda (1963) found the order of abundance of branched-chain acids to be: 12-methyl-C14:0, 14-methyl-C16:0, C15:0 iso, C16:0 iso, C17:0 iso and C14:0. The addition of short-chain acids (butyric, isobutyric, isovaleric and 2-methyl-butyric) to the culture medium resulted in the increased formation of long-chain acids related to these short-chain acids, i.e., C14:0 and C16:0 from butyrate; C14:0 iso and C16:0 iso from isobutyrate; C15:0 iso and C17:0 iso from isovalerate; and 12-methyl-C14:0 and 14-methyl-C16:0 from 2-methylbutyrate. The addition of propionate or valerate to the medium resulted in the formation of two new odd-length fatty acids, C15:0 and C17:0.

A comparison of the results of these various experiments with rumen bacteria or mixed rumen suspensions indicates some differences between the different species with respect to the fatty acid synthesized from a particular VFA. The data clearly indicate that bacteria can readily synthesize the odd-length and branched-chain acids. Perhaps some of the differences observed are related to the differences in requirements of VFA for growth, since *B. succinogenes* is known to require both a straight-chain and branched-chain VFA, whereas *R. albus,* apparently requires only branched-chain acids for growth.

Katz and Keeney (1963, 1966) have studied the occurrence of fatty aldehydes and keto acids in the rumen. Of the aldehydes, the major constituents were identified as palmitaldehyde and 15-carbon branched-chain aldehydes. The analysis for these compounds yielded gas chromatographic patterns similar to that of butter oil, thus implicating the rumen as the site of origin. With respect to the keto acids, about 45 μmol of ketostearic acid were found per g of lipid or 120 μmol/g of long-chain fatty acid. The major keto acid was identified as 16-ketostearic acid which represented 75% of the total. Eight other ketostearic isomers were found. Ruminal synthesis of keto-stearic acid via the oxidation of 12-hydroxy-stearic acid was demonstrated in vitro and, since none was found in the diet, ruminal synthesis would be indicated as the source of these isomers. More recently, Body (1972) has shown that 2,3-cyclopropane fatty acids are found in appreciable concentrations in the phosphatidylethanolamine fraction of rumen lipids.

Hansen (1966) has isolated phytanic acid (3,7,11,15-tetramethylhexadecanoic, C20:0 iso) from rumen bacteria, butterfat, plasma and kidney fat of cattle. This multibranched C20 acid was not detected in the diet, and he suggested that it might be a derivative of dietary chlorophyll.

Viviani and Lenaz (1965) have investigated the synthesis of long-chain fatty acids in the rumen of sheep fed a diet said to be lipid free. The diet was composed of starch, glucose, cellulose, urea, minerals and choline. Saliva contained long-chain fatty acids equivalent to 50 mg/l of C18:0, but the amount found in rumen fluid was ca. 1,400 mg/l. These authors estimated that the main fatty acids synthesized in the rumen were (mg/day): C14:0, 1,333; C15:0, 1,629; C15:0 iso, 649; C16:0, 1,589; C16:1, 709; and C18:2, 423. In other work from this laboratory (Viviani et al, 1967), it was shown that the proportions of C18:2 and C18:3 in rumen fluid decreased with time and those of C18:0 and C15:0 acids increased. Calves on a no hay diet had greater amounts of both unsaturated and branched-chain acids, but it was not known if this was due to reduced absorption or increased synthesis of long-chain acids.

Patton et al (1968, 1970) have shown that methionine was very effective in stimulating the synthesis of long-chain lipids from both acetate and glucose by in vitro cultures of rumen microorganisms. Label from long-chain fatty acids was transferred to other complex lipids. Sklan et al (1971) suggest that rumen bacteria synthesize C18:2 and other data from this laboratory (Sklan et al, 1972; Sklan and Budowski, 1974) show that aerobic fermentations could result in some desaturation of C18:0 or C18:1 acids, although not during anaerobic conditions.

Studies by Sutton et al (1970), Ørskov et al (1971), Bickerstaffe and others (1972), where absorption was determined in the lower GIT, suggest long-chain fatty acid synthesis of 22 g/day on a low-roughage ration, 9-26 g/day and 23 g/day, respectively, in sheep. Czerkawski (1973) suggests that palmate and, to a lesser extent C14:0, may be the major acid, synthesized and his calculations indicate that rumen microorganisms of the sheep could be synthesizing between 10 and 30 g/day when rumen concentrations of C16:0 are high.

The preceding papers reviewed on synthesis of long-chain fatty acids and on composition of the rumen microorganisms indicate that only very small amounts of the polyunsaturated fatty acids are made available to the host animal. It would appear that the amount available is probably considerably less than is considered adequate for monogastric species (i.e., ca. 1% of the caloric intake). Whether the ruminant animal requires less or whether synthesis may take place in body tissues remains to be seen.

Effect of Dietary Fats on Other Rumen Metabolites and Functions

As a general rule some of the data on metabolism of long-chain acids would indicate little metabolic activity other than hydrogenation and isomerization. It does appear, however, that limited quantities of long-chain acids may be metabolized to ketones. Hird et al (1966) demonstrated that long-chain fatty acids could be slowly metabolized by rumen papillae although ketone production was inhibited at higher concentrations of the fatty acids; in addition, small quantities of shorter chain acids — including acetate — were produced. Jackson et al (1968) found that palmitate increased the formation of ketones by rumen and omasal epithelial tissue, thus confirming the data of Hird et al that long-chain acids may be slowly metabolized to produce ketones.

Relatively high levels of oils or fats in ruminant rations, although perhaps resulting in no adverse effect on dry matter digestibility, have been shown to bring about a depression of in vitro cellulose digestibility (Brooks et al, 1954; Davison and Woods, 1960). There will also be a depression in methane production as was previously mentioned. Robertson and Hawke (1964) have studied the effect of plant oils and whale oil on some aspects of rumen metabolism. In general, they found that adding oils to the rumen or in vitro fermentations caused a depression in digestibility of fibrous components, increased ammonia formation, reduced acetate and increased propionate concentration. In further work from this laboratory (Kirk et al, 1971) it was shown that total VFA were increased in short-term fermentations (24 hr), but not in long-term studies (48-72 hr).

The effect of diet on the rumen microbial population is well known. Latham et al (1972) found that changing cattle to a low roughage diet increased the number of lactogenic and propionogenic bacteria and reduced the proportion of *Butyrivibrio* and *Borrelia,* both known to be involved in hydrogenation. It was also noted that hydrogenation of soybean oil was reduced in vitro when the inocula came from cattle fed low-roughage rations. When working with pure cultures, Henderson (1973) observed that addition of oleic acid did not affect growth of *Anaerovibrio lipolytica, Peptostreptococcus elsdenii, Bacteroides ruminicola* and *Selenomonas ruminantium* . However, growth of Butyrivibrio was stimulated by low concentrations of C18:1, C14:0 and C8:0, while higher concentrations were inhibitory. C14:0, C16:0 and C18:0 were inhibitory at all concentrations tested. Production of methane by pure cultures of *Methanobacterium ruminantium* was inhibited by additions of long-chain acids, of which oleic was the most inhibitory.

Storry (1970) points out that addition of lipids to the diet also influences the pattern of rumen fermentation and resultant VFA production. Observed responses differ from experiment to experiment and much of this variation can be attributed to differences in the basal diet, fatty acid composition of the fat supplement and the level and way in which the fat is fed. Results from a variety of different experiments with tallow, cottonseed, safflower and cod-liver oils as well as different long-chain acids show that additions to the diet tend to bring about increased percentages of propionic and valeric acids and decreased percentages of acetic and sometimes butyric acids (Shaw and Ensor, 1959; Nottle and Rook, 1963; Steele and Moore, 1968; Varman et al, 1968; Noble et al, 1969). The effect of linseed oil acids on rumen VFA is illustrated in Fig. 14-2.

More specific examples will be illustrated from more recent research. For example, Steele et al (1971) fed cows 8% soybean oil either in the form of ground beans or added oil. Either form resulted in an increase in percentage of propionic acid, but adding the oil alone caused a decrease in acetic and

total VFA. Nicholson and Sutton (1971) fed fish oils to dairy cows receiving rations varying in roughage content. Decreases in the percentage of acetic acid and increases

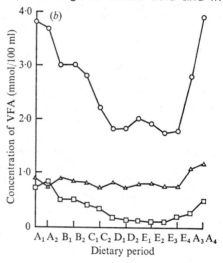

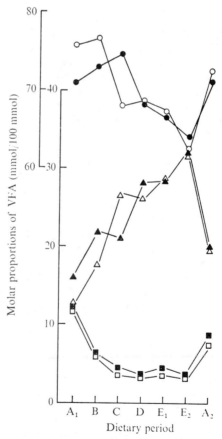

Figure 14-2. Concentration and molar proportions of VFA in the rumen of sheep given linseed oil fatty acids. Diets: A, basal; B,C,D,E, contained 20, 40, 60 and 80 g of fatty acids per day. Values are shown for acetic [O], Propionic [△] and butyric [□] acids. From Czerkawski [1973].

in propionic acid caused by the oil became greater as the amount of oil in the diet increased. However the effect with a low oil intake was greatest on the low roughage diet. On high oil intake, responses were variable, but the effect tended to be greatest on the low roughage rations. Adaptation (in terms of VFA percentage) was shown on the low oil ration during the 2nd and 3rd week of feeding. In another experiment where sheep were given linseed oil acids and rations with 25-75% pelleted grass hay, it was noted that 5% fatty acids caused a decrease in digestibility of crude fiber. With the 50 and 75% hay rations, 5% acids caused a depression in digestibility of dry matter and organic matter and an increase in ruminal propionic acid and reduced butyric acid. When sugar beet pulp was the substrate, addition of small amounts of linseed oil acids had little effect on total gas production, utilization of sugar or molar percentages of the VFA, but methane production was strongly inhibited. Large amounts of the fatty acids temporarily inhibited production of gas and utilization of sugar. With sucrose, even the small amounts of fatty acids had a marked inhibitory effect on production of gas and utilization of sugar (Czerkawski and Breckenridge, 1969).

Conclusions

Published data on rumen metabolism of dietary lipids indicate that rapid hydrolysis of triglycerides or galactosyl glycerol esters occurs in the rumen. Following hydrolysis, a high percentage of unsaturated free fatty acids may be hydrogenated to the saturated analogue. Of those that are not completely saturated, many will have *trans* double bonds, particularly in bacterial cultures. In addition, a variety of positional isomers may be produced. Rumen bacteria contain substantial amounts of odd-length and branched-chain acids, particularly of the C15 acids. Comparative analyses indicate that rumen ciliates contain little of the C15 acids and that bacteria might be the source of these acids. Branched chain and keto acids as well as branched chain and odd length aldehydes and cyclopropane fatty acids may also be found in rumen microorganisms, indicating that the rumen microorganisms are most likely the source of these various isomeric forms that have also been found in blood plasma, milk and body fats. The odd length and branched chain VFA would appear to be the substrates from which the corresponding long chain fatty acids are synthesized. Different bacterial species have been shown to vary somewhat with respect to which long chain acid is synthesized from a given VFA. Quantitative data are inadequate, but research at this point in time indicates some synthesis of C14 and C16 acids in the rumen, with relatively little if any production of the C18 acids.

When fats are added to the diet, most evidence indicates that there is apt to be a reduced percentage of acetic acid and often of butyric acid. Propionate tends to increase, perhaps due to metabolism of glycerol, although there may be a selective effect of different fatty acids on different ruminal bacteria. Methane production tends to be reduced and indications are that part of the hydrogen normally going to methane may be diverted to saturation of polyunsaturated fatty acids.

References Cited

Allen, R.A. and A.A. Kiess. 1955. J. Amer. Oil Chem. Soc. 32:400.
Allison, M.J., M.P. Bryant, I. Katz and M. Keeney. 1962. J. Bact. 84:1084.
Bailey, R.W. 1964. N.Z. J. Agr. 7:417.
Bickerstaffe, R., D.E. Noakes and E.F. Annison. 1972. Biochem. J. 130:607.
Body, D.R. 1972. Febs Letters 27:5.
Brooks, C.C., et al. 1954. J. Animal Sci. 13:758.
Brumby, P.E., J.E. Storry and J.D. Sutton. 1969. Rep. Natn. Inst. Res. Dairy, 1968, 89.
Chalupa, W. and A.J. Kutches. 1968. J. Animal Sci. 27:1502.
Chalupa, W., G.D. O'Dell, A.J. Kutches and R.L. Lavker. 1967. J. Dairy Sci. 50:1002 (abstr).
Clarke, D.G. and J.C. Hawke. 1970. J. Sci. Fd. Agr. 21:446.
Cottyn, B.G., F.X. Buysse and C.V. Boucque. 1972. Nutr. Abstr. Rev. 42:137.

Czerkawski, J.W. 1973. J. Agr. Sci. 81:517.
Czerkawski, J.W. and K.L. Blaxter. 1965. Biochem. J. 96:25C (abstr).
Czerkawski, J.W., K.L. Blaxter and F.W. Wainman. 1966. Br. J. Nutr. 20:349; 485.
Czerkawski, J.W. and G. Breckenridge. 1969. Br. J. Nutr. 23:51.
Davidson, K.L. and W. Woods. 1960. J. Animal Sci. 19:54.
Dawson, R.M.C. 1959. Nature 183:1822.
Dawson, R.M.C. and P. Kemp. 1969. Biochem. J. 115:351.
Felinski, L. and R. Toullec. 1972. Nutr. Abstr. Rev. 42:515.
Garton, G.A. 1960a. Nature. 187:511.
Garton, G.A. 1960b. Nutr. Abstr. Rev. 30:1.
Garton, G.A., P.N. Hobson and A.K. Lough. 1958. Nature. 182:1511.
Garton, G.A., A.K. Lough and E. Vioque. 1959. Biochem. J. 73:43P (abstr).
Garton, G.A., A.K. Lough and E. Vioque. 1961. J. Gen. Microbiol. 25:215.
Hansen, R.P. 1966. J. Dairy Res. 33:333.
Harfoot, C.G., R.C. Nobel and J.H. Moore. 1973. Biochem. J. 132:829.
Hartman, L., F.B. Shorland and I.R.C. McDonald. 1954. Nature 174:185.
Hawke, J.C. 1971. Biochem. Biophys. Acta 248:167.
Hawke, J.C. and J.A. Robertson. 1964. J. Sci. Fd. Agr. 15:283.
Hawke, J.C. and W.R. Silcock. 1970. Biochem. Biophys. Acta 218:201.
Henderson, C. 1973. J. Agr. Sci. 81:107.
Hidiroglou, M. and M. Lepage. 1967. Can. J. Biochem. 45:1789.
Hilditch, T.P. 1956. The Chemical Constitution of Natural Fats. Chapman and Hall, Ltd. (3rd ed).
Hird, F.J.R., R.B. Jackson and M.J. Weidemann. 1966. Biochem. J. 98:394.
Ifkovits, R.W. and H.S. Ragheb. 1968. Appl. Microbiol. 16:1406.
Jackson, H.D., A.M. Preston and J.M. Carter. 1968. J. Animal Sci. 27:203.
Johns, A.T. 1963. N.Z. J. Sci. Tech., 35A:262.
Kaneda, T. 1963. J. Biol. Chem. 238:1229.
Kanegasaki, S. and H. Takahashi. 1968. Biochem. Biophys. Acta 152:40.
Katz, I. and M. Keeney. 1963. J. Dairy Sci. 46:637 (abstr).
Katz, I. and M. Keeney. 1966. J. Dairy Sci. 49:962; 967.
Keeney, M., I. Katz and M.J. Allison. 1962. J. Amer. Oil Chem. Soc. 39:198.
Kepler, C.R., K.P. Hirons, J.J. McNeil and S.B. Tove. 1966. J. Biol. Chem. 241:1350.
Kirk, R.D., D.R. Body and J.C. Hawke. 1971. J. Sci. Fd. Agr. 22:620.
Klopfenstein, T.J., D.B. Purser and W.J. Tyznik. 1966. J. Animal Sci. 25:765.
Kunsman, J.E. 1967. Dissert. Abstr. 27:2978B.
Latham, M.J., J.E. Storry and M.E. Sharpe. 1972. Appl. Microbiol. 24:871.
Macleod, G.K., A.S. Wood and Y.T. Yao. 1972. J. Dairy Sci. 55:446.
Miller, L.G. and D.A. Cramer. 1969. J. Animal Sci. 29:738.
Mills, S.C., T.W. Scott, G.R. Russell and R.M. Smith. 1970. Aust. J. Biol. Sci. 23:1109.
Moore, J.H., R.C. Nobel and W. Steele. 1969. Br. J. Nutr. 23:141.
Nicholson, J.W.G. and J.D. Sutton. 1971. J. Dairy Res. 38:363.
Nobel, R.C., W. Steele and J.H. Moore. 1969. J. Dairy Res. 36:375.
Nottle, M.C. and J.A.F. Rook. 1963. Proc. Nutr. Soc. 22:vii (abstr).
Ogilvie, B.M. and G.L. McClymont. 1961. Nature 190:725.
Oksanen, H.E. and B. Thafvelin. 1965. J. Dairy Sci. 48:1305.
Ørskov, E.R., C. Fraser and I. McDonald. 1971. Br. J. Nutr. 25:225; 243; 26:477.
Patton, R.A., R.D. McCarthy and L.C. Griel. 1968. J. Dairy Sci. 51:1310.
Patton, R.A., R.D. McCarthy and L.C. Griel. 1970. J. Dairy Sci. 53:460.
Polan, C.E., J.J. McNeill and S.B. Tove. 1964. J. Bact. 88:1056.
Reiser, R. 1951. Fed. Proc. 10:236.
Reiser, R. and H.G.R. Reedy. 1956. J. Amer. Oil Chem. Soc. 33:155.
Robertson, J.A. and J.C. Hawke. 1964. J. Sci. Fd. Agr. 15:274; 890.
Scott, T.W., et al. 1970. Aust. J. Sci. 32:291.
Scott, T.W., L.J. Cook and S.C. Mills. 1971. J. Amer. Oil Chem. Soc. 48:358.
Shaw, J.C. and W.L. Ensor. 1959. J. Dairy Sci. 42:1238.
Shorland, F.B., R.O. Weenink, and A.T. Johns. 1955. Nature 175:1129.
Shorland, F.B., R.O. Weenink, A.T. Johns and I.R.C. McDonald. 1957. Biochem. J. 67:328.
Sklan, D. and P. Budowski. 1974. J. Dairy Sci. 57:56.
Sklan, D., P. Budowski and R. Volcani. 1972. Br. J. Nutr. 28:239.
Sklan, D., R. Volcani and P. Budowski. 1971. J. Dairy Sci. 54:515.
Smith, A. and A.K. Lough. 1973. Proc. Nutr. Soc. 32:62A.
Smith, L.M. 1961. J. Dairy Sci. 44:607.
Steele, W. and J.H. Moore. 1968. J. Dairy Res. 35:343; 353; 361.
Steele, W., R.C. Nobel and J.H. Moore. 1971. J. Dairy Res. 38:43.
Storry, J.E. 1970. J. Dairy Res. 37:139.
Sutton, J.D., J.E. Storry and J.W.G. Nicholson. 1970. J. Dairy Res. 37:97.
Tanaka, K. and H. Hayashi. 1972. Nutr. Abstr. Rev. 42:1363.
Tanaka, K., R. Shimuzu and H. Hayashi. 1974. Nutr. Abstr. Rev. 44:316.
Tove, S.B. and G. Matrone. 1962. J. Nutr. 76:271.
Tove, S.B. and R.D. Mochrie. 1963. J. Dairy Sci. 46:686.

Tweedie, J.W., M.G. Rumsby and J.C. Hawke. 1966. J. Sci. Fd. Agr. 17:241.

Ulyatt, M.J., J.W. Czerkawski and K.L. Blaxter. 1966. Proc. Nutr. Sci. 25:xvii (abstr).

Varman, P.N., L.H. Schultz and R.E. Nichols. 1968. J. Dairy Sci. 51:1956.

Viviani, R., A.R. Borgatti, P.G. Monetti and A. Mordenit. 1967. Zentrabl. Vet. Med. 14A:833.

Viviani, R., M.G. Gandolfi and A.R. Borgatti. 1965. Nutr. Abstr. Rev. 35:143.

Viviani, R. and G. Lenaz. 1965. Nutr. Abstr. Rev. 35:82.

Ward, P.F.V., T.W. Scott and R.M.C. Dawson. 1964. Biochem. J. 92:60.

Watanabe, Y., T. Kyuma and H. Murai. 1969. Jap. J. Zootech. Sci. 40:390.

Weenink, R.O. 1959. N.Z. J. Sci. 2:273.

Wegner, G.H. 1962. Ph.D. Thesis, University of Wisconsin, Madison.

Wegner, G.H. and E.M. Foster. 1963. J. Bact. 85:53.

Wilde, P.F. and R.M.C. Dawson. 1966. Biochem. J. 98:469.

Williams, P.P., J. Gutierrez and R.R. Davis. 1963. Appl. Microbiol. 11:260.

Wood, D.R., M.C. Bell, R.B. Grainger and R.A. Teekell. 1963. J. Nutr. 79:62.

Wright, D.E. 1959. Nature 184:875.

Wright, D.E. 1961. N.Z. J. Agr. Res. 4:216.

Wright, D.E. 1969. N.Z. J. Agr. Res. 12:281.

Yokoyama, M.T. and C.L. Davis. 1971. Proc. Fed. Soc. Exptl. Biol. 30:295 (abstr).

Zerebocov, P.I. and A.D. Listunov. 1972. Nutr. Abstr. Rev. 42:936.

CHAPTER 15 — VITAMINS AND MINERALS IN RUMEN FERMENTATION

VITAMINS

It has been known for many years that the vitamin requirements of ruminants are different than those of monogastric species. Barnett and Reid (1961) point out that Theiler and others suggested in 1915 that "the requirements of cattle are so low that they may even be covered indirectly by synthesis carried out by the extensive bacterial flora of the intestines."

Evidence from a variety of laboratories indicates that the tissues of ruminant animals require a number, if not all, of the vitamins known to be required by most monogastric species. This evidence has been obtained by studying the requirements of young animals on liquid diets, or prior to the development of normal rumen fermentative function, or with the use of vitamin antagonists of one kind or another. There is no question that preruminant animals need a dietary supply of the B-complex vitamins (see Ch. 26, Vol. 2). In animals with a functioning rumen, however, there is only some questionable evidence that some of the B-complex vitamins may not be adequate for rapid growth. Most feeding trials with fattening animals or with lactating cows have not given any significant indications of need. Only in the case of animals affected with cerebrocortical necrosis or polioencephalomalacia, where a thiaminase enzyme seems to be involved, is there good evidence of a practical dietary need for a water-soluble vitamin. Thus, this indirect evidence indicates that adequate synthesis of most of the vitamins occurs either in the GIT or in body tissues. Vitamins A, D, and E are exceptions to this statement, of course.

Vitamin Requirements of Rumen Microorganisms

Investigations that have been carried out with pure cultures of individual species or with washed suspensions of mixed species of rumen bacteria indicate that a number of species either require one or more vitamins or that the vitamins are stimulatory (Bryant et al, 1959; Gibbons and Doetsch, 1959; Bryant and Robinson, 1961, 1962; Bryant, 1963; Hungate, 1963; Scott and Dehority, 1965).

Although differences between species and strains of bacteria have been demonstrated, the data generally indicate that biotin is most apt to be an essential vitamin. At times p-aminobenzoic acid has been shown to be required or stimulatory. Cobalamin (B_{12}) sometimes shows a response, although the response can, at times, be eliminated when methionine is included in the medium — probably acting as a methyl donor. The effect of thiamin on metabolic activity has been demonstrated by including thiamin inhibitors (thiopental, hexetidine, pyrithiamin and amprolium), although synthesis is apparently adequate in the absence of inhibitors (Milligen et al, 1968). The omission of biotin from a medium may be expected to result in a marked decrease in cellulose digestion and VFA production with propionate production being decreased about twice as much as acetate production (Milligan et al, 1967).

Some relatively recent evidence indicates that choline may be stimulatory to rumen metabolism. Swingle and Dyer (1970) concluded that the addition of choline to the diet of cattle allowed an increase in bacterial numbers. In vitro data indicated an increase in gas production and VFA concentration without any alteration in gas or VFA composition.

Synthesis of Water-soluble Vitamins

The first factual evidence of vitamin synthesis in the rumen was obtained by Bechdel and coworkers (1926, 1928). These experiments demonstrated, among other things, that rumen digesta would support growth of rats. However, when rats were fed the same ration as the calves which supplied the rumen digesta, growth was very poor. These researchers isolated a rumen bacterium which, when grown on agar, could adequately supplement a B-complex deficient diet for rats.

McElroy and Goss (1940, 1941) and McElroy and Jukes (1940) carried out an extensive series of experiments on vitamin synthesis in the rumen. Some of their findings are mentioned briefly. With respect to riboflavin, they found about 33 µg/g in rumen contents from sheep fed rations containing less than 0.3 μg/g. They estimated that 16-18 mg of riboflavin were secreted/day in milk when animals were on a maximum dietary intake of 1.8 mg. Dried rumen contents from this animal contained ca. 25 μg/g of riboflavin. In the case of pyridoxine (B_6), dried rumen contents were found to contain 10 μg/g on diets containing 1-1.5 μg/g. Milk from a cow fed a deficient ration contained at least as much pyridoxine as milk from cows fed a normal ration. Likewise, with thiamin they found 7 μg/g in dried rumen contents from diets with >0.4 μg/g. They could not detect thiamin in the rumen contents of two fistulated cows fed the same ration but milk contained 2-2.5 μg/g (dry basis). With pantothenic acid, levels in the rumen of sheep were ca. 25 fold those in the diet and 20-30 fold in the case of two cows; biotin was also found to be synthesized from diets low in this vitamin. Other early papers demonstrating synthesis of B-complex vitamins include those of Wegner et al (1941) and Hunt et al (1943).

Hamilton and others (1955) have estimated the synthesis of riboflavin and thiamin by cows fed rations of hay; silage, hay and a dairy ration; and hay, oats and barley. With respect to thiamin, there was a considerable difference in the amount of thiamin in the rations. However, rumen contents were low, indicating rapid destruction of the vitamin. On the other hand, the thiamin content of fecal samples was always higher than that of rumen contents — indicating that an appreciable amount of synthesis probably occurred in the lower GIT. The level of thiamin found in the rumen varied from diet to diet, probably a reflection of the marked differences in dietary thiamin but fecal levels were much less variable. The data obtained in riboflavin indicated a substantial synthesis of this vitamin on all of the rations except silage. Rumen contents ranged from 1.5 to <2-times greater than the diet except for the silage ration. Fecal samples were always lower than rumen samples. Data obtained on calves fed purified diets (Agrawala et al, 1953) indicated that appreciable amounts of riboflavin, pantothenic acid and niacin were synthesized. Virtanen (1963) has also shown this to be the case for lactating cows fed a vitamin-free ration. Analyses indicated that appreciable amounts of thiamin, riboflavin, nicotinic acid, folic acid, biotin, pantothenic acid and pyridoxine were produced; levels in the rumen were at least as high as in control cows fed natural rations.

Yskshsdi et al (1967) found the nicotinic acid content in the rumen of goats to be 25-40 μg/g of dry matter before feeding; this level increased after feeding a diet of hay and concentrate. When extractions of bacteria were made, evidence indicated the presence of 5 or 6 derivatives.

When young lambs were rumen sampled at 3, 6, 10, 14 and 21 days of age, data indicated a decline (in initial levels provided by colostrum) in pantothenic acid, niacin and biotin concentrations to 21 days of age. Riboflavin concentration was increased by creep feeding (Poe et al, 1972).

The fact that animals with functional rumens do not require B-complex vitamins would appear to be adequately explained by the extensive synthesis of many of the important vitamins by rumen micro-organisms and/or intestinal synthesis (thiamin, vitamin K). These results indicate that enough vitamins must be synthesized in the GIT to provide adequately for the host's requirements as well as for those species of bacteria that have a requirement for a given vitamin.

Factors Affecting Synthesis of Water-soluble Vitamins

After the early work cited previously, most of the subsequent research has dealt with variables that influence the amount of vitamin synthesis in the rumen. Some of this research is reviewed briefly in subsequent paragraphs.

Effect of Dietary Nitrogen. Wegner et al (1941) reported that variation in the amount of urea or protein in a supplementary grain mix fed to cattle had very little, if any, effect on the vitamin content of ingesta. Data were presented on thiamin, riboflavin, pyridoxine, pantothenic acid, nicotinic acid and biotin. Pearson et al (1953) observed that a low-N diet did not reduce riboflavin excretion although excretion of niacin and pantothenic acid was reduced. Hollis et al (1954) reported that the addition of N, either as soybean oil meal or urea, along with corn to a basal roughage of prairie hay resulted in a marked increase in synthesis of nicotinic acid, riboflavin and pantothenic acid. Buziassy and Tribe (1960) found that the amounts of riboflavin and nicotinic acid in the rumen were more closely related to the N intake than to the dietary intake of the respective vitamins. Synthesis of thiamin and riboflavin was not affected when casein was partially or completely replaced by urea. Complete withdrawal of protein N did reduce synthesis of nicotinic acid. For that matter, deficiency symptoms of nicotinic acid can be produced in young calves only if the tryptophan and niacin content of the diet are low (Johnson et al, 1947). Buziassy and Tribe further noted that synthesis of the vitamins mentioned previously was greater when the diet was deficient in the vitamins, particularly in the case of young lambs receiving considerable amounts of these vitamins from pasture and ewe's milk. Teeri and Colovos (1963) published data which indicated that fecal excretion (an indirect measure of synthesis) of nicotinic acid, riboflavin and cobalamin generally increased on low-fiber rations as the amount of urea intake increased, but not on high-fiber rations.

More recently Pavel et al (1968) have studied vitamin synthesis in goats fed semipurified diets. On an almost N-free diet there was much synthesis of thiamin which reached a concentration of 4.0 mg/100 g of dry matter 2 hr after feeding. On the same diet very little riboflavin or pyridoxine was found. When soluble urea was added to the diet, riboflavin and pyridoxine were found but thiamin values were low and little or none was present 5 hr after feeding. When a coated urea product was fed, values for all 3 vitamins were low. Addition of urea and lysine stimulated synthesis of riboflavin. In other work sheep were fed semipurified diets containing corn gluten meal which was substituted with urea or soy protein over a 5 day period followed by a 50-day feeding period (Tucker and Fontenot, 1970). No significant differences were observed due to rations, animals or days on trial for choline, B_6, biotin, folic acid, pantothenic acid, niacin or ascorbic acid. There was a gradual decline in B_{12} for both rations during the feeding period and the inositol level was higher for lambs fed the soy protein. Zerebocov et al (1972) have studied ruminal vitamin synthesis in cattle on natural feed ingredients following replacement of digestible N with urea or different ammonium salts. Replacing 20% of the digestible N by urea did not affect synthesis of thiamin and B_{12} but riboflavin synthesis was increased 14%. Increasing the substitution to 30% allowed a moderate increase in thiamin and B_{12}. Replacement of 20% of

digestible N with ammonium acetate resulted in a sharp increase in thiamin and riboflavin but B_{12} was depressed; however an increase to 30% replacement did stimulate B_{12} synthesis. A 30% replacement with ammonium propionate stimulated synthesis of these vitamins, but thiamin and riboflavin fell with 50% replacement. Variable results were seen with ammonium sulfate.

Effect of Dietary Carbohydrates. Hunt et al (1952, 1954) have studied synthesis of some vitamins with in vitro fermentations. They determined that the addition of starch to the fermentation medium resulted in an increased synthesis of riboflavin, niacin and pantothenic acid (especially the latter) when the inoculum was from a timothy hay-fed steer and for these vitamins plus cobalamin when the inoculum was from an alfalfa hay-fed steer. When using washed suspensions of rumen bacteria, Hayes et al (1966) reported that synthesis of riboflavin, niacin and cobalamin was greater when starch was the substrate than when cellulose was the substrate; more niacin was synthesized when the initial pH of the inoculum was 6.8 than when it was 5.5. Values for riboflavin, folic acid and cobalamin indicated little, if any, synthesis when the substrate was cellulose. With goats fed a semipurified diet, replacing starch with sucrose allowed a large increase in production of riboflavin which was even greater when both sucrose and urea were coated with gypsum (Pavel et al, 1968).

Miscellaneous Factors. Endo et al (1962) observed some diurnal variation in vitamin concentration in the rumen. Levels of thiamin, B_6 and pantothothetic acid rose to some extent after feeding, while the amount of biotin decreased slightly after feeding. The response of riboflavin and nicotinic acid was variable. Vitamin levels in the rumen of a goat grazing wild grass was similar to those in a sheep on silage, but biotin was lower and riboflavin was higher in the goat's rumen. Hunt et al (1943) reported that omission of corn from the ration of a steer resulted in a reduction of riboflavin synthesis. Hayes and others (1966) observed that thiamin, pantothenic acid, folic acid, niacin and cobalamin were found in greatest concentrations in ruminal fluid of steers fed all-concentrate rations, while the highest levels of riboflavin were in the rumens of steers that received ground hay in their rations. Hunt et al (1954) noted that the addition of sodium sulfate and methionine stimulated synthesis of riboflavin and cobalamin; however, the addition of sulfur other than in the elemental form inhibited pantothenic acid synthesis. Chlortetracycline appeared to inhibit synthesis of the vitamins studied except for cobalamin. In research with a goat given intraruminal infusions of extracts of dried ladino clover, data indicated that the clover extract stimulated the synthesis of pantothenic acid but inhibited that of nicotinic acid (Takahashi and Goto, 1972).

With regard to cobalamin it has been well established that a deficiency of cobalt will result in a reduced synthesis of this vitamin (Hale et al, 1950) as might be expected since the molecule contains cobalt. Teeri et al (1955) reported that excretion of cobalamin exceeded intake by 40-55 fold in older cattle. Recent reports on B_{12} synthesis indicate that synthesis is reduced in cattle or sheep fed low-roughage diets and that the Co requirement is affected by the intake of digestible dry matter (Walker and Elliot, 1972; Hedrich et al, 1973). Although total B_{12} activity was higher in the serum of cows, much of the activity was due to the presence of B_{12} analogues (see Ch. 20, Vol. 2). Dryden and Hartman (1971) have estimated that rumen contents of heifers contained from 12-663X the amount of B_{12} found in the food. Heifers fed silage had 1.4-2.7X more B_{12} in rumen contents than those fed chopped or pelleted hay. A hay-grain diet resulted in less synthesis, also.

In the case of ascorbic acid (vitamin C), data published by Knight and others (1940) indicated a rapid and pronounced destruction of ascorbic acid in the rumen as determined by analysis of samples of ingesta at regular intervals after a cow had been fed. Erb et al (1947) suggest that such losses may be due to chemical causes as well as microbial degradation. Golubev (1972) determined that ruminal synthesis was increased by supplements of Zn alone or with Cu, B_6 or B_{12} orally or I.M. and synthesis was depressed by adding vitamin A. Ascorbic acid content of liver cells was increased by I.M. B_{12} or oral doses of B_6 or ascorbic acid, but there was no effect of vitamin A.

Field Problems with Thiamin

Polioenchephalomalacia or cerebrocortical necrosis has shown an increasing incidence in recent years, often in animals fed high grain diets. Symptoms similar to it can be induced by feeding amprolium, a coccidiostat used for poultry. Generally, the current evidence indicates a high concentration of thiaminase in the rumen of affected animals. However, affected animals may have normal blood thiamin concentrations although thiamin diphosphate levels may be low. Current evidence indicates that thiamin may be only one, although perhaps the most important, of several factors elaborated or modified by the rumen which results in the disease (Edwin and Lewis, 1971; Loew, 1972; Loew and Dunlop, 1972). Whatever the end results may be, remission of symptoms is often seen following treatment with thiamin. Further information on the symptoms and occurrence of this disease is given in Ch. 24 of Vol. 2.

Fat-Soluble Vitamins

Carotenes and Vitamin A. With respect to the carotenes and vitamin A, there is no evidence indicating synthetic activity in the stomach. However, there is evidence of destruction even though these compounds have conjugated double bonds which are said to be resistant to hydrogenation. Data published by King et al (1962) showed substantial losses of both carotene and vitamin A following in vitro fermentation. Recovery of carotene in nonincubated tubes was 97% as compared to 66% in tubes fermented 9 hr. For vitamin A, comparable values were 81 and 60%, respectively. Santoquin and tocopherol (antioxidants) both reduced losses. Destruction was similar in rumen fluid from cattle or sheep and from cattle fed hay or high-grain rations. Data published by Davison and Seo (1963) also indicated losses of an appreciable amount of carotene during in vitro fermentations. However, Keating and others (1964) presented data which showed no effect of fermentation on loss of carotene, although there was some loss of vitamin A acetate. When rumen liquor was obtained from steers fed a ration with 30% roughage, loss of vitamin A on prolonged fermentation (up to 16 hr) was less than when the inoculum came from steers fed only roughage.

In additional studies with vitamin A at the Kentucky station, it has been reported that incorporation of oxidizing agents such as nitrate failed to increase destruction and dietary supplements of antioxidants such as vitamin E did not eliminate this destruction (Mitchell et al, 1967, 1968). Losses of vitamin A were apparently enhanced when high-concentrate diets were fed (Warner et al, 1970). In animals given a basal diet with 53% hay, it was shown that addition of either 7% corn starch or 7% cottonseed oil (high in unsaturated fatty acids) allowed similar rates of destruction in the stomach of steers and sheep; approximately 62-70% of doses of vitamin A acetate was degraded in the stomach (Long et al, 1971).

It might be of interest to mention a paper by McGillivary (1951). In this research carotene:lignin ratios were determined at different points in the GIT of sheep. McGillivary's evidence indicated that the amount of carotene increased as digesta passed through the intestinal tract, thus indicating synthesis (or loss of lignin) by intestinal microorganisms. Some lignin is partially soluble in the GIT, especially in less mature plants. It may also be that solubility of carotene was increased in the intestinal digesta, thus allowing more complete extraction as suggested by Almendinger and Hinds (1969). It seems unlikely that β carotene would be synthesized in the intestinal tract.

Vitamin K. Early data published by McElroy and Goss (1940) indicated that rumen contents were a good source of vitamin K when animals were on diets practically devoid of this vitamin. Lev (1959) reported that a strain of *Fusiformis* found in the rumen had a requirement for vitamin K. It is assumed that an adequate amount of this vitamin is synthesized in the rumen and/or lower GIT except in situations in which an excess of dicumarol is found in the diet (White et al, 1954).

More recently, Matschiner (1970) has identified vitamin K compounds in the bovine rumen as menaquinones-10, 11, 12 and 13, compounds similar to those which have been isolated from bovine liver; this supports the view that they are of bacterial origin and are absorbed and deposited in the liver.

With respect to the other recognized fat-soluble vitamins, E and D, there appears to be no evidence re rumen metabolism of them although Barnett and Reid (1961, p 221) quote a reference indicating that high concentrations of vitamins A, E, and D_2 were toxic to rumen protozoa.

MINERALS

The major (or macro) minerals in solution in the rumen serve a number of generalized functions in addition to specific functions they may be involved with in cells and tissues. These generalized functions would include maintenance of a physiological pH through the action of buffers — primarily Na and K salts, maintenance of a desirable redox potential, and a desirable osmotic pressure — all factors which have an important effect on growth and metabolic activity of the rumen population.

Some of the early research directed toward the mineral requirements of rumen microorganisms include that of Burroughs et al (1950, 1951), McNaught et al (1950) and Bentley et al (1953). These and many other studies were carried out with crude suspensions of rumen organisms and, as a result, may not have been as precise as if washed suspensions or pure cultures had been used. Nevertheless, they provided some data on an otherwise unknown subject. The past six years have been a productive period for this area of research. Pertinent papers on mineral requirements are reviewed in subsequent paragraphs.

The mineral content of rumen fluid may logically be expected to vary with the diet and in association with factors which might modify salivary secretion, passage out of the rumen or absorption from the rumen. Poutiainen (1970) concluded that rumen concentration of Na and K were not affected by dry matter intake or proportion of long hay but there was an effect of time after feeding as Na decreased while K increased during the first 3 hr after feeding. Dietary factors examined (level of feed intake, proportion of long hay and dosage with NaCl) did not affect concentrations of Ca and Mg in the rumen fluid, but these also were affected by time after feeding. P, on the other hand, increased with decreasing NaCl dosage and decreasing dry matter intake but not with time after feeding.

An example of the relationships between diet, rumen fluid and rumen bacterial concentrations of a variety of different mineral elements is shown in Table 15-1 from data of Martinez (1973). When comparing the major elements in feed and bacteria, note that there is a moderate concentration of K, Na, P and S, but little or none with Ca and Mg. With the required microminerals, maximal concentration in this instance was with Co, followed by Se, Fe, Mo, Zn, Ni, Cu and Mn. The rumen bacteria also concentrate some elements having no known function such as Al, B, Ba, Cd, F and Sr.

Table 15-1. Mineral content of grass hay and rumen fluid and rumen bacteria obtained from a steer fed the hay. [a]

Element	Mineral content			
	Grass hay, dry basis	Rumen fluid, wet basis	Rumen bacteria, dry basis	
			Concentration	Increase over diet, %
Macro elements, %				
Ca	0.66	0.036	0.88	33
K	0.90	0.120	2.10	133
Mg	0.29	0.014	0.29	0
Na	0.54	0.360	3.60	567
P	0.29	0.036	1.90	555
S	0.19	0.0042	0.78	388
Trace elements, µg/g				
Al	46.0	1.30	265.0	476
B	4.3	0.42	16.0	272
Ba	26.0	0.70	37.0	42
Cd	0.10	0.03	0.50	400
Co	0.08	<0.01	3.75	4587
Cr	<3.00	<0.15	<1.50	—
Cu	12.00	0.83	22.0	83
F	22.00	1.52	82.0	273
Fe	66.0	2.00	525.0	695
Mn	170.0	2.90	230.0	35
Mo	1.20	<0.10	6.20	417
Ni	2.0	0.02	7.0	250
Se	0.03	0.0008	0.50	1567
Sr	22.0	2.30	46.0	109
Zn	22.0	0.16	92.0	318

[a] Data from Martinez (1973).

The Macro Minerals

Calcium. Data on Ca are limited and somewhat inconclusive. Burroughs et al (1951) indicated that small amounts of Ca were stimulatory to rumen organisms with respect to digestion of cellulose in vitro. Later work from the same laboratory with washed suspensions (Hubbert et al, 1958) indicated that additions of 50 to 300 µg of Ca/ml of medium gave a small increase in cellulose digestion although statistical analyses showed no consistent response. On the other hand, levels of 450 µg/ml resulted in a slight depression in cellulose digestion. When working with a pure culture of *Bacteroides succinogenes,* an important cellulolytic bacterium, Bryant et al (1959) concluded that this organism did require Ca when cell growth was measured with optical density. In research with rumen protozoa, Uesaka et al (1966) concluded that Ca showed a tendency to increase VFA production.

Magnesium. Burroughs et al (1951), Hubbert et al (1958) and Bryant et al (1959) all reported that Mg was required for maximal cellulose digestion or cell growth of rumen bacteria. However, a later report by Chamberlain and Burroughs (1962) indicated that cellulose digestion by washed suspensions was not reduced by the omission of Mg. In studies with protozoa, Uesaka et al (1966) found that Mg, when at a concentration of 50 µg/ml, stimulated VFA production. Likewise, Ammerman et al (1971) have shown that Mg deficient rations resulted in reduced in vitro digestion of cellulose and a slight decrease using nylon bag procedures accompanied by a marked decrease in feed intake (see Fig. 15-1). In studies using crude rumen suspensions, Martinez (1973) showed only very slight increases in cellulose digestion with addition of Mg in the presence of adequate S and P. Fitt et al (1972) have shown that cell walls of rumen bacteria are capable of binding Mg and suggest that this may be critical during times of minimal intake.

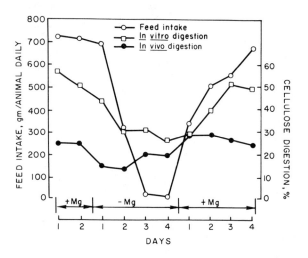

Figure 15-1. **Effect of dietary Mg on voluntary feed intake, in vitro cellulose digestion [Solka Floc] and in vivo cellulose digestion [soybran flakes]. From Ammerman et al [1971].**

Potassium. With respect to K, several reports indicate a requirement of rumen organisms for K (Burroughs et al, 1951; Hubbert et al, 1958; Bryant et al, 1959). Hubbert et al found that the K:Na ratio was of some importance; at high levels of K (100-400 μg/ml), Na tended to increase cellulose digestion. These authors also reported that rubidium could replace about half of the K requirement for in vitro cellulose digestion, whereas Li and Cs were ineffective in this respect. Caldwell and Hudson (1974) have shown that K was required for growth of rumen bacteria in media containing Na, but K could be replaced, for most species, by Rb. However, Uesaka et al (1966) did not observe any effect on VFA production. In studies where purified diets were fed to lambs, Lee and Matrone (1971) observed that supplementation with Na and K increased the molar % of propionate and ruminal lactate was primarily the L (+) isomer; without Na and K, the lactate was primarily

D (-). With high levels of K (to 1,000 mM/l.), Kahn et al (1969) observed depressed utilization of urea and glucose utilization.

Sodium. Burroughs et al (1951) and Bryant et al (1959) found that Na was slightly stimulatory to rumen bacteria. However, Hubbert et al (1958) did not find this to be the case when K levels were adequate. Uesada et al (1966) found that Na stimulated VFA production and Caldwell and Hudson (1974), when working with purified media, determined that Na was a required element for rumen bacteria; removal of Na completely eliminated growth of most species. Na could not be replaced by Rb, Li or Cs.

Chlorine. Although Burroughs et al (1951) indicate that Cl was stimulatory to cellulose digestion, Hubbert et al (1958) found that it was not a limiting factor.

Phosphorus. Data from the work of Burroughs et al, Hubbert et al and Bryant et al clearly indicate that P is required by rumen microorganisms for cellulose digestion or cell growth. Information published by Evans and Davis (1966) adds substantive evidence. Since P is an ubiquitous element in many metabolic reactions and since it is an integral component of many vital compounds such as the nucleoproteins, there can be no doubt that it is a required element. However, it is not always easy to show that it stimulates VFA production or cellulose digestion (Uesada et al, 1966; Martinez, 1973).

Reports from several different laboratories indicate that in vitro rumen techniques can be employed to evaluate the utilization of different sources of P. Anderson et al (1956) used this technique to evaluate microbial utilization of acidulated phosphate, steamed bone meal, Curacaco rock phosphate, colloidal clay and dicalcium phosphate. Hall et al (1961) and Chicco et al (1965) have also used similar methodology to evaluate P sources. Reid et al (1947) demonstrated that phytate P could be utilized in the rumen and Raun et al (1956) and Punj et al (1969) used the in vitro technique to study phytate utilization; their results indicated almost complete utilization. This is in contrast to very poor utilization of phytate P by monogastric species.

Sulfur. Burroughs et al (1951) and Hubbert et al (1958) concluded that S was required for maximal cellulose digestion as did Hunt et al (1954). This is not surprising, of course, in view of the large amount of the S-containing amino acids found in microbial proteins.

Lewis (1954) and Anderson (1956) and others have demonstrated that rumen organisms can rapidly reduce sulfate S to sulfide S. Normal levels of sulfide are said to be on the order of 15-30 µg of S/ml (Anderson, 1956). Absorption is also rapid (Kulwich et al, 1956); experiments with ^{35}S show that rumen sulfide has a half life of 10-22 min (Bray, 1969). Reduction of sulfate to sulfide occurs most rapidly at pH 6.5 and Anderson (1956) has estimated that as much as 12 g of sulfide/day might be produced by rumen contents.

A substantial amount of sulfide may also originate from S-containing amino acids. Australian data indicates that cystine or cysteine infusions resulted in appreciably higher levels of rumen sulfide than methionine (Bird, 1972) or inorganic sulfate sources (Bird and Hume, 1970; Hume and Bird, 1970). Infusion of methionine may also result in the production of CH_3SH.

A number of research studies have shown that labeled S from inorganic sulfate salts can be rapidly incorporated into amino acids and microbial proteins in the rumen (Block et al, 1951; Emery et al, 1957a, b; Hendrickx et al, 1964). Hungate (1966, p 347) cites a reference indicating that protozoa did not take up labeled sulfate. Studies by Paulson et al (1968) and Streeter et al (1969) suggest a gradual incorporation of labeled S into microbial protein, however Bird and Hume (1970) and Hume and Bird (1970) calculate that 55-70% of S coming from the omasum of sheep was protein S and that 42% of rumen S was recycled daily. This suggests active and relatively rapid metabolism of S in the rumen.

Halverson et al (1968) observed that maximal utilization of added sulfate S for protein synthesis occurred when the added sulfate was present at a level of 500 µM. The overall production of sulfide was increased some by casein or methionine and markedly by cystine and these increases resulted in somewhat less utilization of added sulfate-S for protein synthesis (i.e., a dilution effect). Added sulfide S lowered sulfate utilization, indicating that the organisms preferred the sulfide form. In other research on this subject, Emery and others (1957a) published data which indicated that only 5 or 10 cultures of rumen bacteria could utilize a significant amount of inorganic sulfate to synthesize organic S-containing compounds and only 3 cultures incorporated inorganic S

into their microbial proteins when cysteine was present in the medium. With mixed cultures, Hendrickx et al (1964) found that labeled S from sulfate, sulfite or sulfide S was utilized and Trenkle et al (1958) observed that, for a given quantity of S, methionine gave better response in terms of cellulose digestion in vitro than sulfate or sulfite S or cysteine or glutathione. More recent data by Bull and Vandersall (1973), however, suggests that S sources such as sodium sulfate, calcium sulfate, dl-methionone and methionine analog were equal at equal S content in their ability to promote cellulose digestion. Optimal concentration was 0.16-0.24% S; with corn fodder pellets, optimal S was 0.14-0.17% in vitro (Barton et al, 1971). When using crude suspensions, Martinez (1973) did not show any consistent differences in cellulose digestion between 10 and 100 µg/ml of added S. For starch digestion, Kennedy et al (1971) suggest that the requirement is more on the order of 2-2.4 µg/ml when using a simplified medium and 3-5 µg/ml in a complex medium. In work with Na sulfite, Krabill et al (1969) found that methane production was depressed as was acetate production.

It is obvious when summarizing the results of the papers just reviewed that there are differences in terms of utilization of S sources, requirements, and so on. Since the pure culture studies (Emery et al, 1957a, b) indicate some ruminal microorganisms cannot utilize inorganic S sources, and since it was shown that incorporation of inorganic S into organic compounds was faster with rumen fluid from cattle fed high-concentrate rations than from those fed high-roughage rations, it seems likely that diet and adequacy of other nutrients must have a pronounced effect on S utilization in the rumen. This is a subject for further work which is needed for clarification of S metabolism in the rumen.

Comments on Mineral Requirements

It might be worth pointing out that the development of proof of need of a given mineral element, particularly when required in very small amounts, is not easy to obtain. When using crude suspensions of rumen organisms, many nutrients may be carried over in the liquid, feed particles, or cells of the organism. Even if washed suspensions are used, there may be enough of a given trace mineral carried over in the cells to satisfy growth requirements for some time. The mineral requirement of an element can probably best be detected by using very small amounts of inocula, such as one might do with a stab or loop inoculation in normal bacterial procedures. These methods avoid transferring appreciable amounts of the element in question into the medium as can easily be done where massive inoculums are used.

Water supplies, equipment, glass that is slightly soluble, etc., may provide sources of the trace elements. Last, but not least, purified mineral salts are almost never 100% pure sources of the minerals on the label. Consequently, errors may easily be made when concluding that a given mineral element is or is not required.

An example from some of the data of Bryant et al (1959) is shown in Table 15-2. This is based on pure culture studies in which inoculation was done with very small cell numbers. Evaluation of growth was done on the basis of increase in optical density.

Table 15-2.   Effect of deletion of certain minerals on growth of strain S85 of *Bacteroides succinogenes*.[a]

Element deleted	Relative growth
None	93
Phosphate	0
Potassium	0
Magnesium	16
Iron	85
Ammonium	0
Calcium	9
Cobalt	89
Manganese	85

[a] Bryant et al (1959)

Macromineral Interactions

An appreciable amount of information on interactions between the macrominerals is available on different animal species (see Ch. 19, Vol. 2). However, relatively little information is available on rumen metabolism. Evans and Davis (1966) provided some of the first information on this subject, results indicating that S and P gave positive additive effects on cellulose digestion in vitro and that the depression in digestion caused by Cu was lessened by adding S. Kawashima et

al (1968) also showed that the addition of 300 μg/ml of P showed a tendency to inhibit sulfide production; the effect was more pronounced when sulfide production was further depressed by the addition of Mo to the medium. In further work from this laboratory (Uesada et al, 1968), it was shown that addition of 1,500 μg/ml of P into a Ca-free medium caused a depression in cellulose digestion. When 100-800 μg/ml of Ca as the chloride was added, cellulose digestion was not depressed by the added P. When a Mg-free medium was used, addition of 800 μg/ml of Ca depressed cellulose digestion which was counteracted by the addition of 50-400 μg/ml of Mg. Addition of 1,500 μg of P also depressed cellulose digestion with a Mg-free medium, but the depression was reduced by addition of 50-400 μg/ml of Mg. When all three elements were combined, the addition of 800 μg of Ca and 1,500 μg of P depressed cellulose digestion when the medium contained 0-10 μg of Mg, but this depression was completely alleviated by the addition of 100-200 μg/ml of Mg. Martinez (1973) has shown that addition of 200 μg/ml of Ca or Mg depressed cellulose digestion by mixed suspensions of bacteria. The depression caused by Ca was partially alleviated by Mg but Ca only very slightly alleviated the depressing effects of excessive Mg. Other data on interactions of macro-trace elements will be presented in a subsequent section.

Trace Minerals

Data on the quantities of trace minerals in rumen organisms are very limited. Ellis et al (1958) reported that one batch of dried rumen bacteria contained the following amounts (in ppm): Fe, 300; Zn, 200; Cu, 100; and Mo, 10. Sala (1957) has also reported some values for different elements which were (ppm): Fe, 535-990; Mn, 242-400; Zn, 130-220; Mo, 2-5; Cu, 40-72; Ni, 8-15; V, 0.9-2; and Ti, 25-87. Other values are given in Table 15-1.

Iron. McNaught and others (1950) reported that small amounts of Fe (1-2 ppm) produced good growth in rumen microbial suspensions and that increasing amounts of Fe resulted in greater protein synthesis. The organisms could tolerate 100 ppm, but 1,000 ppm was inhibitory to growth and metabolism. As shown in Table 15-2, Bryant et al (1959) could show very little effect by deletion of Fe. Likewise, Hubbert et al (1958) could show no improvement in cellulose digestion by adding Fe and moderate amounts were inhibitory to cellulose digestion. These authors cite a thesis in which the optimum Fe concentration for cellulose digestion was reported to be from 1-8 ppm of Fe. Little et al (1958) studied trace mineral requirements in vitro by first adding a chelating agent (EDTA) and then adding various amounts of the mineral in question. In the case of Fe, the addition of 0.5-12.5 ppm increased cellulose digestion. Although they did not detect any effect on cellulose digestion, Uesada et al (1965) found that added Fe resulted in increased protein and vitamin B_{12} synthesis. More recently, Martinez and Church (1970) have shown Fe to be slightly stimulatory to washed suspensions when evaluation was based on cellulose digestion.

In view of the concentration of Fe found in rumen organisms and the importance of Fe in a number of cellular enzymes known to contain Fe (flavoproteins and cytochromes), it is certain that Fe is required by rumen organisms to carry out metabolic reactions to completion even though requirements may be difficult to demonstrate. The same comments apply to Mn and probably to Zn, as well as to some other elements.

Copper. Hubbert et al (1958) and Little et al (1958) could not demonstrate that Cu had any stimulating effect on cellulose digestion, nor could Martinez and Church (1970) and Martinez (1973). However, Ellis et al (1958) indicated that Cu was stimulatory to cellulose digestion. Uesada et al (1965) found that Cu increased protein synthesis and Zerebocov et al (1971) state that low levels of Cu (1-1.3 ppm) stimulated degradation of protein, deamination of amino acids and utilization of carbohydrates with resulting synthesis of bacterial protein. The data from these papers and that of McNaught et al (1950) and Sala (1957) indicate that very low levels of Cu may be inhibitory to rumen microbes. Levels as low as 2-3 ppm or less may be inhibitory, especially in washed cell suspensions. Crude suspensions appear to be less affected.

Cobalt. Data of Bryant et al (1959) and Hubbert et al (1958) show that very small amounts of Co were stimulatory in some trials and not in others. Little et al (1958) found no effect under the conditions used although Martinez and Church (1970) demonstrated a slight stimulation of cellulose digestion. In other studies no effect on cellulose digetion was shown where crude suspensions were used (McNaught et al, 1950; Salsbury et al, 1956; Sala, 1957), although Zerebicov et al (1971) states that Co stimulated breakdown of protein and carbohydrates, resulting in growth of rumen organisms and increased protein N in rumen fluid. Note that Co is also toxic at relatively low concentrations (Table 15-3).

It is, of course, obvious if rumen organisms synthesize cobalamin (B_{12}) that Co must be required

Table 15-3. Concentrations of different mineral elements that were stimulatory to cellulose digestion and toxic concentrations for rumen bacteria.

Element	Stimulatory concentration,[a] ppm	Toxic concentration, ppm	
		Martinez and Church	Uesada et al[b]
B	0	300	
Ba	0	30	
Br	0	>1000	
Cd	1-7	10	
Co	1-3	7	5
Cr	1-3	10	
Cu	0-0.1	1	5
F	0	0.5	10
Fe	2-5	100	500
I	20	>1000	
Mn	5-30	100	500
Mo	10-200	>500	2500
Ni	0	0.5	
Rb	20-50	>1000	
Se	0	7	
Sr	10-15	200	
V	0	5	
Zn	2-10	20	50

[a]From Martinez and Church (1970); data on washed cell suspensions.
[b]From Uesada et al (1965)

by some of the microflora or microfauna since Co is a constituent of this vitamin. Gall et al (1949) reported that the rumen population of Co-deficient ruminants was dissimilar to that of normal animals when examined microscopically. However, Marston et al (1961) published data which indicated that the production of V FA in the reticulo-rumen of Co-deficient sheep was more of less normal, thus indicating that rumen metabolism was not grossly changed.

Tosic and Mitchell (1948) observed that most of the Co added to deficient diets was rapidly concentrated in the microbial tissue. Comar et al (1946) indicated, when radio-active Co was injected I.V., that none was detected in saliva although Keener and others (1951) detected small amounts of labeled Co in the rumen after parenteral administration; thus, these papers indicate that very little recycling of Co occurs in the rumen. Andrews et al (1958) and others have demonstrated that an adequate supply of Co can be provided to animals on deficient diets by intraruminal administration of pellets made of cobaltic oxide, providing the pellets stay in the rumen. Davis et al (1956) found that the amount of ^{60}Co incorporated into cobalamin in the rumen was greatly influenced by the amount of Mo in the diet. High levels of Mo inhibited Co utilization, resulting in reduced vitamin synthesis. Other data on this topic are discussed in Ch. 20 of Vol. 2.

Manganese. Hubbert et al (1958) and Uesada et al (1965, 1966) could not show that Mn stimulated cellulose digestion by rumen bacteria or protozoa although Little et al (1958) found that 7.5 ppm of Mn increased cellulose digestion after chelating agents had been added to the medium. Chamberlain and Burroughs (1962) showed that omission of Mn resulted in a reduction in cellulose digestion and Martinez and Church (1970) observed a slight stimulus when Mn was added (5-30 ppm) to washed suspensions.

Mn is known to be an important cofactor for many enzymes and the concentration found in rumen bacteria indicates that this is so in these organisms. Mn deficiency has also been reported in ruminants although it is not believed to be a common problem (see Ch. 20, Vol. 2).

Molybdenum. Ellis et al (1958) found that Mo was stimulatory to cellulose digestion in vitro and that the addition of Mo and Cu promoted about the same degree of increased cellulose digestion as did the addition of alfalfa ash. Martinez and Church (1970) have also demonstrated that Mo was stimulatory to cellulose digestion, and Uesada et al (1966) found some stimulus to VFA production by protozoa. Other workers have not noted any effect on rumen bacterial activity (McNaught et al, 1950; Sala, 1957; Uesada et al, 1965).

Zinc. Neither Hubbert et al (1958) nor Sala (1957) could show a response to supplementary Zn and low levels were inhibitory to cellulose digestion. However, Little et al (1958) observed some response after chelating agents had been added and Martinez and Church (1970) observed stimulation of cellulose digestion by adding 2-10 ppm of Zn to washed suspensions. The situation with Zn is similar to that of some other trace minerals in that it is known to be a cofactor for a number of enzymes. Perhaps some of the other divalent ions may be able to replace it totally or partially, although it seems more likely that media used have not been deficient enough to show a response.

Other Microminerals. Little et al (1958) have indicated that Se stimulated cellulose digestion and Hidiroglou et al (1968) have shown with labeled Se that rumen bacteria fix it into microbial protein. In sheep fed a purified diet low in protein, they noted that Se supplementation caused a marked alteration in rumen microorganisms. However, Martinez and Church (1970) could show no effect of Se on cellulose digestion.

In other research, Washburn and Thrall (1961) showed some evidence of a stimulatory effect of vanadium, but this was not confirmed by Martinez and Church (1970). Martinez and Church (1970) have shown some effect of a number of elements on cellulose digestion. These include (see Table 15-3): Cd, Cr, I, Rb and Sr. Further research is required to evaluate the function of these elements in rumen metabolism.

Trace Mineral Interactions

In terms of total body metabolism, there are numerous interactions known between various macro and trace minerals and some between different trace minerals (see Ch. 20, Vol. 2; Underwood, 1971). There is relatively little information on the interaction between these minerals in the rumen. In some of the early work, Davis et al (1956) demonstrated that high levels of Mo interfered with cobalamin synthesis and Evans and Davis

(1966) observed that the addition of Cu or Mo to in vitro fermentations lessened the depressing effect of the other in the presence of P. They also concluded that the depression in cellulose digestion caused by Cu was lessened by added S. Although Ellis et al (1958) suggest an additive effect of Cu and Mo on cellulose digestion, neither Japanese data (Kawashima et al, 1968; Zembahashi et al, 1968) nor Martinez (1973) showed this to be the case for VFA production by protozoa or cellulose digestion by rumen bacteria, respectively. In fact, the combination of Cu and Mo was more apt to intensify the toxicity which was not alleviated by 1000 µg/ml of S. Zembahashi et al (1968) did find that addition of P tended to alleviate toxicity of Mo and Mo + sulfate. Thus, these interactions appear to be different than those seen in the ruminant animal.

Table 15-4. Effect of combinations of Ca and Zn on in vitro rumen cellulose digestion.[a]

Ca added, µg/ml	Zn added, µg/ml				Mean
	0	0.5	5.0	50	
0	62.2	62.4	39.0	8.4	43.0
20	60.7	62.2	56.0	22.5	50.4
40	54.7	53.7	57.3	40.1	51.4
100	40.3	37.3	38.1	40.7	39.1
Means	54.5	53.9	47.6	29.9	

[a]From Martinez (1973)

Other mineral interactions in the rumen include one between, F, Mg and Mn suggested by Chamberlain and Burroughs (1962). Martinez (1973) has identified a number of others: Ca-Zn, Mn-Zn, S-Mg-Ni, P-Mg-Ni, Mg-Co, P-Mg-Co and Mg-Co-Ni. Some of his data on Ca-Zn are shown in Table 15-4. In the other interactions, it was shown that Mg partially reversed the severe depression in cellulose digestion caused by excessive Ni; addition of S and P enhanced this protection. Mg also alleviated the depressing effects of excessive Co, or Ni and Co in combination.

Trace Mineral Toxicity

A number of comments on trace mineral toxicity have already been made and some data presented in Table 15-3. There are, however, several other papers on the subject which are worthy of reviewing. Japanese research (Kawashima et al, 1969; Kim et al, 1969) has shown that toxicities of Co, Cu, Se and Zn were reduced when casein and isolated soy protein were used as N sources, however the toxicities of F and Mo were enhanced, and N source did not affect the toxicity of Fe or Mn on cellulose digestion. They suggested that Co, Cu, Se and Zn probably formed a less toxic chelate with the protein. This was confirmed by adding urea and Na-EDTA as the combination reduced toxicity. Their results also indicated that unsaturated fatty acids may form a complex with some trace elements which may be detrimental to rumen bacteria. For example, the toxicity of Mo and Se was increased by addition of C18:1 and that of Co, Cu, F, Se and Zn by addition of C18:2 and F by corn oil. C14:0, C16:0 and C18:0 had no effect on trace element toxicity.

In research with F, Leemann and Stahel (1972) observed that 80 ppm of Na fluoride caused a marked effect on rumen cilates as did a daily intake of 6 mg of fluoride/kg of body weight to a cow. Based on production of methane or dimethyl sulfide, Salsbury (1973) concluded that 23 ppm Cu, 3 ppm Hg and 380 ppm Pb were not inhibitory. Cu at 50 ppm and Hg at 32 ppm were toxic, although low levels of Hg tended to be stimulatory. Hg also inhibited cellulose digestion at 50 ppm.

References Cited

VITAMINS

Agrawala, I.P., C.F. Huffman, R.W. Leucke and C.W. Duncan. 1953. J. Nutr. 49:631.
Almendinger, R. and F.C. Hinds. 1969. J. Dairy Sci. 52:2044.
Barnett, A.J.G. and R.L. Reid. 1961. Reactions in the Rumen. Edward Arnold LTD.
Bechdel, S.I., C.H. Eckles and S.L. Palmer. 1926. J. Dairy Sci. 9:409.
Bechdel, S.I., H.E. Honeywell, R.A. Dutcher and M.H. Knutsen. 1928. J. Biol. Chem. 80:231.
Bryant, M.P. 1963. J. Animal Sci. 22:801.
Bryant, M.P. and I.M. Robinson. 1961. Appl. Microbiol. 9:91.

Bryant, M.P. and I.M. Robinson. 1962. J. Bact. 84:605.
Bryant, M.P., I.M. Robinson and H. Chu. 1959. J. Dairy Sci. 42:1831.
Buziassy, C. and D.E. Tribe. 1960. Aust. J. Agr. Res. 11:989; 1002.
Davison, K.L. and J. Seo. 1963. J. Dairy Sci. 46:862 (abstr).
Dryden, L.P. and A.M. Hartman. 1971. J. Dairy Sci. 54:235.
Edwin, E.E. and G. Lewis. 1971. J. Dairy Res. 38:79.
Endo, A., K. Kumai, K. Suto and T. Uemura. 1962. Nutr. Abstr. Rev. 32:848.
Erb, R.E., F.N. Andrews and R.E. Nichols. 1947. J. Dairy Sci. 30:673.
Gibbons, R.J. and R.N. Doetsch. 1959. J. Bact. 77:417.
Golubev, L.I. 1972. Nutr. Abstr. Rev. 42:922.
Hale, W.H., A.L. Pope, P.H. Phillips and G. Bohstedt. 1950. J. Animal Sci. 9:414.
Hamilton, P., B.E. Plummer and H.C. Dickey. 1955. Maine Agr. Expt. Sta. Bul. 543.
Hayes, B.W., G.E. Mitchell, C.O. Little and N.W. Bradley. 1966. J. Animal Sci. 25:539.
Hedrich, M.F., J.M. Elliot and J.E. Lowe. 1973. J. Nutr. 103:1646.
Hollis, L., C.F. Chappel, R. MacVicar and C.K. Whitehair. 1954. J. Animal Sci. 13:732.
Hungate, R.E. 1963. J. Bact. 86:848.
Hunt, C.H., O.G. Bentley and T. Hershberger. 1952. Fed. Proc. 11:233.
Hunt, C.H., O.G. Bentley, T.V. Hershberger and J.H. Cline. 1954. J. Animal Sci. 13:510.
Hunt, C.H., et al. 1943. J. Nutr. 25:207.
Johnson, B.C., H.H. Mitchell, T.S. Hamilton and W.B. Nevens. 1947. Fed. Proc. 6:410.
Keating, E.K., W.H. Hale and F. Hubbert. 1964. J. Animal Sci. 23:111.
Kercher, C.H. and S.E. Smith. 1956. J. Animal Sci. 15:550.
King, T.B., T.H. Lohman and G.S. Smith. 1962. J. Animal Sci. 21:1002 (abstr).
Knight, C.A., R.A. Dutcher, N.B. Guerrant and S.I. Bechdel. 1940. Proc. Soc. Exp. Biol. Med. 44:90.
Lev, M. 1959. J. Gen. Microbiol. 20:697.
Loew, F.M. 1972. Rev. Cubana Cienc. Agr. 6:301.
Loew, F.M. and R.H. Dunlop. 1972. Can. J. Comp. Med. 36:345.
Long, R.D., G.E. Mitchell and C.O. Little. 1971. Int. J. Vit. Nutr. Res. 41:327.
Matschiner, J.T. 1970. J. Nutr. 100:190.
McElroy, L.W. and Harold Goss. 1940. J. Nutr. 20:527; 541.
McElroy, L.W. and Harold Goss. 1941. J. Nutr. 21:163; 405.
McElroy, L.W. and T.H. Jukes. 1940. Proc. Expt. Biol. Med. 45:296.
McGillivray, W.A. 1951. Br. J. Nutr. 5:223.
Milligan, L.P., J.M. Asplund and A.R. Robblee. 1967. Can. J. Animal Sci. 47:57.
Milligan, L.P., J.M. Asplund and A.R. Robblee. 1968. Can. J. Animal Sci. 48:99.
Mitchell, G.E., C.O. Little and B.W. Hayes. 1967. J. Animal Sci. 26:827.
Mitchell, G.E. et al. 1968. Int. J. Vit. Res. 38:304.
Pavel, J., J. Zak and J. Tylecek. 1968. Arch. Tierernahrung. 18:264.
Pearson, P.B., L. Struglia and I.L. Lindall. 1953. J. Animal Sci. 12:213.
Poe, S.E., G.E. Mitchell and D.G. Ely. 1972. J. Animal Sci. 34:826.
Scott, H.W. and B.A. Dehority. 1965. J. Bact. 89:1169.
Swingle, R.S. and I.A. Dyer. 1970. J. Animal Sci. 31:404.
Takahashi, N. and M. Goto. 1972. Nutr. Abstr. Rev. 42:1336.
Teeri, A.E. and N.F. Colovos. 1963. J. Dairy Sci. 46:864 (abstr).
Teeri, A.E., H.F. Enos, E. Pomerantz and N.F. Colovos. 1955. J. Animal Sci. 14:268.
Tucker, R.E. and J.P. Fontenot. 1970. J. Animal Sci. 31:256 (abstr).
Virtanen, A.I. 1963. Biochem. Z. 338:443.
Walker, C.K. and J.M. Elliot. 1972. J. Dairy Sci. 55:474.
Warner, R.L., G.E. Mitchell, C.O. Little and N.E. Alderson. 1970. Int. J. Vit. Res. 40:585.
Wegner, M.I., A.N. Booth, C.A. Elvehjem and E.B. Hart. 1941. Proc. Soc. Expt. Biol. Med. 47:90.
White, W.H., J.E.R. Greenshields and W. Chubaty. 1954. Can. J. Agr. Sci. 34:601.
Yskshsdhi, N., K. Kubo and J. Osawa. 1967. Jap. J. Zootech. Sci. 38:339.
Zerebocov, P.I., V.F. Vrakin and A.A. Khodyrev. 1972. Nutr. Abstr. Rev. 42:94.

MINERALS

Ammerman, C.B., et al. 1971. J. Dairy Sci. 54:1288.
Anderson, C.M. 1956. N.Z. J. Sci. Tech. 37A:379.
Anderson, R., E. Cheng and W. Burroughs. 1956. J. Animal Sci. 15:489.
Andrews, E.D., C.E. Isaacs and R.J. Findlay. 1958. N.Z. Vet. J. 6:140.
Barton, J.S., L.S. Bull and R.W. Hemken. 1971. J. Animal Sci. 33:682.
Bentley, O.G., S. Vanecho, C.H. Hunt and A.L. Moxon. 1953. J. Animal Sci. 12:908 (abstr).
Bird, P.R. 1972. Aust. J. Biol. Sci. 25:185.
Bird, P.R. and I.D. Hume. 1970. Aust. J. Agr. Res. 22:443.

Block, R.J., J.A. Stekol and J.K. Loosli. 1951. Arch. Biochem. Biophys. 33:353.
Bray, A.C. 1969. Aust. J. Agr. Res. 20:739.
Brink, M.F. and W.H. Pfander. 1961. J. Animal Sci. 20:966 (abstr).
Bryant, M.P., I.M. Robinson and H. Chu. 1959. J. Dairy Sci. 42:1831.
Bull, L.S. and J.H. Vandersall. 1973. J. Dairy Sci. 56:106.
Burroughs, W., H.G. Headley, R.M. Bethke and P. Gerlaugh. 1950. J. Animal Sci. 9:513.
Burroughs, W., et al. 1951. J. Animal Sci. 10:693.
Caldwell, D.R. and R.F. Hudson. 1974. Appl. Microbiol. 27:549.
Chamberlain, C.C. and W. Burroughs. 1962. J. Animal Sci. 21:428.
Chicco, C.F., et al. 1965. J. Animal Sci. 24:355.
Comar, C.L., et al. 1946. J. Nutr. 32:61.
Davis, G.K., F.H. Jack and J.T. McCall. 1956. J. Animal Sci. 15:1232 (abstr).
Ellis, W.C., W.H. Pfander, M.E. Muhrer and E.E. Pickett. 1958. J. Animal Sci. 17:180.
Emery, R.S., C.K. Smith and L. Fai To. 1957a. Appl. Microbiol. 5:363.
Emery, R.S., C.K. Smith and C.F. Huffman. 1957b. Appl. Microbiol. 5:360.
Evans, J.L. and G.K. Davis. 1966. J. Animal Sci. 25:1010; 1014.
Fitt, T.J., K. Hutton, A. Thompson and D.G. Armstrong. 1972. Proc. Nutr. Soc. 31:100A (abstr).
Gall, L.S., et al. 1949. Science. 109:468.
Hall, O.G., H.D. Baxter and C.S. Hobbs. 1961. J. Animal Sci. 20:817.
Halverson, A.W., G.D. Williams and G.D. Paulson. 1968. J. Nutr. 95:363.
Henderickx, H., J. Martin and L. Baert. 1964. Nutr. Abstr. Rev. 34:156.
Hidiroglou, M., D.P. Heaney and K.J. Jenkins. 1968. Can. J. Physiol. Pharmacol. 46:229.
Hubbert, F., E. Cheng and W. Burroughs. 1958. J. Animal Sci. 17:559; 576.
Hume, I.D. and P.R. Bird. 1970. Aust. J. Agr. Res. 21:315.
Hungate, R.E. 1966. The Rumen and Its Microbes. Academic Press.
Hunt, C.H., O.G. Bentley, T.V. Hershberger and J.H. Cline. 1954. J. Animal Sci. 13:570.
Kahn, B.B., J.G. Nagy, E.W. Kienholz and G.M. Ward. 1969. J. Animal Sci. 29:166 (abstr).
Kawashima, R., S.W. Kim and S. Uesada. 1969. Bul. Res. Inst. Fd. Sci. Kyoto Univ. 32:8.
Kawashima, R., S. Uesada and T. Toyama. 1968. Bul. Res. Inst. Fd. Sci. Kyoto Univ. 31:7.
Keener, H.A., R.R. Baldwin and G.P. Percival. 1951. J. Animal Sci. 10:428.
Kennedy, L.G., G.E. Mitchell and C.O. Little. 1971. J. Animal Sci. 32:359.
Kim, S.W., R. Kawashima and S. Uesada. 1969. Bul. Res. Inst. Fd. Sci. Kyoto Univ. 32:17; 24.
Krabill, L.F., W.S. Alhassan and L.D. Satter. 1969. J. Dairy Sci. 52:1812.
Kulwich, R., L. Struglia and P.B. Pearson. 1956. J. Nutr. 61:113.
Lee, D. and G. Matrone. 1971. J. Nutr. 101:967.
Leemann, W. and O. Stahel. 1972. Fluoride 5:200.
Lewis, D. 1954. Biochem. J. 56:391.
Little, O., E. Cheng and W. Burroughs. 1958. J. Animal Sci. 17:1190 (abstr).
Marston, H.R., S.H. Allen and R.M. Smith. 1961. Nature 190:1085.
Martinez, A. 1973. Ph.D. Thesis. Oregon State Univ., Corvallis, Oregon.
Martinez, A. and D.C. Church. 1970. J. Animal Sci. 31:982.
McNaught, M.L., E.C. Owen and J.B. Smith. 1950. Biochem. J. 46:36.
Paulson, G.D., C.A. Baumann and A.L. Pope. 1968. J. Animal Sci. 27:497.
Poutiainen, E. 1970. Annal. Agr. Fenn. 9:347.
Punj, M.L., A.S. Kochar and I.S. Bhatia. 1969. Indian Vet. J. 46:881.
Raun, A., E. Cheng and W. Burroughs. 1956. J. Agr. Fd. Chem. 4:869.
Reid, R.L., M.C. Franklin and E.G. Hallsworth. 1947. Aust. Vet. J. 23:136.
Sala, J.C. 1957. Ph.D. Thesis. Univ. of Florida, Gainesville, Fla.
Salsbury, R.L. 1973. J. Animal Sci. 37:356 (abstr).
Salsbury, R.L., C.K. Smith and C.F. Huffman. 1956. J. Animal Sci. 15:863.
Streeter, C.L., C.O. Little and G.E. Mitchell. 1969. J. Animal Sci. 29:172 (abstr).
Tosic, J. and R.L. Mitchell. 1948. Nature 162:502.
Trenkle, A., E. Cheng and W. Burroughs. 1958. J. Animal Sci. 17:1191 (abstr).
Uesada, S., R. Kawashima and M. Zembayashi. 1965. Bul. Res. Inst. Fd. Sci. Kyoto Univ. 28:10.
Uesada, S., R. Kawashima and M. Zembayashi. 1966. Bul. Res. Inst. Fd. Sci. Kyoto Univ. 29:21.
Uesada, S., R. Kawashima, M. Zembayashi and K. Fujusawa. 1968. Bul. Res. Inst. Fd. Sci. Kyoto Univ. 31:13.
Undersood, E.J. 1971. Trace Elements in Human and Animal Nutrition. 3rd ed. Academic Press, New York.
Washburn, L.E. and B.E. Thrall. 1961. Proc. West. Sec. Amer. Soc. Animal Sci. 12:87.
Zembayashi, M., R. Kawashima and S. Uesada. 1968. Bul. Res. Inst. Fd. Sci. Kyoto Univ. 31:1.
Zerebocov, P.I., V.F. Vrakin and N.S. Sevelev. 1971. Nutr. Abst. Rev. 41:937.

CHAPTER 16 — RUMEN FERMENTATION OF NATURAL FEEDSTUFFS

The intent of this chapter is to focus attention on some of the factors affecting rumen fermentation that may have been neglected in earlier chapters dealing with specific nutrients. To some extent part of the material covered may be repetitive. However, the discussions should provide a more coordinated picture of rumen fermentation to the reader. The primary material that will be discussed will center around information relating to the volatile fatty acids, rumen pH, rumen gases, rumen volume and adaptation of the rumen microorganisms to ration changes.

Volatile Fatty Acids in the Rumen

Volatile fatty acids (VFA) have been mentioned many times previously, and it has been known for many years that VFA are normal constituents of rumen contents (see Hungate, 1966, p 192) However, data in the literature prior to the late 1940's are sparse due to the fact that analytical methods were tedious and did not always resolve the different acids. With the development of liquid-liquid chromatographic analyses and, subsequently, gas chromatographic methods (see apparatus in Fig. 16-1), many, many investigations relating to VFA have appeared in the literature. Consequently, only a limited number of the available papers will be mentioned in this chapter.

Normal Levels

Acids in the rumen that are normally classed as VFA include formic, acetic, butyric, isobutyric, 2-methylbutyric, propionic, valeric, isovaleric and traces of C6 and C8. Usual molar concentrations are in the order of acetic, propionic and butyric with lesser amounts of isobutyric and isovaleric. Although small amounts of acids other than acetic, propionic and butyric are often found, many writers ignore them or lump them together as "higher" acids.

Shown in Table 16-1 are typical levels and molar ratios that one might expect to find in the rumen of 10 different ruminant species.

Data on the first five examples are from animals grazing green forage or animals which were fed freshly cut forage. Total VFA levels are expressed as means or ranges in means for different animals on the same ration. However, the values are not at all representative of the range of values to be found in the literature. For that matter, a large range might be expected in view of the host of factors which influence rumen fermentation, the different analytical methods utilized, variations in sampling methods and differences in diets. For example, it has been shown that total VFA levels are usually lower when stomach tubes are utilized to sample rumen contents; this is due to dilution of rumen fluid with saliva (Bryant, 1964; Lane et al, 1968). Note that total acids are sometimes expressed as mg% or meq%, but the generally accepted method in recent years has been as μmol/ml or mMol/100 ml.

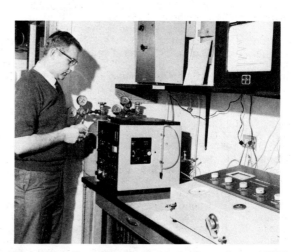

Figure 16-1. Former graduate student carrying out VFA analyses with gas-liquid chromatograph in the author's laboratory.

It is interesting to note how similar the molar percentages are (Table 16-1). Unfortunately, the only species comparisons available in which the animals were fed identical rations seem to be those of Ichhponai and Sidhu (1965) and Pant et al

Table 16-1. Typical quantities and molar ratios of volatile fatty acids found in the rumen of different ruminant species.

Animal	Ration	Time of sampling in relation to eating	Total VFA, μmol/ml	Molar %				
				Acetic	Propionic	Butyric	Valeric	Others
Sheep[1]	ryegrass-clover pasture	unknown	114	64-65	18	12-13	1	4
Cattle [Bos tarus][2]	pasture	7 a.m. to 5 p.m.	131-148	65-67	18-19	11-12	—	3-4
Cattle[3]	ryegrass pasture	after feeding	127-129	60-62	20-21	13-14	1.6-1.7	3-4
Cattle [Bos indicus][4]	green berseem	before feeding	94	60	18-19	14-15	—	—
Asian buffalo[4]	green berseem	before feeding	117	62-63	22-23	15	—	—
Asian buffalo[5]	wheat straw + concentrates	after morning feed of concentrates	62.8					
Sheep[5]	wheat straw + concentrates	after morning feed of concentrates	65.7					
Goats[5]	wheat straw + concentrates	after morning feed of concentrates	73.5					
Black-tailed deer[6]	alfalfa, grain, browse	early morning	90	56	21	19	3	1
Sheep[6]	alfalfa	after morning feed	108	59	20	15	6	—
Red deer[7]	browse and concentrates	unknown	106	67	21	11	1	—
Fallow deer[7]	concentrates	unknown	120	57	29	12	2	—
Mule deer[8]	summer range	unknown	—	63	22	13		2
Pronghorn antelope[9]	early fall range	unknown	117	70	17	9	4	—

[1]Jamieson (1959) [2]Balch and Rowland (1957) [3]Bath and Rook (1965) [4]Ichhponani and Sidhu (1965) [5]Pant et al (1963) [6]Allo et al (1973) [7]Prins and Geelen (1971) [8]Short et al (1966) [9]Nagy and Williams (1969)

(1963). These comparisons do indicate some differences in total acids and molar percentages, but certainly not extreme differences. Thus, we can conclude that these end products of rumen fermentation are remarkably similar in rather diverse ruminant species. Even some of the values on the wild species consuming native browse are not markedly different from values shown for the domestic species.

Of the minor or "higher" acids present in rumen fluid, Gray et al (1952) have reported the presence of formic acid which may, in some cases, be found in hay or forage and el-Shazly (1952) observed that branched-chain acids were found in the rumen of sheep on a variety of diets. Jamieson (1959) found 0-2.0% formic, 1.0-4.5% isobutyric, 0.5-4.0% isovaleric and 0-3.5% 2-methylbutyric present in samples from sheep grazing ryegrass-clover pasture. Bath and Rook (1965) reported molar percentage values for isobutyric acid to be on the order of 0.7-2.3 and isovaleric + 2-methylbutyric to be 0.8-3.6 in dairy cows on a variety of rations. In steers fed purified diets containing isolated soy protein, Oltjen et al (1971) found 13.5% butyric, 1.5% isobutyric, 3.8% valeric and 1.9% of isovaleric + 2-methylbutyric acid. In work with pure cultures of rumen bacteria, Allison and Bucklin (1971) concluded that some species produced branched chain acids and some did not when grown on media containing either enzymatically or acid hydrolyzed casein. Those species that did produce branched chain acids produced more on the enzyme hydrolyzed casein and more 5-carbon than 4-carbon acids.

Effect of Feed Ingestion on VFA Concentration

The quantity of VFA present in the reticulo-rumen fluids is a reflection of microbial activity and of absorption or passage out of the rumen. Following the ingestion of readily fermentable feed, microbial activity increases rapidly, resulting in an increase in VFA concentrations. Data shown in Table 16-2 (from Gray and Pilgrim, 1951) illustrate the changes that might be expected to occur when animals are fed once per day.

The data in the table show a more than twofold increase in total VFA concentration from the initial values before feeding to the peak values (2.74 for alfalfa and 2.36 for wheaten hay). However, it is interesting to note that the molar percentages changed very little for the alfalfa-fed sheep, although there was a substantial change for those fed wheaten hay, resulting in relatively less acetate and proportionately more propionic acid with minor changes in butyric acid.

In contrast to the data of Gray and Pilgrim, data presented by Gray et al (1967) are shown in Fig. 16-2 to illustrate the effect of more

Table 16-2. Change in Rumen VFA concentration and molar percentages after feeding.[a]

Time after feeding, hr	Forage fed to sheep							
	Alfalfa Hay				Wheaten Hay			
	Total VFA, μmol/ml	Molar %			Total VFA, μmol/ml	Molar %		
		Ac	Pr	Bu		Ac	Pr	Bu
0	93	70	15	15	87	68	18	14
0.5	125	71	17	12	94	65	20	15
1	158	71	18	11	112	62	22	16
2	210	70	19	11	141	59	25	16
3	252	69	19	12	144	59	26	15
4	255	69	19	12	182	58	26	16
6	216	70	19	11	205	59	27	14
8	223	71	19	10	136	60	26	14
12	228	73	17	10	152	64	23	13
16	183	73	16	11	132	67	21	12
20	135	71	16	13	114	68	19	13
24	100	69	17	14	90	70	17	13

[a] From Gray and Pilgrim (1951)

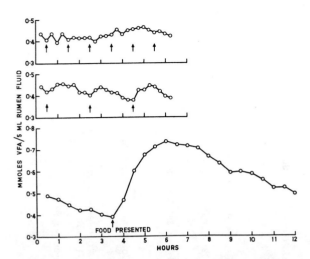

Figure 16-2. Concentration of VFA in the rumen of sheep fed at intervals of 1, 2, and 12 hr. From Gray et al [1967].

frequent feeding, using apparatus similar to that shown in Fig. 16-3. In this case sheep were fed chopped alfalfa hay at hourly intervals from 0800 to 1900. During the period from about 1200 to 2200 hours, the amount of VFA fluctuated very little (from ca. 63 to 78 µmol/ml for acetic acid). Bath and Rook (1963) have also published data on the effect of increasing frequency of feeding on rumen fermentation. They found that increasing the times fed from 1 to 4 for dairy cows had little effect on concentration of VFA (sampled less frequently, however), but it did decrease the range of values observed between feeding. Data from animals fed more than once per day are more typical of those to be expected in grazing animals or those fed dry feed ad libitum, situations which would be much more typical of a ruminant's normal feeding behavior (see Ch. 4).

Other papers reporting rather extensive data on VFA concentrations with time after feeding include those of Phillipson (1952), Emery et al (1956), Balch and Rowland (1957), Stewart et al (1958), Ichhponani and Sidhu (1965), Ghorban et al (1966), Williams and Christian (1966), Weller et al (1967), Ibrahim et al (1969), Omori et al (1969) and Fenner et al (1970).

Effect of Ration Ingredients on Rumen VFA

There have been many, many papers published in the literature which show the effect of different rations on VFA concentration and molar percentage. Excerpts from some of the papers are shown in Table 16-3.

The list in the table is, perhaps, more extensive than necessary to illustrate the effect of diet, however, it is only a small portion of the total available. The reader should remember that comparisons between different experiments may not be warranted, particularly with respect to total VFA present. This is so because animals have been sampled at different times; a variety of analytical techniques have been used; some authors have not analyzed for all the acids present and some papers give ranges whereas others give mean values. Furthermore, total VFA concentrations are generally less reliable values than those for molar percentages. Consequently, the most valid comparisons should be within those published by one author or within one experiment by any given author.

With respect to total VFA, the data are somewhat contradictory because errors in sampling are involved and the time after eating that samples were taken may have varied from experiment to experiment. However, it is probably safe to conclude that ingesting immature grass, increasing amounts of carbonaceous or protein supplements, increasing levels of feed intake, and pelleted roughages tend to result in higher VFA levels. Other factors that have, at times, indicated increased levels of VFA would include buffers, antibiotics and pelleted concentrates.

With respect to the molar distribution of the VFA, high levels of acetate are usually seen with silage, particularly alfalfa, mature hays and mature pastures. A high level of protein intake may be expected to increase the concentration of branched chain acids and of butyric acid. Pelleting or heat treatment of grain will generally result in greater levels of propionic acid, although there are exceptions to this as well as to most of the other conclusions previously noted.

What factors contribute to the differences observed in molar percentages or total VFA when animals are fed different diets? Information is not adequate to specify all the factors involved. However, it is known that drastic changes in the chemical composition of the diet usually result in marked changes in bacterial and protozoal populations and we can presume that moderate changes in the diet will result in moderate shifts in the microbial population. In addition, rumen fermentation may be influenced by the

Table 16-3. Effect of ration on VFA concentration in the reticulo-rumen.

Animal	Ration	Total VFA, μmol/ml	Molar % Acetic	Propionic	Butyric	Others	Authors
Dairy cows	pasture	131-148	65-67	18-19	11-12	3-4	Balch and Rowland (1957)
	poor meadow hay	105-121	69	18	10	3	
	16 lb poor meadow hay and 15 lb dairy cubes	107-137	60	23	13	4	
	good silage	87-130	74	17	7	2	
Dairy cows	spring pasture, ryegrass	138-158	56-58	23-24	15-16	4-5	Bath and Rook (1965)
	hay, timothy/fescue	101-107	70-71	17-18	7-8	3-4	
	hay, alfalfa	88-98	69-70	17-18	7-8	6-7	
	silage, alfalfa	89-97	71-72	14-15	7-8	5-6	
	hay, alfalfa and concentrates	99-104	64-68	18-21	10-11	4-6	
	silage, early cut ryegrass	88	62	19	15	4	
	silage, late cut ryegrass	124	63	17	13	7	
	hay, ryegrass from same field	95	73	17	7	3	
	sugar beet tops	124-140	60-62	17-18	16-18	4-5	
	dried sugar beet pulp	99-105	60-62	17-23	11-19	4-5	
	dried sugar beet pulp and hay	94-101	68-69	17-18	10-11	3-4	
Dairy cows	low protein ration	105	62-63	18-19	14	4-5	Davis et al (1957)
	med. protein rations	114	61-62	19-20	14-15	4-5	
	high protein ration	115	58-59	20-21	15-16	4-6	
Dairy cows	10 lb of 1:1 mix of hay and concentrates	93-97	68-69	15-17	13-15	2	Bath and Rook (1963)
	15 lb of the same	104-108	66-67	16-17	14-16	2	
	20 lb of the same	114-121	65	16-17	16-17	2	
	30 lb of the same	123-126	63-64	17-18	16-18	2-3	
Dairy cows	Alfalfa hay	—	73	17	10		Esdale et al (1968)
	corn silage		64	19	17		
	alfalfa-grain	101	69	21	10		Bauman et al (1971)
	High-grain	122	45	47	8		
Dairy cows	med. ground hay + concentrate	—	64-65	19-20	12-13	3-4	Thomas et al (1968)
	pelleted hay + concentrate	—	65	18-19	13-14	3	
	steamed hay + concentrate	—	65-66	17-18	14-15	2-3	
Dairy cows	ground alfalfa hay, expanded grain	—	53-54	31-32	10-11	4	Colenbrander et al (1967)
	chopped alfalfa hay, cracked grain	—	68-69	17-18	12-13	2-3	
Dairy cows	long alfalfa hay + 16 lb of ground corn	89	60-61	20	17	2-3	Jorgensen and Schultz (1963)
	long alfalfa hay + 16 lb of pelleted corn	107	57-58	22	17-18	3-4	
	pelleted alfalfa hay + 16 lb of ground corn	126	55-56	27	15-16	2-3	
	alfalfa hay + concentrates	—	52	31	13	4	Moody (1971)
	alfalfa hay + concentrates with 6% tallow	—	51	33	12	4	

Animal	Ration	Total VFA, μmol/ml	Molar % Acetic	Propionic	Butyric	Others	Authors
Steers	early summer veld grazing	92-98	68	18	11	3	Topps et al (1965)
	late summer veld grazing	78-91	69-70	18	9	4	
	winter veld grazing	70-84	70-71	20	7	3	
	winter veld grazing + carbohydrate	70-82	67-68	20	9	3	
	winter veld grazing + protein	73-84	69-70	20	8	3	
	winter veld grazing + both	84-97	66-67	18	12	3-4	
Steers	20:80 silage:grain	90-95	62-64	19-21	15	2-4	McCullough and Smart (1968)
	20:80 hay:grain	84-88	67-69	17-18	9-10	5-6	
Steers	pelleted alfalfa, cracked corn	98	55	28-29	11	5-6	Clanton and Woods (1966)
	pelleted alfalfa, pelleted corn	117	51	32	11-12	5-6	
	ground alfalfa, cracked corn	87	50	31	12-13	6-7	
	ground alfalfa, pelleted corn	99	52	29-30	12-13	5-6	
Steers	pelleted corn-soy, molasses	88	42	35	23		Oltjen and Davis (1965)
	same + buffers	128	38	40	22		
	pelleted corn-urea, molasses	115	39	40	21		
	same + buffers	114	50	35	15		
Steers	dehydrated alfalfa meal		65	19	13	1	Weiss et al (1967)
	58% dehydrated alfalfa meal + 38% gr corn, 1% urea		55	22	18	2	
	17% dehydrated alfalfa meal + 69% gr corn, 1% urea		41	37	15	5	
Steers	barley	132	49	33	18		Franks et al (1972)
	corn	121	45	41	14		
	oats	120	49	40	11		
	sorghum	119	49	39	12		
	sorghum, ground	110	47	36	17		
	sorghum, reconstituted	103	43	42	12		
	sorghum, steam flaked	106	38	45	17		
Steers	corn, dry	—	59	27	8		Tonroy and Perry (1974)
	corn, high moisture	—	64	20	8		
	corn, reconstituted	—	64	18	10		
	corn, plus fatty acids	—	61	28	7		
	high corn diet	—	31	47	12	10	Harvey et al (1968)
	high corn + hay	—	38	32	18	12	
	high corn + chlortet-racycline	—	33	38	17	12	

Animal	Ration	Total VFA, μmol/ml	Molar % Acetic	Propionic	Butyric	Others	Authors
Sheep	dried immature ryegrass	110	62	23	11	4	Weston and Hogan (1968)
	dried mature ryegrass	93	66	22	10	2	
	dried immature forage oats	98	70	18	9	3	
	dried mature forage oats	75	71	17	10	2	
Sheep	frozen grass	117-138	54-55	22-24	12-14	3-4	el-Shazly (1952)
	dried grass	135-140	58-64	22-26	8-12	3-4	
	silage	110-145	53-67	24-25	7-11	6-7	
Sheep	crushed corn	63-70	49-53	39-40	4-9	3-4	Judson et al (1968)
	50% alfalfa hay, 50% crushed corn	62-87	62-64	19-25	10-14	3-6	
	⅔ alfalfa hay, ⅓ crushed corn	93-129	62-66	16-22	9-14	3-5	
Sheep	alfalfa and concentrate	131	70	17	12	2	Purser et al (1965)
	same + Aureomycin	125	67	19	13	1	
	same + Tylosin	125	64	23	12	2	
Sheep	long alfalfa hay and concentrate	64	53	32	12	2	Woods and Luther (1962)
	whole ration pelleted	93	41	44	10-11	4	
	concentrate portion pelleted	75	48	38	11	3	
	roughage portion pelleted	88	42	47	8-9	3	
Sheep	80% concentrate, 20% roughage	70	53	26	19	2	Raun et al (1962)
	same + 3%NaHCO₃	79	55	24	17	4	
Sheep	50% concentrate, 50% roughage	89	58	26	15	1	Raun et al (1962)
	same + 0.7% urea	87	62	24	13	1	
	same + chlortetracycline	83	61	20	18	1	
	same + urea + chlortetracycline	92	59	23	17	1	
Sheep	oat straw + urea		70	21	8	1	Faichney (1968)
	oat straw + urea + 45 g sucrose		62	26	10	2	
	oat straw + urea + 90 g sucrose		58	27	13	2	
Sheep	steam-flaked corn		59	22	13	6	Johnson and McClure (1972)
	steam-flaked corn + 6% fat		57	25	13	5	
	high-roughage, low fat		69	17	9	5	
	high-roughage, 6% fat		67	20	9	4	

physical form of the diet, the level and frequency of feeding, feed processing methods which result in heating of starch and protein or gelatinization of starch, by rumen pH, chemical additives and other factors (Thomas and Clapperton, 1972). Furthermore, it is known from pure culture work that the end products from different organisms differ, thus we can assume that the shift in microbial populations may be sufficient to account for many of the observed differences. Further information on production of VFA from specific ration components will be found in subsequent discussions in this chapter or in Ch. 12-14.

Interconversion of Ruminal VFA

Substantial interconversion of the principal VFA occurs during active rumen fermentation. This is a reflection, no doubt, of the fact that an acid that is an end product of one microorganism may be a usable substrate for another species. An example of the distribution of radioactivity after continuous infusion of different individual acids is shown in Table 16-4.

Table 16-4. Distribution of ^{14}C-label following infusion.[a]

Acid infused	% of total ^{14}C in each acid		
	Acetic	Propionic	Butyric
Acetic	84	8	8
Propionic	7	89	4
Butyric	21	3	76

[a]From Weston and Hogan (1968)

When the specific activity of the specified acid and that of the acid infused are known, the transfer of label from the infused acid to another acid can be calculated. Data of this type have been published by several authors and some examples are shown in Table 16-5.

The data shown agree, in general, that appreciable amounts of butyrate (40-80%) may be derived from acetate as a result of condensation of two moles of acetate to form one mole of butyrate. These reports also agree that only negligible amounts of acetate are derived from propionate (0-5%). Substantial amounts of acetate may be derived from butyrate (6-20%). These estimates of propionate formation from acetate vary widely (3-37%) as do those for butyrate formation from propionate (0-18%). With respect to the high estimate of propionate formation from acetate (Knox et al, 1967), the authors speculate that interchange of tritium label on acetate with water and subsequently with propionate may have occurred, although no information was presented on this.

A number of laboratories that have collected data on VFA production have data that would lend themselves to calculations of interconversions of the VFA. Unfortunately they have not published estimates at this time. Consequently, the only feasible conclusion to be made is that further work is required to determine the extent of interconversion and the effect of rations or other factors.

Table 16-5. Estimates on interconversion of ruminal VFA.

Ration	% Ac from		% Pr from		% Bu from		Reference
	Bu	Pr	Ac	Bu	Ac	Pr	
Wheaten hay[a]	6	3	27	4	80	13	Gray et al (1960)
Grass hay	20	4-5	14	4-5	61	4-5	Bergman et al (1965)
Alfalfa chaff	11	0	4	3	47	0.0	Leng and Britt (1966)
Corn, alfalfa	12	0.2	6	3	44	0.2	
Corn, alfalfa	13	1.4	4	3	48	2-3	
Alfalfa, wheat straw	6	0.2	3	2	40	0.3	
Unknown[b]	10	3	37	5	49	18	Knox et al (1967)
Alfalfa hay[b]	18	1	12	5	62	1	Esdale et al (1968)
Corn silage[b]	15	1	14	9	72	1	
alfalfa + concentrate[b]	15	8	17	10	63	7	Wiltrout and Satter (1972)

[a]Approximate values calculated from graphs.
[b]Dairy cows; all others were sheep.

Production of VFA in the Rumen

There has been an appreciable amount of research relating to the production of VFA in the rumen of animals fed natural diets. Aside from the academic interest in the subject, a part of the effort expended has been made to determine the relative contribution of VFA to the energetic needs of ruminant species. For a good review on much of the older literature, the reader is referred to a paper by Warner (1964) in which the different methods and their deficiencies are discussed.

Methods Utilized. The principal methods that have been utilized to measure VFA production (and/or absorption) are those which base the estimate on the change in concentration with time of rumen VFA, methods which depend on measurement of absorbed VFA as a measure of production or a combination of absorption via the rumen veins plus estimates of passage of VFA into the lower GIT, or the use of in vitro fermentations to estimate production.

There are, as might be imagined, a number of complicating factors involved regardless of which method is utilized. It has been pointed out previously that both the concentration and molar percentages may change markedly following the ingestion of readily fermentable feed. Compensation will need to be made for the production of saliva, ingestion of water, changes in pH which affect absorption and any changes in rumen volume. To some extent this can be accomplished by the use of a marker such as PEG. Differential absorption of the various acids (see Ch. 9), interconversion of one acid to another and metabolism of VFA by microorganisms (see Hoover et al, 1963) and by rumen epithelium are also factors that contribute to the problem of accurately measuring VFA production. Not the least of the problems is that of obtaining a representative sample of rumen contents. One method utilized to reduce variability is illustrated in Fig. 16-3 from an experiment in which Gray et al (1967) clearly demonstrated the effect of frequent feeding in reducing the variation in rumen VFA concentration. A second method has been the use of pumps which circulate rumen contents in animals with rumen fistulas in an attempt to provide homogenous ingesta (Sutherland et al, 1962).

If the VFA absorbed are to be the basis of estimates of production, it is necessary to sample blood from the ruminal veins and either the ruminal or peripheral arteries so that the A-V difference can be determined. In addition, it is necessary to know the flow rate of blood in the rumen veins so that estimates can be quantitated over a period of time. Obviously, this involves acute experiments or placement of catheters, either of which may interfere with normal digestive physiology. Another necessary bit of information required is an estimate of the amount of endogenous VFA produced in the tissues, a value which may be rather substantial at times (Annison and White, 1962).

In the case of in vitro experiments, several problems are apparent. The usual in vitro fermentation does not reproduce conditions which are representative of the rumen for any great length of time. Consequently, one must expect some modification in the microbial population which may be reflected, quantitatively and qualitatively, in VFA production. Secondly, in order to utilize small samples, the substrates (feedstuffs) utilized would normally be rather finely ground, producing a relatively large surface area as compared to ingested feedstuffs in the rumen. This could have a substantial effect when estimating rates. Consequently, in vitro results, other than short-time fermentations, are to be regarded with caution when estimating VFA production. However, Gray et al (1965) have reported rather good estimates when using an artificial rumen apparatus with dialyzing membranes.

Recent Estimates. Some of the recent estimates of VFA production in the rumen are listed in Table 16-6. These estimates were made with isotope dilution techniques in which continuous infusions of labeled acids were made over a period of several hours. This method appears to offer the most accurate means of measuring production of the VFA because it requires a minimum of disturbance to the normal physiology of the animal. In practice the technique requires administration of acetic, propionic, and butyric acids, either singly or labeled in different ways if administered together. This is necessary to calculate interconversion of one acid to another, a factor which may result in a substantial error if corrections are not made.

In the first example in the table (Bergman et al, 1965) lambs were fed on a continuous basis and a rumen pump was used to provide

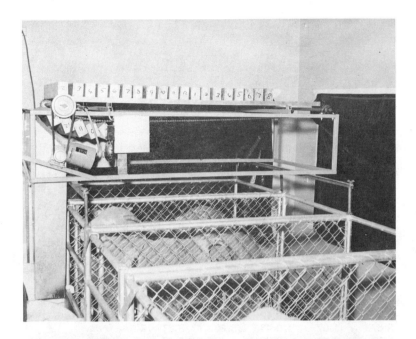

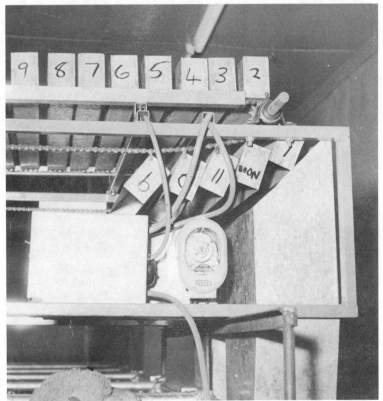

Figure 16-3. Apparatus used to feed sheep at regular intervals, usually every hour. The close-up courtesy of D.J. Minson; the other picture is from Minson and Cowper [1966].

a homogenous material to sample. The other experiments involved feeding at frequent intervals or at 12 hr intervals or, in one case, use of sheep on pasture. As a whole the daily estimates would indicate production of about 4-5.5 moles/day, depending upon the diet fed. An obvious exception to this range is the example from Leng and Brett (1966). However, these authors estimated production during a 12 hr period when the animals were fed every hour and it is undoubtedly an overestimate since the animals were not fed during the interval from 1900 to 0800 hours.

The amount of VFA production that may be produced per unit of feed from a given ration is, obviously, an uncertain value at the present time although there is some evidence that it can be predicted with reasonable certainty. For example, Gray et al (1967) found that 53% of the digestible energy of a diet of alfalfa and wheat hay was accounted for as rumen VFA, a value equivalent to about 246 Kcal/100 g of digestible organic matter. Bergman et al (1965) reported that a pelleted grass ration produced VFA equivalent to 62% of the digestible energy intake, and Weston and Hogan (1968) obtained a high correlation (r = 0.94) between digestible organic matter and VFA production. Their data indicated the production of 0.85 moles or 243 Kcal/100 g of digestible organic matter. In dairy heifers, Whitelaw et al (1970) estimated VFA production in one animal fed 5.1 kg of a high-barley diet, basing estimates on marker changes. Production was calculated to be

Table 16-6.   In vivo production of ruminal VFA as determined by isotope dilution procedures using continuous infusion methods.

Conditions	Daily VFA production, moles				Total/kg of feed intake	Reference
	Acetic	Propionic	Butyric	Total		
Sheep						
900 g grass pellets fed on continuous basis on a belt feeder	3.7	1.05	0.68	5.4	6.0	Bergman et al (1965)
900 g alfalfa chaff fed at hourly intervals from 8 a.m. to 7 p.m.	3.74	0.91	0.71	5.36	5.96	Leng and Leonard (1965)
Fed at hourly intervals from 8 a.m. to 7 p.m.						Leng and Brett (1966)
800 g alfalfa chaff	5.33	1.41	0.42	7.16	8.95	
400 g corn + 200 g alfalfa	3.67	1.07	0.46	5.20	8.67	
300 g corn + 300 g alfalfa	3.28	0.84	0.36	4.48	7.47	
450 g wheaten straw chaff + 50 g alfalfa	1.77	0.49	0.16	2.42	4.03	
1,000 g of 50% alfalfa and 50% wheaten hay chaff fed at 12 hr intervals				4.51	5.00*	Gray et al (1966)
1,000 g of 40% wheaten hay chaff and 60% alfalfa fed at 12 hr intervals	3.87	0.96	0.71		5.54*	Weller et al (1967)
1,000 g of 50% alfalfa and 50% wheaten chaff fed at						Gray et al (1967)
1 hr intervals				4.12	4.8*	
2 hr intervals				4.02	4.45*	
12 hr intervals				4.24	4.9*	
Green pasture	3.1	0.9	0.4	4.4		Leng et al (1968)
Dried ryegrass						Weston and Hogan (1968)
27% crude protein				5.52		
12% crude protein				4.76		
6% crude protein				3.39		
Cows, fed hourly						
alfalfa hay, 3.5 kg of DM daily	19.6	6.7	4.6	30.9	6.8*	Esdale et al (1968)
corn silage, 3.9 kg of DM daily	19.6	5.2	4.6	29.4	8.8*	
Cows						
concentrate and alfalfa dry cows, 9.5 kg DM daily	42	12**	8	62	6.7*	Wiltrout and Satter (1972)
lactating, 17.0 kg DM daily	77	25**	6	108	6.4*	

* Dry feed basis
**Estimates less precise than for C2 and C4 acids.

18.2 moles, equivalent to 36% of digestible energy intake.

VFA production has also been shown to be positively related to VFA concentration in the rumen in some of these studies where continuous infusions were utilized and where sheep were fed at frequent intervals to maintain a steady rate of fermentation. Weston and Hogan (1968) have plotted data of their own and from Bergman et al (1965) and Gray et al (1967) and derived an equation to estimate production. It is: $Y = 0.068X - 1.75$, where Y is the total VFA production (mol/day) and X the total VFA concentration in rumen liquor (mmol/l.). For their own data Weston and Hogan found a correlation of 0.67 between VFA production and rumen concentration. They could obtain a better correlation ($r = 0.81$) between VFA production and rumen VFA pool size (moles of VFA in the rumen).

It has been emphasized that estimates of VFA production are best made under conditions in which a steady rate of fermentation is going on and with the infusion of labeled VFA. Another interesting means of evaluating the production from a single feed or from a specific feedstuff is to produce ^{14}C-labeled feed by growing it in an atmosphere containing labeled carbon dioxide. Yadava et al (1964) and Alexander et al (1965) have carried out experiments with ^{14}C-labeled alfalfa hay. In the first case labeled hay was mixed with the ingesta of normally fed fistulated cows. In the second, the labeled hay was mixed with the ingesta, the cows were fed once and then starved for 48-72 hr. Figure 16-4 shows some of the data presented by Yadava et al. As shown in the graph, there was a very rapid increase in labeled VFA, the peak being reached in about 4 hr after administration. The authors did not find that this method was very accurate for predicting VFA production, but it is probable that refinement of the method might have application in a number of situations.

For the most part, the data cited in Table 16-6 provide estimates of VFA production that are appreciably higher than those cited by Warner (1964) from older experiments. The newer estimates are generally on the order of >4 moles/day for sheep and on the order of 30-40 moles in nonlactating cattle and up to 108 moles in lactating cows. These estimates indicate that ruminal VFA provide 70-80% of the energy requirements of sheep when measured in a calorimeter, values

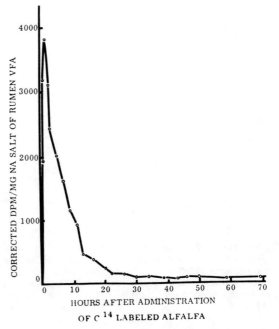

Figure 16-4. Concentration of radioactivity in ruminal VFA following the administration of a single intra-ruminal dose of ^{14}C-labeled alfalfa hay. From Yadava et al [1964].

considerably higher than had been indicated previously.

Rumen pH

There are a considerable number of papers in the literature which include data on rumen pH, however it is probable that much of the data are of little value. This is so because it has been shown that pH varies with location in the reticulo-rumen, with diet, with time after feeding and is greatly affected by saturation of rumen liquor with carbon dioxide (see Ch. 10). Consequently, any meaningful data must take these factors into account.

Diurnal Variations

Johnson and Sutton (1968) have published relatively recent information on methodology required for continuously recording changes in rumen pH. Some of the results of their research are illustrated in Fig. 16-5. This graph illustrates very clearly the changes that would normally be encountered following the ingestion of feed at regular intervals and it probably shows the picture much better than can be done by relatively infrequent ruminal samplings. The recording shows that the cycles are quite similar,

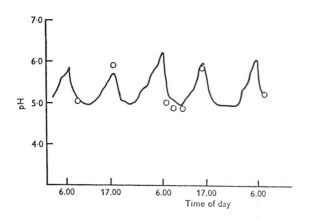

Figure 16-5. Variation in rumen pH in a cow accustomed to a diet with barley which was fed in equal portions at 0600 and 1700 hr. Aspiration samples [o] were taken for comparison near the electrode which was in the ventral sac. After Johnson and Sutton [1968].

although not identical. It would be surprising if recordings were identical in view of the differences noted within and between animals on the same rations (Bath and Rook, 1963; Emmanuel et al, 1969).

Effect of Ration on Rumen pH

There have been a number of reports of experimental results in which pH values have been given on animals fed different rations. A sampling of the literature would include papers by Balch and Rowland (1957), Briggs et al (1957), Reid et al (1957), Bath and Rook (1963, 1965), Bryant (1964), Morris et al (1965), Topps et al (1965), Slanina and Cabadaj (1968), Tremere et al (1968), Emmanuel et al (1969), Fenner et al (1970), Fonnesbeck et al (1970), Rumsey et al (1970), Isahaque et al (1971), Cheng and Hironaka (1973) and Ciszuk (1973). One recent graphical example is shown in Fig. 16-6.

As a general rule, published data indicate that pH will be relatively high in the rumen of animals fed low quality or inadequately supplemented forage. On the other hand, pelleting or grinding of roughage will usually increase microbial activity, resulting in greater VFA production and lower pH. Increasing the daily allowance of hay or concentrates or the frequency of feeding will tend to reduce the range in pH values encountered as does continuous consumption of pasture forage.

Rumen pH tends to be higher when animals are fed rations with alfalfa as compared to wheaten hay, indicating that rumen liquor from alfalfa-fed animals has a higher buffering capacity. Although consumption of silage will usually result in relatively low rumen pH, differences between other roughages of similar quality are minimal.

It is generally true that feeding a diet with a high percentage of concentrates results in a low rumen pH and it tends to be lower with a concentrate diet for a given VFA concentration than with roughage diets (Briggs et al, 1957). In addition, feed processing methods such as grinding or flaking of concentrates tend to produce lower rumen pH values.

Relation of pH to VFA Concentration and Molar Percnetages

Briggs et al (1957) carried out rather extensive investigations with sheep on the effect of a variety of rations on rumen pH and VFA. The rations varied from all roughage (alfalfa or wheaten hay) to rations with over 50% starch. An example of some of their data is shown in Fig. 16-7. In this particular experiment the sheep were fed alfalfa hay, only. The graph illustrates the decline in rumen pH as VFA level increases. On eight different rations the regression of pH on VFA was negative, the regression coefficients varying from -0.049 to -0.213, depending on the diet (indicating an inverse relationship between total VFA and pH). However, in the case of rations that resulted in the production of ruminal lactic acid, there was an equally high relationship between ruminal pH and lactic acid. High levels of lactic acid and lower rumen pH occurred together and high levels of lactic acid usually resulted in lower levels of VFA. Morris et al (1965) have also shown that VFA and rumen pH were inversely related in sheep fed supplemental rations on native range forage, although no statistical comparisons were presented.

In a companion paper to that of Briggs and coworkers, Reid et al (1957) have investigated the relationship of rumen pH and molar percentages of the VFA. They found that on all diets the proportion of propionic acid increased after feeding and reached a peak which coincided with the maximal level of total VFA (and usually the lowest pH except in the presence of lactic acid). The response of butyric was variable, and acetic acid (molar %) declined after feeding. These responses were modified in experiments in which rumen pH fell below 5.0 as a result of lactic acid accumulation. When animals were first fed on such diets, a decline in rumen pH below 5.0-5.5 after feeding was always associated with a pronounced decline in the percent of propionic and butyric acids to levels as low as 8 and 5%, respectively. Continued feeding of the diet did not affect butyric acid but there was, frequently, a substantial increase in propionic acid, in some cases to as high as 39% of the total; presumably, this was as a result of the development of acid-resistant organisms that probably ferment lactic acid to propionic acid.

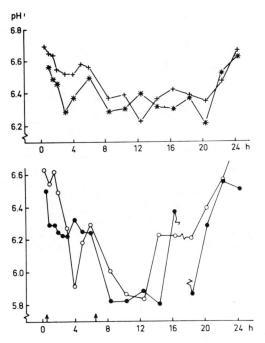

Figure 16-6. Diurnal variations in the pH of the rumen fluid on four different rations. * grass hay, low crude protein, mean of 2 animals; + high temp. dried grass, high crude protein, mean of 2 animals; • hay + grain + soya meal; o hay + grain + urea. Feeding times marked with arrow. interval of 1 day. From Ciszuk [1973].

Rumen Gases

It has been known for many years that carbon dioxide is produced during rumen fermentation and Washburn and Brody (1937) pointed out that methane production in the rumen was shown as long ago as 1875 by a man by the name of Popoff (this name should be good for a pun or two). The effect

of different feedstuffs, processing methods and various additives, and a knowledge of some of the minor gases and similar data have been developed in more recent years. For an extensive review of some of the early literature on gas production by ruminants, the reader is referred to the bulletin by Washburn and Brody.

Gases Found in the Reticulo-Rumen

Data on the composition of rumen gases are shown in Table 16-7. The data presented in the publication of Washburn and Brody (1937) are probably not comparable to that of other authors shown in the table in that their experiments involved feeding animals once per day and then collecting periodic samples until the next feed. They observed a great deal of variation with time in the case of most gases. Some of their findings are mentioned briefly. Carbon dioxide varied from 33.5-48.5% before feeding (one cow, 3 experiments) and increased to 67-80% after feeding. Maximal values generally occurred 1-8 hr after feeding, followed by a gradual decline during the next few hours. Rumen methane, in most cases, was within 30-40% of total gases. A slight decline usually followed feeding. Oxygen levels ranged from 0.0 to 13% with the concentration generally

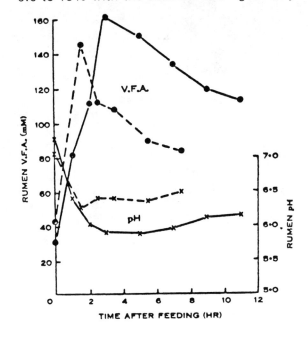

Figure 6-7. Rumen pH and VFA concentration in sheep fed 680 g of chopped alfalfa. All of the hay was consumed within 2 hr. From Briggs et al [1957].

the lowest during periods that would correspond to maximum fermentation rates. Hydrogen values ranged from 0.0 to 5.6%. Nitrogen values (determined by difference and could include H_2S, CO, NH_3 as well as N_2) ranged from 0.0 to a high of 67.8%. Values generally decreased after feeding, reaching low levels at from 2-8 hr after feeding followed by a gradual increase until the next feed. The effect of time of sampling in relation to feeding is also clearly illustrated in the more recent data of Czerkawski and Clapperton (1968). This information shows that CO_2 was low prior to feeding while N was quite high. After feeding CO_2 increased sharply and CH_2 and N decreased sharply.

Pilgrim (1948) states that some of the older information is likely in error since much of it showed relatively large amounts of H_2 in rumen gases. He used two different methods of analysis and could not detect H_2 in the rumen gases of normally fed sheep. In starving sheep, however, H_2 accounted for some of the free rumen gas. When rumen contents of starving sheep were replaced with buffer solutions, H_2 accounted for 22-57% of the free gas; when rumen contents were removed and animals given a drench of 150 ml of rumen contents from a normally fed sheep, H_2 accounted for 2.5-12% of free gas initially but this was rapidly reduced as the animals were given feed.

Table 16-7. Composition of rumen gases.

Author, animal	Volume % composition					
	CO_2	CH_4	O_2	N*	H_2	H_2S
Washburn and Brody (1937) dairy cow, mean range in two trials	47.0-52.2	25.8-34.5	2.2-4.1	13.0-16.7	1.1-3.4	
goat, mean of two trials	40.0	40.5	1.4	13.9	4.3	
Kleiber et al (1943)						
cow fed alfalfa hay	69.0		0.5			0.16
cow fed no hay	66.9	22.1	0.4	10.4		0.09-0.15
cow fed sudan hay	65.7	26.8	1.0	6.4		0.10
cow fed alfalfa, bloating	67.8	28.8	0.2	3.1		0.10
McArthur and Miltimore (1961) cows	65.4	26.8	0.6	7.0	0.2	0.01
Czerkawski and Clapperton (1968) Sheep fed at 0900 hr						
Sampled 0800-0900	24.8	32.5	6.5	36.2	0.01	
Sampled 0900-1000	56.0	18.8	3.1	18.0	4.12	
Sampled 1200-1300	60.2	33.5	1.3	6.0	0.05	
Dougherty (1941, 1942) steers dead of bloat						0.14-0.70
Pilgrim (1948) sheep, 4-8 hr after feeding	63-65	27-29	< 1	6.7		

*These values presumably include N_2 and NH_3, and in the case of data by Washburn and Brody these could include other gases such as H_2S and CO since the values were determined by difference.

Quantity of Gas Produced

Colvin et al (1957) measured gas production by means of a tracheal cannula and a face mask (see Fig. 16-8). Their data indicate that gas production 3-4 hr following a feeding of alfalfa tops was at the rate of about 30 l./hr for animals weighing ca. 450 kg. Dougherty and Cook (1962) measured gas production in the same manner and found a production rate of about 34 l. in one cow and about 49 l./hr in a second cow. On the basis of calorimetry trials, Blaxter and Clapperton (1965) reported that sheep produced an average of 30 l. of methane/day as compared to 154 l./day by cattle, although Blaxter (1962) states that cattle may produce as much as 400 l./day and sheep up to 50 l./day. Further information on quantity is given in the section on prediction of quantity of methane production.

When comparing data of this type, the reader must keep in mind that the type of feed, its solubility and susceptibility to rapid fermentation and the time after feeding at which the measurements are made may all have a pronounced effect on the amount of gas produced by rumen fermentation. Unless these conditions are standardized, comparisons between experiments are not very rewarding.

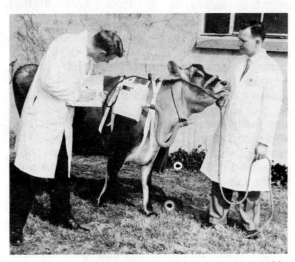

Figure 16-8. An illustration of the use of portable equipment to measure CO2 production in a cow with a cannulated trachea. Similar equipment can be used to measure oxygen consumption when a face mask can be used. Courtesy of P.W.Moe.

Origin of Rumen Gases

Carbon dioxide, of course, has long been known to be an end product of fermentation or respiration. Oxygen in the rumen, which is predominantly anaerobic, is probably derived from oxygen dissolved in water and possibly from some aerobic organisms taken in with feed. Hydrogen sulfide, as pointed out in Ch. 15, can be derived from various inorganic or organic sources of sulfur. Nitrogen and/or ammonia are presumably derived from air taken in with feed and water and from degradation of proteins, hydrolysis of urea, etc. (see Ch. 13), although most of the ruminal ammonia is probably in the liquid phase rather than in the gas phase in the rumen.

In the case of methane, the exact means by which it is produced are less clear although, as pointed out by Washburn and Brody (1937), speculations on its origin have been of interest to ruminant nutritionists for a long time. The interest in methane is partially because it accounts for a rather large amount of energy consumed by ruminants. Washburn and Brody calculated that methane production accounted for 12 or 14.6% of ingested energy in cows fed at a level of ca. 2X maintenance and at a level of slightly above maintenance, respectively. Some of the research relating to methane synthesis is reviewed in subsequent paragraphs.

The suggestion was made quite a few years ago that CH_4 formation results from the chemical reduction of CO_2 (Symons and Buswell, 1933) and this still appears to be the case. In vitro experiments by Beijer (1952) indicated that the addition of formate to rumen contents gave rise to CH_4. Carroll and Hungate (1955) confirmed this and stated that formate was not itself reduced to CH_4 but supplied H_2 to reduce CO_2 and suggested that 4 moles of formate were required to produce one mole of CH_4. Their results also indicated that, when manometric experiments were carried out in an atmosphere with excess hydrogen, much additional CH_4 was produced. McNeill and Jacobson (1955) also found that CH_4 was produced in a hydrogen atmosphere (in vitro) when a source of CO_2 was supplied to mixed suspensions of bovine rumen bacteria. They concluded that the failure to find more than trace amounts of H_2 in the rumen may be due to an extremely active hydrogenase system and further suggested that the lack of H_2 may be a limiting factor in CH_4 production. Carroll and Hungate also presented data which indicated that the conversion of formate to CO_2 + H_2 did not exceed the presumed reaction, CO_2 + $4 H_2 \rightarrow CH_4$ + $2 H_2O$, otherwise H_2 would accumulate. However, Kingwell et al (1959) found that, when the rumen of a cow was continuously gassed with H_2 until free hydrogen accounted for 22% of rumen gas, the formation of CH_4 was not increased, thus tending to refute the hypothesis of McNeill and Jacobson and of Carroll and Hungate. Hungate (1966) contends that this can be explained by the difficulty in dispersing the gas through the rumen contents. Subsequent research by Hungate (1967) indicated that CH_4 synthesis was closely correlated to the concentration of dissolved H. Czerkawski et al (1972) also found that CH_4 formation was related to the amount of H_2 taken up from the gas phase. However, H_2 produced from formate accumulated in the aqueous phase and was not related to CH_4 production.

The culture of pure strains of rumen bacteria that produce CH_4 has not been accomplished with any regularity (see Hungate, 1966). Oppermann et al (1957) reported that they cultured strains which produced CH_4 from formic and acetic acid. When given a choice, the organisms preferentially and completely utilized formic acid before acetic acid was fermented. Some bacterial species such as *Ruminococcus albus*, however, may produce formate but do not degrade it to H_2 and CO_2 (Miller and Wolin, 1973).

Nelson et al (1958) found that stabilized cultures could produce CH_4 from butyric and valeric acids but they could not show production from propionic acid. Butyric acid was oxidized to acetate, CH_4 and CO_2 but the oxidation of valeric acid was not carried to completion, and in such cultures propionic acid accumulated from the partial oxidation of valerate. Acetate, derived from butyrate oxidation, was readily utilized. Their data indicate that butyric and valeric acids serve as reductants with CO_2 as an oxidant for the formation of CH_4 in addition to other pathways. They suggested that reduction of CO_2 with H_2 may predominate during the early period of rapid fermentation and that acetate utilization and the reduction of CO_2 coupled with the oxidation of the higher fatty acids may contribute to CH_4 formation late in the digestion cycle.

Oppermann et al (1959) investigated the formation of CH_4 in vivo after the addition of acetate labeled with ^{14}C in the 1 or 2 positions and with labeled formate. They found that CH_4 and CO_2 became labeled soon after the addition of labeled acetate. The labeling of CO_2 was greater than CH_4 irrespective of the position of the label in the acetate (thus indicating the possibility of reduction of CO_2 to CH_4). Their data indicated that 3-5% of rumen CH_4 was derived directly or indirectly (via butyrate or propionate) from acetate. The addition of labeled formate resulted in the rapid labeling of both CH_4 and CO_2, with the label also appearing in acetate, propionate and butyrate. Labeled formate could not be detected in the rumen after a period of 30-45 min. Free hydrogen was not found during formate decomposition. Knox et al (1969) have also studied transfer of label from the VFA, lactate and barley straw. Only 0.2-3% of the ^{14}C from the VFA and only 2-4% of that from barley straw was recovered in labeled CH_4. They suggested that 40-60% of the carbon in CH_4 originated from the ruminal carbonate pool, but this depended on the substrates involved. In studies involving a wide variety of individual compounds, Czerkawski and Breckenridge (1972) found that CH_4 production was associated only with the fermentation of formate, certain hydroxyacids, pyruvic acid, primary alcohols, glycerol and methyl compounds.

Matsumoto (1962) demonstrated with goats that the addition of 30 g of sodium formate into the rumen resulted in an increase in rumen CH_4 from 40.7 to 51.8% of rumen gases. Vercoe and Blaxter (1965) have studied CH_4 production when formic acid was infused continuously into the rumen of sheep confined in a respiration chamber. The average results showed that CH_4 production increased 4.9 l. and CO_2 by 18.1 l./mole of formic acid given. Their calculations indicated that 4 mole of formic acid should yield 1 mole of CH_4, 3 of CO_2 and 2 of water. Williams et al (1963) have studied CH_4 synthesis by providing labeled CO_2 in the rumen and collecting expired gases via a tracheal cannula. They could show the production of labeled CH_4 but it took 5 hr or longer for eructed CH_4 and CO_2 to become equally labeled, and they suggested that the inflow of CO_2 from the blood (and saliva) into the rumen diluted the rumen CO_2 and thus accounted for this delay. Demeyer and Henderickx (1964) found that washed suspensions of rumen bacteria took up gas when incubated under a H_2-CO_2 atmosphere. When mixed suspensions of protozoa and bacteria were used, there was no difference in gas uptake, and the authors concluded, therefore, that the protozoa did not produce any appreciable amount of CH_4.

Prediction of Quantity of Methane Production

Several authors have published papers giving prediction equations for CH_4 production by ruminants. Two papers will be mentioned here. This topic is of interest if one wishes to calculate the metabolizable energy of a feed or ration and does not have a respirometer to collect expired gases. Bratzler and Forbes (1940) have made such calculations based on 130 different measurements made at the Penn. State Expt. Station with cattle. They found that they could estimate CH_4 production with rather good precision by the formula, $E = 4.012X + 17.68$, where $E = $ g CH_4 produced and $X = $ hundreds of g of carbohydrate digested. This formula was developed on carbohydrate intakes ranging from 900 to 5,800 g/day.

Blaxter and Clapperton (1965) have calculated prediction equations for both sheep and cattle. These equations were derived from more than 2,500 determinations of the daily CH_4 production obtained in calorimeter trials. Analytical error was on the order of 3% for day-to-day variation in the same animal and 7 to 8% for between-animal variation. In each of 48 trials with different feeds, CH_4 production (expressed as Kcal CH_4/100 Kcal feed intake) fell as the level of feeding increased. At the maintenance level CH_4 production varied from 6.2 to 10.8 Kcal/100 Kcal of feed and could be calculated with a rather high accuracy with the equation $C_m = 3.67 + 0.062D$ where $C_m = CH_4$ production in terms of Kcal/100 Kcal of feed energy, and $D = $ apparent digestibility of the energy of the feed. In the case of animals fed over maintenance, CH_4 production could be estimated by the equation: CH_4 production $= 1.30 + 0.112D + L$ $(2.37 - 0.050D)$, where $D = $ digestibility at the maintenance level and $L = $ level of feeding as a multiple of maintenance.

As pointed out, Bratzler and Forbes found that CH_4 production was highly related to the amount of carbohydrate consumed whereas Blaxter and Clapperton found that the amount of digestible energy was closely related to CH_4 production. Methane

production should negatively relate to fat intake since Czerkawski et al (1966) observed that ruminal infusion of fatty acids resulted in reduced CH_4 production (see Ch. 14). Blaxter and Clapperton (1965) did not find any appreciable differences in CH_4 production of sheep and cattle nor between different rations which were similar in digestible energy.

Miscellaneous Information on Rumen Gases

Clapperton and Blaxter (1965) and Blaxter and Clapperton (1965) point out that, irrespective of feeding level with diets with an apparent digestibility of 40% (energy), 15-16% of the energy apparently digested is lost as CH_4. When apparent digestibility was 60%, ca. 12% of digested energy was lost as CH_4 and at a digestibility of 80%, 8-11% of DE was lost as CH_4. Miltimore and McArthur (1962) found that efficiency of feed utilization was negatively correlated with CH_4 concentration and positively with CO_2 concentration or CO_2:CH_4 ratio. They suggested that data on rumen gases might be used to estimate feed utilization or to supplement the data usually obtained.

In contrast to two reports previously mentioned, Johnson (1972) has shown that increasing consumption of a 40% roughage diet from 1X to 2.2X maintenance resulted in a decrease in CH_4 production, as a % of GE, from 8.4 to 5.6%; or, if expressed on the basis of DE, the decline was from 11.7 to 8.4%. Digestible energy (% of GE) was also depressed from 71.5 to 66.9%, a common response seen in ruminant animals as intake is increased. An increasing intake, however, is usually associated with an improved feed conversion even though digestibility declines. Thus, this response may account for the negative correlation between CH_4 concentration and feed efficiency observed by Miltimore and McArthur.

Ogimota et al (1962) found that the general pattern of gas formation (in vitro) was similar from rumen fluid of goats on different feeding regimes. Generally, a peak in gas production occurred several hours after feeding and the second peak occurred at 16-18 hr. VFA production showed a similar trend, reaching peak levels 10-12 hr after feeding. Positive correlations were found between the amounts of gas and VFA produced during in vitro fermentation. Data indicated greater gas production when the goats were fed fresh legumes or legume silage than when fed fresh grass or grass hay. When sheep were given diets with beet pulp or hay, Clapperton and Czerkawski (1969) found that the rate of CH_4 production on both diets increased during feeding and then decreased to a steady value, suggesting that rapid CH_4 production during feeding was associated with fermentation of the more soluble part of the diet. If no food was given, the rate continued to fall exponentially.

Absorption of Fermentation Gases or Other Volatile Gases in the Rumen

Dougherty et al (1964) have studied the transfer of ^{14}C-labeled CO_2 and CH_4 following insufflation into the rumen. In four sheep allowed to inspire eructated gas, radioactive carbon was detected in blood from the carotid artery 4-5 sec after the first rumen eructation contraction following administration of the labeled CO_2. In one sheep and one goat not allowed to inhale eructated gas there was eventual absorption of labeled carbon from the GIT, but at a much lower level. Radioactivity gradually increased in the saliva samples until it was more than double that of blood samples. Labeled CO_2 appeared in milk within 3 min following eructation and reached maximal values within 15 min. In one sheep and two goats insufflated with labeled CH_4, radioactivity in the blood was much less than after intraruminal administration of CO_2.

Dougherty et al (1962) have studied transport of flavors and odors to milk in cows with tracheal cannulas. In the case of onions the cows inhaled air passed through a slurry. This produced no off flavor. When the onions were introduced into the rumen, off flavor was apparent in 30-45 min but was much greater when the cows were allowed to inhale eructated gases, thus indicating that some microbial action was necessary to release the volatiles causing the off flavor although it could not be identified by a taste panel as onion. In contrast, wild leek leaves produced volatiles that could be detected in milk after inhalation (onion or garlic-like). Various compounds such as ethyl and amyl acetates were also picked up on inhalation. Shipe et al (1962) report further research of this nature on components found in silage that could be detected when administered either directly into the lungs or via the rumen when eructed gas was not inhaled.

McCauley and Dziuk (1965) studied gas production in goats when resting or ruminating. Gas production rates were higher during rumination than during rest but were reduced below resting rates during ruminal atony induced by administration of atropine. Three conditions resulting in abrupt increases in gas in the dorsal sac were: ruminal contractions following a period of atony, changing from rest to rumination and vigorous somatic movements. Their observations indicated that reduced eructation rates during periods of rest result from a reduction in gas accumulation in the dorsal sac because of a temporary storage of gas at other sites.

Inhibition of Methane Synthesis

Studies relating to the inhibition of methane have been an active field of research since Czerkawski et al (1966) demonstrated that fatty acids inhibit CH_4 production and as a result of other reports showing that various halogenated CH_4 analogues are powerful inhibitors (see Ch. 14). Research from the Hannah Research Station (Czerkawski et al, 1966; Clapperton and Czerkawski, 1969; Czerkawski and Breckenridge, 1969) indicates that fatty acids or various sulfated C16 and C18 alcohols would inhibit CH_4 synthesis but, the fatty acids did not result in a marked depression of digestibility of the rations or accumulation of H_2. Instead, some of the H_2 appears to be diverted to saturation of unsaturated fatty acids and, apparently, to synthesis of other lipids.

Other reports showing favorable effects of fatty acids or triglycerides include those of Demeyer et al (1967) and Van Nevel et al (1971, 1973). Clapperton and Czerkawski (1972) have also shown that propane-1:2-diol is capable of causing a reduction in CH_4 production accompanied by sharp decrease in acetate (30%) and a marked increase in propionate (60%) concentration.

A wide variety of CH_4 analogues or halogenated compounds has been shown to be effective in inhibiting CH_4 production in the rumen. These include chloroform, carbon tetrachloride, methylene chloride and numerous other CH_4 analogues containing Cl, Br, F, and I (Bauchop, 1967; Rufener and Wolin, 1968; Quaqhebeur and Oyaert, 1971; Trei et al, 1971; Johnson et al, 1972); chloral hydrate or a hemiacetal of chloral and starch (Van Nevel et al, 1969; Johnson, 1972, 1974; Trei et al, 1972) and other compounds such as trichloroacetamide (Trei et al, 1971; Clapperton, 1973), dichlorovinyl dimethyl phosphate (Howes and Dyer, 1968), sodium sulfite (Demeyer and Henderickx, 1967; Van Nevel et al, 1970, 1973), $KMnO_4$ or $KClO_3$ (Demeyer and Henderickx, 1967; Prins, 1970).

In vitro and in vivo studies indicate that most of the halogenated compounds result in a relative increase in molar % of propionate, but total VFA are apt to be reduced. With inhibitors such as di- or trichloroacetamide, evidence shows that rumen microbes become adapted after a period of time (Slyter and Weaver, 1972; Clapperton, 1973).

Although CH_4 production may be completely inhibited (see Table 16-8), there is usually an increase in H_2 production but less than can be accounted for by the reduction in CH_4. Digestibility and energy metabolism studies often show improved digestibility of energy and metabolizable energy may be higher; however there tends to be greater heat production (Table 16-9). Furthermore, although CH_4 production is reduced and ME may be higher, there is usually a reduction in feed intake with the overall effect in the feedlot that gain and feed conversion are not improved (Tables 16-8, 9). At this time it seems obvious that further research is required to determine if CH_4 inhibitors have some practical use. Perhaps, as Czerkawski (1972) suggests, combinations of inhibitors may be useful, depending on the objectives desired in the overall inhibition of CH_4 and formation of ruminal end products.

Table 16-8.   Effect of a methane inhibitor on energy metabolism.[a]

Diet	GE, intake per day	DE	Urinary energy	CH_4	H_2	ME
	$Kcal/kg^{0.75}$			— % of GE —		
low level	150.5	71.5	3.0	8.4	—	60.1
+ HCS*	153.3	73.2	3.1	4.2	1.6	64.3
High level	329.5	66.9	2.2	5.6	—	59.1
+ HCS*	329.0	65.2	2.3	1.0	1.7	60.3

[a]From Johnson (1972)   *A hemiacetal of choral fed at a level of 2 g HCS/kg of diet on the high level and adjusted to that amount on the low level.

Table 16-9. Effect of a methane inhibitor [bromo-chloromethane] on lamb performance and energy metabolism.[a]

Item	BCM level, mg/kg BW/day		
	0	1.5	3.0
Growing lambs			
DM intake, kg/day	1.45	1.33	1.36
Daily gain, kg	0.282	0.245	0.256
Feed conversion	5.13	5.43	5.33
GE/kg of gain, Mcal	22.8	24.1	23.7
Mature wethers			
Energy partition, % of GE			
Fecal E	37.7	28.8	30.6
Methane E	6.1	1.0	0.9
Heat production	43.9	45.0	44.4
Energy balance	8.3	20.8	20.0
Digestible E	62.3	71.2	69.4
Metabolizable E	52.2	66.8	64.4

[a]From Sawyer et al (1974)

Rumen Volume

A substantial amount of information is now available on rumen volume and on factors affecting it, particularly since the development and use of markers such as PEG and Cr-EDTA. One important characteristic of rumen volume is that it is not constant in any given animal and may vary with different factors. At least this is the case for rumen contents of fluid and/or solids, as the amount of fluid present has been the most common method utilized to estimate volume in the living animal. Perhaps the true capacity of the organ when filled completely does not vary so much, but without a doubt the amount of fill varies.

Differences Between Similar Animals

Between animals obvious factors include age, body size and species differences. Within animals, one important factor that has been well identified is the type of diet. Purser and Moir (1966) have reported on experiments in which sheep of similar size (63-75 kg) were fed the same rations. Rumen volume was estimated by dilution of chromic oxide administered intra-ruminally and subsequently by measuring the contents and the volume of the organ by filling with water after slaughter. Some of their data are shown in Table 16-10. It can be seen from these data that volume estimated with Cr_2O_3 overestimated the actual measured volume by a factor of 30-50 + %; since the two varied

found that the rapidity of feed intake was highly related to rumen volume as estimated by Cr_2O_3 dilution. Data from one experiment are shown in Table 16-11. The marked differences observed here in the rapidity with which some of these sheep ate their daily ration as compared to those that ate very slowly would be comparable to once a day feeding versus continuous feeding. The differences in VFA levels in the rumen on such a comparison have already been discussed. Additional data (Purser and Moir, 1966) shown in Table 16-11 show the differences in bacterial and protozoal counts associated with the differences in rumen volume and relative eating rate. Statistical

Table 16-10.   Individual differences in rumen volume and feed consumption.[a]

Sheep No.	Sheep weight, kg	Water filled volume	Cr_2O_3 dilution	Measured contents	Dry matter of rumen contents, %	Rumen tissue wt, g
7	72	18.0	9.1	6.0	7.7	1186
8	76	24.0	9.9	7.6	7.0	1126
9	65	14.0	8.1	4.6	9.2	826
10	62	9.9	3.8	2.5	8.2	854
11	70	17.7	7.0	5.5	6.5	912
12	69	13.8	5.1	3.1	15.3	840
13	71	23.2	9.1	6.5	8.0	986
14	63	13.8	9.1	4.7	11.5	788
15	69	14.4	6.4	5.0	8.0	955
16	71	21.7	9.1	5.3	8.2	1186
17	72	18.7	9.1	6.1	5.4	1030

[a] From Purser and Moir (1966)

directly, the indicator method would seem to be of value in estimating relative variation. The volume estimated by filling the rumen with water was markedly larger, on the order of 3-4 fold the actual measured volume of contents; part of this difference would reflect the difference in rumen gases, of course. Tissue weights have also been shown to be related to rumen volume, but the data from this experiment would indicate a relatively low relationship. It appears that some of these sheep with small rumen volumes (particularly number 12 and 14) compensate by maintaining a higher level of dry matter. A more rapid rumen turnover must also occur.

In a previous experiment with these same animals fed a different ration, the authors

analyses of the data showed that animals with small rumen volumes, slow rates of intake and low water consumption had (generally) greater protozoal concentrations, below average rumen ammonia (data not shown), and usually greater nitrogen retention. Animals with a large rumen volume and rapid eating habits had above average dry matter digestibility together with below average rumen pH.

In studies with lambs fed a pelleted 60% roughage diet, Randall (1974) has developed some interesting correlations. Measurements of feed consumption 30 and 60 min after access to feed was given and an eating rate index (feed consumed/unit of metabolic size) were significantly correlated with total weight gain, daily gain and feed efficiency.

Table 16-11. Rumen volume as related to feed intake, water consumption, and microbial population.[a]

Sheep No.	Estimated rumen volume, l.	Relative eating rate,[b] %	Water consumption, ml	Bacterial concen., 10^9/ml	Protozoal concentration	
					Entodinium 10^3/ml	Holotricha 10^3/ml
7	7.0	99	1340	9.9	1246	62
8	7.0	100	1980	9.5	707	72
9	7.2	77	1920	11.3	1631	36
10	3.9	33	980	10.9	2155	103
11	7.5	97	1940	7.7	797	61
12	3.8	33	360	12.0	1160	134
13	7.7	70	1680	8.4	1030	41
14	2.1	17	1460	9.4	783	34
15	6.0	57	1720	12.7	784	22
16	6.2	99	2740	10.6	1224	47
17	6.7	96	2340	7.9	801	7

[a] From Purser and Moir (1966)

[b] Animals were fed 855 g of a semipurified diet. The relative rate is in terms of the amount consumed in 4 hr after feeding.

Rumen size was correlated to daily gain and feed efficiency, but not to daily feed consumption. Eating rate was positively correlated with weight of abomasal tissues and animal performance was positively associated with tissue weights of the abomasum and small intestine. In older research, Sinclair et al (1958) found a significant correlation between rumen weight of sheep and daily gain, thus providing confirmatory evidence of the physiological significance of rumen volume.

Effect of Diet

The literature contains many references to the effect of ration on rumen fill. Some papers that are particularly pertinent to this discussion will be reviewed briefly. In one example, ewes on different forages were killed and stomach volume measured (Johns et al, 1963). Values on stomach fill were (volume in l.): perennial ryegrass, 20.0; ryegrass + white clover, 19.0; short-rotation ryegrass, 16.0; and short-rotation ryegrass + white clover, 15.4. Ulyatt (1964) also found that rumen volume of ewes and lambs was affected by the type of forage grazed. Ulyatt et al (1967) reported that rumen volume of sheep was similar in three forages of varying digestibility. Reducing intake to 70 or 50% of maximum resulted in some reduction in rumen volume. Weston and Hogan (1967) observed that the rumen volume (indicator

dilution) of sheep was greater in sheep fed ground alfalfa hay as compared to those fed chopped hay. However, the reverse was true in the case of those fed wheaten hay. Egan (1966) estimated fluid volume in the rumen of sheep receiving wheat straw, oat hay and alfalfa hay. Volume before a meal was 3.80, 5.95 and 5.60 l., respectively. After a meal, the volumes were: 4.52, 5.24 and 6.98 l., the data thus showed a marked effect of diet and an increase in rumen size as a result of food consumption. In young lambs (Wilson, 1963) rumen volume and rumen capacity (water filled) was markedly affected by diet. Volume was least on a milk diet, but greatest when shavings were administered. Hay in the diet increased rumen volume about twofold.

With respect to cattle, Balch and Line (1957) observed substantial differences in rumen weight of wet and dry contents in cows grazing a variety of different forages. They also found that rumen volume was greater in animals consuming hay plus concentrates than when grazing on fall pasture. Campling et al (1961) found substantial differences in the wet weight of rumen contents of cows fed at different levels of intake, values ranging from 165 lb to 250 lb (wet weight) in cows fed 10 lb to ad libitum intakes of hay. In the case of steers, Putnam et al (1966) reported that steers fed rations with 25 or 89% hay had a larger rumen volume when fed the 89% hay ration (i.e., 36-40 l. on 25% hay vs 44-58 l. on 89% hay). Feeding the rations in pelleted form appeared to reduce rumen volume and there appeared to be a positive correlation between salivary secretion and amount of rumen fill. It might be noted that it can be demonstrated in the laboratory that pelleted alfalfa does not take up the volume that ground alfalfa does when mixed with water. Perhaps the compression during pelleting ruptures many plant cells and prevents rehydration to the same extent as nonpelleted forages

Other Environmental Factors

Warner and Stacy (1968) calculated that fast-eating sheep — with an initial rumen volume of 3.9 l. — had an expansion in volume during eating of 0.53 l. Slow eaters, on the other hand, had almost no expansion in size as measured by fluid volume (0.06 l.). In another experiment, they calculated an initial volume of 3.94 l. Rumen expansion was 0.4 l. on feeding and contraction post feeding (ca. 6 hr later) was 0.6 l. Changes following drinking ranged from 0.4-1.8 l.

Forbes (1968, 1969) has published data on estimated rumen volume of ewes in various stages of pregnancy based on area measurements of sections of frozen bodies (see Fig. 16-9). In open ewes rumen volume ranged from 7.6 to 9.0 l. for animals weighing from 43.5 to 50.9 kg, or an average of 17.7% of live weight. By mid-pregnancy this value had risen to 19.9%. However, in late pregnancy it had declined to 12.1% accompanied by an increase in uterine volume to about 6-10 l., depending on whether the ewe was carrying single or twin lambs. Thus, it was shown that an increase in rumen volume occurred in the early stages of pregnancy, but volume was eventually diminished due to the volume of the reproductory tract. The author points out that one fat ewe had a rumen volume of only 4.3 l. (others were smaller) and a thin ewe had a rumen volume of 10.2 l. These data would indicate that excessive visceral fatness, by depressing rumen volume and appetite, may be a contributory factor to ketosis. The weight of the rumen epithelia also increases during pregnancy and lactation (Weekes, 1971).

Experiments on variation in rumen volume during the day (Tulloh et al, 1965) indicated minimal volume occurred about 1030 and maximal volume about 1630 in animals with access to pasture at all times except for about an hour morning and evening at milking time. Mean values for four cows

ranged from a low of 29.5 l. to a high of 44.7 l.; thus estimates of rumen volume can be seen to vary considerably during the day. Tulloh (1966) has also shown some minor seasonal differences in rumen volume when basing estimates on weight of rumen contents or when using a balloon in the rumen filled with air or water. During the summer months, particularly, rumen volume of lactating animals was greater than their dry twins which showed only minor seasonal differences. When comparing rumen volume of cows using PEG dilution or weight of rumen contents, Tulloh and Hughes (1965) found that PEG tended to underestimate rumen volume and that the error could be substantial at times. However, their data show that rumen volume was generally considerably higher in lactating cows than in their dry twins (about 32 vs. 40 l. in animals weighing 340-360 kg).

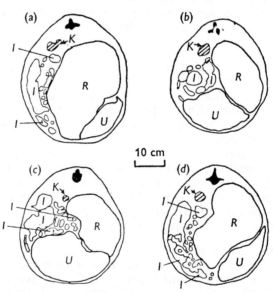

Figure 16-9. Diagrams of the anterior aspect of frozen sections of ewes in the region of the 3rd lumbar vertebra. The diagrams illustrate the marked reduction in rumen volume which occurs during late pregnancy. [a,b,c] ewes 8, 111 and 143 days pregnant with single lambs, respectively. [d] ewe 95 days pregnant with twins. I, intestine; K, kidney; R, reticulo-rumen; U, uterus. From Forbes [1968].

Nagel and Paitkowski (1972) have also shown that there are changes in rumen volume associated with milk production (305 day data). Although mature cows producing 4,752 kg of FCM had rumen volumes averaging 132 l., less than the 142 l. for cows giving 3,528 kg of FCM, their rumens were more elastic as shown by measuring volume at two different pressures. These workers also observed that ruminal capacity in cows increased at a rate of 3.7-4.0 l./year of age.

The data at hand on rumen volume do not permit a complete evaluation of its importance. There appears to be a great flexibility within a given animal from time to time and between similar animals. Data on animals consuming forage would indicate that rumen volume tends to expand to accommodate a greater bulk of less digestible forage, perhaps to allow a longer time for the rumen microorganisms to attack and digest it, without resulting in a drastic reduction in nutrients to the host. Rumen volume appears to be related to rapidity of intake and it seems logical that it may be related to the efficiency of nutrient metabolism. More data of the type published by Purser and Moir are required to establish true relationships and importance.

Importance of Rumen Turnover

Rumen turnover is a term used to indicate the length of time digesta remain in the rumen. Information based on some of the papers discussed in Ch. 7 indicates that rumen turnover time will, obviously, vary considerably depending upon what fraction of the digesta is in question, the method of calculation and the indicators utilized. Rumen turnover time appears to be controlled primarily by resistance of ingesta to microbial fermentation and rate of passage of ingesta through the GIT, which is affected, in turn, by such factors as specific gravity, particle size and level of intake of dry matter. Rumen volume or rumen fill may be of considerable importance in the control of appetite and there is ample evidence of a substantial difference between sheep and cattle in the rate of ingesta passage.

When the level of feed intake of a given ration is increased by one means or another, excretion is more rapid and rumen retention time is usually reduced, resulting in somewhat lower digestibility, although the decline in digestibility will usually be greater for the more fibrous plant parts which are more resistant to digestion. However, the net nutrient yield to the animal will be increased considerably in this situation. In the event that the quality of a ration is improved and the level of intake also increases, the effect will be shown as in Table 16-12. As these data show, rumen retention time was greatest when sheep were fed the poor quality hay which was voluntarily consumed at a rate considerably lower than the other two hays. As the quality of the hay increased, digestibility increased as well as intake accompanied by a reduction in rumen retention; the net result being a yield of digestible energy about 3 times greater on the good hay as compared to the poor hay.

It must be assumed that rumen turnover would eventually reach a point of diminishing returns with respect to nutrient yield. However, Hungate (1966) points out that rumen microorganisms, when compared with in vitro bacterial cultures, represent a stage at which the population is high and the growth rate is decelerating. A faster feed rate at a fixed volume reduces the population, but the specific growth rate increases to keep pace with the new feed rate. If rumen turnover rate is not limiting, as for example in animals on high grain diets, it is likely that other factors may limit the nutrient intake or metabolism by the tissues.

Rumen turnover would also appear to be limited by factors which control appetite (and rumen fill) as well as by a limitation on the amount of effluent that can pass through the lower GIT. In a practical situation it is

Table 16-12. Relationship between intake, digestibility and rumen retention time in sheep.[a]

Ration	Voluntary intake, g/kg wt $.73$	Intake of digestible energy, Kcal/24 hr/kg wt $.73$	Digestible energy, %	Rumen retention time,[b] hr
Poor hay	50.5	101.9	44.7	83
Medium hay	77.2	206.3	58.8	55
Good hay	94.0	318.9	74.2	41

[a]From Blaxter et al (1961)
[b]Estimated as difference between excretion of 5 and 80% of stained particles.

obvious that the value of rapid production which can be achieved by fast rumen turnover by such means as pelleting, grinding or utilization of higher quality feedstuffs at greater expense must be related to the value that can be obtained by a lower level of production when using less costly feeds. It should also be pointed out that the added value of pelleted roughages, for example, is difficult to evaluate when formulating rations. Since rations are usually formulated on the basis of the contribution of energy of individual feedstuffs and since pelleted roughages may be even less digestible than unprocessed roughages, some means of equating the greater intake and more rapid rumen turnover is needed in the practical utilization of such feedstuffs.

Rumen Adaptation to Ration Changes

The ruminant animal in its native state tends to eat a relatively stable diet from day to day. It is true that quite a variety of forage and/or browse may be consumed, but the percentage composition of the total diet does not change markedly from day to day but, rather, gradually as seasonal changes occur in availability and chemical composition of plants. This is quite a different pattern than may occur in many monogastric species. Humans, for example, prize a diet with variability and diversity. Presumably, factors (whatever they may be) controlling taste and appetite in ruminants may account for the constancy of diet. In view of the nature of the GIT of ruminants, this is obviously beneficial to the animal. This is so because of the complex nature of the microbiota in the stomach. Many of the microorganisms are quite adaptable and able to metabolize different substrates. However, the typical microflora and fauna found in an animal consuming hay will be quite different than that found in one consuming high levels of readily available carbohydrates. Thus, a sudden shift in diet can be expected to have a detrimental effect on the rumen microorganisms and, in many cases, on the metabolism of the host (see Ch. 17). The net result is that a period of adaptation is required which gives the microorganisms a chance to adapt to a different substrate (feedstuff). This is usually accomplished in practice by a gradual change in the diet selected by free grazing animals or by a gradual shift in ration ingredients when animals are managed by man.

Effect of Ration Changes on Rumen Microorganisms

Specific examples involving bloat, acute indigestion, nitrate and urea toxicity are mentioned in Ch. 17. Other pertinent and recent papers on adaptation are reviewed in subsequent paragraphs.

Gouws and Kistner (1965) have studied the predominant cellulolytic bacteria in the rumen of sheep when each was successively conditioned to alfalfa hay, abruptly changed to teff hay, conditioned to teff hay, abruptly changed back to alfalfa hay, conditioned to alfalfa hay, and changed back to teff hay. *Ruminococcus albus* strains were the predominant cellulose digesters when the sheep were fully conditioned to alfalfa. On changing from this diet to teff hay, *Butyrivibrio* species became established as the most numerous organisms within 2 wk in one sheep, while this required 4 wk in another and was not completed in 5 wk in the third sheep. On returning the sheep to alfalfa hay, *R. albus* again became predominant in the rumen of all three sheep within 2 wk after the change. In the periods immediately following the changes in diet, cocci giving rise to atypical colonies and zones of cellulolysis transiently occurred as the most abundant cellulose digesters. When sheep were abruptly changed from alfalfa pellets to a concentrate diet to rice straw or rice straw to a 1:1 mixture of alfalfa hay and concentrate, Sasaki et al (1973) found that rumen protozoa decreased each time there was an abrupt change. Lowest counts were reached within 3-5 days. Later the ciliates increased gradually and attained values typical for the particular feed in 30-35 days.

Warner (1962) published data on one sheep changed from a ration of hay to hay plus concentrates. Graphical data presented showed a marked increase in holotricha sp. and flagellate protozoa. Total bacteria also increased substantially. His data indicate that essentially stable levels had been reached 10 days following the change in ration. Giesecke et al (1966) have investigated the effect of changing sheep from a hay diet to pelleted diets. They noted little change in bacterial cultural counts in cows changed abruptly from a ration of alfalfa hay, corn silage and a concentrate mixture to corn silage, alfalfa hay or a grain-concentrate mixture. Their data indicated a linear decrease in bacteria from a beginning level of about 10^{10} to between 10^6 and 10^7 on the fifth day. This was followed by a gradual increase in bacterial numbers but they had not attained the original values by 21 days, thus indicating a rather long adaptation period for a ration change that was much less drastic than other reports mentioned.

Oltjen et al (1966) have studied rumen changes in twin cattle using a reversal trial technique in which the cattle were fed alfalfa hay for 4 wk, changed over to a ration containing 63% cracked corn during a 2-wk period and then maintained on the corn ration (or a purified ration) for a 6-wk period. Bacterial culture counts averaged 1.4 bil. after 4 wk on the hay diet. These counts had declined to 0.46 bil. during the first wk of the changeover and had risen to 0.73 bil. by the first day that cattle received only the experimental ration. The counts reported were quite variable during the 6-wk period and were as follows by weeks: 6.9, 0.83, 3.6, 1.1, 5.9, and 2.1 bil./ml. Thus, these data would indicate that the rumen population had not stabilized or that the counting technique did not give representative values. Direct counts of *Entodinium* protozoa showed a rise and fall during the changeover period, a decline in numbers after 3 wk on the corn ration, followed by an increase to peak levels after 5 wk (21,450/ml). *Isotricha* species followed similar trends although they were present at much lower levels after 5 wk (910/ml).

Effect of Ration Changes on Rumen Metabolites

In the paper by Nilson et al (1967), it was shown that niacin and pyridoxine concentration in rumen fluid reached peak values about 7-10 days following the ration changes. Oltjen et al (1966) found that ammonia N levels reached a low in the 4th wk after a gradual change from alfalfa hay to a corn-based ration (6 wk after corn first fed), followed by a gradual increase in the next 2 wk. Rumen pH was apparently stabilized by about 2 wk on the natural ration but required about 4 wk on a purified diet. Total VFA levels were somewhat erratic on both the natural and purified diets but molar percentages were pretty well stabilized by the 3rd wk after the changeover. Ryan (1964) studied some aspects of rumen chemistry in sheep gradually switched from a hay diet to a hay and grain diet. During the transitional period

there were transitory increases in ruminal concentrations of lactic, succinic, valeric and butyric acids and of glucose. Ruminal glucose and succinic acid tended to reach peak values about 3-4 wk after the start of wheat feeding and tapered off afterwards. Annison et al (1959) investigated some changes occurring in animals transferred from various diets to pasture. They found that there was a sustained rise in the concentration of VFA and ammonia in the rumen when transferred to pasture. In the rumen the initial and final lactic acid (22 days later) concentrations were similar but two sheep showed high concentrations on different days. As a whole, their data indicated rapid adaptation to the change in diet — essentially that adaptation had occurred within a week.

In more recent research on this topic, Lister et al (1971) have studied ruminal changes when steers were switched from low quality hay or hay + barley to pasture or pasture plus hay or barley. All steers showed an increase in ruminal ammonia, blood urea and plasma lactic acid on the first day and a decrease in plasma Ca and Mg on the second day on pasture. These blood values had not returned to prepasture levels by 21 days. Feeding supplemental hay tended to reduce ruminal ammonia. When dairy cows initially fed grass hay which was replaced stepwise with corn silage, Fenner et al (1970) concluded that a complete replacement of hay with silage did not change the ruminal pH or total VFA. Total bases and the molar % of propionate, isovalerate, valerate and n-caproate were increased. However, combinations of hay and silage decreased the molar % of propionate and increased total VFA.

Bide et al (1973) have studied blood profiles (similar to those used in human medicine) of cattle during a changeover from hay to a high grain diet. Of the blood minerals, there was no effect on Na; K increased, mean values being higher than starting values between 20 and 40 days. On the other hand, Ca levels dropped, reaching minimal values by 30 days and then increased slightly. Cl increased between the 10th and 40th days and then declined slightly, and inorganic P increased slightly over the first 40 days of feeding. With organic components, plasma creatinine increased between days 40 and 60. Urea N levels were essentially unaltered until after 80 days on feed, when they increased.

Plasma glucose was unchanged in the early period but declined slightly during the latter stages of the feeding period. Cholesterol showed a sharp decline during the first 10 days and then returned to normal levels until 70 days and increased thereafter. Plasma protein showed an initial decline and then increased gradually after 40 days. As a result of these studies, the authors concluded that metabolic adaptation requires at least 40 days following the start of grain feeding. Satter and Bringe (1969) have studied the effect of abrupt ration changes accompanied by a shift of rumen contents. One cow was fed a normal dairy herd ration (concentrate, alfalfa hay) and another a fat-depressing ration (75% pelleted concentrate, 25% alfalfa hay). After the rations and rumen contents were abruptly switched they concluded that feed intake was not altered, but 5-6 days were required to effect a change in the level of milk fat following this change. Thus, this technique shows that moderate changes can be made rapidly if the rumen population is changed at the same time but a longer time may be required for adaptation of the body. It appears obvious that further information is needed on this topic. Relatively little information is available on the effect of sudden ration changes on the lower GIT and liver, but the organs and tissues involved must be stressed considerably at times.

General Considerations

A number of experiments (for example Ryan, 1964; Nilson et al, 1967; Tremere et al, 1968) indicate that a rapid change from a forage type diet to one with appreciable quantities of readily available carbohydrates will result in a rather rapid increase in feed intake for a few days followed by a period of inappetence, thus indicating a disturbance in the metabolism of the animal, presumably from the changes going on in the rumen. The changes that occur in the VFA, pH (see Fig. 16-10), the production of lactate and succinate, etc., may also require some adaptation in the abomasum and by intestinal enzymes and tissues, as there are data indicating an adaptive response with some of the carbohydrase enzymes (see Ch. 9). Data from experiments on digestibility by the total GIT also show that a period of adaptation is required. Graphical data from Lloyd et al (1956) are shown in Fig. 16-11). In these experiments, sheep were transferred directly from pasture to a ration of grass hay. The

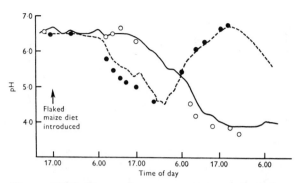

Figure 16-10 Change in rumen pH in two different cows when their diet was abruptly changed from hay to flaked corn. Each ration offered at 0600 and 1700 hr. The • or o represent samples taken by aspiration; the line was from a recording pH meter. From Johnson and Sutton [1968].

graphs indicate that a substantial amount of time was required before digestibility of dry matter, protein, fiber, ether extract and NFE were stabilized, although the authors concluded that a 10-day preliminary period was an adequate adjustment period. Nicholson et al (1956) observed considerable fluctuation in calculated digestion coefficients when rations were changed, particularly when the amount of hay and grain varied.

As indicated, published data on time required for adaptation of ruminant animals to a drastically different diet would appear to vary with circumstances. A general conclusion would be that time required for adaptation for a shift from one forage to another would tend to be relatively short, perhaps on the order of 10 days to 2 wk; however, when increasing levels of concentrates are the major change, the data seem to indicate that a period of 4-6 wk may not always allow complete adaptation. Further work on this problem is certainly warranted.

Control of Rumen Fermentation

This subject has received more and more attention in recent years, and a symposium on the topic was held in England in 1972. Some of the papers resulting from the meeting may be of interest to some readers. They would include those by Hobson (1972), Hutton (1972), Singleton (1972) and Thomas and Clapperton (1972). In addition, there have been numerous references in many of the chapters in this book which have referred to factors which may result in some alteration in rumen fermentation. Thus, perhaps it will be of some advantage, particularly to

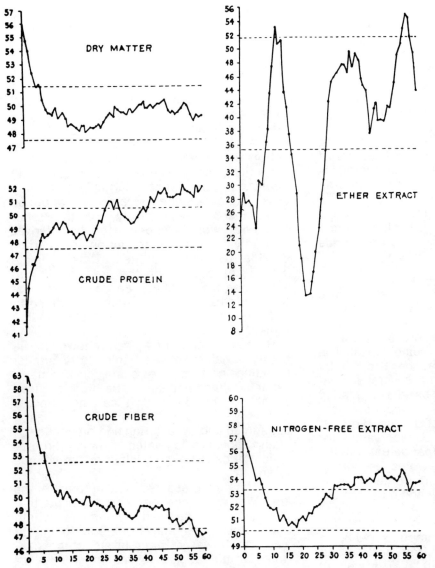

Figure 16-11 Change in apparent digestibility of fractions of an all-roughage ration when fed to sheep. Sheep were placed on hay after grazing grass. Data were calculated from 10-day fecal collections. That is, digestibility on day 0 reflects analyses of feed and feces collected for the first 10 days, etc. From Lloyd et al [1956].

undesirable problems such as toxicity, bloat and acute indigestion or to speed adaptation of the rumen and the animal's tissues to ration changes.

Alteration of the end products (VFA primarily) can be achieved by changing the ration content of readily available carbohydrates, by pelleting forages, heat treatment of high starch feedstuffs and by appropriate use of buffers. Thus various combinations of these procedures can be utilized in appropriate situations. Normal rumen fermentative action can be prevented on some proteins by treatment with materials such as aldehydes and tannins and fat can be protected from hydrogenation by preparing casein-fat emulsions and treating with aldehyde. In addition, the use of methane inhibitors results in some alteration of the end products, hopefully with some improvement in energy utilization. Other examples could be cited.

Ration preparation methods such as pelleting or cubing of roughages usually allow

students, if some of this information is summarized briefly.

The objectives in manipulating rumen fermentation might be several. One aim might be to alter the end products, such as changing the molar % of acetate and propionate, which have some influence on utilization of energy for maintenance, gain or milk fat production. A second aim might be to increase the efficiency of utilization of feedstuffs and nutrients. Others could include alteration of rations in order to increase feed consumption, to prevent

a considerably greater intake accompanied by some changes in molar % of the VFA. As a result of the increased consumption, gross energetic efficiency and feed conversion may be greatly improved. Chemical treatments, such as treatment of straw with NaOH, may greatly increase digestibility of low quality roughage and also allow greater consumption. With the feed grains, ration preparation methods such as steam process flaking usually result in greater efficiency although consumption may not be altered.

In order to prevent urea toxicity, urea can

be combined with starch in a form that results in slower release, thus reducing the likelihood of toxicity. Antibiotics and other additives can be used to reduce bloating as can various surface active compounds and buffers offer the potential of reducing the incidence of acute indigestion when animals are abruptly changed from forage to high grain diets.

In each of these examples, there is some alteration of rumen metabolism in terms of reaction rates or a change in the microflora or microfauna which causes some overall alteration in rumen metabolism. Thus, it is apparent that there are a number of options which can be utilized to alter rumen metabolism and, ultimately, the performance of the animal.

Conclusions

Literature reviewed in this chapter shows rather clearly that the VFA will vary in concentration in the rumen, attaining maximum values on the order of 3-6 hr following the ingestion of a single meal. The concentration of VFA may be affected by ration ingredients, with the general indication that rations high in protein or readily available carbohydrates will produce higher concentrations than most forage diets. It would be difficult to give average values for VFA, but we might say that values on the order of 80-150 µmol/ml would be normal depending upon the diet, the time samples were obtained after feeding and other factors such as rumen volume. An appreciable amount of interconversion of ruminal VFA occurs, with substantial amounts (40-80%) of butyrate being derived from acetate and acetate from butyrate (6-20%). The amount of VFA produced in the rumen would appear to vary considerably, but it seems safe to conclude that sheep probably produce on the order of 4-5.5 mol/day and lactating dairy cows as much as 110 mol/day, although the latter estimate is a less reliable value.

Rumen pH has been shown to fluctuate with feed intake and is inversely related to VFA concentration. The pH tends to be much lower (4.5-5.0) on rations with high levels of readily available carbohydrates, whereas alfalfa tends to exert a greater buffering action than some other forages.

Rumen gases are known to be produced in substantial quantities, particularly carbon dioxide and methane which average about 65 and 26-28%, respectively, of the total. Methane would appear to be derived primarily from the reduction of carbon dioxide by free hydrogen. Data indicate average production on the order of 30 and 150 l. per day by sheep and cattle, respectively. Methane production can be related to digestible carbohydrate or digestible energy intake.

Rumen volume has been shown to be highly variable between animals of similar breeding and in the same environment. Rumen volume appears to be high in sheep which eat rapidly and it can be affected markedly by the nature of the ration consumed and by lactation and pregnancy. It would appear to be related to rumen turnover which tends to be rapid when rumen volume is small.

Information presented on adaptation of the animal to ration changes would indicate that adaptation may be relatively complete within 2 wk when changing from one forage to another; however, high levels of concentrates would appear to require 4-6 wk or longer for adaptation to be complete.

References Cited

Alexander, C.L., E.F. Bartley, J.L. Morrill and R.M. Meyer 1965. J. Dairy Sci. 48:924.
Allison, M.J. and J.A. Bucklin. 1971. J. Animal Sci. 33:274 (abstr).
Allo, A.A., J.H. Oh, W.M. Longhurst and G.E. Connolly. 1973. J. Wildl. Mgt. 37:202.
Annison, E.F., D. Lewis and D.B. Lindsay. 1959. J. Agr. Sci. 53:34.
Annison, E.F. and R.R. White. 1962. Biochem. J. 84:546.
Balch, C.C. and C. Line. 1957. J. Dairy Res. 24:11.
Balch, D.A. and S.J. Rowland. 1957. Br. J. Nutr. 11:288.
Bath, I.H. and J.A.F. Rook. 1963. J. Agr. Sci. 61:341.
Bath, I.H. and J.A.F. Rook. 1965. J. Agr. Sci. 64:67.
Bauchop, T. 1967. J. Bacteriol. 94:171.
Bauman, D.E., C.L. Davis and H.F. Bucholtz. 1971. J. Dairy Sci. 54:1282.
Beijer, W.H. 1952. Nature 170:576.
Bergman, E.N., et al. 1965. Biochem. J. 97:53.

Bide, R.W., W.J. Dorward and M.E. Tumbleson. 1973. Can. J. Animal Sci. 53:697.
Blaxter, K.L. 1962. The Energy Metabolism of Ruminants. Hutchinson Pub. Co., London.
Blaxter, K.L. and J.L. Clapperton. 1965. Br. J. Nutr. 19:511.
Blaxter, K.L., F.W. Wainman and R.S. Wilson. 1961. Animal Prod. 3:51.
Bratzler, J.W. and E.B. Forbes. 1940. J. Nutr. 19:611.
Briggs, P.K., J.P. Hogan and R.L. Reid. 1957. Aust. J. Agr. Res. 8:674.
Bryant, A.M. 1964. N.Z. J. Agr. Res. 7:694.
Campling, R.C., M. Freer and C.C. Balch. 1961. Br. J. Nutr. 15:531.
Carroll, E.J. and R.E. Hungate. 1955. Arch. Biochem. Biophys. 56:525.
Cheng, K.J. and R. Kironaka. 1973. Can. J. Animal Sci. 53:417.
Ciszuk, P. 1973. Swedish J. Agr. Res. 3:167.
Clanton, D.C. and W. Woods. 1966. J. Animal Sci. 25:102.
Clapperton, J.L. 1973. Proc. Nutr. Soc. 32:57A (abstr).
Clapperton, J.L. and K.L. Blaxter. 1965. Proc. Nutr. Soc. 24:xvi (abstr).
Clapperton, J.L. and J.W. Czerkawski. 1969. Br. J. Nutr. 23:813.
Clapperton, J.L. and J.W. Czerkawski. 1972. Br. J. Nutr. 27:553.
Colenbrander, V.F., et al. 1967. J. Dairy Sci. 50:1966.
Colvin, J.W., J.D. Wheat, E.A. Rhode and J.M. Boda. 1957. J. Dairy Sci. 40:492.
Czerkawski, J.W. 1972. Proc. Nutr. Soc. 31:141.
Czerkawski, J.W., K.L. Blaxter and F.W. Wainman. 1966. Br. J. Nutr. 20:349; 485.
Czerkawski, J.W. and G. Breckenridge. 1969. Br. J. Nutr. 23:51.
Czerkawski, J.W. and G. Breckenridge. 1972. Br. J. Nutr. 27:147.
Czerkawski, J.W. and J.L. Clapperton. 1968. Laboratory Practice 17:994.
Czerkawski, J.W., C.G. Harfoot and G. Breckenridge. 1972. J. Appl. Bact. 35:537.
Davis, R.F., N.S. Woodhouse, M. Keeny and G.H. Back. 1957. J. Dairy Sci. 40:75.
Demeyer, D. and H. Henderickx. 1964. Arch. Internat. Physiol. 72:1.
Demeyer, D. and H. Henderickx. 1967. Arch. Internat. Physiol. 75:157.
Demeyer, D., H. Henderickx and C. Van Nevel. 1967. Arch. Internat. Physiol. 75:555.
Dougherty, R.W. 1941. J. Amer. Vet. Med. Assoc. 99:110.
Dougherty, R.W. 1942. Amer. J. Vet. Res. 3:401.
Dougherty, R.W., M.J. Allison and C.H. Mullenax. 1964. Amer. J. Physiol. 207:1181.
Dougherty, R.W. and H.M. Cook. 1962. Amer. J. Vet. Res. 23:997.
Dougherty, R.W., et al. 1962. J. Dairy Sci. 45:472.
Egan, A.R. 1966. Aust. J. Agr. Res. 17:741.
el-Shazly, K. 1952. Biochem. J. 51:640.
Emery, R.S., C.K. Smith and C.F. Huffman. 1956. J. Animal Sci. 15:854.
Emmanuel, B., M.J. Lawlor and D.M. McAleese. 1969. Br. J. Nutr. 23:805.
Esdale, W.J., G.L. Broderick and L.D. Satter. 1968. J. Dairy Sci. 51:1823.
Faichney, G.J. 1968. J. Agr. Sci. 19:803.
Fenner, H., R.A. Damon and H.D. Barnes. 1970. J. Dairy Sci. 53:1568.
Fonnesbeck, P.V., L.E. Harris and C.W. Cook. 1970. J. Animal Sci. 30:283.
Forbes, J.M. 1968. J. Agr. Sci. 70:171.
Forbes, J.M. 1969. J. Agr. Sci. 72:119.
Franks, L.G., J.R. Newsom, R.E. Renbarger and R. Totusek. 1972. J. Animal Sci. 35:404.
Ghorban, K.Z., K.L. Knox and F.M. Ward. 1966. J. Dairy Sci. 49:1515.
Geisecke, D., M.J. Lawlor and K. Walser-Karst. 1966. Br. J. Nutr. 20:383.
Gouws, L. and A. Kistner. 1965. J. Agr. Sci. 64:51.
Gray, F.V., G.B. Jones and A.F. Pilgrim. 1960. Aust. J. Agr. Res. 11:383.
Gray, F.V. and A.F. Pilgrim. 1951. J. Exptl. Biol. 28:83.
Gray, F.V., A.F. Pilgrim, H.J. Rodda and R.A. Weller. 1952. J. Exptl. Biol. 29:57.
Gray, F.V., R.A. Weller and G.B. Jones. 1965. Aust. J. Agr. Res. 16:145.
Gray, F.V., R.A. Weller, A.F. Pilgrim and G.B. Jones. 1966. Aust. J. Agr. Res. 17:69.
Gray, F.V., R.A. Weller, A.F. Pilgrim and G.B. Jones. 1967. Aust. J. Agr. Res. 18:625.
Harvey, R.W., M.B. Wise, T.N. Blumer and E.R. Barrick. 1968. J. Animal Sci. 27:1438.
Hobson, P.N. 1972. Proc. Nutr. Soc. 31:135.
Hoover, W.H., E.M. Kesler and R.J. Flipse. 1963. J. Dairy Sci. 46:733.
Howes, A.D. and I.A. Dyer. 1968. Proc. West. Sec. Amer. Soc. Animal Sci. 19:19.
Hungate, R.E. 1966. The Rumen and Its Microbes. Academic Press.
Hungate, R.E. 1967. Arch. Microbiol. 59:158.
Hutton, K. 1972. Proc. Nutr. Soc. 31:151.
Ibrahim, E.A., J.R. Ingalls and G.D. Phillips. 1969. Can. J. Animal Sci. 49:399.
Ichhponani, J.S. and G.S. Sidhu. 1965. Indian J. Vet. Sci. 35:316.
Isahaque, M., P.C. Thomas and J.A.F. Rook. 1971. Nature New Biol. 231:253.
Jamieson, N.D. 1959. N.Z. J. Agr. Res. 2:314.
Johns, A.T., M.J. Ulyatt and A.C. Glenday. 1963. J. Agr. Sci. 61:201.
Johnson, D.E. 1972. J. Animal Sci. 35:1064.
Johnson, D.E. 1974. J. Animal Sci. 38:154.
Johnson, E.D., A.S. Wood, J.B. Stone and E.T. Moran. 1972. Can. J. Animal Sci. 52:703.
Johnson, R.R. and K.E. McClure. 1972. J. Animal Sci. 34:501.
Johnson, V.W. and J.D. Sutton. 1968. Br. J. Nutr. 22:303.

Jorgensen, N.A. and L.H. Schultz. 1963. J. Dairy Sci. 46:437.
Judson, G.J., E. Anderson, J.R. Luick and R.A. Leng. 1968. Br. J. Nutr. 22:69.
Kingwill, R.G., R.A. Oppermann, W.O. Nelson and R.E. Brown. 1959. J. Dairy Sci. 42:912 (abstr).
Kleiber, M., H.H. Cole and S.W. Mead. 1943. J. Dairy Sci. 26:929.
Knox, K.L., A.L. Black and M. Kleiber. 1967. J. Dairy Sci. 50:1716.
Knox, K.L., A.L. Black and M. Kleiber. 1969. J. Dairy Sci. 52:484.
Lane, G.T., et al. 1968. J. Dairy Sci. 51:114.
Leng, R.A. and D.J. Brett. 1966. Br. J. Nutr. 20:541.
Leng, R.A., J.L. Corbett and D.J. Brett. 1968. Br. J. Nutr. 22:57.
Leng, R.A. and G.J. Leonard. 1965. Br. J. Nutr. 19:469.
Lister, E.E., et al. 1971. Can. J. Animal Sci. 51:179.
Lloyd, L.E., H.E. Peckham and E.W. Crampton. 1956. J. Animal Sci. 15:846.
Matsumoto, T. 1962. Nutr. Abstr. Rev. 32:793.
McArthur, J.M. and J.E. Miltimore. 1961. Can. J. Animal Sci. 41:187.
McCauley, E.H. and H.E. Dziuk. 1965. Amer. J. Physiol. 209:1152.
McCullough, M.E. and W.G. Smart. 1968. J. Dairy Sci. 51:385.
McNeill, J.J. and D.R. Jacobson. 1955. J. Dairy Sci. 55:608 (abstr).
Miller, T.L. and M.J. Wolin. 1973. J. Bacteriol. 116:836.
Miltimore, J.E. and J.M. McArthur. 1962. Nature 196:288.
Minson, D.J. and J.L. Cowper. 1966. Br. J. Nutr. 20:575.
Moody, E.G. 1971. J. Dairy Sci. 54:1817.
Morris, J.G., L.E. Harris, J.E. Butcher and C.W. Cook. 1965. J. Animal Sci. 24:1152.
Nagel, S. and B. Paitkowski. 1972. Arch. fur Tierernahrung. 22:449.
Nagy, J.G. and G.L. Williams. 1969. J. Wildl. Mgt. 33:437.
Nicholson, J.W.G., E.H. Haynes, R.G. Warner and J.K. Loosli. 1956. J. Animal Sci. 15:1172.
Nilson, K.M., F.G. Owen and C.E. Georgi. 1967. J. Dairy Sci. 50:1172.
Ogimoto, K., F. Shibata and C. Furusaka. 1962. Nutr. Abstr. Rev. 32:793.
Oltjen, R.R., J. Gutierrez, R.P. Lehmann and R.E. Davis. 1966. J. Animal Sci. 25:521.
Oltjen, R.R., L.L. Slyter, E.E. Williams and D.L. Kern. 1971. J. Nutr. 101:101.
Omori, S., T. Kobayashi and A. Kawabata. 1969. Bul. Nat. Inst. Animal Ind. 19:33.
Oppermann, R.A., W.O. Nelson and R.E. Brown. 1957. J. Dairy Sci. 40:779.
Oppermann, R.A., W.O. Nelson and R.E. Brown. 1959. J. Dairy Sci. 42:913 (abstr).
Pant, H.C., M.D. Pandey, J.S. Rawat and A. Roy. 1963. Indian J. Dairy Sci. 16:29.
Phillipson, A.T. 1952. Br. J. Nutr. 6:190.
Pilgrim, A.F. 1948. Aust. J. Scient. Res., Series B. 1:130.
Prins, R.A. 1970. Nutr. Abstr. Rev. 40:1508.
Prins, R.A. and M.J.H. Geelen. 1971. J. Wildl. Mgt. 35:673.
Purser, D.B., T.J. Klopfenstein and J.H. Cline. 1965. J. Animal Sci. 24:1039.
Purser, D.B. and R.J. Moir. 1966. J. Animal Sci. 25:509; 516.
Putnam, P.A., D.A. Yarns and R.E. Davis. 1966. J. Animal Sci. 25:1176.
Quaghebeur, D. and W. Oyaert. 1971. Zbl. Vet. Med. 18:55; 64.
Randall, R.P. 1974. Ph.D. Thesis, Oregon State Univ., Corvallis.
Raun, N.S., W. Burroughs and W. Woods. 1962. J. Animal Sci. 21:838.
Reid, R.L., J.P. Hogan and P.K. Briggs. 1957. Aust. J. Agr. Res. 8:691.
Rufener, W.H. and M.J. Wolin. 1968. Appl. Microbiol. 16:1955.
Rumsey, T.S., P.A. Putnam, J. Bond and R.R. Oltjen. 1970. J. Animal Sci. 31:608.
Ryan, R.K. 1964. Amer. J. Vet. Res. 25:653.
Sasaki, M., Y. Yamatani and I. Otani. 1973. Nutr. Abstr. Rev. 43:707.
Satter, L.D. and A.N. Bringe. 1969. J. Dairy Sci. 52:1776.
Sawyer, M.S., W.H. Hoover and C.J. Sniffen. 1974. J. Animal Sci. 38:908.
Shipe, W.F., et al. 1962. J. Dairy Sci. 45:477.
Short, H.L., D.E. Medin and A.E. Anderson. 1966. J. Wildl. Mgt. 30:466.
Sinclair, H.H., et al. 1958. J. Animal Sci. 17:1220 (abstr).
Singleton, A.G. 1972. Proc. Nutr. Soc. 31:147.
Slanian, L. and R. Cabadaj. 1968. Nutr. Abstr. Rev. 38:802.
Slyter, L.L. and J.M. Weaver. 1972. J. Animal Sci. 35:275 (abstr).
Steward, W.E., D.G. Stewart and L.H. Schultz. 1958. J. Animal Sci. 17:723.
Sutherland, T.M., W.C. Ellis, R.S. Reid and M.G. Murray. 1962. Br. J. Nutr. 16:603.
Symons, G.E. and A.M. Buswell. 1933. J. Amer. Chem. Soc. 55:2028.
Thomas, G.D., E.E. Bartley, H.B. Pfost and R.M. Meyer. 1968. J. Dairy Sci. 51:869.
Thomas, P.C. and J.L. Clapperton. 1972. Proc. Nutr. Soc. 31:165.
Tonroy, B.R. and T.W. Perry. 1974. J. Animal Sci. 38:676.
Topps, J.H., W.D.C. Reed and R.C. Elliott. 1965. J. Agr. Sci. 64:397.
Trei, J.E., R.C. Parish, Y.K. Singh and G.C. Scott. 1971. J. Dairy Sci. 54:536.
Trei, J.E., G.C. Scott and R.C. Parish. 1972. J. Animal Sci. 34:510.
Tremere, A.W., W.G. Merrill and J.K. Loosli. 1968. J. Dairy Sci. 51:1065.
Tulloh, N.M. 1966. N.Z. J. Agr. Res. 9:252; 999.
Tulloh, N.M. and J.W. Hughes. 1965. N.Z. J. Agr. Res. 8:1070.
Tulloh, N.M., J.W. Hughes and R.P. Newth. 1965. N.Z. J. Agr. Res. 8:636.
Ulyatt, M.J. 1964. N.Z. J. Agr. Res. 7:713.

Ulyatt, M.J., K.L. Blaxter and I. McDonald. 1967. Anim. Prod. 9:463.

Van Nevel, C.J., D.I. Demeyer, B.G. Cottyn and H.K. Henderickx. 1970. Nutr. Abstr. Rev. 40:1339.

Van Nevel, C.J., D.I. Demeyer, B.G. Cottyn and C.V. Voucque. 1973. Nutr. Abstr. Rev. 43:1032.

Van Nevel, C.J., D.I. Demeyer and H.K. Henderickx. 1971. Appl. Microbiol. 21:365.

Van Nevel, C.J., H.K. Henderickx, D.I. Demeyer and J. Martil. 1969. Appl. Microbiol. 17:695.

Vercoe, J.E. and K.L. Blaxter. 1965. Proc. Nutr. Soc. 24:xvii (abstr).

Warner, A.C.I. 1962. J. Gen. Microbiol. 28:129.

Warner, A.C.I. 1964. Nutr. Abstr. Rev. 34:339.

Warner, A.C.I. and B.D. Stacy. 1968. Br. J. Nutr. 22:389.

Washburn, L.E. and S. Brody. 1937. Mo. Agr. Expt. Sta. Res. Bul. 263.

Weekes, T.E.C. 1971. Res. Vet. Sci. 12:373.

Weller, R.A., F.V. Gray, A.F. Pilgrim and G.B. Jones. 1967. Aust. J. Agr. Res. 18:107.

Weston, R.H. and J.P. Hogan. 1967. Aust. J. Agr. Res. 18:789.

Weston, R.H. and J.P. Hogan. 1968. Aust. J. Agr. Res. 19:419.

Weiss, R.L., B.R. Baumgardt, G.R. Barr and V.H. Brungardt. 1967. J. Animal Sci. 26:389.

Whitelaw, F.G., J. Hyldgaard-Jensen, R.S. Reid and M.G. Kay. 1970. Br. J. Nutr. 24:179.

Williams, V.H. and K.R. Christian. 1966. J. Agr. Sci. 67:59.

Williams, W.F., D.R. Waldo, W.P. Flatt and M.J. Allison. 1963. J. Dairy Sci. 56:992.

Wilson, A.D. 1963. Aust. J. Agr. Res. 14:226.

Wiltrout, D.W. and L.D. Satter. 1972. J. Dairy Sci. 55:307.

Woods, W. and R. Luther. 1962. J. Animal Sci. 21:809.

Yadava, I.S., et al. 1964. J. Dairy Sci. 47:1346.

CHAPTER 17 — NUTRITIONAL PROBLEMS RELATED TO THE GASTRO-INTESTINAL TRACT

The ruminant animal is subject to a number of severe maladies due to the nature of its digestive tract and, partly, to complicating factors introduced by management or nutritional practices in modern day agriculture. Those primarily involved with rumen function are bloat, acute indigestion, urea toxicity and nitrate toxicity. Other problems such as displaced abomasum will be discussed briefly.

Bloat is a problem that may be assumed to be mainly a result of man's modern agriculture practices. Since it is primarily a result of consumption of certain leguminous plants, man's efforts to propagate legumes are a major factor. In the same manner, acute indigestion and urea toxicity result from the use of feeding practices which are intended to increase the productivity of animals and the quality of the product or to reduce the cost of production. Nonetheless, whether these problems are natural or are artifacts, they may be very severe. Literature pertaining to them is reviewed in subsequent pages. Other important maladies affecting ruminants such as milk fever, ketosis and grass tetany are discussed in detail in Vol. 2 of this series.

Bloat [Tympanites]

Bloat is characterized primarily by a distension of the reticulo-rumen due to the accumulation of excessive amounts of fermentation gases. It is an important factor in the production of domestic ruminants since losses (death and morbidity) are probably well over $100 million/year in the USA. Death losses in cattle are estimated at > 0.5% of the cattle population.

No doubt bloat has been a problem in modern man's domestic ruminants for many centuries, since bloat was described as long ago as 60 A.D. by a Roman author. Bloat would seem to be one of the penalties associated with modern agriculture since most of the death losses are associated with the consumption of legume hay or forage. The author is unaware of information as to the severity of bloat in wild ruminants. However, it would seem unlikely to be a major problem except possibly in situations where such animals might intensively graze fields of tame legumes cultured by man for his domestic animals.

As a consequence of the high losses sustained from bloat, a tremendous amount of research has been carried out and there is a large volume of literature available, some of it dating back many years. Of the numerous reviews, some of relatively recent vintage that might be recommended include Johns (1956, 1958), Cole and Boda (1960) and Ayre-Smith (1971). In addition, Hungate (1966, pp 442-454) also has a section in his book that is recommended reading.

Etiology of Bloat

Many different factors have been implicated at one time or another as contributing to bloat in ruminants and, as a result, different authors have used various schemes of classifying bloat based on the nature of the bloat or on the probable cause. For example, Cole et al (1956) classified bloat as chronic, subacute and acute. As so classified, chronic bloat is restricted to conditions not related to diet. Subacute bloat is defined as that resulting from a specific regimen such as succulent legumes. Acute bloat is similar to subacute bloat except that the condition is further advanced and distressing symptoms are manifested by the affected animal. Bloat has also been classified as free-gas bloat or frothy bloat by Hungate (1966) as well as by other writers. This seems to be a more logical classification to this author since most cases of subacute or acute bloat appear to be related to the presence of froth in the reticulo-rumen. Observations on bloated animals also show that bloat classified as subacute may frequently turn into acute bloat; consequently, this distinction seems to have little physiological meaning in so far as the etiology of the condition is concerned. Frothy bloat is often referred to as pasture or feedlot bloat. Unfortunately, published observations indicating the extent of froth formation in feedlot bloat are inadequate. It should be clearly understood, however, that all types of bloat have one thing in common — namely, that bloat results from a failure to get rid of fermentation gases as rapidly as they are formed. Note in Fig. 17-1 the amount of ruminal distension in a bloated bovine.

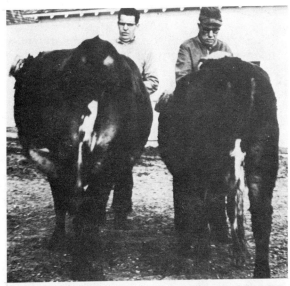

Figure 17-1. An example of the amount of ruminal distension which may occur in a severely bloated animal. Courtesy of E.E. Bartley.

Free-Gas Bloat

Several factors have been identified as being primary causes of bloat where no froth or foam is commonly found in the reticulo-rumen. Some of these are listed and discussed briefly.

Overfilling of the Reticulo-Rumen. Dougherty (1940) and Weiss (1953) have both demonstrated that filling the reticulo-rumen with liquids and elevation of the hindquarters of the animal tends to inhibit eructation although other reports by Quin (1953) and Dziuk and Sellers (1955) indicated less effect. Weiss (1953) reported on experiments in which water was withheld from both cattle and sheep for periods up to 24 hr after which they were turned onto alfalfa pasture. The incidence and severity of bloat was considerably higher among the watered groups than among the controls. In another case, water was withheld from sheep which were given alfalfa hay. When the sheep were insufflated with air after both feed and water were available for 2 hr, the ability to eructate the added air was reduced, being proportional to the combined food and water intake.

An example of the effect of overfilling witnessed by the author occurred in a calf withheld from water for a few hours on a hot day. The calf drank a relatively large quantity of water and was dead of bloat (presumably) within half an hour, most likely due to overfilling of the reticulo-rumen.

Acidosis of the Reticulo-Rumen. Ash (1959) and Ash and Kay (1959) reported that buffered solutions of volatile fatty acids at pH of 3.5-5.0 inhibited stomach contractions as did vapor from fatty acids. It was concluded that the effect was not simply caused by local pH changes (since the vapor changed pH very little) but due to the rapid penetration of fatty acid vapor into the epithelium. In these reports there was no reference to bloat and inhibition of eructation.

Hungate (1966) and other writers make reference to acidic conditions as a possible cause of bloat and a number of reports agree with the results of Ash that acidic conditions in the rumen tend to reduce the frequency as well as the amplitude of stomach contractions. Data indicating that low pH is a direct cause of bloat are inconclusive, particularly since some studies indicate that eructation can still occur when the stomach has been immobilized with drugs.

Miscellaneous Factors. Some dwarf calves are habitual and chronic bloaters, apparently because of some physiological or anatomical defect which interferes with eructation (Hafez et al, 1959; Fletcher and Hafez, 1960). With respect to different chemical factors, it has been shown that large doses of alkali may cause ruminal paralysis and inhibit eructation (Clark and Lombard, 1951; Weiss, 1953). A variety of drugs and/or toxins such as K cyanide, atropine, histamine, adrenalin, saponins and toxic factors in rumen microorganisms have been implicated at one time or another (Cole and Boda, 1960) and field observations indicate that bloat may develop after consumption of spoiled or mouldy feed. Carbamylocholine and veratrine, both stimulatory agents, result in spasms of the rumen musculature and appear to interfere with eructation as a result (Weiss, 1953).

Mechanical injury or obstruction of the esophagus or reticulitus resulting from ingestion of hardware, etc., are said to be factors that may frequently result in bloat. In addition, there is occasionally evidence of abnormal growths which may cause chronic bloating (Benson, 1957). Traumatic reticulitis and peritonitis may cause damage to vagal nerves and chronic bloating (Weiss, 1953).

Distension of the abomasum, duodenum, ileum and cecum have been shown to inhibit flow of digesta from anterior parts of the GIT, eventually resulting in reduced reticular motility. Consequently, we might anticipate that trauma or disease in any of these parts might result in bloat. Weiss (1953) found this to be the case in animals with appreciable amounts of digesta in the reticulo-rumen. In the empty organ, eructation was inhibited very little.

It seems likely in animals prostrated suddenly by milk fever or other maladies which have a sudden onset, that a number of affected animals may die of bloat although it may be a secondary cause of death. Unfortunately, information on this subject is entirely inadequate to evaluate its importance, but field observations indicate that bloat may sometimes be relieved by I.V. administration of Ca and Mg solutions.

This listing, by no means a complete one, indicates clearly that many factors other than the ingestion of legumes may result in bloat at one time or another. Some of these factors such as overfilling of the stomach may also be important in legume bloat. The relative importance of these factors in unknown but is presumed to be of minor importance as compared to frothy bloat resulting primarily from consumption of legumes. Some of these factors have undoubtedly served to confuse the bloat picture and made an understanding of the etiology of bloat more difficult to the uninformed, particularly when an adequate diagnosis was not available.

Frothy Bloat

Legume Bloat. Observation on rumen-fistulated animals bloating on legumes indicates that froth is usually present in the dorsal sac. In some cases very little free gas space remains (Quin, 1943; Clark, 1948; Hungate et al, 1955; as well as other papers). Quin (1943) found that many of the gas bubbles were trapped in the ingesta, a situation resembling that of rising bread. He reported that foamy ingesta (from sheep) kept standing at room temperature required several hours before gas bubbles collapsed and he demonstrated similar effects with pressed alfalfa juice and water extracts of alfalfa hay. However, Boda et al (1956) point out that some free gas was almost invariably

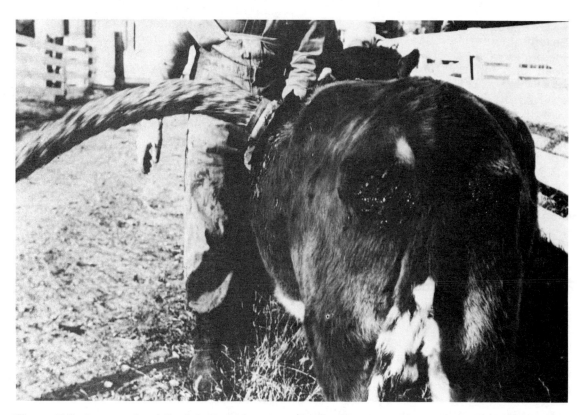

Figure 17-2. An example of the intraruminal pressure involved in severe bloat. Courtesy of E.E. Bartley.

found in the dorsal sac of cows bloating on alfalfa as determined by passage of a stomach tube. Examination of a cow that died of bloat revealed that a "large amount" (estimated at several cubic feet) of free gas escaped when the rumen was punctured with a trocar and cannula immediately before death and that further opening of the rumen with a knife allowed a mass of foamy ingesta to escape. Walker (1960) reported observations on a number of dairy cows observed shortly before and after death. He found that cows dying of bloat invariably had froth in the rumen; however, rumen contents of animals dead several hours frequently did not contain froth — thus probably accounting for some of the uncertainty on this subject. Mills and Christian (1970) observed similar changes in cattle known to have died of bloat. Thus, these and other observations seem to establish without much doubt that froth is a primary characteristic of legume bloat. Examples of the type of froth and an indication of the pressure involved are shown in Fig. 17-2, 3.

Physiological Changes Occurring During Bloat

Clinical Symptoms. Antemortem signs observed in bloated cattle include: gaseous distension of the left flank and of the abdomen (Fig. 17-1), uneasiness as indicated by stamping of the feet, frequent urination and defecation, extension of the head and neck, dyspena (labored breathing), slight protrusion of the tongue and, finally, collapse and death almost without a struggle. Examination of rumen contents shortly after death nearly always shows froth. Post mortem signs: generalized symptoms include extreme congestion of the lymphoid tissues of the head and neck with absence of congestion in the muscles and lymph nodes of the hind quarters, extensive petechiation into the mucosa of the trachae and congestion of large areas of the ventral sacs in the rumen. Purplish-pink edema of connective tissues is not associated with lesions of muscle tissues; rumen contents of animals dead several hours may not contain froth (Cole and Boda, 1960; Walker,

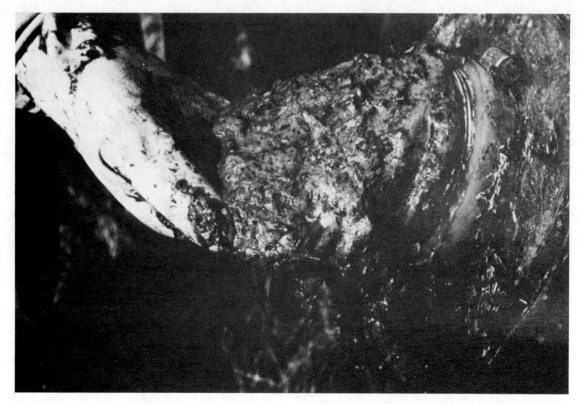

Figure 17-3. An illustration of the very foamy digesta in the rumen of a bovine with pasture bloat. Courtesy of E.E. Bartley.

1960). In a more recent paper, Mills and Christian (1970) note that the lungs were compressed; there was congestion and hemorrhages in the cervical esophagus and the thoracic portion of the esophagus was pale and blanched. Gas was frequently noted in the intestines. They suggest that partial or complete occlusion of the abdominal aorta occurs and, as a result of reduced blood flow to the kidney, that hyperkalemia (high blood K) may be a contributing factor to death.

Intraruminal Pressure and Motility. In the normal animal intraruminal pressure is near atmospheric pressure when the rumen is at rest. During severe cases of bloat, pressures may be as high as 70 mm of Hg (Boda et al, 1956; Colvin et al, 1958). Data reported by Boda et al and Dougherty et al (1955) indicate that a considerable difference may be noted between individuals on the amount of intraruminal pressure they can tolerate. Dougherty and coworkers reported that one sheep could tolerate intraruminal pressures up to 100 mm of Hg when insufflated with oxygen gas; however, when inflated with CO_2 at 60 mm of Hg, the animal collapsed in less than 3 min. Observations and postulations by Quin (1943), Dougherty et al (1955), Walker (1960) and Davis et al (1965) indicate that the increased intraruminal pressure results in an increased absorption of CO_2 into the blood and restricts the return of venous blood through the vena cava vein back to the heart. In experimental studies with goats, it has been shown that rumen insufflation to pressures of 40 mm of Hg results in increased blood pressure but decreased cardiac output, presumably due to increased peripheral resistance caused by obstruction of venous blood return (Reschly and Dale, 1970). The net effect is that the animal probably dies of suffocation.

Observations on rumen contractions of bloated animals (Weiss, 1953; Boda et al, 1956; Colvin et al, 1958) indicate that the initial stages of bloat may result in some hypermotility. There is quite a bit of variability in the proportion of primary to secondary contractions in normal animals from the same herd on the same ration (see Ch. 6). However, data on bloated animals indicate that there is apt to be an increase in secondary contractions (Weiss, 1953; Colvin et al, 1958). Even in animals no longer able to eructate, the contractions may still be quite vigorous (Weiss, 1953).

Effect of Bloat on Salivary Production. A number of reports (Ash and Kay, 1959; Phillipson and Reid, 1958; Phillipson and Mangan, 1959; Davis et al, 1965) show that inflation of the rumen with gas or balloons may affect salivary flow in conscious or anesthetized sheep. The results generally show that a modest amount of pressure (5-20 mm Hg) will cause increased production by the parotid glands. Higher pressures (15-40 mm of Hg) result in inhibition of the response. Increased pressures may also result in an increase (up to 5 fold) in the mucoprotein content of submaxillary saliva (Phillipson and Mangan, 1959). However, Mendel and Boda (1961) did not find any significant differences in salivary mucin between bloating and nonbloating cows fed alfalfa tops. They also found that susceptible cows secreted less saliva during rest and feeding and it had a higher concentration of bicarbonate than saliva from nonsusceptible animals.

Changes in Rumen Microorganisms and Rumen Contents. A good many writers have speculated that the rumen microbial population of bloating animals may differ from that of nonbloaters. This is a logical and reasonable assumption in view of the fact that oral or parenteral administration of antibiotics will, at least temporarily, reduce the incidence of bloat (see later section). Marked differences, however, have been difficult to demonstrate. Quin (1943) reported that a strain of false yeast, *Schizosccharomyces ovis,* was present in large numbers in sheep pastured on alfalfa and he speculated that this organism produced more gas than more typical organisms. Bryant and others (1960) studied the bacteria in bloating and nonbloating steers pastured on ladino clover. They found no significant differences between these groups of cattle in counts of cellulolytic or total anaerobic bacteria or in the occurrence of 11 different bacterial groups. When the bloating animals were treated with penicillin, counts of facultative anaerobic streptococci were depressed, but no other change was apparent. Mangan et al (1959) and Wright (1961) suggest that antibiotics are effective because they inhibit bacterial degradation of chloroplasts, thus permitting an increase in antifoaming activity of rumen liquor. There is good evidence that bloaters have a higher concentration of mucinolytic bacteria than nonbloaters (Fina et al, 1961). In studies with two mucinolytic strains of *Streptococcus bovis,* Mishra (1969) found that administration of these organisms resulted in more bloat in cows grazing alfalfa or those fed freshly cut alfalfa or a bloat causing diet of concentrate and alfalfa. Since *S. bovis* is often found in high numbers in the rumen of animals fed concentrates, Mishra suggests that it is an important factor in feedlot bloat.

There is also evidence that more slime formers are found in bloating animals (Hungate et al, 1955; Gutierrez et al, 1959, 1963) although Bryant et al (1960) found no differences between bloaters and non-bloaters in slime or bacteria producing slime. Both Mishra (1969) and Clarke et al (1969) suggest that bloat is partially correlated with protozoal populations, but Clarke and Hungate (1971) did not find any consistent patterns in bacterial populations which differed between bloaters and nonbloaters fed red clover forage.

With few exceptions studies indicate that common end products in the rumen are very similar in bloating and nonbloating animals. Three reports showing slight differences will be mentioned. Snyder and Underbjerg (1964) used twins to study bloat. In one experiment one twin was given penicillin and the other was not treated. The treated animal had rumen fluid with less urea and ammonia N, the pH was higher and the contents were darker (due to lack of bubbles in the ingesta). More recently, Essig et al (1972) have studied rumen pH and VFA concentrations in rumen samples from cattle taken before and after grazing Ladino clover. The change in VFA concentration was greater in bloaters than in nonbloaters. Ruminal pH was also lower in bloaters. Medication with penicillin or poloxalene tended to decrease ruminal VFA. McArthur and Miltimore (1969) also point out that severe legume bloat only occurred when ruminal pH was in the range of 5.2 to 6.0. Other studies on blood or tissue metabolites indicate only minor differences which will not be discussed here.

Froth Formation

Quite a number of compounds have been shown to have some potential as frothing agents in the rumen. Data at this point in time indicate that frothing in the rumen is likely to be caused by multiple factors resulting from interactions between animal factors, rumen microbiological differences and due to differences in plant biochemistry. That animal differences are involved are shown by studies which indicate that bloat susceptibility is partially inherited in cattle (Johns, 1954).

Proteins. At the present time much of the recent research indicates that plant proteins are a major factor in froth formation. Boda et al (1957) were among the first to demonstrate that proteins could be a factor in foam formation in the rumen, although the possibility had been suggested by other writers. These researchers fed or added fresh eggwhite to the rumens of cattle fed dehydrated alfalfa hay and produced stable foam. Mangan (1959) demonstrated that salivary mucoproteins would produce relatively stable foams in vitro; however, Van Horn and Bartley (1961) and Bartley and Yadava (1961) demonstrated that mucins from saliva, other animal mucins and plant mucins possessed antifoaming activity in vitro or in vivo. Bartley explained this contradiction by suggesting that saliva serves as a foam inhibiting and foam breaking agent when associated with the foam forming constituents of bloat provoking legumes. This was demonstrated in vitro using saponin solutions. More recent information indicates that salivary mucoprotein produces a very persistent foam of low compressive strength and that the foam was unaffected by changes in pH over the range of 4.0 to 7.0 (Jones and Lyttleton, 1972).

Clarke (1965) suggested that cell contents of rumen protozoa may be a contributing factor to formation of stable foam. Jones and Lyttleton (1972) confirmed this, showing that holotrich protozoal proteins produced very rigid foams, some of the proteins becoming insoluble as a result of surface denaturation at pH 5.8. Maximum presistence of the foams occurred within the pH range 5.5 to 6.5. Buckingham (1970) has also shown that pH and protein concentration are important factors in the stability of cytoplasmic plant protein foams.

There is a substantial amount of evidence showing that cytoplasmic proteins from bloat producing plants are a major factor in producing stable foams in the rumen. This was first shown by Mangan (1959) with red clover. This was followed up by research of Pressey et al (1963b), who showed that foaming properties of alfalfa were associated primarily with the leaves. The stability of the foam was dependent on the pH and temperature. They also demonstrated that foam inhibitors were present and suggested that the plant contains a complex system of foaming agents, inhibitors and stabilizers and that the bloat potential might be a net effect of a delicate balance of these different components.

McArthur et al (1964) published data substantiating the effect of cytoplasmic proteins of alfalfa and suggested that a protein identified as 18S was related to the formation of foam. This protein, believed to be an enzyme, is presumed to be derived from the chloroplasts in plant cells. Bloat has been shown to be related to the protein content of forage (Meyer et al, 1965) and, more specifically, to the content of the 18S fraction which increases foam viscosity (Miltimore et al, 1970). A concentration of 1.8% of the fraction was shown to be the critical level in bloat production. Although the Canadian workers first thought that only the 18S fraction was related to bloat, later work indicated that two protein fractions were involved (McArthur and Miltimore, 1969; Miltimore et al, 1970).

Stifel et al (1968) have shown that total and soluble leaf chloroplast protein levels were related to severity of bloat in both cattle and sheep, the highest correlation being between fraction I (18S) and bloat. When going from forage causing no problems to high bloat-provoking forage, the percentage of soluble protein in chloroplasts increased from 45 to 77%.

New Zealand data have shown that both fraction I (high molecular weight) and fraction II (low molecular weight) proteins produced strong foams over normal ruminal pH ranges. The incidence of bloat was also shown to be related to the presence of protein precipitants, the level of soluble proteins released when the plants were extracted and the nature of foams generated in vitro from extracts. Their more recent research has shown that the presence of protein precipitants in nonbloating legume pastures is correlated with the presence of flavanols in the leaves of these plants. These compounds were shown to be present in medium amounts in white and red clover petals with only trace amounts in the stems and extremities. They appear to act by forming insoluble protein complexes which prevent foam formation from surfactants such as cytoplasmic leaf proteins and protozoal proteins (Jones and Lyttleton, 1969, 1971, 1973; Jones et al, 1970; 1973; Ross and Jones, 1974).

Lipids. Most of the early data indicated that lipids are apt to be more related to foam dispersal than to foam stability (Mangan, 1959; Cole and Boda, 1960; Hungate, 1966). However, research by Stifel et al (1968a, b) indicated that chloroplast lipids were inversely related to bloat. They concluded that stable foam is produced by an imbalance of protein and lipid chloroplast components since large lipid granules were seen in the nonbloat chloroplasts. Other data from this laboratory showed that more Ca and Mg were bound to the fraction I chloroplast protein in forage which caused a high incidence of bloat. Lecithin was shown to decrease Ca binding to fraction I protein as did palmitic acid.

Pectins. Conrad et al (1958) found that plant pectins resulted in a substantial increase in the amount of gas produced in vitro and that added pectin decreased the amount of plant material required to form a stable foamy mass. They suggested that the combined effects of the physical structure of green alfalfa fiber, pectic substances, galacturonic acid obtained on hydrolysis of pectic substances and reducing sugars normally present were capable of causing the formation of stable foam. Subsequent work by Head (1959) tended to confirm the possible importance of a pectin or hemicellulose in froth formation. Wright (1961) reported that rumen bacteria and protozoa contain pectin methylesterase and polygalacturonase and that the galacturonic acid produced by these enzymes was utilized in the formation of gas and various acids. Gupta and Nichols (1962) published evidence indicating that the hydrophilic colloidal properties of higher molecular weight polymers of pectic substances were produced chiefly by demethylation with pectin methylesterase. The stability of froth produced by rumen liquor to which the polymers were added was markedly greater than that of controls. Furthermore, pectic acid, formed by adding pectin methylesterase to a solution of pectin containing bicarbonate and Ca^{++}, slowly released CO_2 from the bicarbonate which was trapped as small bubbles in the gel formed. In the absence of the enzyme no gelling or CO_2 formation occurred. The enzyme was demonstrated to be in an aqueous extract of fresh alfalfa and ruminal fluid. A subsequent report by Nichols and Deese (1966) indicated that, on bloating days, the alfalfa fed was lower in dry weight and higher in pectin methylesterase activity than on nonbloating days. Enzyme intake on bloating days was estimated to have been about twice that of nonbloating days. Another report by Nichols (1963) demonstrated that bloat in cows fed fresh legume chop could be inhibited by feeding alkyl aryl sulfonate, a compound that inhibits pectin methylesterase, and which was reported to be 97% effective on legume pasture. Although Pressey et al (1963a) found that legumes had much higher levels of pectic substances than grass such as bromegrass, their data did not show a correlation between water soluble and total pectins and bloat potential in alfalfa.

Further evidence on the relationship between pectin methyl esterase activity of fresh alfalfa and bloat was published by Nichols et al (1968). The esterase activity was shown to be higher on bloating days in each of two different years. In addition, Clark (1972) has reported that plants known to have a high bloat producing capacity were found to contain large amounts of histamine and pectin methyl esterase.

Minerals. Minerals have been implicated in several reports. Cooper and Woodle (1957) reported that a high Ca-low P ratio tends to cause bloat as well as a high N-low P ratio and that a liberal fertilization program was an effective means of preventing bloat. Smith and Woods (1962) found that a foliar spray of Ca or Mg carbonate increased the severity of bloat in lambs grazing alfalfa, as did drenching with these two mineral compounds. A paper by Harris and Sebba (1965) indicated that the stability of foam from alfalfa samples could be increased substantially by the addition of nickel sulfate to the medium and Miltimore et al (1970) have shown that the content of Ca, Ni and Zn in alfalfa were significantly associated with bloat.

Other Plant Components. A number of earlier papers had indicated that saponins (steroid or triterpene glycosides) might have some relationship to bloat (Lindahl et al, 1957a; Gutierrez et al, 1958; Gutierrez and Davis, 1962). Tannins have also been implicated. It seems likely that the work of Jones and others (see section on protein) may be related to tannins as Jones et al (1973) point out the flavanols are synonymous with condensed tannins.

Plant Toxins as a Factor in Bloat

From time to time there have been adherents to the theory that bloat might be caused by toxins found in plants which might be released during rumen fermentation. Some of the early work indicated that histamines might be a factor since relatively high levels were reported in the rumens of bloated animals. Hydrogen sulfide, likewise, has been implicated on the same basis. The administration of large amounts of saponins can produce bloat by inhibition of eructation (Lindahl et al, 1957b) and other extracts from bloat producing forages or from the rumens of bloated animals have been shown to inhibit activity of smooth muscle or respiration (Parsons et al, 1955; Shaw and Jackson, 1957; Jackson et al, 1962). Hydrocyanic acid in legumes has also been suggested, but data do not indicate that it is an important factor (Clark and Quin, 1945).

At the present time it is not known if these factors (or other unmentioned ones) are important in legume bloat. However, one of the best arguments against toxins is the fact that relief of the pressure in bloated animals is nearly always followed by recovery. Another argument against toxins would be the fact that only some of the animals may be affected by bloat at any given time. If a toxin were universally present in the forage, the assumption would be that most of the animals would be affected to some degree.

Other Miscellaneous Environmental Factors

Legume bloat differs from feedlot bloat in that the occurrence of bloat may be quite unpredictable on legumes whereas feedlot bloat tends to develop more slowly and may frequently become more severe with time. Consequently, there have been a number of investigations in which researchers have attempted to relate various factors to the incidence of legume bloat. Some of these are reviewed briefly.

A paper by Quin (1943) some years ago showed that sheep tend to bloat more severely in the afternoon as compared to the morning. This was confirmed in a report of an experiment in which lambs were fed alfalfa soilage cut about 0800 and 1400 hr (Stifel and Vetter, 1967). The lambs bloated more in the afternoon regardless of the amount of soilage consumed. In a subsequent trial when lambs were fed "low" or "high" levels of soilage in morning and afternoon, lambs on high-high and low-high levels bloated more than those receiving low-low or high-low levels. Nichols and

Deese (1966) reported that, on bloating days, alfalfa was lower in dry weight (and higher in pectin methyl esterase activity) than on nonbloating days and Meyer et al (1964) pointed out that as the water content of feed increased that salivation decreased. Brown et al (1957) studied the incidence of legume bloat as related to various weather observations (temperature, relative humidity, rainfall, cloudiness, wind velocity and moisture on the forage). They found that bloat severity usually increased about one day after rain and decreased during hot weather. Other weather measurements were not closely correlated with bloat.

As a result of very extensive studies on legume bloat, Jones and Lyttleton (1973) have concluded that the main factors relating to rumen foam are modified salivary mucoproteins, soluble leaf proteins, and lipid (reduction of) components. This appears to be a reasonable evaluation as of this time.

Experimental Production of Bloat

As the reader may have concluded, the study of bloat is frequently hampered by the sporadic occurrence in animals on legume or legume-grass pastures. In order to produce bloat more consistently, the practice of stall-feeding fresh alfalfa tops (the upper part of the plant) from immature plants has been used with a high degree of success (see Cole and Boda, 1960). In the case of feedlot bloat, a ration developed at the Michigan Experiment Station (Smith et al, 1953) has been used successfully there and at other laboratories (Lindahl et al, 1957a) to consistently produce bloat. This ration consists of 61% barley, 16% soybean oil meal, 22% alfalfa meal, and 1% salt. Practical observations in the feedlot indicate that a barley-alfalfa combination is apt to be a bloat-prone combination.

Much less published information is available on feedlot bloat than on legume bloat because of less research. This is partly due to the fact that feedlot bloat tends to develop into a severe problem over a period of time and some animals that bloat never do have to be treated; whereas in the case of legume bloat it may strike without warning resulting in the sudden death of many animals. Another factor regarding feedlot bloat is that animals are more confined and can be observed with greater convenience, consequently treatment can be provided

more easily than in the case of animals on pasture.

Lindahl et al (1957a) found that feedlot bloat produced on the ration of Smith et al (1953) was of a frothy type. Some free gas was always found in the rumen, however. Some of the free gas could be released with a stomach tube directed toward the dorsal blind sac and gas could always be released from a fistulated animal by opening the fistula. Further data indicated that bloat could not be correlated to eating habits nor was the severity related to an increase in feed consumption. Jacobson et al (1957) reported that both total and stable froth formation were noted following the removal of rumen contents from cattle on bloat producing diets. No correlation was found between the percent dry matter of rumen contents and bloat or between a consistency index and bloat.

Some changes have been noted in rumen microbial populations in bloated animals. Jacobson et al (1957) reported an increase in encapsulated bacteria in bloated animals and more slime was found in the rumen fluid. Gutierrez et al (1959) also reported that bloated animals showed an increase in a small short chain encapsulated streptococcus and much slime in isolated cultures which were believed to be similar to *Streptococcus bovis*. A large organism, designated as *Peptostreptococcus elsdenii*, was also cultured. Bryant et al (1961) reported that *P. elsdenii* disappeared from the rumens of animals treated with penicillin and that *S. bovis* was not found in large numbers. More recent information on this topic tends to confirm that *S. bovis* organisms are not related to feedlot bloat (Hironaka et al, 1973).

Rumen pH does not appear to be a predominant factor since Elam and Davis (1962) found that the administration of synthetic salivary salts increased rumen pH yet they could show no significant correlation between rumen pH and the incidence of bloat. Other research indicates that rumen pH tended to be lower in twin cattle fed rations which caused a higher incidence of bloat. In these studies (Hironaka et al, 1973), cattle were fed all concentrate rations differing in feed particle size. Their results showed that the particle size affected ruminal pH, soluble carbohydrate content and viscosity of rumen fluid. They suggested that the chemical substances responsible for the foam may be protozoal or microbial in origin. Previously, Kodras (1966) had suggested that rumen protozoa may contribute substantially to gas production in bloating animals on high grain rations.

In other research on feedlot bloat, Meyer and Bartley (1972) point out that froth production was best correlated with surface tension and viscosity of rumen fluids. Low froth production was related to low surface tension and high relative viscosity. Other work from this station (Meyer and Bartley, 1971) indicated that viscosity was related to cell free glucose and rhamnose, the latter probably derived from capsular material of slime producing bacteria (Hobson and Mann, 1955).

Prevention of Bloat

It is obvious that prevention of bloat is desirable from the point of view of reducing death losses. However, bloat may also affect productivity, most likely due to a reduction in feed intake (Wolfe and Lazenby, 1972). The effect of bloat on daily gain was demonstrated by Miller and Frederick (1966) in studies with Holstein and Shorthorn cattle. On a variety of rations, correlations between gain and bloat ranged from -0.44 to -0.67. Shorthorns (on a different ration) bloated more than Holsteins.

The prevention of pasture bloat can be accomplished with a high degree of certainty by not allowing ruminants access to leguminous forage since grasses have only rarely been implicated as a causative factor in bloat. This method is, unfortunately, frequently undesirable since legumes are highly rated as forage and valued for their soil building properties. Various means of preventing bloat can logically be divided into management practices, the use of antibiotics and the use of a variety of antifoaming agents.

Management Practices. The way in which pastures are managed can have a bearing on the amount of bloat. For example, fertilization to stimulate grasses in the grass-legume mixture, strip-grazing to force animals to eat most of the plant material rather than just the succulent top growth, control of legumes with herbicides and clipping of pastures to induce new growth of grasses (Ayre-Smith, 1971). Another possibility might be the practice of grazing sheep and cattle together. Some data indicate that sheep tend to choose a diet predominantly of legumes, at least in some forage mixtures and at some seasons of the year; whereas cattle tend to choose more grass on the same mixtures (Bedell, 1967). Whether grazing sheep and cattle together will reduce bloat is unknown, but the possibility should be explored.

Cole et al (1943) and Colvin et al (1958) have demonstrated that bloat in cattle on alfalfa pasture can be reduced by feeding dry forage such as sudan or oat hay. The feeding of soilage apparently reduced bloat as compared to pasture (Cole and Boda, 1960). We would assume that these methods may be effective because drier feeds promote a greater flow of saliva during ingestion and rumination or because, with soilage, the animal is forced to consume more of the stems, the part of the plant which has less cytoplasmic protein. In the case of the hay, dilution of froth-forming components in rumen contents might be a factor.

Use of Antibiotics. A great deal of interest was evident in the use of antibiotics after Barrentine and coworkers (1956) first reported that penicillin would prevent bloat on ladino clover. Control of bloat with penicillin and other antibiotics was confirmed by a number of other workers (for example, Brown et al, 1958; Johns et al, 1959). Unfortunately, data indicate that continued feeding of one or a mixture of antibiotics tends to result in a gradual loss of protection against bloat (Brown et al, 1958; Johnson et al, 1960). The feeding of a mixture of antibiotics or the use of single antibiotics in rotation appears to be more effective than the continued use of a single antibiotic; in fact, data reported by Van Horn et al (1963) indicated relatively good control of legume bloat during the grazing season when using four different antibiotics in a mixture.

Antibiotics have most frequently been fed in a concentrate mixture or in salt-mineral mixtures and most of the research has been with animals on pasture. The effect on the rumen organisms is uncertain since Bryant et al (1960) found little difference in various types of organisms by administration of antibiotics and Van Horn et al (1963) observed no marked differences in the numbers of gram-positive or gram-negative organisms. Miller and Jacobson (1961) reported that rumen contents of alfalfa-fed cattle, when treated with penicillin, produced appreciably less gas than when penicillin was not administered. It would be presumed that antibiotics prevent bloat by modifying slightly the relative numbers of different organisms and/or by changing some of the end products produced so that fewer froth-forming products are formed.

Use of Antifoaming Agents. In contrast to the action of antibiotics, antifoaming agents apparently act by reducing the surface tension of rumen liquids enough so that a stable froth does not form. Possibly some act indirectly as in the case of an inhibitor for pectin methylesterase reported by Nichols (1963). This inhibitor (alkyl aryl sulfonate), which appears to be very effective in reducing the incidence of legume bloat, apparently prevents the release of pectin derivatives which promote formation of stable foam.

Many surface active agents have been used experimentally for the prevention of bloat. A sampling of the literature shows the variety of compounds used. These would include: vegetable oils, lecithin, animal fats, whale oil, mineral oils, liquid paraffins paraffin-wax emulsions, detergents, turpentine, diethyl ether, silicones, glycerol, plant and animal mucins and, more recently, synthetic polymers designated as poloxalene or pluronics (Reid and Johns, 1957; Brown et al, 1958; Johnson et al, 1958; Colvin et al, 1959; Bartley and Yadava, 1961; Reid et al, 1961; Elam and Davis, 1962; Bartley, 1965; Essig and Shawver, 1968; Lippke et al, 1969; Miltimore and McArthur, 1970; Wright, 1971). Other materials such as copper sulfate and dioctyl sodium sulfosuccinate or dimetridazole, compounds which are anti-protozoal, have been used with limited success but intake tends to be reduced (Willard and Kondras, 1967; Clarke and Reid, 1969; Davis and Essig, 1971).

When evaluating compounds effective against feedlot bloat, Meyer and Bartley (1972) found that none of the drugs tested (235 compounds) completely prevented froth production in vitro. Some of their evidence indicates that quarternary ammonia was one of the more effective compounds.

One of the chief problems in controlling bloat with surface active agents is that of maintaining an adequate concentration in the rumen. Liquids may pass out of the rumen rapidly; consequently, the protection may be of short duration. Various methods of administration have been tried such as addition of water dispersible oils to the water supply, feeding in a salt supply or spraying on forage in the case of pasture studies. Some products used have not been palatable

and water or salt consumption may be very irregular with the result that these methods have met with variable success. Probably the most certain method of bloat control on legume pastures is to spray oils on the forage (Reid and Johns, 1957; Johnson et al, 1958; Reid, 1958). This has worked very well, particularly when strip grazing has been used. It is not an inexpensive method, however, and has not found wide application in most problem areas, although its use is apparently widespread in New Zealand where intensive pasture production systems are widely utilized (Ayre-Smith, 1971). At the present time poloxalene or the pluronics generally are more widely utilized for control of pasture bloat than other compounds. These are available in supplemental blocks that can be made available to animals on pasture. These compounds are not, however, as effective for feedlot bloat control.

Ayre-Smith (1971) mentions one method of administration of antifoaming agents which was devised by Laby. He devised a plastic capsule which is administered by a tube into the stomach. On entering the rumen it changes shape, thus ensuring its retention. From the exposed surfaces of the capsule a detergent then diffuses at a steady rate from a detergent-ethylcellulose gel; this appears to be an effective method of sustained release for a period of several weeks. Australian results for this method are apparently very encouraging.

Treatment of Bloat

Methods used in treatment of bloated animals are varied in nature depending on the severity of the individual case. Seemingly, they have progressed relatively little since ancient times, since a remedy attributed to a Roman writer in 60 A.D. included "pouring vinegar through the left nostril (could it be better than the right?) and putting two ounces of grease in the jaws" (Anonymous, 1958). The usual modern methods include:

In mild cases of feedlot or pasture bloat, feeding some scabrous feed if the animal will still eat, kneading of the rumen or enforced vigorous exercise frequently are effective. Presumably such treatment helps to clear the cardia and increases the amount of free gas in the rumen. The author has had relatively good success, in mild cases of feedlot bloat, with administration of intramuscular doses of penicillin. Apparently enough of the antibiotic is recycled to the rumen to help control organisms promoting froth formation. Administration of an antifoaming agent by drenching, stomach tube or with a syringe intraruminally will usually be effective for a short time. In slightly more severe cases it may be necessary to relieve intraruminal pressure by passage of a stomach tube. In very severe cases, it may be necessary to puncture the rumen to allow escape of froth and gases.

Prevention of bloat can be achieved in some instances by altering the diet. With pasture bloat, sometimes different pastures are much less prone to cause bloat. In the feedlot, the inclusion of less fine material, a change in feed ingredients, use of silages or changing antibiotics where routinely utilized may all be effective at times. With animals which bloat frequently and persistently, the best management procedure is to put them on rations containing relatively large amounts of coarse nonlegume forage.

Conclusions

The majority of reports which provide adequate observations clearly indicate that legume or feedlot bloat is a result of formation of stable froth in the rumen. Normal gas eructation is inhibited. There may be more gas formation than in nonbloaters, but there is no reason to believe the excess gas could not easily be eructated if the reflex were not inhibited.

Froth formation may apparently be increased by reduced salivation when the animals are consuming succulent feeds, by cytoplasmic plant proteins and plant pectins. It also appears to be related to a reduced content of flavonals and chloroplast lipids. Protozoa also appear to contribute to formation of stable foams. Hungate pointed out in 1966 (and it is still the case) that it is not possible to evaluate the relative importance of these various factors unless they are all investigated under the same circumstances. Hopefully, research in the near future will aid in more completely evaluating the different factors.

Pasture bloat caused by legumes can be prevented with a relatively high rate of success with a variety of surface active agents which inhibit froth formation, temporarily by administration of antibiotics and with at least one enzyme inhibitor. The chief problem with these methods is that of maintaining an adequate concentration of the antifoaming agent in the rumen.

Acute Indigestion

There are a number of situations in which rumen fermentation may deviate from the accepted normal pattern with resultant detrimental effects on the health and well being of the animal. Names commonly used to describe rumen dysfunction and symptoms resulting from it include acute indigestion, acidosis, over eating disease, cereal poisoning, founder and acute impaction. For further reading on the topic, the reader is referred to the chapter by Fox (1970) or the book by Jensen and Mackey (1971). This area has been an active field of research in the past few years and, as a result, a number of recent papers are available.

Primary Causes

In the case of young suckling ruminants, excessive amounts of milk in the reticulo-rumen may result in lactic acid type fermentations which are believed to contribute to the development of scours. However, this is a special case which will be discussed in more detail elsewhere (Ch. 28, Vol. 2).

Indigestion in ruminants is usually associated with the ingestion of larger than normal amounts of readily fermented carbohydrates, primarily starches and di- or monosaccharides. However, Broberg (1956) points out that cattle (examined at a veterinary clinic in Norway), with abnormal rumen odors and/or abnormal rumen microflora, developed the abnormal fermentations due to the following causes: excess protein with poor hygiene in the barn; brewer's grains; bad silage; contaminated water (i.e., water from pails used to feed pigs); and rotten potatoes. Most cases were attributed to the ingestion of poor silage and dirty water.

The cereal grains, especially wheat, have probably been the most common offenders in cases involving cattle or sheep in the USA. Other feedstuffs that have been implicated include apples and apple pulp, mangolds, potatoes, green corn and other similar crops. In some cases a sudden change from a dry ration to new grass may also result in rumen dysfunction. The fact that this latter group of feedstuffs, all of which can be very useful feeds, cause problems is a reflection of the fact that the rumen microbial population needs some time to adapt to new substrates, otherwise an excess of one byproduct or another may be produced which may be detrimental to the animal. However, spontaneous cases frequently develop which often are not closely related to the amount of readily available carbohydrate consumed (Hyldgaard-Jensen and Simesen, 1967).

Morris (1971) reports that abruptly changing cattle from rolled sorghum to rolled wheat caused high death losses. When changed from sorghum to barley, death losses were also sustained, but less than when changed to wheat. A change from wheat to barley did not cause any deaths. Ørskov (1973) observed that rumen pathology was more severe in sheep fed pelleted barley and rolled barley than whole grain, and Tutt (1972) found that changing cows from one silage to another with a high lactic acid level resulted in many cases of enteritis.

Although indigestion, particularly that resulting from consumption of cereal grains, is more of a problem in animals during the early stages of adaptation to high grain diets, Klatte (1970) points out that it may occur in cattle that have been on feed over 90 days and that it can occur in cattle on pasture and, less often, in cattle on high roughage feeding programs. He also points out that alterations in the feeding program may increase the incidence. Factors known to be related to increased indigestion include: outright removal of feed as occurs in the normal marketing processes; restriction of intake due to weather changes; change in palatability of feed or change in the character of feed which may be due to milling problems or a change in certain toxic constituents without a change in ration ingredients (i.e., aflatoxins, oxalic acid, molds, and bacterial toxins). It is an important problem in feedlots as animals with indigestion, founder and abscessed livers do not do as well as healthy animals (Elam, 1969).

Clinical Signs

Fox (1970) suggests that indigestion should be classified into 3 types: simple indigestion, indigestion with toxemia and indigestion with impaction. As described by this author, simple indigestion occurs in individual animals or, less commonly, as a herd problem. The animal will be partially or completely anorectic (no appetite) and have normal to slightly elevated pulse and respiratory rates and, with rare exceptions, a normal temperature. When the problem is due to green feed, grain or moderately fermented feed, the feces may be watery. Rumen contractions tend to be weaker or less

frequent than normal. He states that indigestion with impaction is less common and nearly always associated with ingestion of poor quality roughage or lack of water. General signs are the same but rumen contents are firm and doughy with weak and infrequent rumen contractions.

In experimental animals with acute indigestion, the time required to develop clinical symptoms varies and may be as short as 2 to 3 hr or as long as 2 to 3 days and death losses may occur as early as 6 to 7 hr or after an interval of several days (Huber et al, 1962; Ryan, 1964; Fox, 1970; Jensen and Mackey, 1971). Most reports indicate that sheep are more apt to die from acute indigestion than are cattle but the losses in cattle may be very high at times (Morris, 1971).

Clinical symptoms include anorexia (loss of appetite), loss of rumen motility, severe diarrhea, lethargy, craving for roughage and ulceration of the abomasum. A high pulse rate, ataxia and low skin temperature often occur. The blood picture changes rapidly, indicating dehydration as evidenced by increased values for hemoglobin, hematocrit (up to 140% increase) and total blood protein. Blood bicarbonate tends to decrease and chloride may fall sharply before death. Blood lactate and inorganic P rise but there is little effect on blood Ca, Na or K. Blood glucose tends to rise to very high values towards the end. Urine pH may fall to as low as pH 5; volume and specific gravity increase with excess excretion of inorganic P, protein and glucose (Ryan, 1964; Hyldgaard-Jensen and Simesen, 1967; Uhart and Carroll, 1967; Lane, 1968; Brawner et al, 1969; Jensen and Mackey, 1971).

Rumenitis

Chronic cases as well as acute cases often develop rumenitis. Jensen et al (1954) reported that 38% of the stomachs of 1,535 fat cattle examined had lesions in the rumen and 5.5% showed traumatic reticulitis. In rumenitis the epithelia of the rumen exhibits localized or generalized superficial necrosis, edema and hemorrhages. Swollen papillae are round, friable and dark brown. Many papillae may be detached. Histologically, the epithelium shows necrosis, vesicles and colonies of bacteria, including *Spherophorus necrophorus* , which may penetrate injured tissue. Subepithelial tissue may show a strong inflammatory reaction, necrosis, bacteria and edema. Chronic rumenitis is characterized grossly by depigmentation, loss of papillae, scars, ulcers, pits and nodules (Fig. 17-4; Plate 17-1, 2). Hyperkeratosis is also found in many animals.

More recent research in Britain (Fell et al, 1968, 1972; Kay et al, 1969) indicates that young calves fed a high barley diet start to show changes in ruminal epithelia by the time they have been on these diets for two weeks. Symptoms were progressive up to 12 wk, but not as severe as indicated from the work of Jensen et al (1954). Similar findings were noted in older animals examined after slaughter (Rowland et al, 1969). In these studies many animal hairs were observed in the interpapillary spaces and there were numerous lesions due to the penetration of the tissues by both animal and vegetable hairs. Furthermore, the addition of cattle hair to the diet of sheep increased the number of inflammatory lesions in the rumen wall and these workers concluded that animal hairs may be an important factor in rumenitis. Data from one experiment also suggest that the fall in ruminal pH is a contributing factor to the changes seen in the rumen, as one experiment of a limited nature showed that addition of bicarbonate to the diet prevented most of the typical changes (Kay et al, 1969). Typical microscopic changes seen were: stiffening and hardening of walls of the rumen, generalized hyperkeratosis of the epithelium and thickening and clumping of the papillae. The clumps often contained dry food particles and matted hair. Most of the papillae were hard and opaque, but isolated, inflamed papillae occurred irregularly throughout the ruminal epithelia. Ulcers were seen in the epithelia of the cranial pillars and the dorsal sac was checkered with dark areas in which the epithelium was necrotic and covered with adherent debris. The iron content of the papillae was also quite high. Limited information indicates that rumen parakeratosis may be reversed in as short a time as 8 days after changing cattle from an all concentrate diet to one containing 30% ground hay (Cunningham et al, 1969).

Jensen and Mackey (1971) point out that animals with rumenitis are prone to have abscesses of the liver, presumably resulting from invasion of the blood stream of organisms such as *S. necrophorus* which lodge in the liver and set up a secondary site of infection (necrobacillosis). These writers also point out that many nonfatal cases of acute indigestion in cattle result in laminitis (founder), a condition in which tissue fluid accumulates in the connective tissue in the hooves, resulting in lameness. In addition, they state that congestion and inflamation may be present in the abomasum and small intestines. Serosal surfaces commonly contain petechial and ecchymotic hemorrhages.

Rumen Microbiology

In the rumen of sheep given doses of cereal grains via fistulas or sheep which have consumed large amounts of grain, protozoa and cellulolytic organisms decreased markedly and *S. bovis* multiplied rapidly, often becoming, by far, the most abundant organism (Hungate et al, 1952). In the case of animals given doses of lactose, there was a gradual rise in numbers of gram-positive *Streptococci* but little change in numbers of cellulolytic bacteria which could be cultured or in the general appearance of rumen flora

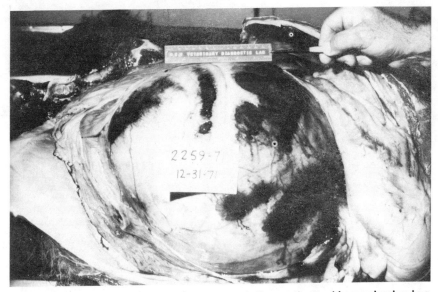

Figure 17-4. The exterior of the rumen showing inflammation and hemorrhaging in a rumenitis case. Courtesy of Don Helfer, Diagnostic Laboratory, Oregon State University.

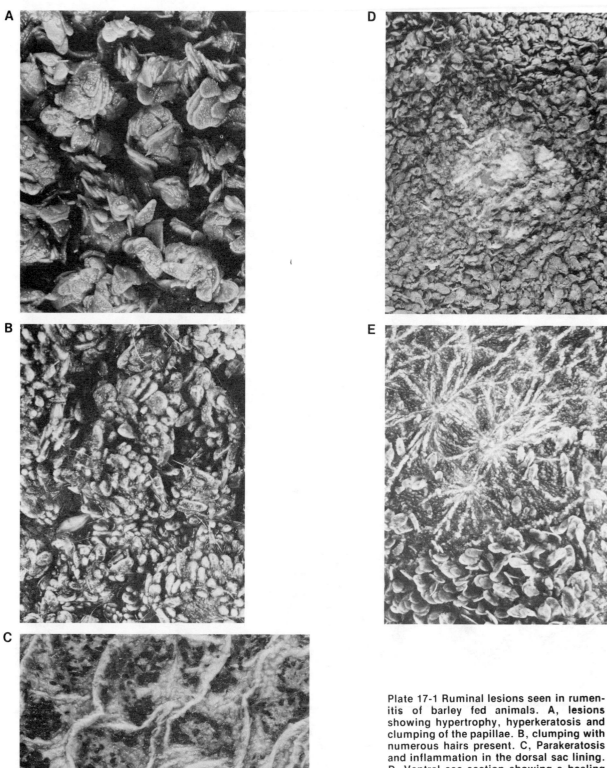

Plate 17-1 Ruminal lesions seen in rumenitis of barley fed animals. A, lesions showing hypertrophy, hyperkeratosis and clumping of the papillae. B, clumping with numerous hairs present. C, Parakeratosis and inflammation in the dorsal sac lining. D, Ventral sac section showing a healing ulcer with depigmentation. E, Ventral sac section showing stellate scars and areas denuded of papillae. Courtesy of Alan C. Rowland, Veterinary Field Station, U. of Edinburgh.

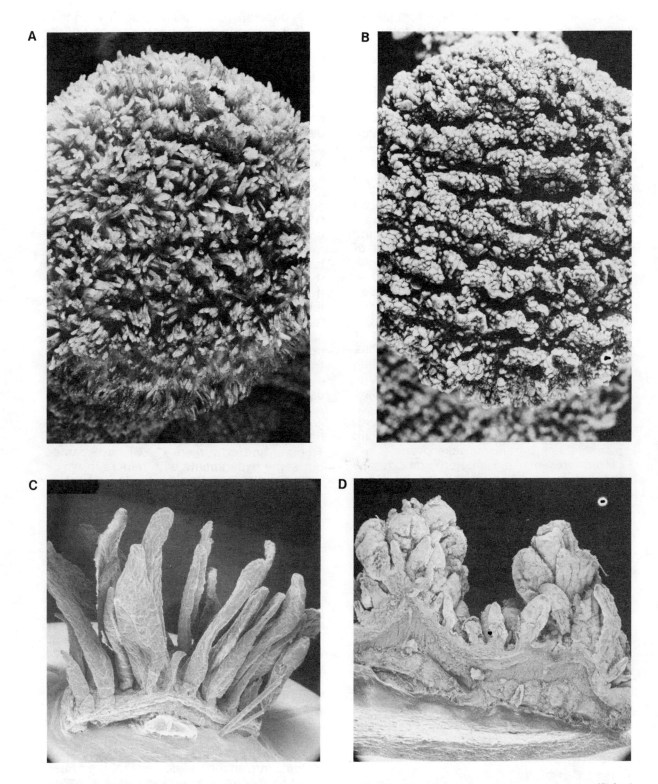

Plate 17-2. Abnormal papillary development in the rumen of calves 4-6 wk of age which were fed insufficient roughage. A, cranial sac with normal papillae. B, cranial sac showing clumping and a tendency to arrange in rows [13-15X]. C, scanning electron microscope photos showing normal development and D, scanning electron microscope photo showing the abnormal rumen papillae. [1.5X]. Courtesy of M.D. McGavin and J.L. Morrill, Kansas State University.

and fauna. Sheep could tolerate from 600 to 1,200 g/day of lactose. When the tolerated dose was exceeded, there was a rapid drop in pH and in numbers of cellulolytic bacteria and gram-positive cocci and a rapid rise in numbers of lactobacilli. The normal protozoal and bacterial population disappeared. Similar results were found when sucrose was given in excess, although tolerance for sucrose was generally lower than for lactose (Krogh, 1960). In the case of starch, sheep could tolerate wheat starch in increasing amounts up to about 900 g/day. When that amount, or more, depending on the rate of increase, was given, there was a sudden change in the rumen flora and acute acid indigestion developed. At the point of change a large population of lactobacilli developed in the rumen, the pH dropped and the normal flora and fauna disappeared (Krogh, 1960, 1961).

Hungate (1966) points out that *S. bovis* is usually found in relatively large numbers in hay fed animals and that this organism has an extremely rapid growth potential. When the animal is dosed or allowed to eat a large amount of carbohydrate, the initial marked increase by *S. bovis* can thus be explained. Later, as the rumen becomes more acid, such conditions favor growth of lactobacilli sp. and these organisms take over.

More recent information on rumen bacteriology has been presented by Mann (1970). When large amounts of barley were fed to a heifer, there were gross changes in rumen microbes. Lactobacilli increased to the point where they comprised 60-65% of the count, displacing the usual organisms (*Bacteroides* and gram negative vibrio types). In similar studies with sheep, streptococci numbers increased sharply, peaking at 18 hr and lactobacilli, which were undetectable at 0 hr, peaked at 48 hr (Chaplin and Jones, 1973). Also, in cases of acidosis, rumen protozoa usually disappear (Dash et al, 1972). In the cecum of sheep dosed with wheat, Allison et al (1972) observed increases in number of lactobacilli, streptococci, coliforms and *Clostridium perfringens.* Concentrations of these organisms were consistently higher in the cecum than in the rumen.

Rumen Chemistry

In the rumen, acute indigestion is characterized by the development of a very acid digesta, the pH frequently being 4.5 or lower (Hungate et al, 1952; Ryan, 1964; also many

other papers). Total titratable acidity tends to increase sharply but a substantial part of the increase appears to be due to a marked increase in lactic acid. Ryan (1964) found that lactate might be as high as 13.5 mmol/ml (equivalent to 338 mg%) in sheep given 6 lb of cracked wheat. As the condition developed the volatile acids generally decreased and lactic acid increased, accounting for 50-90% of total acids. In cases where analyses were carried out, succinic acid tended to increase (to 7-39% of total acids). Formic acid was also present in appreciable amounts in some samples. Ryan (1964) also studied changes in sheep gradually adapted to a wheat-containing ration. He found that the quantity of D(-) lactate gradually increased in relationship to the amount of L(+) lactate. He further found that ruminal glucose and succinic acid tended to increase as feed intake increased, reaching peak values about 3 to 4 wk after the start of feeding. Thereafter, these components gradually decreased. He speculated that the low pH found in the rumen discouraged growth of organisms that usually metabolize glucose and lactate. Allison et al (1964a) showed that a ration containing crushed apples or wheat also resulted in substantial levels of ethanol. Tremere and coworkers (1968) have carried out some experiments with heifers in which increasing increments of ground wheat or mixed concentrates were given to animals accustomed to hay. Their data indicated that high levels of wheat almost invariably resulted in the development of high levels of ruminal lactic acid, whereas the feeding of mixed concentrates did not. An example of some of their data is shown in Fig. 17-5. As shown in the figure, high levels of lactic acid in wheat fed animals occurred after 4-5 days and were associated with low rumen pH.

Other reports showing similar responses in pH and lactic acid production include those of Lane (1968), Patton (1970), Telle and Preston (1971), Chaplin and Jones (1973) and Wilson et al (1973a). In more chronic cases with animals fed high grain rations, data indicate that ruminal pH may be low but there may be no increase in the amount of lactic acid (Fell et al, 1968).

Some information indicates that the rumen is apt to accumulate large amounts of water, cations and bicarbonate, possibly as a result of its high osmotic pressure but also in an attempt to neutralize the excess acid present

(Jones, 1965). Even though this occurs, body tissues are apt to be dehydrated, diarrhea usually occurs and acidemia develops as a result of the rumen acids and transfer of bicarbonate to the rumen. In research studies with sheep, Huber (1970) determined that rumen contents were hypertonic to serum (it is usually hypotonic). Ruminal concentration of Na, K and Cl were reduced and that of lactic acid was greatly elevated. On the other hand, Telle and Preston (1971) reported that ruminal K decreased while Na remained relatively constant.

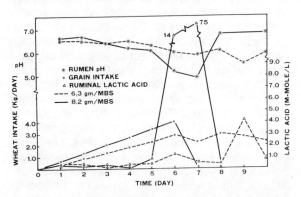

Figure 17-5. Effect of increasing amount of grain intake by cattle on rumen pH and ruminal lactic acid level. From Tremere et al [1968].

Dain et al (1955) found that histamine was produced in large quantities in sheep given large feeds of wheat or corn. Histamine and tyramine were both believed to be toxic agents and the authors state that the illness of the sheep was found to be directly correlated with the level of histamine in the ingesta. Histamine levels increased as pH dropped. Below pH 5, the levels of histamine reached values greater than 70 μ/ml of rumen ingesta and animals became fatally ill. Sanford (1963) reported similar results with in vitro fermentations, pointing out that histamine content appeared to depend on a fall in pH, although marked increases usually required some 24 hr or more, thus suggesting that a change in microflora was required. Some years before Rodwell (1953) found that lactobacillus organisms could produce large amounts of histamine during in vitro fermentations. Shinozaki (1957) observed that histamine and methylamine were present in the rumen fluid of grazing goats and sheep, although very little histamine was absorbed via a rumen pouch and it had no apparent effect on rumen contractions or eructation.

In other research involving histamine, Taylor et al (1969) found that they could produce rumen lesions by administration of lactic acid, but none were caused by histamine and a combination of histamine and lactic acid did not change the type or severity of lesions. Similar results were noted by Aherns (1967). In studies with cows, Fuquay et al (1969) did not find any relationship between ruminal histamine and pH nor between blood histamine levels and health disorders related to experimental treatments. Long et al (1971) have demonstrated that infusions of soluble proteins such as casein result in an increase in ruminal histamine production and Sjaastad (1967) has shown that some histamine is excreted in urine and feces and a substantial amount of it may be inactivated by tissues of the forestomach and intestinal tract. Dickinson and Huber (1972) have also studied catabolism or orally administered histamine. Current evidence does not clearly indicate that histamine is a specific toxic factor.

Miscellaneous Information

A number of investigators have studied the influence of acids on development of rumenitis or typical symptoms of acute indigestion. Jensen et al (1954) found that the feeding of acetic acid or Na acetate failed to produce rumenitis. Hungate et al (1952) also found that administration of acetic or lactic acids to sheep resulted in only transitory effects, although Matscher (1959) reported that administration of acid (pH 2) reduced rumen pH from 5.7 to 3.1 in an experimental sheep. The animal made two attempts to ruminate, but swallowed regurgitated material without chewing. The rumen was atonic and feed was refused until rumen pH rose to 6 (3rd day). Ash (1959) has also demonstrated that acid solutions would inhibit rumen contractions. Results of Ahern (1967) and Taylor et al (1969) have been mentioned previously. Thus, it appears that the pronounced decrease in rumen pH is the primary causative factor in rumenitis.

In other studies, Juhasz and Szegedi (1969, 1970) have observed that similar metabolic changes were caused when large amounts of grain or glucose were given orally or lactic acid infused via a rumen fistula. The increasing acid load and corresponding fall of rumen pH brought about tachycardia, accelerated respiration rates and reduction of rumen contractions before a rise in blood lactic acid occurred. Increasing blood lactic acid was accompanied by a fall in blood pH and bicarbonate. A compensated acidosis developed which progressed to uncompensated acidosis. Blood glucose, pyruvic acid and inorganic P, hematocrit and plasma protein increased while blood Na and Cl decreased. At times rumen fermentation of grain or glucose resulted in high levels of alcohol. When pH of the rumen was reduced, the output of saliva increased and it became more alkaline. At the same time volume of urine fell and it became more acid. Na and K increased in saliva. When animals died, death was attributed to asphyxia caused by paralysis of the respiratory center of the brain.

In the blood of sheep, Telle and Preston (1971) observed that K increased while Na, Ca and Mg were relatively constant. In urine, lactate increased rapidly in the early hours after infusions and then decreased and Na, Mg and Ca excretion increased within 3 hr and then decreased rapidly. Urinary ammonia N concentration and excretion showed a marked and steady increase during a 10 hr period.

Bruce and Huber (1973) report that both the intravenous infusion of secretin and duodenal infusion of lactic acid inhibited amplitude and frequency of rumen contractions of sheep. Results indicated that a hormone other than secretin may also be involved. With respect to renal function, Huber (1969a) has reported that lactic acidosis reduced renal blood flow and kidney filtration rate.

Some research evidence indicates that rumen fermentation during acute indigestion results in the production of both D and L-lactic acid (Ryan, 1964; Dunlop and Hammond, 1965). Infusion studies with these isomers indicate that D-lactate levels persisted longer in the blood, but L-lactate resulted in larger changes in such parameters as arterial blood pH and plasma bicarbonate, suggesting that the L isomer is likely to be more toxic (Braide and Dunlop, 1969). Huber (1969b) also found that the L isomer was oxidized more rapidly than a racemic mixture of lactate.

Mullenax et al (1966) suggest that toxins produced by some gram-negative bacteria may be partially responsible for some of the symptoms noted in acute indigestion. They extracted rumen fluid and rumen bacteria and injected the extract into sheep or cattle. The extract produced a number of toxic reactions. Wilson et al (1973b) have also shown that rumen fluid from cattle with acidosis was toxic to mice, but considerably fewer deaths resulted than from rumen fluid of apparently healthy cattle on high grain rations or those succumbing to the sudden death syndrome.

Prevention and Treatment

Reports from a good many sources indicate that prevention of acute indigestion is best accomplished by limiting the amount of readily fermentable carbohydrates in the ration of ruminants or by gradual adaptation to diets containing large amounts of such carbohydrates. The effect of gradual adaptation to diets containing wheat was shown by Allison and coworkers (1964a). In this experiment 8 lambs were fed cracked wheat via ruminal fistulas. Four of the lambs had been previously inoculated intraruminally with ruminal contents from sheep that had been adapted to a diet containing wheat. Following the feeding of wheat via the fistula, the inoculated lambs did not become sick, while 3 of 4 lambs not inoculated exhibited typical symptoms of acute indigestion. Patton (1970) observed that rumen inoculations reduced the incidence of acidosis in both lambs and steers when suddenly switched to high grain diets, and Huber (1973) observed that inoculation with 400 ml of rumen fluid prevented acidosis in lambs. Lypholyzed organisms, however, were not effective. Satter and Brunge (1969) have shown that an abrupt ration change accompanied by switching rumen contents did not affect feed intake of cows, but did reduce milk fat. However, blood acetate and glucose indicated some time was required for adaptation of the tissues.

With respect to prevention, Jensen and others (1954) found that feeding 1 lb of $CaCO_3$ to cattle did not have any protective value in experimental cattle fed rations high in barley and corn. In sheep, Huber et al (1962) found that feeding $Al(OH)_3$ to lambs resulted in some protection, although 1 of 4 lambs died when dosed with 2.5 to 3.5 lb of glucose. However, the survivors were eating hay the next day. In less acute experiments, Raun and others (1962) found that feeding $NaHCO_3$ at levels of 1.5-3% to sheep tended to increase rumen pH although buffering capacity was not altered. Data by Tremere et al (1968) indicated that wheat feeding could be increased at a rate of about 6 g/unit of metabolic size (weight $^{0.75}$) per day without resulting in acute symptoms of indigestion. Increasing the frequency of feeding from 1 to 2 or 3 times/day resulted in a delay in the time development of indigestion and allowed a greater intake of concentrates before indigestion occurred. Feeding or intra-ruminal infusion of $NaHCO_3$ tended to keep rumen pH from dropping as low as it otherwise did, however it did not prevent the animals from going off feed. Other reports dealing with the use of buffers include those of Nicholson et al (1960, 1963), Lassiter et al (1963), Oltjen and Davis (1963), Wise et al (1965), Urhart and Carroll (1967), Patton (1970) and Shelton and Calhoun (1970). An example is shown in Table 17-1 of changes to be expected in feed intake and in the rumen when animals are abruptly shifted from a high roughage to a high concentrate ration. Note that feed intake was drastically reduced within two days following the ration change and that ruminal lactic acid was markedly increased.

Table 17-1. Effect of an abrupt ration change on feed consumption and on ruminal parameters.[a]

Item	Treatment	
	High barley	+6% $NaHCO_3$
Feed intake, lb/head		
Day 1	24.3	17.8
Day 2	1.7	23.3
Day 10	20.0	27.0
Rumen pH		
Before ration change	6.82	6.45
Day 2	6.09	6.19
Day 7	5.89	5.98
Rumen lactic acid, μmg/ml		
Before change	3.8	5.4
Day 2	1320	4.2
Day 7	23.1	10.5
Rumen VFA, μM/ml		
Before change	98.6	108.0
Day 2	46.7	114.4
Day 7	99.6	97.6

[a]Data from Patton (1970). [b]Steers fed alfalfa-grass hay pellets prior to trial, then abruptly changed to a ration containing 93% concentrate.

Reports from feedlot managers indicate that Glaubers salts ($Na_2SO_4 \cdot 10 H_2O$) and dolomitic limestone are effective in preventing acidosis under feedlot conditions. Certainly, further research on effective methods of prevention is needed.

Treatment of sick animals, as suggested by Jensen and Mackey (1971), includes evacuation of the rumen, administration of mineral oil or drugs to depress absorption of acids and/or toxins and accelerate evacuation of the intestines. These authors also recommend treatment of cattle with $NaHCO_3$ to restore the acid-base balance as do Hyldgaard-Jensen and Simesen (1967) and Raz and Landau (1970). Schotman (1971) suggests that I.V. administration of Na bicarbonate is the method of choice in the treatment of metabolic acidosis although Krogh (1960) reported that neutralizing rumen contents of sheep with Na bicarbonate resulted in aggravation of the indigestion. Lamberth (1969) recommends the use of Mg sulfate where there is dessication of rumen contents and suggests that in these circumstances it exerts its influence by drawing water into the rumen. He questions its use when acidosis is due to ingestion of grain and suggests that it should not be given without giving water also. Fox (1970) suggests use of boluses of milk of magnesia and, where toxemia is indicated, administration of Ca gluconate if ruminal contractions are weak or absent with additional treatment of blood transfusion, glucose or electrolyte solutions and, in some cases, antihistamines.

Other Abnormalities Often Related to Diet

Numerous other problems which affect the GIT occur in ruminants from time to time. Of these only a few will be mentioned here. For additional information, refer to sources such as Blood and Henderson (1968), Gibbons et al (1970), Jensen and Mackey (1971) or Jensen (1974).

Miscellaneous Problems

Ruminants are well equipped to regurgitate food, but vomiting (emesis) is not commonly seen. Fox (1970) states that it appears to occur more frequently in recent years and is often a herd problem. He attributes most of it to greater consumption of grass silage. More specific causes have been identified as toxins from some weeds, spoiled food or highly acid feeds. Other causes may be diaphragmatic hernia, foreign bodies in or near the esophageal hiatus, impaction of the abomasum or nonspecific gastritis.

For many years abomasal ulcers have also been known to occur. Fox suggests that the increased incidence may be caused by hyperacidity related to the feeding of large amounts of concentrates and the feeding of more silage than used to be the custom. Young calves may also have an appreciable incidence of abomasal ulcers (Groth and Berner, 1972).

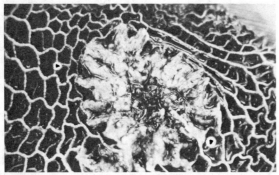

Figure 17-6. Reticulitus in the bovine caused by a fungus infection. Courtesy of D. Helfer, Diagnostic Laboratory, Oregon State U.

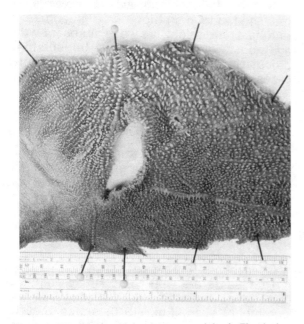

Figure 17-7. Damaged bovine omasal leaf. The hole, which had a well healed edge, was presumably caused by some relatively sharp object.

Traumatic gastritis (reticulitis, peritonitis) is the condition which develops following perforation of the stomach wall, usually the reticulum, by sharp objects (Fox, 1970). Cattle will often ingest nails, wire and other similar objects which may be trapped by the cells of the reticulum and eventually puncture the stomach wall and damage adjacent tissues. The use of magnets which will attract ferous metals has been used in many herds with apparent success in preventing or reducing the incidence of this problem. Reticulitis may also be caused by infections of fungi (Mullen, 1970; Fig. 17-6). Damage to many parts of the GIT may occur following ingestion of sharp objects, for example that illustrated in Fig. 17-7 with an omasal leaf.

Impaction of the abomasum is rare. It is apparently caused by foreign materials such as hairballs or placental tissues (Fox, 1970). Omasal impaction sometimes occurs, but its incidence must also be rare (McDonald and Witzel, 1968; Ramakrishna and Rama-chandraiah, 1973).

Abomasal Displacement

Displacement of the abomasum has been encountered with increasing incidence in cattle, particularly in dairy cows in recent years (Fox, 1970; Coppock, 1974). In one case the incidence ranged from 2 to 12% of the milking cows during a 39 mo. period (Robertson, 1968). The most common displacement of the abomasum is a leftward and upward shift from its normal position (Fig. 17-8) although it may also be displaced to the right in which case the abomasum extends dorsally and caudally. Abomasal torsion (twisting) also occurs, but less commonly (Whitlock, 1969). Left displacement is more of a chronic, although serious, problem than the other types.

Abomasal displacement is detrimental because it results in marked reduction in feed consumption and milk production. The animal resembles one with chronic ketosis but the condition can be distinguished by palpation of the rumen, differences in fecal consistency, use of ketone tests, and typical sounds heard in affected animals (Fox, 1970).

There is not unanimous agreement on the causes. Most reports indicate that the majority of cases occur by 6 wk after calving and the incidence tends to be high in cows fed silage and/or large amounts of grain, especially prior to calving. On the other hand, Martin (1972) points out that the incidence increases with age and successive pregnancies and it was highest during the spring and early summer months. He also presents evidence indicating a genetic relationship, but did not find, on the basis of survey data, that diet, housing, calving site

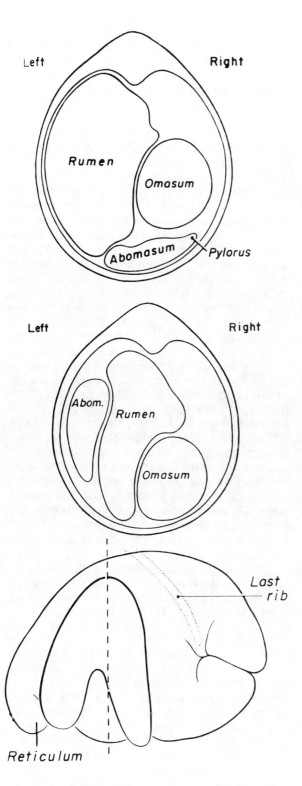

Figure 17-8. Diagram of normal stomach position. Top, section through the 11th thoracic vertebra of a 7 yr. old cow. Middle, body of the abomasum displaced to left. Bottom, left side of rumen with displaced abomasum. Broken like indicates plane of section in the middle diagram. From Fox [1970].

or milk production were highly related to the disorder. However, Coppock (1974) discounts the genetic factor.

Sack and Svendsen (1970) have examined the position of the abomasum in healthy cows fed either a high roughage or high concentrate ration for 2-3 wk. When dissected, there was not a clear cut effect of either ration on size and position of the abomasum, but the abomasums of the cows fed the high concentrate ration tended to be slightly larger and more to the right and their pyloruses were more caudal. Other work, however, indicates a closer relationship to relatively high levels of concentrate feeding prior to calving (Coppock, 1974) and Svendsen (1970) has shown that the VFA may contribute to this, resulting in an inhibition of abomasal motility and an increase in gas production in the abomasum. Other factors causing loss of muscle tonus (milk fever, ketosis, metritis) may contribute to the incidence (Fox, 1970; Coppock, 1974).

Coppock et al (1972) have investigated the effect of forage and concentrate on the incidence of abomasal displacement in cows. Prior to and after calving cows were fed rations with 75, 60, 45 and 30% forage where the forage was provided by equal dry matter from corn silage and alfalfa-bromegrass silage. The incidence of abomasal displacement, when 10 cows were used/treatment, was 0, 2, 4 and 4; thus, the greater intake of concentrate was related to an increased incidence. They also pointed out that many of the affected cows had concurrent problems such as metritis. In addition to a good herd health program, preventative measures such as minimum grain and silage prepartum with other forage ad libitum are indicated at this time (Coppock, 1974).

Urea [or Ammonia] Toxicity

It has been known for many years that rumen microorganisms are capable of utilizing N sources from NPN compounds such as urea. In fact, ammonia was shown by Bryant and Robinson (1962) to be required by about 25% of a number of isolated strains of bacteria. However, the feeding of urea or other NPN compounds may result in toxicity and death at times, particularly when poorly mixed feeds are given to hungry animals. Examples of several cases of this nature have been reported by Bullington et al (1955) as well as by other authors. It should be pointed out however, that urea has been used in a number of cases to provide the sole source of N in purified diets without difficulty, due largely to the fact that such rations are usually unpalatable with the result that consumption at any one time is restricted.

Clinical Symptoms of Urea Poisoning

Toxicity symptoms from over consumption of urea develop rapidly, usually within 30-60 min after ingestion of the feed, although symptoms may appear within 10 min or less following a drench (Word et al, 1969). The rapidity with which symptoms develop is a reflection of the high urease activity of rumen liquor (Jones et al, 1964). In cattle, symptoms include uneasiness, staggering and kicking at the flank at which point they tend to go down. Other symptoms include dyspnea (labored breathing), incoordination, tetany, slobbering and bloating (Dinning et al, 1948; Whitehair et al, 1955; Davis and Roberts, 1959). Clark et al (1951) reported somewhat similar symptoms in sheep. There was dullness and severe muscular twitches over the whole body and moderate to severe bloating followed by severe tetanic spasms of the skeletal musculature of the whole body. The animal went down with the legs stiffly extended. Stimulation by touch or sound caused a marked increase of the tetanic spasms — a situation resembling strychnine poisoning. Dyspnea developed and regurgitation of ruminal contents occurred just before death. Post mortem examination indicated that the cause of death was acute circulatory collapse. Ruminal contents had a strong smell of ammonia.

Although symptoms of urea toxicity are usually acute, sublethal doses may have some effect on rumen motility. Moderate doses of urea have been shown to inhibit rumen contractions (Annicolas et al, 1956; LeBars and Simonnet, 1959; Coombe et al, 1960). Levels up to 0.3 g/kg of body weight generally had little effect, but 0.5 g/kg inhibited contractions completely. In contrast, large doses injected slowly I.V. increased contractions (LeBars and Simonnet, 1959).

Toxic Compounds

The general opinion prevails that the ammonium ion is the toxic factor, whether urea or other NPN compounds are involved since a rapid increase in blood ammonia is noted in toxicity of a wide variety of different compounds. Although some of the earlier research with ammonia compounds indicated that animals were apt to go into a coma without the usual tetany and related symptoms (Clark et al, 1951; Lewis and coworkers, 1957), more recent research indicates similar if not identical symptoms to those from urea. For example, Singer and McCarty (1971) used ammonium Cl, sulfate and a mixture of ammonium salts in studies with sheep. Signs of poisoning included muscular trembling, tonic muscle spasms and convulsions, ruminal stasis, rapid pulse, labored breathing and high body temperature. Death was due to respiratory collapse in all but one animal which died of cardiovascular collapse. Blood and urine analyses indicated severe acidosis, hyperglycemia, sharp increases in amino acid and urea concentrations, hematuria and albuminuria.

Repp and others (1955) investigated the toxicity of a number of NPN compounds when given to sheep. Fairly extensive tests showed that the ammonium salts of acetic, formic and propionic acids were about as toxic as urea (comparable N basis) and resulted in symptoms similar to those reported by Clark et al (1951). However, propionamide, ammonium succinate, formamide, biuret, casein and glycine were not toxic at comparable levels. Guanidine carbonate resulted in death, but symptoms were different than those from the other compounds. The lack of toxicity of some of the NPN sources, particularly the amides, is presumed to reflect a low amidase activity in the rumen. Lewis (1960) has studied the toxicity of ammonium acetate and chloride as compared to urea. The ammonium acetate and chloride ions were unquestionably toxic, but data obtained indicated a somewhat different pattern of metabolism. Lewis points out that the specific site of toxicity may be in brain tissue, suggesting that the tissue may fix some of the ammonia by changing α-ketoglutarate to glutamate and, by interfering with the tricarboxylic acid cycle, account for the toxicity.

Several years ago there was some interest in the use of products ammoniated under heat and pressure to provide a source of NPN compounds. However, some reports (Tillman et al, 1957) showed that relatively small amounts of ammoniated molasses (about 0.25 lb for sheep and 2 lb for steers) resulted in a "peculiar" stimulation after feeding for about a week. Cattle would become aroused and run blindly into fences or other objects. Death loss occurred in some lambs, the cause being attributed to lesions in the heart. The type of toxicity resulting from the feeding of ammoniated products is apparently different from that resulting from urea; presumably, the toxicity is due to some of the ammoniated carbohydrates found in the product fed.

Rumen and Blood Changes

Normal levels of rumen ammonia are on the order of 10 to 45 mg%, depending on the ration and method of analysis used for ammonia. When studying toxicity, Lewis et al (1957) found that rumen ammonia levels were paralleled by changes in portal blood, although portal levels were much lower (0.3-0.5 mmol/l. in portal vs. 20-40 mmol/l. in the rumen) and there was a lag of about 2 hr before high rumen levels were reflected in high portal blood values. They found that rumen ammonia levels as high as 60 mmol/l. (ca. 108 mg% NH_4) could be attained without resulting in any increase in ammonia in peripheral blood. When rumen concentration increased from 60 to 100 mmol/l., a slow "leakage" of ammonia occurred into peripheral blood. Thus, their data would indicate that the liver could handle levels up to about 60 mmol/l. in the rumen. Above this level, the capacity of the liver to convert ammonia to urea was exceeded and blood levels built up, reflecting the inability of the kidneys to excrete ammonia rapidly enough to prevent an increase in blood.

Blood ammonia levels which are indicative of toxicity may be affected by such factors as susceptibility of the animals, analytical methods used and other items. Representative data on this topic indicate that blood ammonia levels >1 mg% are apt to result in acute toxicity (Repp et al, 1955; Lewis et al, 1957; Holzschuh and Wetterau, 1962; Word et al, 1969; Webb et al, 1972).

Studies with monogastric species have indeed confirmed the suggestion of Lewis that blood glutamate levels rise during urea toxicity. When ruminal infusions were given, Bartik et al (1971) observed increases in blood ammonia, glutamine and urea, peak values occuring in 30-90, 60-120 and 420 min, respectively. Soar et al (1973) also found that plasma glutamine increased ca. 50%, but plasma amino acids remained constant or were depressed. Blood urea showed no marked change, but blood glucose rose from 48 to 109 mg% at the onset of acute toxicity when ammonium acetate was infused. Blood Mg did not change, but plasma K rose slightly during infusion and fell sharply when the infusion was stopped, suggesting that ammonia interferes with K interchange and that this might be the underlying cause of ammonia toxicity. Data on liver enzymes suggest that tolerance to ammonia toxicity is partly a function of the activity of the urea cycle enzymes (Payne and Morris, 1969). There appears to be only a small reserve capacity of enzymes and ammonia may cause derangements in the enzymes in liver and other tissues (Chalupa et al, 1970).

Fatal Levels of Urea

The amount of urea which an animal can consume without toxicity and death is affected by a number of factors. With poorly fed or starved animals, data indicate that ingestion or dosage with 0.4-0.5 g/kg of body weight with a time span of ca. 30 min is required for lethal effects. When animals have been fed better rations, doses more on the order of 0.65-0.75 g/kg of weight may be required. Published data indicate that blood levels of ca. 4 mg% are nearly always fatal (Dinning et al, 1948; Clark et al, 1951; Whitehair et al, 1955; Davis and Roberts, 1959; Yoshida et al, 1957; Word et al, 1969). Data from a number of experiments show that ammonia can be absorbed rapidly by the small intestine (see Ch. 9). This has been shown in sheep in which hydrolyzed casein was administered via a duodenal cannula. Felinski (1959) found that urea introduced into the large intestine of lambs was much less toxic than when placed in the rumen. Its effect was intermediate when placed in the duodenum.

Prevention and Treatment

As suggested, research from a variety of locations has demonstrated that the amount of urea or other NPN required to kill an animal may be modified by various factors. The rapidity of consumption is one of the most critical factors. It has been demonstrated many different times that ruminants can exist on NPN compounds without any source of preformed protein. Provided consumption is spread throughout the day, toxicity does not develop.

The chief problems on the farm or ranch are poor mixing and sudden and rapid consumption by hungry or fasted animals, particularly animals that are not adapted to a diet containing urea. Thus, preconditioning an animal to urea lessens the risk of toxicity as does the practice of feeding urea along with a soluble or readily available carbohydrate (McBarron and McInnes, 1968). For example Webb et al (1972) showed that simultaneous administration of molasses with either urea or ammonium acetate reduced rumen ammonia concentrations, rumen pH and markedly reduced blood ammonia and urea. Data indicate that feeding a high protein diet reduces the risk of toxicity (Payne and Morris, 1969), possibly because of better adaptation of liver enzymes which convert ammonia to urea. For that matter, any dietary component which reduces ruminal pH, which in turn reduces ruminal ammonia absorption (see Ch. 9), will likely reduce toxicity.

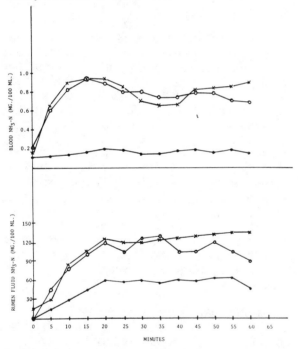

Figure 17-9. Effect of three levels of intraruminal urea administration on ruminal fluid and plasma ammonia-N levels.●—●,11; ○—○, 22; x—x, 0.33 g/kg body wt. From Word et al [1969].

A report by Cunningham and Anthony (1967) indicates that sheep treated with vitamin A were less susceptible to urea toxicity. Copper, Cr, and oxytetracycline, known to inhibit urease activity, were given along with urea and some evidence was obtained indicating partial protection for

animals given lethal doses of urea. Kromann et al (1971) concluded that withholding feed up to 24 hr had no effect on toxicity but toxicity was higher in lambs than in ewes. It was also said that a low protein ration (3.8% DP) with high concentrates (85% concentrates) caused the most toxicity, results somewhat different than those usually indicated with high concentrate rations. The source of the concentrate may have some effect as McBarron and McInnes (1968) noted that wheat-urea caused some deaths in sheep while molasses-urea was well tolerated, even with much higher urea intake.

Data from a variety of sources indicate that treatment of urea toxicity can be successfully carried out with acetic acid administered orally provided treatment is given before tetany develops. Repp et al (1955) reported that one lamb drenched with 80 g of acetic acid along with 40 g of urea remained off feed for about 24 hr although no symptoms of urea toxicity appeared. These authors also found that administration of acetic acid I.V. had no protective effect in contrast to the report of Clark et al (1951).

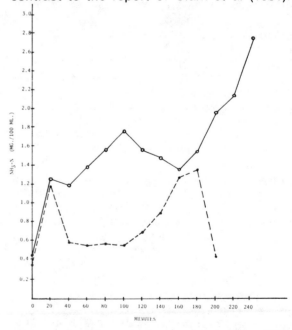

Figure 17-10. Effect on blood ammonia-N levels of treating with acetic acid 15 and 180 min after dosing with a lethal urea dose.○—○ cow which died;●--● av. value of 5 surviving cows. From Word et al [1969].

More recently, similar experiments have been carried out by Word et al (1969). Figure 17-9 illustrates the effect on blood urea when cows were dosed with different levels of urea. Figure 17-10 shows the effect of treatment with acetic acid when cows were given lethal doses of urea. The cows were fed poor quality grass hay and 4 hr prior to dosing were given some ground grain sorghum. Urea was given at a level of 0.44 g/kg of body weight. Fifteen min after dosing with urea, acetic acid was given at a level of 2 mol/mol of urea and again (1 mol/mol) after 180 min. Four of 5 cows survived without ill effect. While this method appears to be effective, it is obvious that one is not likely to have a large amount of acetic acid at hand when needed to treat urea toxicity, as timing is rather critical.

Nitrate-Nitrite Toxicity

Plants may accumulate large amounts of nitrate in some instances (up to 10% or more KNO_3). A variety of different weeds are known to be accumulators as well as many of the cultivated grass plants such as sorghum, corn, millet, wheat and barley. Nearly all of the accumulation is in the vegetative portion with little or none in grain (NAS, 1972). The nitrate content of plants may increase sharply after high levels of N fertilizer are applied and dangerous concentrations may occur, particularly during the first two weeks after application of fertilizer. Weather has an effect on accumulation, as George et al (1971) have shown that an extended period of cool temperature and low light intensity decreased dry matter production and increased nitrate accumulation in sudangrass. Although Buchman et al (1966) did not find any effect of Mo on nitrates when applied as a fertilizer to millet, Liebenow (1972) reports that forage nitrate was decreased by addition of Mo and Mn or urea Mo and Mn, particularly where the Mo/Cu ratio was unfavorable.

Water may also be a significant source of nitrate for livestock (Olson et al, 1971; NAS, 1972), although there is little agreement on what concentrations are toxic. There are, at this point in time, many differences in opinion as to how serious the problem may be, granted that it is well accepted that nitrate toxicity can be very severe at times (Turner and Kienholz, 1972).

Clinical Symptoms

Symptoms seen in acute toxicity include labored breathing (dyspena) grinding of the teeth, uneasiness, excessive salivation, prostration and death (Blood and Henderson, 1968; Dollahite and Holt, 1969, 1970). Urine

nitrate is apt to be quite high and Dollahite and Holt (1969) suggest that blood K, packed cell volume, hemoglobin and total serum protein may be in the low range of normal. The outstanding characteristic is the production of large amounts of methemoglobin which is chocolate brown in color. In acute cases methemoglobin may comprise 60-80% of total hemoglobin. Methemoglobin is formed by nitrite binding to hemoglobin and the complex is more stable than oxyhemoglobin, thus resulting in anoxia.

In the process of studying oat hay poisoning, Bradley et al (1939) demonstrated that NO_3 was the toxic factor and that most of it was present in the straw. No nitrites were found. Subsequent research (Bradley et al, 1940) showed that methylene blue offered protection to animals poisoned with nitrate by allowing a rapid conversion of methemoglobin to oxyhemoglobin. This is still the standard treatment for acutely affected animals.

Nitrates, themselves, are relatively nontoxic when administered I.V., since it is the nitrite ion (or hydroxylamine) which results in methemoglobin formation (Winter, 1962). For that matter, the conversion of hemoglobin to methemoglobin may not be the chief factor leading to death. Holtenius (1957) found that I.V. administration of nitrite resulted in an increase in O_2 consumption and increased CO_2 production, indicating that anoxia may not be so important as previously thought. He reported that up to 65% of total hemoglobin could be in the form of methemoglobin and that his experimental animals could be lying in a coma without any decrease in consumption of O_2 being recorded. He suggested that the vasodilator effect of nitrite (with an associated decrease in blood pressure) might be of primary importance. Sheep generally do not develop as much methemoglobin after dosing with nitrate as cattle and are generally thought to be more resistant to poisoning, although few comparative studies are available (Bradley et al, 1939; Setchell and Williams, 1962; Miyazaki and Umezawa, 1968).

Chronic nitrate toxicity is less well defined and understood. In cattle, research evidence has shown that abortion can be induced (Simon et al, 1959), but there appears to be little evidence for reduced productivity, milk production or growth (Davison et al, 1964; Jones et al, 1966; Arora et al, 1968; Turner et al, 1969; Farra and Satter, 1971; George et al, 1972; Murdock et al, 1972). Jainudeen et al (1965) showed that cattle adapt to chronic nitrate intake by increasing the number of circulating erythrocytes and blood volume. Subsequent research indicated that the pituitaries from nitrate-fed heifers were slightly enlarged and contained more growth hormone than controls, but there was no effect on other pituitary hormones or on thyroid weight or function (Jainudeen et al, 1965). Arora et al (1971) have shown that thyroid uptake of ^{131}I was less in sheep adapted to nitrate than in unadapted animals.

There have been numerous other suggestions that nitrates or nitrites may cause chronic problems including such things as diarrhea in baby calves, vitamin A deficiency, reduced milk production, reproductive failure and other nonspecific problems (Olson et al, 1972; Turner and Kienholz, 1972). However, it has not been shown under research conditions that nitrate is this much of a problem.

Lethal Dose

The amount of nitrate or nitrite that is lethal is highly dependent upon the time factor as there is ample evidence to show that a slow and gradual intake may cause few problems but, if the nitrate is consumed in a short period of time, toxicity may result. For example, Dollahite and Holt (1970) found that feeding hay with 2.1% nitrate did not cause toxicity when it was fed free choice but it readily produced toxicity when large amounts were force fed through a rumen fistula within 4 hr. As much as 1.13 g of nitrate/kg of body wt was consumed in 24 hr without signs, but as little as 0.32 g/kg produced acute signs and death within 4 hr when force fed. Up to 6% nitrate has been fed to dairy cows without any effects other than reduced feed intake (Farra and Satter, 1971) and up to 7.8% to lambs without ill effect (Sokolowski et al, 1961). A number of other examples of this type are also available in the literature.

As a general recommendation, it is said that forage levels above 0.5% nitrate and water levels of 200 ppm are potentially hazardous to young or pregnant animals (Buck, 1969); however, it is obvious that these values are subject to a wide range of latitude.

Rumen Fermentation of Nitrates and Nitrites

The reducing capacity of rumen contents has been well documented (see Ch. 10). However, in the case of nitrates, the reduction to nitrites which are toxic could be considered as very undesirable and probably penalizes the ruminant more than monogastric species.

Sapiro et al (1949) were the first to demonstrate nitrate reduction in the rumen with in vitro studies, showing that nitrate and nitrite disappeared from the ingesta. Lewis (1951a, 1951b) carried out more extensive studies with fistulated sheep. Evidence clearly indicated that nitrate was reduced to nitrite as peak nitrate levels preceded nitrite levels by 2-3 hr. When 10 g of nitrite were administered, he found that rumen NH_3 levels rose from 4 mg% to 11 mg% over a period of 6 hr, thus providing evidence of further reduction of nitrite to ammonia. An oral dose of 25 g of $NaNO_3$ was found to be roughly equivalent to 10 g of $NaNO_2$ or 2 g of $NaNO_2$ given I.V. When oral doses were increased to more than 22.5 g of $NaNO_3$, the capacity of the rumen to reduce NO_2 to NH_3 was exceeded, resulting in an accumulation of nitrite, although nitrate could still be reduced to nitrite. Wang et al (1961) carried out studies with ^{15}N-labeled KNO_3 and found that nitrate, nitrite and ammonium ions were absorbed in considerable amounts from the rumen. Labeled ammonia reached a peak 3-4 hr after dosing with nitrate. The maximum label in the nitrate-nitrite fraction appeared in the blood after 5-6 hr followed by peak values for labeled N in the urine an hour later. No evidence for conversion of nitrate to nitrite in blood was observed. Setchell and Williams (1962) observed that I.V. doses of nitrate resulted in accumulation of some nitrate in the rumen, but no information was presented on the route of entry. Other papers showing evidence of reduction of nitrate to nitrite in the rumen include Jamieson (1959), Sinclair and Jones (1964), Bryant (1965), Tillman et al (1965), Farra and Satter (1971), Jones (1972) and Carver and Pfander (1974). Jones (1972) found that the rate of nitrate and nitrite reduction was affected by the presence of different hydrogen donors. The ranking in order of decreasing effectiveness was formate > hydrogen > glucose > lactate > succinate. In addition to normal ruminal microorganisms, some fungi isolated from the rumen are capable of reducing nitrate (Holtenius and Nielsen, 1958).

Rumen pH has an effect on nitrate reduction, although data are conflicting to some extent. Lewis (1951b) observed that a pH of 6.5 was optimum for nitrate reduction as compared to 5.6 for nitrite and 6 to 7 for hydroxylamine. Holtenius (1957) found that the least nitrite was present in samples at pH 6.6 after the addition of nitrate, thus indicating an optimum pH for nitrate and nitrite reduction. Nitrate reduction, itself, was slowest at pH 5.7 and 7.8. Nitrite breakdown was most rapid over the pH range 6.1 to 6.9 and was inhibited when the pH was reduced to 5.7, but very little at pH 8.0. Perhaps the differences noted for nitrite reduction may be due to differences in rations fed the donor animals.

Holtenius (1957) observed that nitrates inhibited the production of VFA and of CO_2. Jamieson (1959) also found that nitrates caused marked changes in VFA. His data indicate that acetate was decreased accompanied by compensatory changes in the percentages of propionic and, to a smaller extent, n-butyric and branched chain acids. He postulated that the reduced amount of acetate might be due to the utilization of some compounds to provide hydrogen to reduce nitrate — compounds that otherwise might be fermented to acetate; such compounds could include formate, succinate, lactate, citrate and glucose (Lewis, 1951b). However, in contrast to Jamieson's data, Bryant (1965) reported that nitrate addition to in vitro fermentations increased the production of acetic acid with a general decrease in amounts of propionic and butyric acids. Glucose was used at the same rate whether nitrate was present or not, although there was less lactate formed in the presence of nitrate. Farra and Satter (1971) found changes in ruminal VFA similar to those noted by Bryant when nitrate was included in high grain rations fed to cows. Cellulose digestion in vitro has been shown to be decreased by nitrate (Hall et al, 1960) and methane production is decreased (Jones, 1972).

Effect of Diet on Nitrates

There are a number of papers showing the effect of various rations, supplements or soil treatment on nitrate toxicity or metabolism. For example, Holtenius (1957) reported that glucose, fructose, lactate, pyruvate and glycine stimulate nitrite reduction and Sapiro et al (1949) and Emerick et al (1965) also found that glucose increased nitrate and nitrite disappearance. Tillman et al (1965) found that Mo stimulated the reduction of nitrate to nitrite, and Sokolowski et al (1969) reported that increasing the S content of rations to 0.5% reduced nitrate toxicity and improved the utilization of nitrate N by sheep.

Sinclair and Jones (1964) found that rumen ingesta of sheep accustomed to a grass hay diet which contained 0.5% nitrate could reduce nitrate more rapidly than rumen ingesta of sheep consuming a nitrate-free hay, thus indicating adaptation of rumen microbiota to increased utilization of nitrates. As with glucose, Emerick et al (1965) found that feeding corn to sheep offered a large degree of protection against formation of methemoglobin, but replacement of part of the corn with soybean meal reduced protection. Since there was no ration effect when nitrite was given I.V., the authors concluded that protection was due to metabolism in the GIT (presumably the reticulo-rumen). Sokolowski et al (1961) also found that complete rations offered more protection against nitrates than did a poor quality alfalfa hay, and Holtenius (1957) found that penicillin stimulated reduction of nitrite in the rumen.

More recent research from the Missouri Experiment Station (Clark et al, 1970; Carver and Pfander, 1973, 1974) has provided information on supplemental N sources and nitrate utilization. Their results indicate that sheep could utilize up to 4% KNO_3 and urea in combination without ill effects. Based on blood data, they suggest that rumen microorganisms may utilize nitrate before utilizing urea N. With cattle, data indicated that cattle fed high nitrate hay (3.2%) and soybean meal did not adapt completely to this combination and two animals died when fed this hay in combination with urea. Adaptation to nitrate and urea was greater than with nitrate-soybean meal combination.

References Cited

Aherns, F.A. 1967. Amer. J. Vet. Res. 28:1335.

Allison, M.J., J.A. Bucklin and R.W. Dougherty. 1964a. J. Animal Sci. 23:1164.

Allison, M.J., R.W. Dougherty, J.A. Bucklin and E.E. Synder. 1964b. Science 144:54.

Allison, M.J., I.M. Robinson, J.A. Bucklin and R.W. Dougherty. 1972. J. Animal Sci. 35:259 (abstr).

Annicolas, D., H. LeBars, J. Nugues and H. Simonnet. 1956. Bul. Acad. Vet. France 29:263.

Anonymous. 1958. Agra Data 2(3):1. Published by Chas. Pfizer & Co., Inc.

Arora, S.P., et al. 1968. J. Animal Sci. 27:1445.

Arora, S.P., E.E. Hatfield, U.S. Garrigus and F.E. Romack. 1971. Ind. J. Nutr. Dietet. 8:204.

Ash, R.W. 1959. J. Physiol. 147:58.

Ash, R.W. and R.N.B. Kay. 1959. J. Physiol. 149:43.

Ayre-Smith, R.A. 1971. Aust. Vet. J. 47:162.

Bartik, M., I. Risival and K. Zwick. 1971. Acta. Vet. Brno 40:285.

Benson, J.A. 1957. Vet. Rec. 69:412.

Barrentine, B.F. 1960. Proc. 5th Conf. Rumen Function, Chicago.

Barrentine, B.F., C.B. Shawver and L.W. Williams. 1956. J. Animal Sci. 15:440.

Bartley, E.E. 1965. J. Dairy Sci. 48:102.

Bartley, E.E. and I.S. Yadava. 1961. J. Animal Sci. 20:648.

Bedell, T.E. 1967. Ore. Agr. Expt. Sta. Sp. Rpt. 234, p 22.

Blood, D.C. and J.A. Henderson. 1968. Veterinary Medicine. 3rd ed. Williams and Wilkins, Baltimore.

Boda, J.M., P.T. Cupps, H.W. Colvin and H.H. Cole. 1956. J. Amer. Vet. Med. Assoc. 128:532.

Boda, J.M., B.S. Silver, H.W. Colvin and H.H. Cole. 1957. J. Dairy Sci. 40:759.

Bradley, W.B., H.F. Eppson and O.A. Beath. 1939. J. Amer. Vet. Med. Assoc. 94:541.

Bradley, W.B., H.F. Eppson and O.A. Beath. 1940. J. Amer. Vet. Med. Assoc. 96:41.

Braide, V.B.C. and R.H. Dunlop. 1969. Amer. J. Vet. Res. 30:1281.

Brawner, W.R., et al. 1969. J. Animal Sci. 28:126 (abstr).

Broberg, G. 1956. Nutr. Abstr. Rev. 27:604.

Brown, L.R., et al. 1957. J. Animal Sci. 16:1083 (abstr).

Brown, L.R., R.H. Johnson, N.L. Jacobson and P.G. Homeyer. 1958. J. Animal Sci. 17:374.

Bruce, L.A. and T.L. Huber. 1973. J. Animal Sci. 36:213 (abstr).

Bryant, A.M. 1965. N.Z. J. Agr. Res. 8:118.

Bryant, M.P., et al. 1960. J. Dairy Sci. 43:1435.

Bryant, M.P. and I.M. Robinson. 1962. J. Bact. 84:605.

Bryant, M.P., I.M. Robinson and I.L. Lindahl. 1961. Appl. Microbiol. 9:155.

Buchman, D.T., et al. 1966. J. Animal Sci. 25:249 (abstr).

Buck, W.B. 1969. J. Amer. Vet. Med. Assoc. 155:1937.

Buckingham, J.H. 1970. J. Sci. Fd. Agr. 21:441.

Bullington, T.H., C.E. Byrd and T.W. Harris. 1955. N. Amer. Vet. 36:107.

Carver, L.A. and W.H. Pfander. 1973. J. Animal Sci. 36:581.

Carver, L.A. and W.H. Pfander. 1974. J. Animal Sci. 38:410.

Chalupa, W., J. Clark, P. Opliger and R. Lavker. 1970. J. Nutr. 100:170.

Chaplin, R.K. and G.A. Jones. 1973. J. Dairy Sci. 56:671 (abstr).

Clark, G.E. 1972. J. Animal Sci. 34:357 (abstr).

Clark, J.L., et al. 1970. J. Animal Sci. 31:961.

Clark, R. 1948. Onderstepoort J. Vet. Sci. Animal Ind. 23:389.

Clark, R. and W.A. Lombard. 1951. Onderstepoort J. Vet. Sci. 25:79.

Clark, R., W. Oyaert and J.I. Quin, 1951. Onderstepoort J. Vet Sci. 25:73.

Clark, R. and J.I. Quin. 1945. Onderstepoort J. Vet. Sci. Animal Ind. 20:209.

Clarke, R.T.J. 1965. N.Z. J. Agr. Res. 8:1.

Clarke, R.T.J. and R.E. Hungate. 1971. N.Z. J. Agr. Res. 14:108.

Clarke, R.T.J. and C.S.W. Reid. 1969. N.Z. J. Agr. Res. 12:437.

Clarke, R.T.J., C.S.W. Reid and P.W. Young. 1969. N.Z. J. Agr. Res. 12:446.

Cole, H.H., et al. 1956. Natl. Res. Council. Publ. 388.

Cole, H.H. and J.M. Boda. 1960. J. Dairy Sci. 43:1585.

Cole, H.H. and M. Kleiber. 1948. J. Dairy Sci. 31:1016.

Cole, H.H., S.W. Mead and W.M. Regan. 1943. J. Animal Sci. 2:285.

Colvin, H.W., J.M. Boda and I. Wegner. 1959. J. Dairy Sci. 42:333.

Colvin, H.W., P.T. Cupps and H.H. Cole. 1958. J. Dairy Sci. 41:1557; 1565.

Conrad, H.R., W.D. Pounden, O.G. Bentley and A.W. Fetter. 1958. J. Dairy Sci. 41:1586.

Coombe, J.B., D.E. Tribe and J.W.C. Morrison. 1960. Aust. J. Agr. Res. 2:347.

Cooper, H.P. and H.A. Woodle. 1957. Plant Food Rev. 3:7.

Coppock, C.E. 1974. J. Dairy Sci. 57:926.

Coppock, C.E., et al. 1972. J. Dairy Sci. 55:783.

Cunningham, J.P. and W.B. Anthony. 1967. J. Animal Sci. 26:219 (abstr).

Cunningham, J.P., W.B. Anthony and J.G. Starling. 1969. J. Animal Sci. 29:155 (abstr).

Dain, J.A., A.L. Neal and R.W. Dougherty. 1955. J. Animal Sci. 14:930.

Dash, P.K., S.K. Misra and G.P. Mohanty. 1972. Indian Vet. J. 49:672.

Davis, G.K. and H.F. Roberts. 1959. Fla. Agr. Expt. Sta. Bul. 661.

Davis, J.D. and H.W. Essig. 1971. J. Animal Sci. 32:377 (abstr).
Davis, L.E., B.A. Westfall and H.E. Dale. 1965. Amer. J. Vet. Res. 26:1403.
Davison, K.L., et al. 1964. J. Dairy Sci. 47:1065.
Dickinson, J.O. and W.G. Huber. 1972. Amer. J. Vet. Res. 33:1789.
Dinning, J.S., et al. 1948. Amer. J. Physiol. 153:41.
Dollahite, J.W. and E.C. Holt. 1969. Southwestern Vet. 23:23.
Dollahite, J.W.and E.C. Holt. 1970. S. Afric. Med. J. 44:171.
Dougherty, R.W. 1940. J. Amer. Vet. Med. Assoc. 96:43.
Dougherty, R.W., R.E. Habel and H.E. Bond. 1958. Amer. J. Vet. Res. 19:115.
Dougherty, R.W., C.D. Meredith and R.B. Barrett. 1955. Amer. J. Vet. Res. 16:79.
Dunlop, R.H. and P.B. Hammond. 1965. Ann. New York Acad. Sci. 119:1109.
Dziuk, H.E. and A.F. Sellers. 1955. Amer. J. Vet. Res. 16:499.
Elam, C.J. 1969. Feedstuffs 41(15):20.
Elam, C.J. and R.E. Davis. 1962. J. Animal Sci. 21:237; 568.
Emerick, R.J., L.B. Embry and R.W. Seerley. 1965. J. Animal Sci. 24:221.
Essig, H.W., C.E. Rogillio, R. Hagan and W.J. Drapala. 1972. J. Animal Sci. 34:653.
Essig, H.W. and C.B. Shawver. 1968. J. Animal Sci. 27:1669.
Farra, P.A. and L.D. Satter. 1971. J. Dairy Sci. 54:1018.
Felinski, L. 1959. Roczniki Nauk Rolniczych 74B:165. Cited by Stangel, H.J., R.R. Johnson and A. Spellman. 1963.
    Urea and Non-Protein Nitrogen in Ruminant Nutrition. Allied Chem. Co.
Fell, B.F., et al. 1972. Res. Vet. Sci. 13:30.
Fell, B.F., M. Kay, F.G. Whitelaw and R. Boyne. 1968. Res. Vet. Sci. 9:458.
Fina, L.R., C.A. Hay, E.E. Bartley and B. Mishra. 1961. J. Animal Sci. 20:654.
Fletcher, D.W. and E.S.E. Hafez. 1960. Appl. Microbiol. 8:22.
Fox, F.H. 1970. In: Bovine Medicine & Surgery. Amer. Vet. Pub. Inc.
Fuquay, J.W., E.M. Kesler and Z. Zarkower. 1969. J. Dairy Sci. 52:1781.
George, J.R., et al. 1972. Agron. J. 64:24.
George, J.R., C.L. Rhykerd and C.H. Noller. 1971. Agron. J. 63:413.
Gibbons, W.J., E.J. Catcott and J.F. Smithcors (ed.). 1970. Bovine Medicine and Surgery. Amer. Vet. Pub., Inc.
Groth, W. and H. Berner. 1972. Nutr. Abstr. Rev. 42:793.
Gupta, J. and R.E. Nichols. 1962. Amer. J. Vet. Res. 23:128.
Gutierrez, J. and R.E. Davis. 1962. J. Animal Sci. 21:819.
Gutierrez, J., R.E. Davis and I.L. Lindahl. 1958. Science 127:335.
Gutierrez, J., R.E. Davis, I.L. Lindahl and E.J. Warwick. 1959. Appl. Microbiol. 7:16.
Gutierrez, J., H.W. Essig, P.O. Williams and R.E. Davis. 1963. J. Animal Sci. 22:506.
Hafez, E.S.E., M.E. Ensminger and W.E. Ham. 1959. J. Agr. Sci. 53:339.
Hall, O.G., C.D. Gaddy and C.S. Hobbs. 1960. J. Animal Sci. 19:1305 (abstr).
Harris, P.J. and F. Sebba. 1965. Nature 208:869.
Head, M.J. 1959. Nature 183:757.
Hironaka, R., et al. 1973. Can. J. Animal Sci. 53:75.
Hobson, P.N. and S.O. Mann. 1955. J. Gen. Microbiol. 13:420.
Holtenius, P. 1957. Acta Agr. Scand. 7:113.
Holtenius, P. and N. Nielsen. 1958. Nutr. Abstr. Rev. 28:218.
Holzschuh, W. and H. Wetterau. 1962. Arch. Tierernaehr. 12:161.
Howarth, R.E., J.M. McArthur, M. Hikichi and S.K. Sarkar. 1973. Can. J. Animal Sci. 53:439.
Huber, T.L. 1969a. J. Animal Sci. 28:98.
Huber, T.L. 1969b. J. Animal Sci. 29:612.
Huber, T.L. 1970. Amer. J. Vet. Res. 32:887.
Huber, T.L. 1973. J. Animal Sci. 36:226 (abstr).
Huber, T.L., G.E. Mitchell and C.O. Little. 1962. J. Animal Sci. 21:1025 (abstr).
Hungate, R.E. 1966. The Rumen and Its Microbes. Academic Press.
Hungate, R.E., R.W. Dougherty, M.P. Bryant and R.M. Cello. 1952. Cornell Vet. 42:423.
Hungate, R.E., D.W. Fletcher, R.W. Dougherty and B.F. Barrentine. 1955. Appl. Microbiol. 3:161.
Hyldgaard-Jensen, J. and M.H. Simesen. 1967. Nutr. Abstr. Rev. 37:312.
Jackson, H.D., et al. 1962. J. Animal Sci. 21:235.
Jacobson, D.R., et al. 1957. J. Animal Sci. 16:515.
Jainudeen, M.R., W. Hansel and K.L. Davison. 1965. J. Dairy Sci. 48:217; 1382.
James, D.D. and H.W. Essig. 1971. J. Animal Sci. 32:377 (abstr).
Jamieson, N.D. 1959. N.Z. J. Agr. Res. 2:66; 314.
Jensen, R. 1974. Diseases of Sheep. Lea & Febiger, Philadelphia.
Jensen, R., et al. 1954. Amer. J. Vet. Res. 15:202; 425.
Jensen, R. and D.R. Mackey. 1971. Diseases of Feedlot Cattle. 2nd ed. Lea & Febiger.
Johns, A.T. 1954. N.Z. J. Sci. Tech. 36A:289.
Johns, A.T. 1956. Vet. Rev. Annot. 2:107.
Johns, A.T. 1958. Vet. Rev. Annot. 4:17.
Johns, A.T., F.H. McDowall and W.A. McGillivray. 1959. N.Z. J. Agr. Res. 2:62.
Johnson, R.H., et al. 1960. J. Animal Sci. 19:735.
Johnson, R.H., L.R. Brown, N.L. Jacobson and P.G. Homeyer. 1958. J. Animal Sci. 17:893.
Jones, G.A. 1972. Can. J. Microbiol. 18:1783.

Jones, G.A., R.A. MacLeod and A.C. Blackwood. 1964. Can. J. Microbiol. 10:371.
Jones, I.R., et al. 1966. J. Dairy Sci. 49:491.
Jones, L.M. 1965. In: Veterinary Pharmacology and Therapeutics. 3rd ed. Iowa State Univ. Press.
Jones, W.T., L.B. Anderson and M.D. Ross. 1973. N.Z. J. Agr. Res. 16:441.
Jones, W.T. and J.W. Lyttleton. 1969. N.Z. J. Agr. Res. 12:31.
Jones, W.T. and J.W. Lyttleton. 1971. N.Z. J. Agr. Res. 14:101.
Jones, W.T. and J.W. Lyttleton. 1972. N.Z. J. Agr. Res. 15:267; 506.
Jones, W.T. and J.W. Lyttleton. 1973. N.Z. J. Agr. Res. 16:161.
Jones, W.T., J.W. Lyttleton and R.T.J. Clarke. 1970. N.Z. J. Agr. Res. 13:149.
Juhasz, B. and B. Szegedi. 1969. Nutr. Abstr. Rev. 39:1016.
Juhasz, B. and B. Szegedi. 1970. Nutr. Abstr. Rev. 40:141.
Kay, M., B.F. Fell and R. Boyne. 1969. Res. Vet. Sci. 10:181.
Klatte, F.J. 1970. Feedstuffs 42(15):23.
Kodras, R. 1966. Amer. J. Vet. Res. 27:629.
Krogh, N. 1960. Acta Vet. Scand. 1:383.
Krogh, N. 1961. Acta Vet. Scand. 2:103; 357.
Kromann, R.O., A.E. Joyner and J.E. Sharp. 1971. J. Animal Sci. 32:732.
Laby, R.H. and R.O. Weenink. 1966. N.Z. J. Agr. Res. 9:839.
Lamberth, J.L. 1969. Aust. Vet. J. 45:223.
Lane, G.T. 1968. Dissert. Abstr. 29:824B.
Lassiter, J.W., M.K. Hamdy and P. Buranamanas. 1963. J. Animal Sci. 22:335.
LeBars, H. and H. Simonnet. 1959. Ann. Zootech. 8:81.
Lewis, D. 1951a. Biochem. J. 48:175.
Lewis, D. 1951b. Biochem. J. 49:149.
Lewis, D. 1960. J. Agr. Sci. 55:111.
Lewis, D., K.J. Hill and E.F. Annison. 1957. Biochem. J. 66:587.
Liebenow, H. 1972. Arch. Tierernaehr. 22:85.
Lindahl, I.L., et al. 1957b. USDA Tech. Bul. 1161.
Lindahl, I.L., R.E. Davis, D.R. Jacobson and J.C. Shaw. 1957a. J. Animal Sci. 16:165.
Lippke, H., R.L. Vetter and N.L. Jacobson. 1969. J. Animal Sci. 28:819.
Long, R.D., et al. 1971. J. Animal Sci. 32:385.
Mangan, J.L. 1959. N.Z. J. Agr. Res. 2:47.
Mangan, J.L., A.T. Johns and R.W. Bailey. 1959. N.Z. J. Agr. Res. 2:342.
Mann, S.O. 1970. J. Appl. Bact. 33:403.
Martin, W. 1972. Can. Vet. J. 13:61.
Matscher, R. 1959. Nutr. Abstr. Rev. 29:511.
McArthur, J.M. and J.E. Miltimore. 1969. Can. J. Animal Sci. 49:59; 69.
McArthur, J.M., J.E. Miltimore and M.J. Pratt. 1964. Can. J. Animal Sci. 44:200.
McBarron, E.J. and P. McInnes. 1968. Aust. Vet. J. 44:90.
McDonald, J.S. and D.A. Witzel. 1968. J. Amer. Vet. Med. Assoc. 152:638.
Mendel, V.E. and J.M. Boda. 1961. J. Dairy Sci. 44:1881.
Meyer, R.M. and E.E. Bartley. 1971. J. Animal Sci. 33:1018.
Meyer, R.M. and E.E. Bartley. 1972. J. Animal Sci. 34:234.
Meyer, R.M., E.E. Bartley and C.W. Deyoe. 1965. J. Dairy Sci. 48:213.
Meyer, R.M., E.E. Bartley, J.L. Morrill and W.E. Stewart. 1964. J. Dairy Sci. 47:1339.
Miller, K.P. and E.C. Frederick. 1966. J. Animal Sci. 25:1254 (abstr).
Miller, W.M. and D.R. Jacobson. 1961. J. Animal Sci. 20:961 (abstr).
Mills, J.H.L. and R.G. Christian. 1970. J. Amer. Vet. Med. Assoc. 157:947.
Miltimore, J.E. and J.M. McArthur. 1970. Can. J. Animal Sci. 50:651.
Miltimore, J.E., J.M. McArthur, J.L. Mason and D.L. Ashby. 1970. Can. J. Animal Sci. 50:61.
Mishra, B. 1969. Nutr. Abstr. Rev. 39:1375; 1376.
Miyazaki, A. and I. Umezawa. 1968. Jap. J. Zootech. Sci. 39:20.
Morris, J.G. 1971. Aust. Vet. J. 47:129.
Mullen, P.A. 1970. Vet. Rec. 86:587.
Mullenax, C.H., R.F. Keller and M.J. Allison. 1966. Amer. J. Vet. Res. 27:857.
Murdock, F.R., A.S. Hodgson and A.S. Baker. 1972. J. Dairy Sci. 55:640.
NAS. 1972. Accumulation of Nitrate. Nat. Acad. Sci., Washington, D.C.
Nichols, R.E. 1963. Amer. Vet. Med. Assoc. 143:998.
Nichols, R.E. and D.C. Deese. 1966. Amer. J. Vet. Res. 27:623.
Nichols, R.E., D. Deese and J. Lang. 1968. Amer. J. Vet. Res. 29:2005.
Nicholson, J.W.G., H.M. Cunningham and D.W. Friend. 1963. J. Animal Sci. 22:368.
Nicholson, J.W.G., J.K. Looski and R.G. Warner. 1960. J. Animal Sci. 19:1071.
Olson, J.R., F.W. Oehme and D.L. Carnahan. 1971. Vet. Med. Sm. Animal Clin. 67:257.
Oltjen, R.R. and R.E. Davis. 1963. J. Animal Sci. 22:842.
Ørskov, E.R. 1973. Res. Vet. Sci. 14:110.
Parsons, A.R., A.L. Neumann, C.K. Whitehair and J. Sampson. 1955. J. Animal Sci. 14:403.
Patton, W.R. 1970. Ph.D. Thesis. Oregon State University, Corvallis.
Payne, E. and J.G. Morris. 1969. Biochem. J. 113:659.
Phillipson, A.T. and J.L. Mangan. 1959. N.Z. J. Agr. Res. 2:990.
Phillipson, A.T. and C.S.W. Reid. 1958. Nature 181:1722.

Pressey, R., et al. 1963a. Agr. Fd. Chem. 11:396.
Pressey, R., et al. 1963b. J. Animal Sci. 22:970.
Quin, J.I. 1943. Onderstepoort J. Vet. Sci. Animal Ind. 18:91; 113.
Ramakrishna, P. and S.V. Ramachandraiah. 1973. Indian Vet. J. 50:96.
Raun, N.W., W. Burroughs and W. Woods. 1962. J. Animal Sci. 21:838.
Raz, A. and M. Landau. 1970. Refuah. Veterinarith. 27:143.
Reid, C.S.W. 1958. N.Z. J. Agr. Res. 1:349.
Reid, C.S.W. and A.T. Johns. 1957. N.Z. J. Sci. Tech. 38A:908.
Reid, C.S.W., A.T. Johns and P. Vlieg. 1961. N.Z. J. Agr. Res. 4:476.
Repp, W.W., W.H. Hale, E.W. Cheng and W. Burroughs. 1955. J. Animal Sci. 14:118.
Reschly, L.J. and H.E. Dale. 1970. Amer. J. Vet. Res. 31:279.
Robertson, J. McD. 1968. Amer. J. Vet. Res. 29:421.
Rodwell, A.W. 1953. J. Gen. Microbiol. 8:224.
Ross, M.D. and W.T. Jones. 1974. N.Z. J. Agr. Res. 17:191.
Rowland, A.C., M.F. Wieser and T.R. Preston. 1969. Animal Prod. 11:499.
Ryan, R.K. 1964. Amer. J. Vet. Res. 25:646; 653.
Sack, W.O. and P. Svendsen. 1970. Amer. J. Vet. Res. 31:1539.
Sanford, J. 1963. Nature 199:829.
Sapiro, M.L., S. Hofluend, R. Clark and J.I. Quin. 1949. Onderstepoort. J. Vet. Sci. 22:357.
Satter, L.D. and A.N. Bringe. 1969. J. Dairy Sci. 52:1776.
Schotman, A.J.H. 1971. Neth. J. Vet. Sci. 4:5.
Setchell, B.P. and A.J. Williams. 1962. Aust. Vet. J. 38:58.
Shaw, R.A. and H.D. Jackson. 1957. J. Animal Sci. 16:711.
Shelton, M. and M.C. Calhoun. 1970. Proc. West. Sec. Amer. Soc. Animal Sci. 21:207.
Shinozaki, K. 1957. Tohoku J. Agr. Res. 8:149.
Simon, J., et al. 1959. J. Amer. Vet. Med. Assoc. 135:311; 315.
Sinclair, K.B. and D.I.H. Jones. 1964. J. Sci. Fd. Agr. 15:717.
Singer, R.H. and R.T. McCarty. 1971. Amer. J. Vet. Res. 32:1229.
Sjaastad, O.V. 1967. Acta Vet. Scand. 8:136; 176.
Smith, C.K., J.R. Brunner, C.F. Huffman and C.W. Duncan. 1953. J. Animal Sci. 12:932.
Smith, K.J. and W. Woods. 1962. J. Animal Sci. 21:798.
Snyder, J.W. and G.K.L. Underbjerg. 1964. Amer. J. Vet. Res. 25:1451.
Soar, J.B., P.J. Buttery and D. Lewis. 1973. Proc. Nutr. Soc. 32:77A (abstr).
Sokolowski, J.H., E.E. Hatfield and U.S. Garrigus. 1961. Illinois Vet. 4:55.
Sokolowski, J.H., E.E. Hatfield and U.S. Garrigus. 1969. J. Animal Sci. 28:391.
Stifel, F.B. and R.L. Vetter. 1967. J. Animal Sci. 26:385.
Stifel, F.B., R.L. Vetter and R.S. Allen. 1968. Agr. Fd. Chem. 16:500.
Stifel, F.B., R.L. Vetter, R.S. Allen and H.T. Horner. 1969. Phytochem. 7:355.
Svendsen, P. 1970. Nord. Vet. Med. 22:571.
Taylor, D.R., J.F. Hentges, F.C. Neal and J.E. Moore. 1969. J. Animal Sci. 28:126.
Telle, P.P. and R.L. Preston. 1971. J. Animal Sci. 33:698.
Tillman, A.D., et al. 1957. J. Animal Sci. 16:179; 419.
Tillman, A.D., G.M. Sheriha and R.J. Sirny. 1965. J. Animal Sci. 24:1140.
Tremere, A.W., W.G. Merrill and J.K. Loosli. 1968. J. Dairy Sci. 51:1065.
Turner, C.A. and E.W. Kienholz. 1972. Feedstuffs 44(49):28.
Turner, D.O., D.K. Nelson and H.W. Magnuson. 1969. J. Dairy Sci. 52:920 (abstr).
Tutt, J.B. 1972. Vet. Rec. 90:91.
Uhart, B.A. and F.D. Carroll. 1967. J. Animal Sci. 26:1195.
Van Horn, H.H., et al. 1963. J. Animal Sci. 22:399.
Van Horn, H.H. and E.E. Bartley. 1961. J. Animal Sci. 20:85.
Walker, D.M. 1960. Aust. Vet. J. 36:17.
Wang, L.C., J. Garcia-Rivera and R.H. Burris. 1961. Biochem. J. 81:237.
Webb, D.W., E.E. Bartley and R.M. Meyer. 1972. J. Animal Sci. 35:1263.
Weiss, K.E. 1953. Onderstepoort. J. Vet. Res. 26:251.
Whitehair, C.K., et al. 1955. Okla. Agr. Expt. Misc. Pub. 43:92.
Whitlock, R.H. 1969. J. Amer. Vet. Med. Assoc. 154:1203.
Willard, F.L. and R. Kondras. 1967. Appl. Microbiol. 15:1014.
Wilson, J.R., et al. 1973a. J. Animal Sci. 37:361 (abstr).
Wilson, J.R., et al. 1973b. J. Animal Sci. 37:360 (abstr).
Winter, A.J. 1962. Amer. J. Vet. Res. 23:500.
Wise, M.B., et al. 1965. J. Animal Sci. 24:388.
Wolfe, E.C. and A. Lazenby. 1972. Aust. J. Expt. Agr. An. Husb. 12:119.
Word, J.D., et al. 1969. J. Animal Sci. 29:786.
Wright, D.E. 1961. N.Z. J. Agr. Res. 4:203; 216.
Wright, D.E. 1971. J. Dairy Res. 38:303.
Yoshida, J., K. Nakame and R. Nakamura. 1957. Jap. J. Zootech. Sci. 28:185.

DATE DUE
